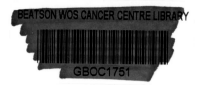
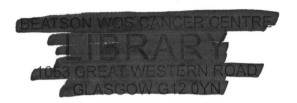

Cognition and Cancer

Cognition and Cancer

Edited by

Christina A. Meyers

Professor and Chief
Section of Neuropsychology
Department of Neuro-Oncology
The University of Texas M. D. Anderson Cancer Center
Houston, Texas, USA

James R. Perry

Tony Crolla Chair in Brain Tumour Research
Head, Division of Neurology
Sunnybrook Health Sciences Centre and Odette Cancer Centre
University of Toronto
Toronto, Ontario, Canada

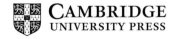

CAMBRIDGE
UNIVERSITY PRESS

CAMBRIDGE UNIVERSITY PRESS

Cambridge, New York, Melbourne, Madrid, Cape Town, Singapore, São Paulo, Delhi

Cambridge University Press
The Edinburgh Building, Cambridge CB2 8RU, UK

Published in the United States of America by Cambridge University Press, New York

www.cambridge.org
Information on this title: www.cambridge.org/9780521854825

First published 2008

Printed in the United Kingdom at the University Press, Cambridge

A catalog record for this publication is available from the British Library

Library of Congress Cataloging in Publication data

Cognition and cancer / edited by Christina A. Meyers.
   p. ; cm.
Includes bibliographical references and index.
ISBN 978-0-521-85482-5 (hardback)
1. Cancer–Complications.   2. Cancer – Treatment – Complications.
3. Cognition disorders – Etiology.   I. Meyers, Christina A.
[DNLM: 1. Neoplasms – complications.   2. Neoplasms – therapy.
3. Antineoplastic Agents – adverse effects.   4. Cognition Disorders – diagnosis.
5. Cognition Disorders – etiology.   6. Neuropsychological Tests. QZ 266 C676 2008]   I. Title.

RC262.C539   2008
616.99′406 – dc22   2008024825

ISBN 978-0-521-85482-5 hardback

Contents

Color plate section will be found between page 32 and 33.

Contributors

Ralph d'Agostino, Jr., Ph.D.
Professor, Department of Biostatistical Sciences
Division of Public Health Sciences
Wake Forest University School of Medicine
Winston-Salem, North Carolina, USA

Tim A. Ahles, Ph.D.
Department of Psychiatry and Behavioral Sciences
Director, Neurocognitive Research Laboratory
Memorial Sloan Kettering Cancer Center
New York, New York, USA

Eduardo Bruera, M.D.
Professor and Chair
Department of Palliative Care & Rehabilitation
  Medicine
The University of Texas M. D. Anderson Cancer Center
Houston, Texas, USA

Jerome Butler, M.D.
Department of Radiation Oncology
Wake Forest University School of Medicine
Winston-Salem, North Carolina, USA

Robert W. Butler, Ph.D., ABPP-Cn
Department of Pediatrics
Hematology/Oncology
Oregon Health & Science University
Portland, Oregon, USA

L. Douglas Case, Ph.D.
Professor, Department of Biostatistical Sciences
Division of Public Health Sciences
Wake Forest University School of Medicine
Winston-Salem, North Carolina, USA

Jane H. Cerhan, Ph.D., ABPP-Cn
Department of Psychiatry and Psychology
Mayo Clinic College of Medicine
Rochester, Minnesota, USA

Robert Collins, Ph.D.
Clinical Neuropsychologist
Neurology Care Line
Michael E. DeBakey Veterans Affairs Medical Center
Houston, Texas, USA

John W. Conlee, Ph.D.
Department of Oncology
Huntsman Cancer Institute
University of Utah School
Salt Lake City, Utah, USA

Denise D. Correa, PhD, ABPP-Cn
Department of Neurology
Memorial Sloan Kettering Cancer Center
New York, New York, USA

Edward Dropcho, M.D.
Professor
Department of Neurology
Indiana University Medical Center
Indianapolis, Indiana, USA

Adrian Dunn, Ph.D.
Professor
Department of Psychology
Pacific Biosciences Research Center
University of Hawaii at Mānoa
Honolulu, Hawaii, USA

Elana Farace, Ph.D.
Associate Professor of Neurosurgery and Public Health
  Sciences
Director of Clinical Research, Department of
  Neurosurgery
Program Co-Leader, Cancer Prevention and Control,
  Penn State Cancer Institute
Pennsylvania State University
Hershey, Pennsylvania, USA

Mercedes Fernandez, Ph.D.
Department of Psychology
Carlos Albizu University
Miami, Florida, USA

Melissa Friedman, Ph.D.
Division of Psychiatry
Department of Medicine
Mount Sinai Medical Center
Miami Beach, Florida, USA

Michael J. Glantz, M.D.
Professor of Oncology, Neurosurgery and Neurology
Huntsman Cancer Institute
University of Utah School of Medicine
Salt Lake City, Utah, USA

John Gleason, Jr., B.A.
Wake Forest University School of Medicine
Winston-Salem, North Carolina, USA

Bebe Guill, M.Div.
Director, Survivorship Programs & Services
The Preston Robert Tisch Brain Tumor Center
Duke University Medical Center
Durham, North Carolina, USA

Edward Ip, Ph.D.
Professor
Departments of Biostatistical Sciences and Social
  Sciences and Health Policy
Division of Public Health Sciences
Wake Forest University School of Medicine
Winston-Salem, North Carolina, USA

Sterling Johnson, Ph.D.
Associate Professor of Medicine
University of Wisconsin
Madison, Wisconsin, USA

Anne E. Kayl, Ph.D.
Assistant Professor
Section of Neuropsychology
Department of Neuro-Oncology
The University of Texas M. D. Anderson Cancer Center
Houston, Texas, USA

Deepak Khuntia, M.D.
Assistant Professor
Department of Human Oncology
Radiation Oncology
University of Wisconsin
Madison, Wisconsin, USA

Dona E. C. Locke, Ph.D., ABPP-Cn
Mayo Clinic Arizona
Division of Psychology
Scottsdale, Arizona, USA

James F. Malec, PhD, ABPP-Cn,Rp
Professor and Co-chair
Division of Tertiary Psychiatry and Psychology
Department of Psychiatry and Psychology
Mayo Clinic College of Medicine
Rochester, Minnesota, USA

Beela S. Mathew, M.D.
Associate Professor
Regional Cancer Centre
Trivandrum, India

Brenna C. McDonald, Psy.D., M.B.A.
Assistant Professor of Radiology and Neurology
IU Center for Neuroimaging
Division of Imaging Sciences
Department of Radiology
Indiana University School of Medicine
Indianapolis, Indiana, USA

Minesh P. Mehta, M.D.
Chairman, Department of Human Oncology
Radiation Oncology
University of Wisconsin
Madison, Wisconsin, USA

Christina A. Meyers, Ph.D., ABPP-Cn
Professor and Chief
Section of Neuropsychology
Department of Neuro-Oncology
The University of Texas M. D. Anderson Cancer Center
Houston, Texas, USA

Bartlett D. Moore, III, Ph.D.
Professor and Chief
Section of Behavioral Pediatrics
Division of Pediatrics
The University of Texas M. D. Anderson Cancer Center
Houston, Texas, USA

H. Stacy Nicholson, M.D., MPH
Professor of Pediatrics
Chief, Division of Pediatric Hematology/Oncology
Oregon Health & Science University
Portland, Oregon, USA

Charles G. Niël, M.D.
Reinier de Graaf Groep
Department of Radiation Oncology
Delft, The Netherlands

Louise Penkman Fennell, Ph.D., ABPP-Cn
Assistant Professor and Director of Internship Training
Argosy University, Hawaii Campus
Consulting Neuropsychologist
Kapiolani Behavioral Health Specialists
Kapiolani Women and Children's Hospital
Honolulu, Hawaii, USA

James R. Perry M.D., FRCPC
Tony Crolla Chair in Brain Tumour Research
Head, Division of Neurology
Sunnybrook Health Sciences Centre and Odette
    Cancer Centre
University of Toronto
Toronto, Ontario, Canada

Stephen R. Rapp, Ph.D.
Professor and Head, Section of Psychology
Department of Psychiatry and Behavioral Medicine
Wake Forest University School of Medicine
Winston-Salem, North Carolina, USA

Renee H. Raynor, Ph.D.
Clinical Neuropsychologist
Director of Clinical Operations
The Preston Robert Tisch Brain Tumor Center
Duke University Medical Center
Durham, North Carolina, USA

Jill B. Rich, Ph.D.
Department of Psychology
York University & Baycrest Centre for Geriatric Care
Toronto, Ontario, Canada

Mike E. Robbins, Ph.D.
Professor and Head, Section of Radiation Biology
Department of Radiation Oncology
Wake Forest University School of Medicine
Winston-Salem, North Carolina, USA

Paul Saconn, M.D.
Department of Radiation Oncology
Wake Forest University School of Medicine
Winston-Salem, North Carolina, USA

Andrew J. Saykin, PsyD, ABPP-Cn
Professor of Radiology
Director, IU Center for Neuroimaging
Division of Imaging Sciences
Department of Radiology
Indiana University School of Medicine
Indianapolis, Indiana, USA

Sanne Schagen, Ph.D.
Department of Psychosocial Research and
    Epidemiology
Netherlands Cancer Institute/Antoni van
    Leeuwenhoek Hospital
Amsterdam, The Netherlands

Christien Schilder, M.Sc.
Department of Psychosocial Research and
    Epidemiology
Netherlands Cancer Institute/Antoni van
    Leeuwenhoek Hospital
Amsterdam, The Netherlands

Edward G. Shaw, M.D.
Professor and Chairman
Department of Radiation Oncology
Wake Forest University School of Medicine
Winston-Salem, North Carolina, USA

John M. Slopis, M.D., M.P.H.
Associate Professor of Child Neurology and Cancer
    Genetics
Department of Neuro-Oncology and Division of
    Pediatrics
The University of Texas M. D. Anderson Cancer Center
Houston, Texas, USA

Jennifer A. Smith, Ph.D.
Biostatistics
Geron Corporation
Menlo Park, California, USA

Martin J. B. Taphoorn, M.D.
Medical Center Haaglanden
Department of Neurology/Neuro-Oncology
The Hague, The Netherlands

Angela K. Troyer, Ph.D.
Department of Psychology
Baycrest Centre for Geriatric Care
Toronto, Ontario, Canada

Alan Valentine, M.D.
Professor
Department of Psychiatry
University of Texas M. D. Anderson Cancer Center
Houston, Texas, USA

Frits van Dam, Ph.D.
Department of Psychosocial Research and
    Epidemiology
Netherlands Cancer Institute/Antoni van
    Leeuwenhoek hospital
Amsterdam, The Netherlands

Jeffrey S. Wefel, Ph.D.
Assistant Professor
Section of Neuropsychology
Department of Neuro-Oncology
The University of Texas M.D. Anderson Cancer Center
Houston, Texas, USA

Preface

This volume is different from anything that has been published in the fields of oncology and neurosciences. The study of cognitive function in cancer patients is in its infancy, and far behind the research in other diseases. However, cognitive impairment and other adverse symptoms associated with cancer are becoming increasingly important to patients and are identified as a major source of concern for survivors. To date there is no comprehensive text that brings together the basic research and clinical perspectives of the many disciplines involved in understanding the impact of cancer and cancer treatment on brain function. Thus, we felt there was a growing need to address cognitive function across cancers and treatments as a resource for oncologists and other professionals who treat cancer patients and those who are involved in translational research that has an impact on cancer-related symptoms. We are pleased that we have brought together the research and views of the most prominent professionals in the field of cognition and cancer. The book is intended to be accessible to a diverse audience: research and clinical neuropsychologists, neuroscientists, medical and neuro-oncologists, surgeons, radiation oncologists, palliative care health teams, nurses, nurse practitioners and physician assistants, and postgraduate trainees and fellows in these disciplines.

We would like to acknowledge the contributions made by our colleagues and our patients from whom we learn daily. We also appreciate the help of Lori Bernstein, Ph.D, who was involved in the conceptual development of the book in its early stages, as well as the tireless support and enthusiasm of Betty Fulford and Laura Wood of Cambridge University Press. We would also like to acknowledge the leadership of Sunnybrook Health Sciences Centre and the University of Toronto for having the foresight and wisdom to embrace an interdisciplinary approach to neurosciences, including cross-programmatic collaboration, which this book embodies. We also acknowledge our families for their patience and unselfish support of projects that take us away from them.

As the book cover implies, solving the disorders of the brain and mind in cancer patients is multifaceted, challenging and at times frustrating, but, in the end, solvable. We hope that this text serves to enhance the quality of life of cancer patients and stimulates awareness, research, and knowledge transfer in the area of cognition and cancer.

Cognition and the brain: measurement, tools, and interpretation

Introduction

Christina A. Meyers and James R. Perry

Cancer patients experience a number of adverse symptoms, including cognitive impairment, fatigue, pain, sleep disturbance, and others often in combination rather than alone. Fortunately detailed symptom assessment is becoming increasingly recognized as a part of routine patient care by physicians, allied health care providers, and accrediting agencies. Cancer treatment may only be considered successful if these symptoms are managed, but successful management is hampered by insufficient knowledge of mechanisms.

Cognitive dysfunction occurs in the majority of cancer patients on active therapy, and is not infrequently a symptom that heralds the diagnosis. In addition, it persists in a substantial number of patients long after treatment is discontinued. In some situations this type of cognitive dysfunction is popularly termed "chemobrain" or "chemofog" although cognitive impairment can be due to a large number of factors (Table 1.1), many of which are discussed in detail throughout this text.

The components of cognitive dysfunction will vary as a result of the specific etiology, but there are several core cognitive domains that appear to be differentially affected. Cancer patients with cognitive dysfunction often present with complaints of memory disturbance. However, objective testing of memory generally demonstrates a restriction of working memory capacity (e.g., the person is able to learn less information, and learning may be less efficient), and inefficient memory retrieval (e.g., spontaneous recall may be somewhat spotty). However, the ability to consolidate or store new information is generally intact, so that the memory disturbance observed in cancer patients is vastly different from that observed in neurodegenerative disorders such as Alzheimer's disease, and is often subtle and relative to the individual's pre-illness level of function. Additional common symptoms include periodic lapses of attention, distractibility, and slowed cognitive processing speed. In general, reasoning and intellectual functions are not affected, but patients often have difficulty performing their normal work due to cognitive inefficiencies.

The effect of these symptoms on daily life can be quite profound, depending upon the demands present in the individual's work and home life. Many patients observe that they can no longer multi-task, and that they may become overwhelmed when too much is happening at once. They are often easily distracted, and find that they may go from project to project without getting them done. Cognitive processing speed is generally diminished, so the person is slower to perform their usual activities. Finally, patients note that it takes increased mental effort to perform even routine tasks. This contributes to the fatigue that is often a co-existing symptom. In fact, cognitive impairment generally does not occur

Table 1.1. Potential causes of cognitive impairment in cancer patients

- Primary or metastatic cancer in the brain
- Indirect effects of non-brain cancer
- Neurotoxic effects of treatment
- Chemotherapy
- Radiation therapy
- Immunotherapy
- Hormonal therapy
- Surgery
- Effects of adjuvant medications
- Co- or pre-existing neurologic and psychiatric illness
- Reactive mood and adjustment disorders
- Sensory impairment and general frailty
- Secondary gain

Table 1.2. Predictors of cognitive impairment

- Soil (host-related factors)
  - Genetic factors
  - Immune reactivity
  - Nutrition
  - Cognitive reserve
- Seed (disease-related factors)
  - Tumor genetic mutations
  - Paraneoplastic disorders
  - Cytokines
- Pesticides (treatment-related factors)
  - Cytokines
  - Poisons
  - Specific mechanisms of action
- Interactions between host-, disease-, and treatment-related factors

in isolation, but interacts in a negative way with fatigue, pain, sleep disturbance, etc.

The impact of cognitive dysfunction on cancer patients depends upon their developmental stage of life, the type of work they do, and their pre-illness lifestyle. For instance, the symptoms described above may not significantly impact the quality of life of an older retired person who can take things at his or her own pace. However, those symptoms may be disabling to an attorney in a court-room setting, and may necessitate changing jobs or going on disability.

Assessment of cognitive function in cancer patients is becoming more routine. For many patients, addressing cognitive problems that exist before treatment begins is important, and the underlying cause can be proactively addressed. In addition, cognitive testing is increasingly becoming an endpoint in clinical trials. In this way, the effect of new agents or treatments on brain function can be evaluated. New studies are incorporating advances in neuroimaging and biomarkers to help improve understanding of the mechanisms by which cognitive dysfunction and other symptoms develop. A number of possible mechanisms are being studied, including the inflammatory response (Lee *et al.*, 2004; Meyers *et al.*, 2005), autoimmune phenomena (Dropcho, 2005), hormonal influences (Wefel *et al.*, 2004), and direct

neurotoxicity of specific agents (Meyers *et al.*, 1997; Scheibel *et al.*, 2004). These will guide the interventions to be offered to minimize the impact of cognitive dysfunction on patients' lives.

Cognitive dysfunction in cancer patients can be thus conceptualized as a result of the interaction between the seed (cancer), the soil (the individual), and pesticides that are offered as treatment (Table 1.2). New intervention strategies are being developed, to improve patient function and quality of life as well as to provide valuable information for clinical trials. This is an exciting time for researchers who are interested in the effect of cancer and cancer treatment on brain function. Understanding the mechanisms of cognitive impairment and the development of efficacious interventions will require a multidisciplinary approach, including oncology, neuropsychology, cognitive neuroscience, genomics, proteonomics, molecular epidemiology, functional neuroimaging, neuroimmunology, animal models, and drug discovery.

This book represents the first attempt to bring together clinicians and scientists to address the effect of cancer and cancer treatment on cognitive function, and the intervention strategies that may be helpful for patients. We hope that the reader will take away our firm belief that optimizing the quality of life of cancer patients is possible, essential, and should be on equal footing with antineoplastic therapy.

REFERENCES

Dropcho EJ (2005). Update on paraneoplastic syndromes. *Curr Opin Neurol* 18(3): 331–336.

Lee BN, Dantzer R, Langley KE *et al.* (2004). A cytokine-based neuroimmunological mechanism of cancer-related symptoms. *Neuroimmunomodulation* 11: 279–292.

Meyers CA, Kudelka AP, Conrad CA, Gelke CK, Grove W, Pazdur R (1997). Neurotoxicity of CI-980, a novel mitotic inhibitor. *Clin Cancer Res* 3: 419–422.

Meyers CA, Albitar M, Estey E (2005). Cognitive impairment, fatigue, and cytokine levels in patients with acute myelogenous leukemia or myelodysplastic syndrome. *Cancer* 104: 788–793.

Scheibel RS, Valentine AD, O'Brien S, Meyers CA (2004). Cognitive dysfunction and depression during treatment with interferon-alpha and chemotherapy. *J Neuropsychiatry Clin Neurosci* 16: 185–191.

Wefel JS, Lenzi R, Theriault RL, Davis RN, Meyers CA (2004). The cognitive sequelae of standard dose adjuvant chemotherapy in women with breast cancer: results of a prospective, randomized, longitudinal trial. *Cancer* 100: 2292–2299.

2

Clinical neuropsychology

Jill B. Rich and Angela K. Troyer

Neuropsychology is a specialized area of study within the field of psychology that focuses on brain–behavior relations, most particularly involving structural–functional connections between the nervous system and mental behavior. Outside of psychology, its closest allies are behavioral neurology, functional neuroanatomy, neuropsychiatry, speech and language pathology, and, more recently, cognitive neuroscience. A distinction may be made between clinical and experimental neuropsychology, although these branches are complementary, as evidenced by a large number of neuropsychologists who identify themselves as clinical researchers and work as true scientist practitioners. For example, neuropsychological rehabilitation generally includes diagnosis and treatment (both clinical) as well as outcome studies (research) assessing the efficacy of various interventions. *Clinical neuropsychology* refers to the practice of neuropsychological evaluation of individuals with known or suspected brain damage. Clinical neuropsychologists typically work in hospital settings or private clinics where they administer standardized, clinical neuropsychological measures to patients referred by physicians, school systems, or insurance companies. *Experimental neuropsychology* is the descriptive term for the academic branch of neuropsychology that focuses on research rather than clinical service delivery. Experimental neuropsychologists typically work in

universities or teaching hospitals where they may develop their own test stimuli and procedures or administer clinical neuropsychological instruments either to healthy individuals with presumptively normal cognition or to patients with known or suspected brain damage. When experimental neuropsychologists administer clinical instruments to patients, however, it is most often to advance understanding of the cognitive processes involved in performing a particular task or for the comparison of cognitive processes in different patient groups rather than for diagnostic purposes.

This chapter focuses on the basic principles of clinical neuropsychology. Following a brief overview of the historical background that gave rise to modern clinical neuropsychology, we review the primary goals of neuropsychological evaluation and detail the procedures common to most evaluations. The remainder of the chapter provides an annotated list of frequently used neuropsychological tests organized by the behavioral domain (cognitive, motor, mood) that they are purported to assess. Our list of tests and our definitions of cognitive constructs are necessarily selective, as there are literally hundreds of published neuropsychological tests now available to clinicians. Interested readers are encouraged to consult some of the excellent compendia that describe test stimuli and administration procedures in detail (e.g., Lezak *et al.*, 2004; Strauss *et al.*, 2006). In contrast to the comprehensiveness of those texts, which are invaluable to actual practitioners in the field, our intent is merely to introduce health care professionals to the scope and general purposes of clinical neuropsychology. Specifically, after reading this chapter, one should have an idea of when it might be appropriate to refer a patient for a neuropsychological evaluation and be sufficiently familiar with concepts and tests to understand a neuropsychological report.

Historical background

Neuropsychology has a long history but only a short past as a formalized field of study. The Edwin Smith Surgical Papyrus, which has been dated to around 2500 BC, documents 48 cases of individuals suffering from traumatic lesions of the head, neck, and other parts of the body, contains the first known record of a word for "brain," and is the first written record demonstrating an awareness of localization of function (Walsh, 1978). Around 2000 years later in Classical Greece, Hippocrates and other physicians observed an association between damage on one side of the brain and spasms or convulsions on the other. By 200 AD, the Greeks and Romans recorded atheoretical observations about aphasias, alexias, and other types of functional loss following head injuries but with no analysis of the underlying cognitive schema. The 1500s brought descriptions of focal symptoms and syndromes involving speech loss following brain damage, unlike previous reports, which had been limited to diffuse problems such as dementia, anoxia, or clouding of consciousness. Building on these observations, clinical descriptions of nearly all the major neuropsychological syndromes appeared over the next 300 years (see Benton, 2000; Gibson, 1969). However, prior to 1800, there was very little theory and virtually no attempt to correlate these syndromes with particular brain regions.

The late nineteenth century brought significant advances in brain–behavior relations. Arguably, the most significant contribution was the French neurologist Paul Broca's demonstration in 1861 of the importance of the "anterior lobe" to the faculty of articulate speech (Benton, 2000). Although Broca himself acknowledged the much earlier work of Bouillaud (1825) for the identification of this association, the year 1861 has been heralded as the beginning of modern neuropsychology as a formalized field of study (Benton & Joynt, 1960). Further advances came in short order, including works on receptive aphasia by Wernicke in 1874, a model of sensory and perceptual processing (the agnosias) by Lissauer in 1889, Dejerine's reports of alexia with and without agraphia in 1891 and 1892, and Liepmann's distinction between apraxia and agnosia in 1900. Thus, the neuropsychological disorders with the longest history of systematic observation and taxonomic categorization are generally characterized by loss of specific functions following cerebrovascular accidents.

The Second World War produced an unfortunate boon to neuropsychology as large numbers of head-injured veterans returned to society. In the intervening years leading up to the present, neuropsychologists have moved away from discrete mapping of isolated brain structures with simple or complex behaviors in favor of seeking patterns of interconnections in distributed systems or networks. For example, amnesia has been associated with three general brain regions: diencephalon [(Korsakoff's syndrome), mesial temporal lobe damage (as represented by the patient HM (Scoville & Milner, 1957) who developed a permanent anterograde amnesia following bilateral surgical resection of the medial temporal lobes for intractable epileptic seizures], and posterior cerebral artery stroke (which serves the hippocampus). More complex disorders, including dementia, schizophrenia, closed-head injuries (i.e., non-penetrating injuries caused by rotational forces of the brain as occur in motor vehicle accidents), and those with undetected (or undetectable) brain damage (which is sometimes the case with irradiation or chemotherapy), are even less localizable. In sum, the history of neuropsychology may be traced from mentioning the brain in an ancient Egyptian papyrus to documentation of associations between a localized brain lesion and loss of a specific cognitive function, to the identification and expectation of the involvement of complex brain systems and networks in complex behaviors and syndromes.

Goals of assessment

The original goal of assessment was *localization of function* for its own sake. Tests were designed to assess the functional integrity of specific anatomical regions. Thus, the inability to identify shapes when palpated with one's right hand while blindfolded would lead to a "diagnosis" of left parietal brain damage, specifically in the "hand" region of the left postcentral gyrus or somatosensory strip. With the advent of brain imaging, of course, neuropsychologists have been called upon less and less to identify the presence and localization of brain lesions that can routinely be obtained by computed tomography (CT) or magnetic resonance imaging (MRI) scanning. Nevertheless, neuropsychology continues to play this role when imaging is contraindicated or otherwise not available and for lesions that are difficult to discern with imaging. For example, a neurosurgeon may refer an epileptic patient for evaluation of language and memory functions prior to surgical resection of a suspected seizure focus in the left mesial temporal lobe. In such cases, the specific seizure focus may be unknown.

More typically, however, neuropsychological evaluations are requested for other purposes, most of which vary according to the clinical setting. The goal for any particular evaluation may be determined on the basis of a mutual understanding arising from an established relationship between the physician and neuropsychologist, by a specified request in the written referral, or, when the referral question is unclear, by contacting the physician to determine the purpose of the referral. In other words, the neuropsychologist requires a contextual framework in order to design the evaluation and report the results. Some of the more common evaluation goals are discussed below.

Differential diagnosis is one of the most common goals of neuropsychological evaluation in cases where the underlying disease is unknown. In memory clinics and some general hospital settings the primary referrals come from neurologists or geriatricians to assist in differential diagnosis of dementia for elderly patients with reported memory problems. The evaluation can determine whether the patient has dementia (or mild cognitive impairment or normal aging or amnesia, for example), and, if so, what the most likely cause may be (Alzheimer's disease, frontal lobar degeneration, subcortical vascular disease, alcoholism, or a potentially reversible dementia syndrome of depression). A very different type of diagnosis may be sought with younger populations, especially in university or other academic settings where neuropsychologists may be called upon to assess individuals with poor academic achievement. In these cases, the objective may be to help determine whether the learning difficulties are primarily attributable to a learning disability as opposed to environmental circumstances. Neuropsychological evaluations are also frequently requested following closed-head injuries sustained in motor vehicle accidents. Even when there is a documented concussion, it may be unclear whether the person has sustained structural brain damage. A thorough neuropsychological evaluation including assessment of both cognitive and personality variables can help determine whether poor concentration and attention following the accident, for example, are likely due to brain damage, psychological factors, or even the medications that the person may be taking for physical injuries sustained in the accident.

When the diagnosis is not in question, such as with a genetic disorder (Huntington's disease, Wilson's disease), medical disorder [infection with human immunodeficiency virus (HIV), epilepsy, multiple sclerosis, Parkinson's disease], documented brain lesion (neoplasm, aneurysm, arteriovenous malformation), or trauma (closed- or open-head injury, electrical injury), an evaluation may nevertheless be requested to provide a *descriptive report* of the patient's cognitive strengths and weaknesses. This evaluative purpose can serve a variety of goals, including treatment planning, workers' compensation and other employment issues requiring vocational guidance, long-term care planning, or documentation of a baseline against which to gauge future abilities. Importantly, many diseases have widely varying behavioral expressions, much as there are multiple phenotypes of a single genotype. Thus, two individuals with the same type of brain tumor may have completely non-overlapping symptoms or may have similar symptoms with differing magnitudes that leave one person functionally intact and the other compromised. Individual differences in pre-existing abilities and different occupational or social demands also lead to different functional outcomes among individuals with the same disease. Neuropsychological evaluation in these cases may be helpful in contextualizing the impact of the brain disease in that person's life.

Neuropsychologists are also called upon to conduct *serial assessments* to document changes over time in response to behavioral or drug interventions (in the case of clinical trials) or when naturalistic changes may be expected that would affect care needs, such as degenerative dementias, chronic progressive disease (e.g., multiple sclerosis), or rapidly growing tumors. Many neuropsychological measures are highly sensitive to practice effects. In fact, stable performance (i.e., with no practice-associated improvement) from initial to repeated administration on some measures may actually indicate the progression of a disease or a decline in function. Practice effects make the selection of tests and interpretation of performance particularly important for serial assessments. Among the armamentarium of tests outlined below are a number of measures with alternate versions of equivalent difficulty specifically designed for serial testing (e.g., Hopkins Verbal Learning Test-Revised; Brandt & Benedict, 2001).

Neuropsychological evaluations are also sought to help *clarify the outcome of a surgical intervention.* Many neurosurgeons routinely refer their patients for neuropsychological evaluations both pre- and post-operatively to assess comparative outcomes from surgical and cognitive perspectives. This is particularly true for surgeries with high morbidity rates or in vulnerable brain regions, where the potential for adverse cognitive outcomes would add to the "cost" in a risk-benefit analysis of whether to perform the surgery (e.g., carotid endarterectomy, pallidotomy for Parkinson's disease, certain brain tumors, shunt placement for normal pressure hydrocephalus in elderly patients or those with severe dementia).

There are a number of situations in which neuropsychological evaluation may be particularly useful or relevant *for the care of cancer patients.* The actual cognitive profiles associated with various brain cancers and the cognitive effects of various cancer treatments are described in subsequent chapters. Below, we briefly sketch some of the circumstances that might lead an oncologist to refer a cancer patient for a neuropsychological evaluation:

- When there are subjective complaints from the patient of (1) cognitive declines, such as poor concentration, slowed thinking, word-finding difficulties, trouble making decisions, right-left confusion, short-term memory problems, difficulty performing calculations, becoming lost in familiar areas; (2) sensory or perceptual changes, such as visual field cuts, anosmia (loss of sense of smell), inability to recognize faces or some other class of objects (cars, buildings); (3) motor changes, such as a change in handwriting, difficulties with balance, gait, or fine-motor skill; or (4) psychological changes, such as irritability, depression, excessive anxiety.

- When there are external reports from friends or family members of any of the above symptoms or of any of the following symptoms that may indicate compromised integrity of the frontal lobes (and which may be unnoticed or denied by the patient): (1) abrupt changes in personality (e.g., lack of empathy, depression, becoming enraged easily); (2) uncharacteristic behaviors, such as making inappropriate sexual remarks, spending large sums of money, engaging in strange or rit-ualistic eating habits; (3) declines in self-care or hygiene; or (4) hypersomnolence or insomnia.

- In cases where the primary tumor is rapidly changing.
- To determine potential cognitive or mood effects of radiation treatment.
- To determine potential cognitive or mood effects of chemotherapy.
- To document possible neuropsychological seque-lae that may have been incurred from destruc-tion of healthy tissue during neurosurgical tumor resection.

Standard neuropsychological evaluation procedures

The clinical neuropsychological evaluation com-prises several discrete sections, including history taking, test selection, the clinical interview, test administration (also called the assessment), inter-pretation of results, and the dissemination of find-ings and conclusions. The *history taking* begins with the referral question. In many cases, the referral itself may include several reports, such as a neuro-logical examination, radiological reports from brain imaging, bloodwork results, other medical reports, or even an entire hospital record. This part of the history review takes place before the assessment and may be done several days or weeks in advance. If the patient has undergone a previous evaluation, as is often the case for patients referred by insurance companies and/or involving a legal claim, reports from those evaluations are typically reviewed as part of the history. This is particularly important when the prior assessment was conducted within the past year (or even within the past month, such as when evaluating a patient pre- and post-surgically), as it will likely affect the selection of tests for the current evaluation.

Historically, clinical neuropsychologists could be divided into two camps in terms of *test selection*: those who used fixed batteries and those who opted for a flexible approach. The most widely known and commonly used battery of tests is the Halstead–Reitan Battery (Reitan & Wolfson, 1993), which was originally developed as a sensitive diagnostic mea-sure of patients with frontal lobe or lateralized brain lesions. Currently, many neuropsychologists use a "core" battery of tests to tap functions in several key functional domains, including general mental sta-tus or intelligence, attention, visual perception, con-struction, language, memory, executive function, and mood, personality, or emotional status. This core battery is then supplemented by additional measures as warranted by the referral question, the patient's capacity for testing, the patient's abil-ities as ascertained throughout the assessment, and the clinical setting. For example, even "Halstead–Reitanners" who use the current version of the orig-inal Halstead–Reitan Battery generally supplement their assessment with one of the Wechsler scales of intelligence as well as tests of memory and other specific functional domains. Some brief evaluations of very elderly patients or those with severe brain damage may include only a single mental status examination that encompasses a minimal sample of several of the domains listed above (e.g., Mattis Dementia Rating Scale; Mattis, 2001). Other general-purpose batteries (e.g., Kaplan–Baycrest Neurocog-nitive Assessment; Leach *et al.*, 2000; The Repeat-able Battery for the Assessment of Neuropsycho-logical Status; Randolph *et al.*, 1998) have been developed for use as contained measures when a brief assessment is appropriate. However, these same measures, as well as brief screening instru-ments such as the Mini-Mental State Examina-tion (Folstein *et al.*, 1975), may be used in longer assessments as a preliminary measure to guide the selection of tests for subsequent evaluation of spe-cific functional domains (many of which are listed below).

The *clinical interview* is typically conducted with the patient alone, especially for inpatients, although permission may be requested to contact a spouse or caregiver separately by phone. When secondary sources are present, as is often the case with out-patients, they may be interviewed together with the patient, especially when the patient may be an unreliable historian, or separately (with the patient's permission in most settings). When a child is being tested, he or she is typically interviewed briefly, though the parents are often asked to report such things as the timing of developmental milestones in addition to current symptoms or problems. Depending on the setting and availability of ancillary records, the clinical interview can take from 10 min to an hour or more. At a minimum, the neuropsychologist ascertains critical demographic variables that may affect test interpretation, such as the patient's age, education, native language, and handedness, as well as social variables, such as highest and most recent occupational attainment, current living situation (including language spoken at home), medical history and current medical status, and the patient's understanding of the reason for the referral.

In general, even when the patient suffers from dementia, the interview will provide useful information, such as whether the patient is aware of his or her deficits and other aspects of insight. It also provides an opportunity to assess spontaneous or conversational speech, including length and appropriateness of responses to open-ended questions. Behavioral observations, such as eye contact, impulsivity, distractibility, and inattention are made during the interview and throughout the assessment. Although there are specific tests to assess for malingering (used frequently in medicolegal contexts), the examiner also tries to gauge the patient's motivation level and fatigue to determine whether the results obtained represent the patient's true abilities.

The actual *neuropsychological assessment* entails the test administration component of the evaluation. This may be done by the neuropsychologist, but more typically the assessment is carried out by a psychometrist (trained technician) or clinical trainee (such as a predoctoral intern or postdoctoral fellow). In the latter cases, the neuropsychologist makes or approves of the test selection and supervises the test administration and scoring accuracy. Commonly used tests for various functional domains are listed in the next section.

Published tests include strict guidelines for standardized test administration, and this is critical for subsequent *interpretation of results*. For example, inexperienced examiners may "coach" patients or give extra cues in an effort to help them get the right answer. Alternatively, the overly rigid examiner may refuse to repeat a question that the patient didn't hear because of poor auditory acuity, a competing public address announcement, or a sneeze. Either of these approaches could yield unrepresentative test results. Among the data to be interpreted are the summary scores obtained on the various tests administered, the qualitative responses that led to those scores, the consistency of performance on multiple measures of the same domain, relative strengths and weaknesses observed across domains, the degree to which the test environment conformed to or deviated from optimal conditions, the patient's co-operation with the test procedures, normative expectations for individuals with similar demographic and social backgrounds, and any motor, visual, auditory, comprehension, or verbal expressive difficulties that may have impacted the patient's ability to perform the presented tasks. Qualitative interpretation of quantitative data is essential. Consider, for example, the many ways in which a score of 0 may be obtained on a single item, such as the identification of a line drawing: (1) no response; (2) identification of the item at the superordinate level of taxonomic categorization (animal for rhinoceros); (3) identification of an exemplar from the same class (hippopotamus for rhinoceros); (4) phonemic paraphasic response (rhinosteros); (5) neologism (pinder); (6) misperception of gestalt, with focus on a single detail (horn for rhinoceros); or (7) correct response after the time limit. These responses have differing interpretive significance, which is why a test score in isolation may be misleading.

Following test selection appropriate to the specified purpose, accurate test administration and scoring, and interpretation of the obtained results in the context of the history, presenting symptoms, and testing circumstances, the final step in the evaluation is *dissemination of the findings*. This most often takes the form of a written report to the referring physician and/or a verbal report given to multidisciplinary teams in hospital settings. The length of the report varies widely across settings and depends primarily on the familiarity and interest of the referring physician. Reports to insurance companies for head-injured patients involved in litigation may be 15–20 pages long. At the other end of the continuum, a two-paragraph chart note may be made in an inpatient record at a nursing home for a patient with severe dementia who could not undergo much testing. Between these extremes is a standard report of three to six pages, which is a typical length for outpatient evaluations. In many clinic and hospital settings, the neuropsychologist will schedule a verbal feedback session with the patient and/or the patient's family or caregivers. Although patients are entitled to receive a copy of their full written report, it is undesirable to merely send them a copy in the mail with no supplemental explanations. Instead, many neuropsychologists offer to provide the patient with a summary of the results after they review it together in the feedback session.

Commonly used neuropsychological tests by domain assessed

Most of the tests described below have alternative versions, modifications, or other corollary measures developed specifically for children. In some cases, modified instruments have been developed for use with other populations, such as the elderly or individuals with severe impairments who are not capable of completing many of the measures described here.

Intelligence

Intelligence is a multidimensional construct that comprises many cognitive abilities. Clinical tests of intelligence, such as the Wechsler Adult Intelligence Scale – III (WAIS-III; Wechsler, 1997a) and the Stanford-Binet Intelligence Scale (Roid, 2003), contain multiple subtests tapping a variety of abilities. Tests of *verbal* intelligence assess vocabulary, general factual knowledge, verbal abstraction, or social judgment. Tests of *non-verbal* (or performance) intelligence assess visual abstraction, visual construction, detection of visual details, or arrangement of pictures to tell a story. Often, the purpose of administering intelligence tests is to obtain an estimate of a person's overall level of cognitive ability, rather than to determine performance on the various subcomponents of intelligence. To achieve the former, only a subset of intelligence tests need be administered (Wechsler, 1999). On the WAIS-III, Verbal IQ is most highly correlated with performance on the Vocabulary subtest, and Performance IQ is most highly correlated with performance on the Matrix Reasoning (visual abstraction) subtest.

Attention and processing speed

Attention is the ability to focus or concentrate on specific stimuli. It comprises selective, sustained, divided, and alternating attention and plays a large role in working memory. *Selective attention* is the ability to focus on information relevant to the task at hand and to filter out irrelevant information. Most people automatically display auditory selective attention for the sound of their name being spoken in a crowded room with a lot of background noise. Tests of visual selective attention may require the search for target stimuli while scanning arrays of target and non-target stimuli (e.g., Ruff 2 & 7; Ruff & Allen, 1996). *Sustained attention* is the ability to maintain attention on a task over an extended time, such as watching a long movie or reading a book. It is tested by having the patient perform a relatively simple task for several minutes at a time, such as hitting a key every time a particular number appears on a screen or a letter is spoken on an audiotape (Test of Everyday Attention; Robertson *et al.*, 1994). *Divided attention* is the ability to focus on multiple tasks simultaneously, such as watching a child and talking on the telephone. It is tested by having the patient perform two concurrent tasks, such as scanning a stimulus array and counting tones.

Alternating attention is the ability to switch attention between two or more sources of information, such as going back and forth between recipes when preparing different parts of a meal. It is most frequently tested by the Trail Making Test (Reitan & Wolfson, 1993; Delis *et al.*, 2001), which requires one to alternate between number and letter sequences (e.g., 1–A–2–B–3–C). It is important to keep in mind that most attention tests tap more than one component of attention. For example, sustained attention almost always requires selective attention. The Trail Making Test includes two subtests: the one described above and a simple numeric sequencing subtest (1–2–3–4). Both tasks require visual scanning, sequencing, and psychomotor control of a pencil, but only the alphanumeric subtest requires cognitive set shifting from one sequence to the other. Thus, the ability to alternate attention can be assessed by comparing performance on the two tasks.

Working memory refers to the ability to manipulate information being held in memory for a short period, such as calculating the tip on a restaurant or taxi bill. Working memory certainly requires attention, and some neuropsychologists characterize it as a type of attention, although others report on this function in the memory section of their reports. Working memory may be tested by asking the patient to perform mental arithmetic (Arithmetic subtest of the WAIS-III; Wechsler, 1997a), to listen to strings of digits and repeat them in backward sequence (Digit Span subtest of the WAIS-III), to listen to strings of randomized digits and letters and repeat back the numbers first in numeric order followed by the letters in alphabetic order (Letter-Number Sequencing subtest of the Wechsler Memory Scale-III; WMS-III; Wechsler, 1997b), or to listen to a series of digits and add each digit to the previously presented one (Paced Auditory Serial Addition Test; Gronwall, 1977).

Processing speed refers to the ability to quickly process and respond to new information, such as slamming on one's brakes when the car ahead stops suddenly. It can be measured by tests requiring patients to rapidly transcribe symbols paired with numbers or to scan series of symbols for the presence of target symbols (Digit-Symbol Substitution subtest and Symbol Search subtest of the WAIS-III; Wechsler, 1997a).

Visual ability

Assessment of visual ability typically involves testing object and spatial perception as well as visual construction. *Object perception* is an ability used in everyday life to recognize such things as household items and people's faces. It may be measured by the identification of missing visual details from a line drawing (Picture Completion subtest of the WAIS-III; Wechsler, 1997a), matching a photograph of a face from an array containing the target face along with different faces or of the same face photographed from different views (Benton Facial Recognition Test; Benton *et al.*, 1983), the identification of pictures of objects (Boston Naming Test; Kaplan *et al.*, 1983, although this task also measures naming ability), discrimination of real from nonsense figures, or the identification of incomplete objects, rotated objects, objects embedded in complex arrays, or overlapping figures (see Lezak *et al.*, 2004; Warrington & James, 1991). *Spatial perception* is the ability to appreciate the physical location of objects either alone or in relation to other objects. This ability underlies many everyday motor activities, such as walking through a doorway rather than into the door frame, reaching for a desired object in the refrigerator, and buttoning one's clothes. Spatial perception may be measured by the comparison and matching of line segments drawn at varying angles (Judgment of Line Orientation; Benton *et al.*, 1983), the discrimination of relative spatial positions of objects (Visual Object and Space Perception Test; Warrington & James, 1991), and mental rotations (Standardised Road Map; Money, 1976).

Visual construction is the ability to put together individual parts to make a coherent whole, such as assembling a new appliance from a box of parts (with or without an instruction manual). This skill requires visual perception, integration of visual details, and a motor response. Visual construction may be measured by having patients arrange colored blocks into designs (Block Design subtest of the WAIS-III; Wechsler, 1997a), assemble puzzle pieces to create an object (Object Assembly subtest of the WAIS-III; Wechsler, 1997a), or copy a detailed geometric figure (Rey–Osterrieth Complex Figure Test; Strauss *et al.*, 2006).

Language

Assessment of language functioning typically includes evaluation of both receptive and expressive abilities. Comprehensive batteries of language tests such as the Boston Diagnostic Aphasia Examination (Goodglass & Kaplan, 1972) contain multiple tests of language ability and are useful for characterizing severe language impairments. *Receptive language* refers to the ability to understand orally or visually presented verbal information and is necessary for following a conversation or reading a book. It may be assessed with a multiple-choice test of vocabulary (e.g., Peabody Picture Vocabulary Test – III; Dunn & Dunn, 1997) or a sentence-comprehension test requiring the patient to follow simple verbal commands (e.g., Token Test; see Strauss *et al.*, 2006). *Expressive language* refers to the ability to generate words or sentences, as used for speaking and writing in everyday life. It may be measured by asking patients to name line drawings of common and low-frequency objects (Boston Naming Test; Kaplan *et al.*, 1983), to generate words in a limited time (typically 60 s) according to specified rules, such as words beginning with a given letter or belonging to a specific semantic category (Verbal Fluency subtest of the Delis–Kaplan Executive Function Scale, or D-KEFS; Delis *et al.*, 2001), to define words (Vocabulary subtest of the WAIS-III; Wechsler, 1997a), or to describe a complex scene depicted on a card (Cookie Theft Picture subtest of the Boston Diagnostic Aphasia Examination; Goodglass & Kaplan, 1972).

Memory

Memory is a complex cognitive ability to measure because it can be broken down into individual components along several dimensions, including temporal span, sensory modality, and stage or process. The majority of clinical memory tests measure *short-term* and *long-term memory* for information that was presented seconds to hours ago, as opposed to *remote* memory for events from many years ago. In everyday life, these types of memory correspond to remembering a phone number long enough to dial it, remembering what you had for breakfast this morning, and remembering your high school graduation. In addition, most tests measure *episodic memory* for new information presented during the assessment (such as a story or a list or words, designs, or faces) as opposed to *semantic memory* for previously known general facts (e.g., the capital of Norway).

A thorough memory assessment typically includes measurement of both verbal and nonverbal memory. *Verbal memory* may be assessed by asking the patient to remember lists of words, such as the California Verbal Learning Test (Delis *et al.*, 2000) or Hopkins Verbal Learning Test-Revised (Brandt & Benedict, 2001), series of word pairs (e.g., Verbal Paired Associates subtest of the WMS-III; Wechsler, 1997b), or prose passages (Logical Memory subtest of the WMS-III). *Non-verbal memory* may be assessed by asking the patient to remember geometric figures (e.g., Brief Visuospatial Memory Test; Benedict, 1997; Rey–Osterrieth Complex Figure Test; Strauss *et al.*, 2006) or new faces (e.g., Family Pictures subtest and Faces subtest of the WMS-III). Memory can be tested with several procedures, including *free recall* of the information without any hints or cues from the examiner and *recognition* of previously presented items randomly dispersed among non-presented items.

The typical procedure of many clinical memory tests involves: (1) multiple presentations of the information to be remembered, with each presentation followed by free recall; (2) an intervening period of 20–30 min during which the individual engages in unrelated tasks; (3) delayed free recall of the information; and (4) delayed recognition of the information. Using this procedure, memory can be parsed into several processes. *Acquisition* is the ability to encode new information into memory and is measured by level of recall after the initial presentations. *Learning* is the ability to benefit from repeated presentation of the information and is measured by the increase in items recalled from the first to the last trial of the initial presentations. Generally, recollection improves with successive presentations. *Retention* is the ability to hold newly acquired information in memory over a delay. Retention is often represented as a proportion of initial acquisition, calculated as the number of items recalled after the delay divided by the number of items recalled after the initial presentations. *Retrieval* is the ability to recall information that has been stored in memory. A retrieval problem is suspected when free recall is significantly poorer than recognition, because this pattern indicates that the information was stored in memory but was not properly accessed.

Executive function

Executive functions are defined as higher order cognitive abilities that are necessary for appropriate, socially responsible, and effective conduct (Goodwin, 1989). They encompass many different types of cognitive ability, including planning, abstract thinking, response inhibition, and switching.

Planning involves the abilities to formulate and weigh alternative approaches to a task and to carry out an effective approach to achieve a goal. Everyday tasks that require planning include packing a suitcase, preparing a meal, and mapping out a transportation route (Shallice, 1982). It can be measured by examining the way in which patients accomplish complex tasks in which impulsive, early steps may slow down the ultimate goal attainment. For example, patients may be asked to copy a detailed geometric figure (e.g., using the Boston Qualitative Scoring System for the Rey–Osterrieth Complex Figure Test; Stern *et al.*, 1999) or to rearrange a given structure to match a target structure using a minimum number of responses in accordance with fixed rules (e.g., Tower subtest of the D-KEFS; Delis *et al.*, 2001).

Abstract thinking is the ability to form generalized concepts from discrete instances. Tests of abstract thinking require the individual to describe similarities between words (e.g., Similarities subtest of the WAIS-III; Wechsler, 1997a), to select the missing component of visual sequences arranged in simple to complex patterns (e.g., Matrix Reasoning subtest of the WAIS-III; Wechsler, 1997a), to sort cards according to various principles (e.g., Card Sorting subtest of the D-KEFS; Delis *et al.*, 2001; Wisconsin Card Sorting Test; Heaton *et al.*, 1993), or to interpret proverbs (Proverbs subtest of the D-KEFS).

Response inhibition is the ability to inhibit an automatic response in favor of a more unusual response. For example, experienced drivers who are conditioned to go when a traffic light is green must instead stop when an ambulance or funeral procession is coming by. A classic measure of response inhibition is the Stroop (1935) paradigm, which involves presenting color names printed in dissonant colors (e.g., the word "red" is written in blue ink) and asking the patient to state the ink color. Because reading the word is an automatic process for fluent readers, this task requires inhibition. Standardized Stroop tests include Stroop Color and Word (Golden, 1978), Victoria Stroop (Strauss *et al.*, 2006), and D-KEFS Color–Word Interference (Delis *et al.*, 2001). Inhibition can also be measured with a sentence-completion task requiring the patient to provide a word that is unrelated to the sentence, such as the Hayling Sentence Completion Test (Burgess & Shallice, 1997).

Switching, also known as cognitive set shifting, is the ability to alternate between different types of information or different categories of response. Switching may be measured by asking the patient to alternately sequence numbers and letters (as in tests of alternating attention; Trail Making Test; Delis *et al.*, 2001; Reitan & Wolfson, 1993), to switch between sorting principles on card sorting tasks (D-KEFS Card Sorting; Delis *et al.*, 2001; Wisconsin Card Sorting Test; Heaton *et al.*, 1993), to generate words from alternating semantic categories on a verbal fluency task (Verbal Fluency subtest of the D-KEFS; Delis *et al.*, 2000), or to switch between color naming and word reading on a Stroop task (D-KEFS; Color–Word Interference subtest; Delis *et al.*, 2001).

Sensorimotor ability

Gross measures of sensory and motor ability are often included in neuropsychological assessment, both to provide information about the functional integrity of specific brain regions and to detect any right/left asymmetries that may indicate lateralized brain dysfunction. Measurement of *sensory ability* may include simple tests of detection of visual, auditory, or tactile stimuli on the left and right sides of the body (Bilateral Simultaneous Sensory Stimulation; Reitan & Wolfson, 1993). Measurement of manual *motor ability* may include assessment of fine-motor speed (Finger Tapping, also called Finger Oscillation Test; Reitan & Wolfson, 1993), strength of hand grip (Grip-Strength Dynamometer; Reitan & Wolfson, 1993), and fine-motor dexterity (Grooved Pegboard; Kløve, 1963).

Mood and personality

Assessment of mood and/or personality is sometimes included in a neuropsychological evaluation because brain dysfunction can cause changes in either emotional responsiveness or even longer term temperament. Evaluation can provide information about symptoms of depression or anxiety, level of stress, somatic complaints, paranoid thoughts, substance abuse, aggressive behaviors, and interpersonal styles. Mood and personality are usually measured with self-report questionnaires, such as the Beck Depression Inventory-II (Beck *et al.*, 1996), Beck Anxiety Inventory (Beck & Steer, 1990), Hospital Anxiety and Depression Scale

(Snaith & Zigmond, 1994), Personality Assessment Inventory (Morey, 1991), and the Minnesota Multiphasic Personality Inventory (MMPI-2; Butcher *et al.*, 1989).

As can be gleaned from this brief review of the history, purpose, procedure, and basic principles of clinical neuropsychology, a number of varying conditions will generally determine the exact nature of a particular neuropsychological evaluation. In addition to the compendia by Lezak *et al.* (2004) and Strauss *et al.* (2006) considered critical for the practice of neuropsychology, the interested beginner reader is referred to the undergraduate text by Kolb and Whishaw (2003) or a standard graduate text edited by Heilman and Valenstein (2003). Several other edited and authored volumes elaborate on the topics touched upon here (e.g., Adams *et al.*, 1996; Bradshaw & Mattingley, 1995; Grant & Adams, 1996; Ogden, 1996).

REFERENCES

Adams RL, Parsons OA, Culbertson JL, Nixon SJ (1996). *Neuropsychology for Clinical Practice: Etiology, Assessment, and Treatment of Common Neurological Disorders.* Washington, DC: American Psychological Association.

Beck AT, Steer RA (1990). *Beck Anxiety Inventory.* San Antonio, TX: Psychological Corporation.

Beck AT, Steer RA, Brown GK (1996). *Beck Depression Inventory-II.* San Antonio, TX: Psychological Corporation.

Benedict RHB (1997). *Brief Visuospatial Memory Test-Revised.* Lutz, FL: Psychological Assessment Resources.

Benton A (2000). *Exploring the History of Neuropsychology: Selected Papers.* New York: Oxford University Press.

Benton AL, Joynt RJ (1960). Early descriptions of aphasia. *Arch Neurol* 3: 205–222.

Benton AL, Hamsher K de S, Varney NR, Spreen O (1983). *Contributions to Neuropsychological Assessment: A Clinical Manual.* New York: Oxford University Press.

Bouillaud JB (1825). Recherches cliniques propres à démontrer que la perte de la parole correspond à la lésion des lobules antérieurs du cerveau, et à confirmer l'opinion de M. Gall sur le siège de l'organe du langage articulé. *Arch Generales Med* 8: 25–45.

Bradshaw JL, Mattingley JB (1995). *Clinical Neuropsychology: Behavioral and Brain Science.* San Diego, CA: Academic Press.

Brandt J, Benedict RHB (2001). *Hopkins Verbal Learning Test-Revised.* Lutz, FL: Psychological Assessment Resources.

Burgess PW, Shallice T (1997). *The Hayling and Brixton Tests.* Bury St. Edmunds: Thames Valley Test Company.

Butcher JN, Dahlstrom WG, Graham JR, *et al.* (1989). *Minnesota Multiphasic Personality Inventory-2 [Manual].* Minneapolis, MN: University of Minnesota Press.

Delis DC, Kramer JH, Kaplan E, *et al.* (2000). *California Verbal Learning Test-II.* New York: Psychological Corporation.

Delis DC, Kaplan E, Kramer JH (2001). *Delis-Kaplan Executive Function System.* New York: Psychological Corporation.

Dunn LM, Dunn LM (1997). *Peabody Picture Vocabulary Test – III.* Circle Pines, MN: American Guidance Service.

Folstein MF, Folstein SE, McHugh PR (1975). "Mini-mental State": a practical method for grading the cognitive state of patients for the clinician. *J Psychiatr Res* **12**: 189–198.

Gibson WC (1969). The early history of localization in the nervous system. In PJ Vinken & GW Bruyn (eds.) *Handbook of Clinical Neurology* (Vol. 2, pp. 4–14). Amsterdam: North-Holland Publishing Co.

Golden CJ (1978). *Stroop Color and Word Test: A Manual for Clinical and Experimental Uses.* Chicago, IL: Stoelting Company.

Goodglass H, Kaplan E (1972). *The Assessment of Aphasia and Related Disorders.* Philadelphia, PA: Lea & Febiger.

Goodwin DM (1989). *A Dictionary of Neuropsychology.* New York: Springer-Verlag.

Grant I, Adams KM (eds.) (1996). *Neuropsychological Assessment of Neuropsychiatric Disorders* (2nd edn.). New York: Oxford University Press.

Gronwall DMA (1977). Paced Auditory Serial-Addition task: a measure of recovery from concussion. *Percept Motor Skills* **44**: 367–373.

Heaton RK, Chelune GJ, Talley JL, *et al.* (1993). *Wisconsin Card Sorting Test (WCST) Manual Revised and Expanded.* Odessa, FL: Psychological Assessment Resources.

Heilman KM, Valenstein E (eds.) (2003). *Clinical Neuropsychology* (4th edn.). New York: Oxford University Press.

Kaplan EF, Goodglass H, Weintraub S (1983). *The Boston Naming Test* (2nd edn.) Philadelphia, PA: Lea & Febiger.

Kløve H (1963). Clinical neuropsychology. *Med Clin North Am* **47**: 1647–1658.

Kolb B, Whishaw IQ (2003). *Fundamentals of Human Neuropsychology* (5th edn.). New York: Worth Publishers.

Leach L, Kaplan E, Richards B, *et al.* (2000). *Kaplan-Baycrest Neurocognitive Assessment.* San Antonio, TX: Psychological Corporation.

Lezak MD, Howieson DB, Loring DW (2004). *Neuropsychological Assessment* (4th edn.). New York: Oxford University Press.

Mattis S (2001). *Dementia Rating Scale-2* (Manual). Odessa, FL: Psychological Assessment Resources.

Money J (1976). *A Standardised Road-Map Test of Direction Sense Manual.* San Rafael, CA: Academic Therapy Publications.

Morey LC (1991). *Personality Assessment Inventory.* Odessa, FL: Psychological Assessment Resources.

Ogden JA (1996). *Fractured Minds: A Case-Study Approach to Clinical Neuropsychology.* New York: Oxford University Press.

Randolph C, Tierney MC, Mohr E, *et al.* (1998). The Repeatable Battery for the Assessment of Neuropsychological Status (RBANS): preliminary clinical validity. *J Clin Exp Neuropsychol* **20**: 310–319.

Reitan RM, Wolfson D (1993). *Halstead-Reitan Neuropsychological Battery.* Tucson, AZ: Neuropsychology Press.

Robertson IH, Ward T, Ridgeway V, *et al.* (1994). *The Test of Everyday Attention.* Bury St Edmunds: Thames Valley Test Company.

Roid GH (2003). *Stanford-Binet Intelligence Scale* (5th edn.) Itasca, IL: Riverside Publishing.

Ruff RM, Allen CC (1996). *Ruff 2 & 7 Selective Attention Test.* Lutz, FL: Psychological Assessment Resources.

Scoville WE, Milner B (1957). Loss of recent memory after bilateral hippocampal lesions. *J Neurol Neurosurg Psychiatry* **20**: 11–21.

Shallice T (1982). Specific impairments of planning. *Philosoph Trans Soc London B* **298**: 199–209.

Snaith RP, Zigmond AS (1994). *The Hospital Anxiety and Depression Scale.* Windsor: NFER-Nelson.

Stern RA, Javorsky DJ, Singer EA, *et al.* (1999). *The Boston Qualitative Scoring System for the Rey-Osterrieth Complex Figure.* Odessa, FL: Psychological Assessment Resources.

Strauss E, Sherman EM, Spreen O (2006). *A Compendium of Neuropsychological Tests: Administration, Norms, and Commentary* (3rd edn.). New York: Oxford University Press.

Stroop JR (1935). Studies of interference in serial verbal reaction. *J Exp Psychol* **18**: 643–662.

Walsh KW (1978). *Neuropsychology: A Clinical Approach.* New York: Churchill Livingstone.

Warrington EK, James M (1991). *Visual Object and Space Perception Battery.* Bury St Edmunds: Thames Valley Test Company.

Wechsler D (1997a). *The Wechsler Adult Intelligence Scale – III.* San Antonio, TX: Psychological Corporation.

Wechsler D (1997b). *The Wechsler Memory Scale – III.* San Antonio, TX: Psychological Corporation.

Wechsler D (1999). *The Wechsler Abbreviated Scale of Intelligence.* San Antonio, TX: Psychological Corporation.

3

Brain imaging investigation of chemotherapy-induced neurocognitive changes

Brenna C. McDonald, Andrew J. Saykin, and Tim A. Ahles

Introduction

Structural and functional neuroimaging techniques provide a unique opportunity to examine the neural basis for cognitive changes related to cancer and its treatment. While the link between cognitive dysfunction and central nervous system (CNS) cancers (e.g., primary brain tumors, primary CNS lymphoma, brain metastases of cancer in other organ systems, etc.) or non-CNS cancers treated with prophylactic whole-brain radiation seems clear, our understanding of the causes for cognitive changes following chemotherapy for other non-CNS cancers remains much more limited. Research using a variety of neuroimaging modalities has begun to delineate the brain mechanisms for cognitive changes related to cancer and chemotherapy, across a number of cancer subtypes. This chapter will briefly summarize the cognitive domains most likely to be affected following chemotherapy, review the available data relating cognitive performance and structural and functional neuroimaging changes in various cancer populations, and suggest avenues for future work in this area.

As clinical efficacy of cancer treatment has improved survivorship, increased awareness has arisen of issues critical to the functioning and quality of life of cancer survivors. Specifically, cognitive impairment related to cancer and its treatment, including radiation, chemotherapy, and hormone therapies, has been a topic of increasing study for 20 years. While more detailed discussion of cognitive studies of changes in function related to cancer treatment can be found elsewhere in this volume, these issues will be briefly summarized here, as they form a major component from which subsequent neuroimaging research has grown. Cross-sectional and longitudinal neuropsychological studies of cancer survivors (Ahles *et al.*, 2002; Brezden *et al.*, 2000; Castellon *et al.*, 2004; Schagen *et al.*, 1999; Shilling *et al.*, 2005; Tchen *et al.*, 2003; Van Dam *et al.*, 1998; Wefel *et al.*, 2004b; Wieneke & Dienst, 1995) have contributed to a growing body of literature suggesting detrimental effects of chemotherapy on cognitive performance, although some studies have not found such an effect (Donovan *et al.*, 2005; Jenkins *et al.*, 2006). The cognitive changes associated with chemotherapy are typically subtle, with patients often showing mildly (though statistically significant) reduced functioning relative to control groups, though overall performance remains within normal limits by clinical standards. Changes related to chemotherapy have been reported across several cognitive domains, including working memory, executive function, and processing speed (Ahles & Saykin, 2002; Anderson-Hanley *et al.*, 2003; Ferguson & Ahles, 2003; Tannock *et al.*, 2004). Acutely, cognitive symptoms are often reported during chemotherapy (Ahles & Saykin, 2002; Ferguson & Ahles, 2003), but appear to persist

Cognition and Cancer, eds. Christina A. Meyers and James R. Perry. Published by Cambridge University Press.
© Cambridge University Press 2008.

post-treatment only in a smaller subset of patients, with estimates ranging from 17% to 34%. These effects were observed even after accounting for variables which may be related to negative cognitive outcomes as well as to cancer and its treatment, including psychological factors such as depression or anxiety, or side-effects of cancer treatments such as fatigue. Studies have also found a higher than expected incidence of impaired cognitive performance in cancer patients at baseline (i.e., before exposure to chemotherapy) (Ahles *et al.*, 1998; Meyers *et al.*, 2005; Wagner *et al.*, 2006; Wefel *et al.*, 2004a), and a history of cancer has been suggested as a potential risk factor for cognitive impairment and Alzheimer's disease in the elderly (Heflin *et al.*, 2005). To date, chemotherapy-related cognitive changes (independent of the effects of cranial irradiation) have been studied most extensively in breast cancer patients; however, there are reports in the literature suggesting that patients with other non-CNS cancers (e.g., lung cancer, lymphoma) may also demonstrate cognitive changes related to cancer and/or chemotherapy (e.g., Ahles *et al.*, 2002; Kanard *et al.*, 2004; Komaki *et al.*, 1995; Meyers *et al.*, 1995; Van Oosterhout *et al.*, 1996).

While studies like those cited above have documented cognitive changes that appear related to chemotherapy, the neural mechanism underlying these changes is as yet poorly understood, though several possible biological pathways have been proposed to account for cognitive changes related to both chemotherapy and cancer itself (Ahles & Saykin, 2007). These include genetic factors which increase risk for both cancer and cognitive impairment, and the potential interaction of these factors with chemotherapy and hormonal cancer treatments. In summary, research to date suggests that cognitive changes associated with chemotherapy need to be examined within the broader context of genetic and other risk factors and biological processes associated with the development of cancer. Significant cognitive changes likely occur only in a subset of chemotherapy-treated patients as a result of these risk factors. It may also be the case

that shared factors interact to increase the risk of cancer itself, as well as cognitive decline more generally, where the presence of such factors might account for the observed baseline impairment in some cancer patients. In the presence of such risk factors, one would perhaps expect to observe exacerbation of cognitive deficits following chemotherapy. From a neuropsychological perspective, an important avenue of research to pursue is the delineation of changes in brain structure and function associated with the cognitive abnormalities observed following chemotherapy, changes which may be related to risk factors for cancer and cognitive decline.

Structural and functional neuroimaging methods

Recent advances in neuroimaging technologies permit investigation of cognitive changes related to cancer and chemotherapy *in vivo*. Examples of these brain imaging methods are briefly reviewed here, and are illustrated in Figure 3.1. Structural magnetic resonance imaging (MRI) can be used to provide a high-resolution picture of neuroanatomical details and atrophy (T1-weighted scans), and visible pathology such as microvascular and inflammatory lesions [T2-weighted scans; fluid-attenuated inversion recovery (FLAIR) scans]. Semi-automated or manual methods can be used to segment or classify the structural images into the main brain tissue compartments (Figure 3.1a), including gray and white matter (GM and WM) and cerebrospinal fluid (CSF), as well as to delineate hyperintense lesions, which can reflect microvascular changes or areas of demyelination. Volume and other characteristics of each tissue type can then be quantitated and compared using imaging and statistical software. Prior to the development of MRI, computerized axial tomography (CAT or CT) scanning was the predominant method of structural brain imaging. CT methodology involves computerized integration of multiple X-ray images to generate cross-sectional views of the brain. Due to its

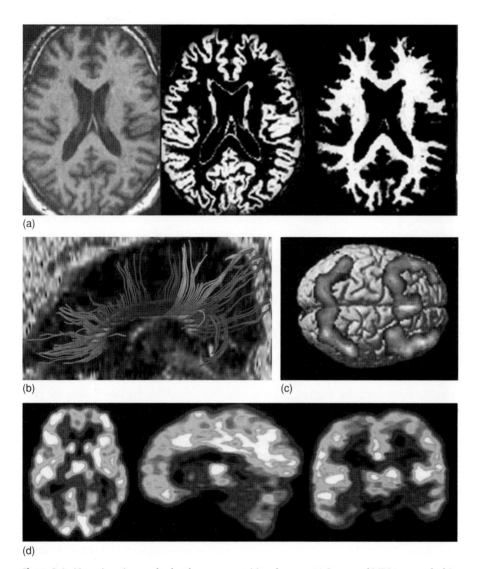

Figure 3.1. Neuroimaging methods relevant to cognitive changes. (a) Structural MRI (gray and white matter atrophy); (b) diffusion tensor imaging (white matter connectivity); (c) functional MRI (brain activity), and (d) PET (brain metabolism). Reprinted with permission from Ahles and Saykin (2007). See color version in color plate section.

much lower intracerebral tissue contrast and the exposure to radiation involved in the technique, however, CT is much less commonly used than MRI for most neuroimaging research related to cancer chemotherapy, though CT remains the optimal method for some purposes (e.g., imaging of bone or acute hemorrhage).

Voxel-based morphometry (VBM) is a recently developed method for analyzing structural MRI data to quantitatively evaluate atrophy and other changes on a voxel-by-voxel basis throughout the entire brain (Ashburner & Friston, 2000, 2001; Good et al., 2001). Unlike the above-noted morphological methods that involve manual segmentation of selected structures, VBM is a fully automated procedure for examining tissue integrity, providing the ability to assess regional volume and density of brain tissue compartments. VBM utilizes statistical parametric mapping procedures similar to those employed for analysis of functional neuroimaging data. Because VBM assesses signal intensities across every voxel in the brain relative to a user-defined *a priori* statistical threshold, it provides an unbiased, comprehensive, and highly reliable assessment of tissue volume that is sensitive to local changes. VBM has been used in a small number of studies, discussed below, to investigate brain changes related to chemotherapy.

Diffusion tensor imaging (DTI) is a recently developed technique that capitalizes on variation in the degree and directionality of diffusion of water molecules in different brain tissue types as an indicator of tissue integrity. Diffusion of water molecules in GM and CSF is largely isotropic (random), but is directionally restricted by axonal membranes and myelin. Therefore, in aggregate, WM fiber bundles are normally highly non-random in diffusion characteristics. By measuring the degree and orientation of anisotropy of diffusion, DTI can demonstrate the directionality of fiber tracts (Figure 3.1b) (Le Bihan *et al.*, 2001), and can demonstrate neuroanatomic connectivity of fiber pathways among brain regions involved in a particular network (Basser *et al.*, 1994; Pierpaoli *et al.*, 1996), thus showing great promise for investigating subtypes of WM pathology. The integrity of WM pathways is also quantitatively indicated by the degree of anisotropy, while pathological changes in GM can be detected by examining differences in mean diffusivity of tissue. Further, DTI can be combined with functional MRI (see below) to relate anatomical connectivity to functional brain activation patterns related to cognitive or motor tasks, and to recovery from brain injury or insult (Werring *et al.*, 1998, 1999). Therefore, DTI shows great promise for investigating subtypes of structural brain pathology, particularly in WM. Although DTI has been used to document abnormalities in other clinical populations where WM disease is a hallmark on neuroimaging, as yet no published reports have used this technique to examine the potential effects of chemotherapy independent of radiation therapy. However, DTI appears to have a great deal of promise for closer study of the WM abnormalities that have been demonstrated after chemotherapy using other structural neuroimaging methods.

Magnetic resonance spectroscopy (MRS) utilizes the differing magnetic properties of biochemical compounds in the brain to allow graphic representation of metabolite concentration, synthesis rates, and relative volumes in neural tissue, *in vivo* and without exposure to radioactivity. Recent developments in MRS allow measurement of specific brain neurotransmitters, including glutamate, glycine, and gamma-amino butyric acid (GABA), among others, in addition to other metabolite markers of neuronal status and integrity such as *N*-acetyl-aspartate (NAA), creatine, choline, and *myo*-inositol.

Functional MRI (fMRI) employs detection of increases in local signal intensity (Belliveau *et al.*, 1992; Kwong *et al.*, 1992) to assess the activation of cortical and subcortical regions during the performance of cognitive or sensorimotor tasks in the scanner [Figure 3.1c; for details of key fMRI methods, see Bandettini & Wong (1997), Rosen *et al.* (1998), and Moonen and Bandettini (2000)]. The differing magnetic susceptibilities of oxyhemoglobin (diamagnetic) and deoxyhemoglobin (paramagnetic) permit deoxyhemoglobin to act as an endogenous contrast agent sensitive to blood oxygenation (Ogawa *et al.*, 1998). This has become known as blood oxygen level dependent (BOLD) contrast. It has been hypothesized that microvascular changes are specific to the dynamic activity of local neural circuits, and recent evidence confirms this model (Logothetis *et al.*, 2001). The change in signal intensity is induced by local field gradients which result from the intravascular compartmentalization of the endogenous contrast agent (Lai *et al.*, 1993). The onset of detectable change in signal intensity is time dependent and occurs maximally at 5–8 s post-activation, with drop off approximately 5–9 s post cessation of stimulation (Bandettini *et al.*, 1993). Fast acquisition capability can take advantage of this rapid change in blood flow. Neuronal activity and local cerebral blood flow, volume, and parenchymal oxygenation are normally tightly coupled, but this may be altered by disease processes and possibly aging (D'Esposito *et al.*, 1999; Johnson *et al.*, 2001; Ross *et al.*, 1997).

In contrast to the MRI-based measures described above, molecular imaging methods such as positron emission tomography (PET) use radiotracers to provide data on cerebral blood flow or specific neurotransmitter/receptor systems (Figure 3.1d). PET utilizes short-lived radioisotopes to examine brain function either at rest or during task performance, most commonly by measuring levels of blood flow (e.g., with ^{15}O-labeled water) or glucose metabolism (e.g., using ^{18}F-fluorodeoxyglucose, or FDG). More recent applications allow targeted examination of specific neurotransmitter systems, including the dopaminergic, cholinergic, and serotonergic systems. Tracers have likewise been developed to study receptor binding for opioids and benzodiazepines. A highly promising area is the development of targeted PET probes for molecular pathology of disease, such as amyloid imaging for Alzheimer's disease and other dementias (e.g., Klunk *et al.*, 2004).

Neuroimaging of cognitive changes related to cancer and chemotherapy

Toga and Mazziotta (1996) provide an overall review of structural and functional neuroimaging methodologies and their application to brain disorders (Mazziotta *et al.*, 2000). Very limited systematic neuroimaging research has been conducted with patients undergoing chemotherapy for non-brain cancers in the absence of radiation therapy (RT), with much of the available literature reflecting case series, convenience samples, or retrospective studies. In addition, the literature is largely restricted to structural neuroimaging studies, with only a few studies utilizing functional neuroimaging techniques. Functional neuroimaging methods

have not yet been examined in systematic, prospective studies of chemotherapy-induced or cancer-associated cognitive changes, but these approaches hold promise for identifying the neural bases of such changes. While the available neuroimaging literature examining chemotherapy effects is somewhat limited, some relevant clinical observations have been published.

MRI studies of childhood leukemia

Structural MRI has been demonstrated to be sensitive to abnormalities in children treated with chemotherapy for acute lymphoblastic leukemia (ALL) (for review, see Reddick *et al.*, 2007). While considerable work has examined the effects of chemotherapy in conjunction with RT, a growing number of neuroimaging studies have also examined the independent effects of chemotherapy by studying children treated for ALL who did not receive RT. Ciesielski, Lesnik and colleagues (Ciesielski *et al.*, 1999; Lesnik *et al.*, 1998) used MRI morphometry to study 10 children who underwent neurotoxic intrathecal chemotherapy with methotrexate but not RT for ALL before age five. In a study focused on the development of brain regions important for memory, Ciesielski *et al.* (1999) found significant volume reductions in the mammillary bodies and prefrontal cortices (PFC), and non-significant reductions in the caudate nuclei in ALL patients relative to healthy controls. In another study using the same patient and control groups, this team found smaller volumes in the PFC and cerebellar lobuli VI–VII, and neuropsychological deficits in visuospatial attention, short-term memory, and visuomotor organization and co-ordination, implicating cerebellar-frontal system alterations in the cognitive changes following chemotherapy in this population (Lesnik *et al.*, 1998).

Harila-Saari *et al.* (1998) found MRI abnormalities in 8 of 32 patients 5 years after RT and/or chemotherapy for ALL. Only 2 of 15 patients who received chemotherapy without RT demonstrated abnormalities (WM changes) however, and one of these subjects had been born prematurely, perhaps indicating a predisposing factor for WM change. Kingma *et al.* (2001) studied 17 ALL patients treated with chemotherapy only with neuropsychological assessment and MRI, and compared this group to children who also received RT and to healthy controls. While structural MRI abnormalities were less frequent in the chemotherapy-only group relative to patients who had also received RT (38% vs. 63%), definite abnormalities were noted in 3 of 16 children with available MRI scans who were treated with chemotherapy without RT, with probable abnormalities noted in another 3 cases. These abnormalities reportedly included WM changes and/or atrophy. In this small sample, the presence of an MRI abnormality was unrelated to other cognitive or academic variables for either ALL group.

Most recently, Reddick *et al.* (2006) studied a large cohort of children who had been treated for ALL with chemotherapy alone ($n = 84$) or with chemotherapy and RT ($n = 28$), in comparison to healthy sibling controls ($n = 33$). Neurocognitive testing demonstrated significant differences relative to normative performance expectations in both cancer groups. Patients treated with RT showed the most significant declines, with cognitive impairment consistent with prior reports. Patients treated with chemotherapy alone also demonstrated statistically significant declines relative to age norms across most neurocognitive tasks, though level of impairment was less severe than for patients treated with RT. For most measures, performance in the chemotherapy-only group was within broad normal limits; however, clinically meaningful impairment (>1.0 SD lower than normative mean) was seen on measures of attentional functioning. A similar pattern was observed for brain WM volume on MRI. Patients treated with RT showed the greatest reduction in WM volume, with significantly smaller volumes than both other groups. The chemotherapy-only group also showed a significant reduction in WM volume relative to controls however, consistent with the studies noted above showing reduced brain volumes in other structures following chemotherapy without RT for ALL.

Reddick *et al.* (2006) also examined the relationship between WM volume and neurocognitive performance within the ALL patients, and found significant inverse correlations for nearly all measures examined, including estimated intellect, academic achievement, and attentional functioning. These findings suggest that chemotherapy and RT likely have both independent and interacting negative effects in terms of structural brain changes and cognitive performance following treatment.

Neuroimaging in osteosarcoma

Early case reports of radiologic abnormalities following chemotherapy for osteosarcoma utilized CT scanning. Packer *et al.* (1983) reported the first case of abnormal CT findings in a child treated with high-dose methotrexate followed by citrovorum rescue in 1983. Another early case study also noted transient encephalopathy and CNS toxicity related to high-dose methotrexate treatment for metastatic osteosarcoma (Fritsch & Urban, 1984), with accompanying CT abnormalities including periventricular hypodensity, particularly around the frontal horns, as well as a hypodense left temporal lesion. These abnormalities were noted to be persistent even 14 months after the acute symptom onset, though cognitive and neurological function was reportedly normal 5 years post-illness, aside from absent deep tendon reflexes. Another case study similarly noted the onset of leukoencephalopathy during high-dose methotrexate treatment with calcium leucovorin rescue for osteosarcoma (Glass *et al.*, 1986), with head CT showing bilateral non-enhancing symmetric hypodensities in the periventricular WM and centrum semiovale. In earlier related work, Allen *et al.* (1980) noted diffuse WM hypodensity (five patients) and atrophic changes (five patients) in individuals treated with high-dose methotrexate with leucovorin rescue without RT for bone or soft-tissue sarcomas who developed leukoencephalopathy.

Later studies utilized MRI to detect abnormalities in osteosarcoma patients with greater anatomic resolution. In a sample of eight patients, mostly adolescents, treated with single-agent high-dose methotrexate without RT, Ebner et al. (1989) observed brain abnormalities on CT or MRI in four, including chronic edema, multifocal WM necrosis, and deep atrophy. Interestingly, while two of these four became encephalopathic, the other two did not manifest clinically evident cognitive abnormalities concurrent with the noted brain abnormalities. Lien et al. (1991) reported MRI findings in 22 patients treated for osteosarcoma with a chemotherapy regimen which included high-dose methotrexate with citrovorum factor rescue, cisplatin, doxorubicin HCl, bleomycin, cyclophosphamide, and actinomycin D. Ten patients who received cisplatin-based treatment for testicular cancer were used as a control group. In the osteosarcoma group, 14 patients showed WM lesions on T2-weighted imaging, which appeared related to time since treatment, as they were observed in 12 of 14 subjects whose MRI scan occurred within 2 years of chemotherapy, but in only 2 of 8 patients who had later MRI studies. Lesions were bilateral in all but one patient, and were most commonly adjacent to the lateral ventricle, though they were also noted in the centrum semiovale and corpus callosum. No MRI abnormalities were observed in the testicular cancer group, suggesting that cisplatin was unlikely to be the major agent responsible for such changes, and arguing that high-dose methotrexate was the most probable cause, though an interactive effect with cisplatin could not be ruled out. In this sample, no CNS symptoms were apparent, though detailed neurological and psychiatric examinations were not conducted.

Other MRI reports of chemotherapy-induced leukoencephalopathy in adults

Development of multifocal gadolinium-enhancing inflammatory brain WM lesions has been reported after treatment with adjuvant 5-fluorouracil and levamisole for adenocarcinoma of the colon (Hook et al., 1992). Biopsy in two of three cases was consistent with active demyelination, with axonal sparing and perivascular lymphocytic inflammation. All

three patients improved with corticosteroid therapy after chemotherapy ended. This study suggested that inflammatory mechanisms may play an important role in the pathophysiology of 5-fluorouracil neurotoxicity, though the authors noted that they could not rule out an effect of levamisole. Subsequently, this group of investigators (Kimmel et al., 1995) reported similar MRI and clinical findings in a patient receiving adjuvant levamisole therapy for malignant melanoma, which again improved after discontinuation followed by corticosteroid therapy. This suggests that levamisole may have been a key factor in the previously reported cases.

Structural and functional MRI studies of chemotherapy-related cognitive changes in breast cancer

Studies that have incorporated neuroimaging techniques have reported structural and functional changes in the brain associated with chemotherapy (Saykin et al., 2003b; Stemmer et al., 1994). A reduction in the volume of brain structures important for cognitive functioning (such as the frontal cortex) and changes in the integrity of WM tracts that connect brain structures have been associated with changes in cognitive functioning, and have been seen using structural MRI in patients after chemotherapy. Stemmer et al. (1994) reported WM changes in 9 of 13 breast cancer patients (stage II–IV) following treatment with high-dose cyclophosphamide, cisplatin, carmustine, and autologous bone marrow support. Based on neuroradiological ratings, four of these patients had severe WM changes, four had moderate changes, and one had mild changes. It is important to recognize that – despite at times extensive structural brain abnormalities, particularly of the WM – many of the studies cited in this chapter note that these changes appear to be "clinically silent," with no noted deficits on neurological examination or cognitive, psychological, or functional complaints reported by their study participants.

In a very recent study using VBM in female breast cancer survivors, Inagaki et al. (2007) compared patients who had been treated with chemotherapy (C+) to those who had not (C−), and to a healthy control group. Groups were compared at two time points, labeled 1 and 3 years post-chemotherapy, though it should be noted that the mean post-treatment interval for the "1 year" sample was about 4 months, while the mean for the "3-year" sample was about 3.25 years. The samples were partially overlapping, but the study was not longitudinal as such. At the 1-year time point, the C+ group was found to demonstrate decreased GM and WM volume relative to the C− group, including prefrontal, parahippocampal, cingulate gyrus, and precuneus regions. No significant intergroup (C+ vs. C−) differences were apparent at the 3-year time point. Despite the finding of smaller regional brain volumes in the C+ relative to the C− group at the 1-year time point, when all cancer patients were compared to healthy controls, no significant volume differences were apparent at either time point. Correlational analyses demonstrated a significant relationship between prefrontal, parahippocampal, and precuneus volumes and indices of attention-concentration and/or visual memory from the Wechsler Memory Scale, Revised (WMS-R) at the 1-year time point.

The lack of significant differences between C+ and C− groups at the 3-year time point was consistent with prior work by this group (Yoshikawa *et al.*, 2005), in which they compared hippocampal volumes obtained using a manual tracing technique between C+ and C− patients who were all more than 3 years post-surgery, and found no between-group differences. They likewise found no group differences in WMS-R memory performance, though attention-concentration performance was significantly weaker in the C+ group.

As noted by the authors themselves and in other commentary, there are methodological issues that affect interpretation of these results. As noted by Eichbaum *et al.* (2007), the majority of patients in the Inagaki *et al.* (2007) study did not receive a recommended standard chemotherapy regimen. Groups were also confounded by hormonal treatment status (significantly more patients received hormonal treatment in the

C+ than the C− group) in both studies, and the possible presence of baseline cognitive deficits in the cancer patients was not taken into consideration. The rationale behind some of the comparisons presented by Inagaki *et al.* (2007) was also unclear. It does not appear that the C+ and C− groups were independently compared to the control group, which would have been informative. It is also unclear whether correlational analyses between cognitive performance and brain volume were done across groups, or just within the C+ group. Attention to such issues will be important in future research.

In contrast to the findings from Inagaki *et al.* (2007), VBM studies in our laboratory have demonstrated smaller regional brain volumes in breast cancer patients who received chemotherapy compared to those who did not and to healthy control participants. In a study of long-term (>5 years post-diagnosis) breast cancer and lymphoma survivors, we utilized VBM to study 12 women treated with chemotherapy compared to 12 demographically matched healthy control subjects (Saykin *et al.*, 2003a, 2003b). Relative to controls, the C+ group showed local bilateral reduction of neocortical GM and cortical and subcortical WM volume in several regions. There were no brain regions in which control subjects demonstrated volume reduction relative to cancer patients. These results provided preliminary evidence of distributed structural changes in GM and WM many years after treatment with chemotherapy, in a relatively diffuse neuroanatomic pattern generally consistent with the relatively diffuse profile of neuropsychological declines noted above and described elsewhere in this volume.

Our laboratory is currently undertaking a longitudinal, prospective study of the neural mechanisms of cognitive changes related to breast cancer and its treatment, utilizing a comprehensive assessment battery including neurocognitive evaluation, structural and functional MRI, and blood biomarker and genotyping analysis. Breast cancer patients treated with (C+) and without (C−) chemotherapy are being compared to healthy control subjects prior to adjuvant treatment and 1 and 12 months after completion of chemotherapy (or yoked intervals).

Preliminary data (Saykin *et al.*, 2007) have shown a pattern of reduced brain activation in frontal areas on fMRI during a working memory task 1 month after chemotherapy, suggestive of dysfunction in circuitry crucial for normal working memory functioning. Unpublished data from VBM analysis of the structural MRI data in this cohort have indicated decreased frontotemporal GM 1 month after breast cancer chemotherapy relative to pre-chemotherapy baseline in C+ patients relative to C− patients and to healthy controls. These data suggest that structural and functional changes in the brain can be detected quite soon after systemic chemotherapy; analysis of the data from the 12-month assessment will help determine the natural course of these changes over time.

Another fMRI study of breast cancer patients is noted in a recent review article (Castellon *et al.*, 2005), though it does not as yet appear to have been published independently. In this study (Wagner *et al.*, 2004), ten cancer patients, most of whom reportedly had breast cancer and who were identified as demonstrating cognitive impairment on formal neuropsychological testing, were compared to a group of demographically matched healthy control participants. Cancer patients were reportedly within 6 months of completion of chemotherapy, and demonstrated deficits in three or more of the neuropsychological domains evaluated, including cognitive efficiency, working memory, visuospatial skills, and delayed memory. All subjects were right-handed. Participants completed a blocked, visual, non-verbal n-back paradigm, with 0-, 1-, and 2-back conditions. In contrast to other functional neuroimaging studies, this group of patients reportedly did not demonstrate differences in task performance or brain activation relative to controls, with the exception of greater activation in the control group in the right cerebellum and dentate nucleus (task condition unspecified in the available citations).

In a case report (Ferguson *et al.*, 2007), we describe differences in structural and functional MRI data in identical twins discordant for breast cancer and chemotherapy treatment. These 60-year-old, right-handed sisters participated in a comprehensive battery of cognitive assessment and structural and fMRI measures, and completed detailed self-report inventories. While cognitive functioning was not meaningfully different between the twins as measured by standardized neuropsychological tests, Twin A, who was treated with adjuvant chemotherapy and hormone therapy for stage II breast cancer, self-reported a much greater level of cognitive concerns than Twin B, who had never had breast cancer. MRI measures showed notable differences between the two subjects. Twin A showed a higher volume of WM hyperintensities on FLAIR imaging (9800.68 mm^3 vs. 6241.11 mm^3) than Twin B; these hyperintensities were read as of uncertain clinical significance by the study neuroradiologist. Twin A also demonstrated an expanded spatial extent of activation during working memory processing on an auditory-verbal "n-back" fMRI paradigm, despite comparable task performance to her sister. These findings illustrate a potential explanation for the commonly seen discrepancy between self-reported cognitive symptoms following chemotherapy and lack of objective findings of cognitive impairment on formal neuropsychological assessment. The expanded extent of brain activation demonstrated in Twin A – which is similar to that we have seen in other clinical populations, including those with multiple sclerosis, traumatic brain injury, and mild cognitive impairment (McAllister *et al.*, 2001; Saykin *et al.*, 2004; Wishart *et al.*, 2004) – may reflect compensatory recruitment of additional brain regions in order to perform the task successfully. This may be perceived by patients as increased task effort, or as tasks becoming more difficult than they were previously. Data from the ongoing longitudinal study noted above will aid in coming to a more detailed understanding of the neural substrate of cognitive changes related to breast cancer and its treatment.

As yet only one published study has examined neural effects of chemotherapy using PET (Silverman *et al.*, 2007). In this study, 16 women who were 5–10 years post breast cancer chemotherapy were compared to a concurrent sample of 8 controls (5 non-cancer healthy controls, 3 women with a history of breast cancer but no chemotherapy treatment), and to a previously acquired sample of 10 healthy controls. ^{15}O-water PET was used to evaluate blood flow related to memory processing, while ^{18}F-FDG PET was used to examine resting cerebral metabolism. During short-term verbal recall, modulation of blood flow in specific frontal and cerebellar regions was significantly altered in the chemotherapy-treated group relative to controls, most significantly in the left inferior frontal gyrus (LIFG). In the chemotherapy-treated patients only, LIFG resting metabolism was observed to correlate directly with performance on a short-term memory task previously found by this group (Castellon *et al.*, 2004) to be impaired in chemotherapy-treated patients. Examination of the effects of hormone treatment on cerebral metabolism demonstrated that patients treated with chemotherapy and tamoxifen (11 of the 16 studied) showed significantly decreased basal ganglia metabolism relative to those who received chemotherapy but did not receive tamoxifen, or those not treated with chemotherapy. These findings offer further evidence of alterations in brain function related to breast cancer treatment, and highlight the importance of further study of the independent and interactive effects of cytotoxic chemotherapy and hormonal treatment.

Proton MRS can reveal neurochemical changes in brain cellular metabolism that appear to be highly relevant for understanding pathophysiological changes after chemotherapy. Relevant data from several small studies have been reported. Brown *et al.* (1998) prospectively attempted to determine the time course for development of WM changes induced by high-dose chemotherapy (HDC). Advanced (stage II–IV) breast cancer patients ($n = 8$) were studied with serial MRI and MRS before chemotherapy throughout the 12 months after treatment [carmustine, cyclophosphamide, and cisplatin, with autologous hematopoietic progenitor cell support (AHPCS)]. MRI appeared normal in all eight subjects at baseline, and in all six patients for whom scans were available

after induction chemotherapy. WM changes were apparent in one of these patients 2 months after HCD/AHPCS. At 3 months and beyond, three of four patients remaining in the study showed an increasing volume of WM changes that stabilized in the 6- to 12-month post-treatment phase. Maximal volumes of abnormal WM ranged from 73 to 166 cm^3. Despite the clear WM abnormalities, few neurochemical changes were detected by MRS, although the ratio of NAA to creatine (Cr) suggested a transient treatment-related decrease (Brown *et al.*, 1998). In an earlier post-treatment study, this group (Brown *et al.*, 1995) compared MRI and MRS in 13 patients undergoing bone marrow transplant for advanced breast carcinoma relative to 13 controls. Extensive HDC-induced WM changes were measured in 10 of 13 patients, with an average volume of abnormal WM of 49 cm^3. NAA/Cr and NAA/choline ratios were not abnormal despite these prominent late-stage structural changes, leading the authors to conclude that chemotherapy-induced WM disease is predominantly a water space and possibly an extra-neuronal process rather than a primary neuronal/axonal disease. These authors also emphasized the complementary nature of information from MRS and MRI in understanding the pathophysiology of chemotherapy effects.

Conclusion

At present, the data regarding the cognitive effects of cancer chemotherapy are somewhat limited. Most studies to date have been conducted post-treatment, and many are confounded by concomitant cranial radiation therapy. The available evidence suggests that multiple neuroimaging modalities are sensitive to the effects of cancer treatment on brain structure and function. There is evidence for both GM and WM structural changes, as well as altered metabolic and activation profiles on functional neuroimaging. Systematic research is needed to determine which neuroimaging modalities are most sensitive and specific for chemotherapy, hormonal therapy, and radiation effects, as well as interactions among these interventions. Further integration of genetics and other biomarkers is also likely to yield important new information. Finally, structural and functional neuroimaging can be expected to play a role in evaluating interventions such as cognitive rehabilitation and medication for treatment of cognitive changes related to cancer and its treatment.

ACKNOWLEDGMENTS

This work was supported by grants from the National Cancer Institute (5R01CA087845 & 5R01CA101318) and a National Institutes of Health Roadmap Grant (U54EB005149).

REFERENCES

Ahles TA, Saykin AJ (2002). Breast cancer chemotherapy-related cognitive dysfunction. *Clin Breast Cancer* **3**(3): 84–90.

Ahles TA, Saykin AJ (2007). Candidate mechanisms for chemotherapy-induced cognitive changes. *Nature Rev* **7**(3): 192–201.

Ahles TA, Silberfarb PM, *et al.* (1998). Psychologic and neuropsychologic functioning of patients with limited small-cell lung cancer treated with chemotherapy and radiation therapy with or without warfarin: a study by the Cancer and Leukemia Group B. *J Clin Oncol* **16**(5): 1954–60.

Ahles TA, Saykin AJ, *et al.* (2002). Neuropsychologic impact of standard-dose systemic chemotherapy in long-term survivors of breast cancer and lymphoma. *J Clin Oncol* **20**(2): 485–493.

Allen JC, Rosen G, *et al.* (1980). Leukoencephalopathy following high-dose iv methotrexate chemotherapy with leucovorin rescue. *Cancer Treat Rep* **64**(12): 1261–73.

Anderson-Hanley C, Sherman ML, *et al.* (2003). Neuropsychological effects of treatments for adults with cancer: a meta-analysis and review of the literature. *J Int Neuropsychol Soc* **9**(7): 967–982.

Ashburner J, Friston KF (2000). Voxel-based morphometry – the methods. *NeuroImage* **11**(6 Pt 1): 805–821.

Ashburner J, Friston KJ (2001). Why voxel-based morphometry should be used. *NeuroImage* **14**(6): 1238–1243.

Bandettini PA, Wong EC (1997). Magnetic resonance imaging of human brain function. Principles, practicalities, and possibilities. *Neurosurg Clin North Am* **8**(3): 345–371.

Bandettini PA, Jesmanowicz A, *et al.* (1993). Processing strategies for time-course data sets in functional MRI of the human brain. *Magn Res Med* **30**(2): 161–173.

Basser PJ, Mattiello J, *et al.* (1994). MR diffusion tensor spectroscopy and imaging. *Biophys J* **66**(1): 259–267.

Belliveau JW, Kwong KK, *et al.* (1992). Magnetic resonance imaging mapping of brain function. Human visual cortex. *Invest Radiol* **27**(Suppl 2): S59–S65.

Brezden CB, Phillips KA, *et al.* (2000). Cognitive function in breast cancer patients receiving adjuvant chemotherapy. *J Clin Oncol* **18**(14): 2695–2701.

Brown MS, Simon JH, *et al.* (1995). MR and proton spectroscopy of white matter disease induced by high-dose chemotherapy with bone marrow transplant in advanced breast carcinoma. *AJNR Am J Neuroradiol* **16**(10): 2013–2020.

Brown MS, Stemmer SM, *et al.* (1998). White matter disease induced by high-dose chemotherapy: longitudinal study with MR imaging and proton spectroscopy. *AJNR Am J Neuroradiol* **19**(2): 217–221.

Castellon SA, Ganz PA, *et al.* (2004). Neurocognitive performance in breast cancer survivors exposed to adjuvant chemotherapy and tamoxifen. *J Clin Exp Neuropsychol* **26**(7): 955–969.

Castellon SA, Silverman DHS, *et al.* (2005). Breast cancer treatment and cognitive functioning: current status and future challenges in assessment. *Breast Cancer Res Treat* **92**(3): 199–206.

Ciesielski KT, Lesnik PG, *et al.* (1999). MRI morphometry of mammillary bodies, caudate nuclei, and prefrontal cortices after chemotherapy for childhood leukemia: multivariate models of early and late developing memory subsystems. *Behav Neurosci* **113**(3): 439–450.

D'Esposito M, Zarahn E, *et al.* (1999). The effect of normal aging on the coupling of neural activity to the bold hemodynamic response. *NeuroImage* **10**(1): 6–14.

Donovan KA, Small BJ, *et al.* (2005). Cognitive functioning after adjuvant chemotherapy and/or radiotherapy for early-stage breast carcinoma. *Cancer* **104**(11): 2499–2507.

Ebner F, Ranner G, *et al.* (1989). MR findings in methotrexate-induced CNS abnormalities. *Am J Roentgenol* **153**(6): 1283–1288.

Eichbaum MHR, Schneeweiss A, *et al.* (2007). Smaller regional volumes of gray and white matter demonstrated in breast cancer survivors exposed to adjuvant chemotherapy. *Cancer* **109**(1): 146–156.

Ferguson RJ, Ahles TA (2003). Low neuropsychologic performance among adult cancer survivors treated with chemotherapy. *Curr Neurol Neurosci Rep* **3**: 215–222.

Ferguson RJ, McDonald BC, *et al.* (2007). Brain structure and function differences in monozygotic twins: possible effects of breast cancer chemotherapy. *J Clin Oncol* **25**(25): 3866–3870.

Fritsch G, Urban C (1984). Transient encephalopathy during the late course of treatment with high-dose methotrexate. *Cancer* **53**(9): 1849–1851.

Glass JP, Lee YY, *et al.* (1986). Treatment-related leukoencephalopathy. A study of three cases and literature review. *Medicine* **65**(3): 154–162.

Good CD, Johnsrude IS, *et al.* (2001). A voxel-based morphometric study of ageing in 465 normal adult human brains. *NeuroImage* **14**: 21–36.

Harila-Saari AH, Paakko EL, *et al.* (1998). A longitudinal magnetic resonance imaging study of the brain in survivors in childhood acute lymphoblastic leukemia. *Cancer* **83**(12): 2608–2617.

Heflin LH, Meyerowitz BE, *et al.* (2005). Re: Cancer as a risk factor for dementia: a house built on shifting sand. *J Nat Cancer Inst* **97**(20): 1550–1551.

Hook CC, Kimmel DW, *et al.* (1992). Multifocal inflammatory leukoencephalopathy with 5-fluorouracil and levamisole. *Ann Neurol* **31**(3): 262–267.

Inagaki M, Yoshikawa E, *et al.* (2007). Smaller regional volumes of brain gray and white matter demonstrated in breast cancer survivors exposed to adjuvant chemotherapy. *Cancer* **109**(1): 146–156.

Jenkins V, Shilling V, *et al.* (2006). A 3-year prospective study of the effects of adjuvant treatments on cognition in women with early stage breast cancer. *Br J Cancer* **94**(6): 828–834.

Johnson SC, Saykin AJ, *et al.* (2001). Similarities and differences in semantic and phonological processing with age: patterns of functional MRI activation. *Aging, Neuropsychol Cogn* **8**(4): 307–320.

Kanard A, Frytak S, *et al.* (2004). Cognitive dysfunction in patients with small-cell lung cancer: incidence, causes, and suggestions on management. *J Support Oncol* **2**(2): 127–132.

Kimmel DW, Wijdicks EF, *et al.* (1995). Multifocal inflammatory leukoencephalopathy associated with levamisole therapy. *Neurology* **45**(2): 374–376.

Kingma A, van Dommelens RI, *et al.* (2001). Slight cognitive impairment and magnetic resonance imaging abnormalities but normal school levels in children treated for acute lymphoblastic leukemia with chemotherapy only. *J Pediatr* **139**(3): 413–420.

Klunk WE, Engler H, *et al.* (2004). Imaging brain amyloid in Alzheimer's disease with Pittsburgh Compound-B. *Ann Neurol* **55**(3): 306–319.

Komaki R, Meyers CA, *et al.* (1995). Evaluation of cognitive function in patients with limited small cell lung cancer prior to and shortly following prophylactic cranial irradiation. *Int J Radiat Oncol, Biol Physics* **33**(1): 179–182.

Kwong KK, Belliveau JW, *et al.* (1992). Dynamic magnetic resonance imaging of human brain activity during primary sensory stimulation. *Proc Nat Acad Sci USA* **89**(12): 5675–5679.

Lai S, Hopkins AL, *et al.* (1993). Identification of vascular structures as a major source of signal contrast in high resolution 2D and 3D functional activation imaging of the motor cortex at 1.5T: preliminary results. *Magn Reson Imaging Med* **30**: 387–392.

Le Bihan D, Mangin JF, *et al.* (2001). Diffusion tensor imaging: concepts and applications. *J Magn Reson Imaging* **13**(4): 534–546.

Lesnik PG, Ciesielski KT, *et al.* (1998). Evidence for cerebellar-frontal subsystem changes in children treated with intrathecal chemotherapy for leukemia: enhanced data analysis using an effect size model. *Arch Neurol* **55**(12): 1561–1568.

Lien HH, Blomlie V, *et al.* (1991). Osteogenic sarcoma: MR signal abnormalities of the brain in asymptomatic patients treated with high-dose methotrexate. *Radiology* **179**(2): 547–550.

Logothetis NK, Pauls J, *et al.* (2001). Neurophysiological investigation of the basis of the fMRI signal. *Nature* **412**: 150–157.

Mazziotta JC, Toga AW, *et al.* (2000). *Brain Mapping: The Disorders*. San Diego, CA: Academic Press.

McAllister TW, Sparling MB, *et al.* (2001). Differential working memory load effects after mild traumatic brain injury. *NeuroImage* **14**(5): 1004–1012.

Meyers CA, Byrne KS, *et al.* (1995). Cognitive deficits in patients with small cell lung cancer before and after chemotherapy. *Lung Cancer* **12**(3): 231–235.

Meyers CA, Albitar M, *et al.* (2005). Cognitive impairment, fatigue, and cytokine levels in patients with acute myelogenous leukemia or myelodysplastic syndrome. *Cancer* **104**(4): 788–793.

Moonen CTW, Bandettini PA (eds.) (2000). *Functional MRI.* Berlin: Springer.

Ogawa S, Menon RS, *et al.* (1998). On the characteristics of functional magnetic resonance imaging of the brain. *Annu Rev Biophys Biomol Struct* 27: 447–474.

Packer RJ, Grossman RI, *et al.* (1983). High dose systemic methotrexate-associated acute neurologic dysfunction. *Med Pediatr Oncol* 11(3): 159–161.

Pierpaoli C, Jezzard P, *et al.* (1996). Diffusion tensor MR imaging of the human brain. *Radiology* 201(3): 637–648.

Reddick WE, Shan ZY, *et al.* (2006). Smaller white-matter volumes are associated with larger deficits in attention and learning among long-term survivors of acute lymphoblastic leukemia. *Cancer* 106(4): 941–949.

Reddick WE, Laningham FH, Glass JO, Pui CH (2007). Quantitative morphologic evaluation of magnetic resonance imaging during and after treatment of childhood leukemia. *Neuroradiology* 49: 889–904.

Rosen BR, Buckner RL, *et al.* (1998). Event-related functional MRI: past, present, and future. *Proc Natl Acad Sci USA* 95(3): 773–780.

Ross MH, Yurgelun-Todd DA, *et al.* (1997). Age-related reduction in functional MRI response to photic stimulation. *Neurology* 48(1): 173–176.

Saykin AJ, Ahles TA, *et al.* (2003a). Mechanisms of chemotherapy-induced cognitive disorders: neuropsychological, pathophysiological, and neuroimaging perspectives. *Semin Clin Neuropsychiatry* 8(4): 201–216.

Saykin AJ, Ahles TA, *et al.* (2003b). Gray matter reduction on voxel-based morphometry in chemotherapy-treated cancer survivors. *J Int Neuropsychol Soc* 9: 246.

Saykin AJ, Wishart HA, *et al.* (2004). Cholinergic enhancement of frontal lobe activity in Mild Cognitive Impairment. *Brain* 127(7): 1574–1583.

Saykin AJ, McDonald BC, *et al.* (2007). *Alterations in Brain Activation during Working Memory in Patients with Breast Cancer: Relation to Treatment Modality, Cancer Status and Task Performance.* Available on CD-Rom in NeuroImage, Chicago, IL.

Schagen SB, van Dam FSAM, *et al.* (1999). Cognitive deficits after postoperative adjuvant chemotherapy for breast carcinoma. *Cancer* 85(3): 640–650.

Shilling V, Jenkins V, *et al.* (2005). The effects of adjuvant chemotherapy on cognition in women with breast cancer – preliminary results of an observational longitudinal study. *The Breast* 14: 142–150.

Silverman DHS, Dy CJ, *et al.* (2007). Altered fron-tocortical, cerebellar, and basal ganglia activity in adjuvant-treated breast cancer survivors 5–10 years after chemotherapy. *Breast Cancer Res Treat* 103(3): 303–311.

Stemmer S, Stears J, *et al.* (1994). White matter changes in patients with breast cancer treated with high-dose chemotherapy and autologous bone marrow support. *Am J Neuroradiol* 15(7): 1267–1273.

Tannock IF, Ahles TA, *et al.* (2004). Cognitive impairment associated with chemotherapy for cancer: report of a workshop. *J Clin Oncol* 22(11): 2233–2239.

Tchen N, Juffs HG, *et al.* (2003). Cognitive function, fatigue, and menopausal symptoms in women receiving adjuvant chemotherapy for breast cancer. *J Clin Oncol* 21(22): 4175–4183.

Toga AW, Mazziotta JC (1996). *Brain Mapping: The Methods.* San Diego, CA: Academic Press.

Van Dam FSAM, Schagen SB, *et al.* (1998). Impairment of cognitive function in women receiving adjuvant treatment for high-risk breast cancer: high-dose versus standard-dose chemotherapy. *J Nat Cancer Inst* 90(3): 210–218.

Van Oosterhout AG, Ganzevles PG, *et al.* (1996). Sequelae in long-term survivors of small cell lung cancer. *Int J Radiat Oncol Biol Physics* 34(5): 1037–1044.

Wagner LI, Sweet JJ, *et al.* (2004). *Performance of Cognitively Impaired Oncology Patients and Normal Controls on Functional MRI Tasks.* American Society of Clinical Oncology Annual Meeting, New Orleans, LA.

Wagner L, Sweet J, *et al.* (2006). Trajectory of cognitive impairment during breast cancer treatment: a prospective analysis. *J Clin Oncol Suppl* 24: 8500.

Wefel JS, Lenzi R, *et al.* (2004a). "Chemobrain" in breast carcinoma?: a prologue. *Cancer* 101(3): 466–475.

Wefel JS, Lenzi R, *et al.* (2004b). The cognitive sequelae of standard-dose adjuvant chemotherapy in women with breast carcinoma: results of a prospective, randomized, longitudinal trial. *Cancer* 100: 2292–2299.

Werring DJ, Clark CA, *et al.* (1998). The structural and functional mechanisms of motor recovery: complementary use of diffusion tensor and functional magnetic resonance imaging in traumatic injury of the internal capsule. *J Neurol Neurosurg Psychiatry* 65: 863–869.

Werring DJ, Clark CA, *et al.* (1999). A direct demonstration of both structure and function in the visual system: combining diffusion tensor imaging with functional magnetic resonance imaging. *NeuroImage* **9**(3): 352–361.

Wieneke MH, Dienst ER (1995). Neuropsychological assessment of cognitive functioning following chemotherapy for breast cancer. *Psycho-Oncology* **4**: 61–66.

Wishart HA, Saykin AJ, *et al.* (2004). Brain activation patterns associated with working memory in relapsing-remitting MS. *Neurology* **62**: 234–238.

Yoshikawa E, Matsuoka Y, *et al.* (2005). No adverse effects of adjuvant chemotherapy on hippocampal volume in Japanese breast cancer survivors. *Breast Cancer Res Treat* **92**(1): 81–84.

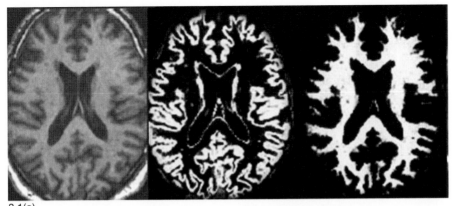

3.1(a)

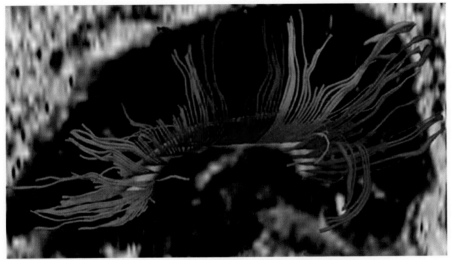

3.1(b)

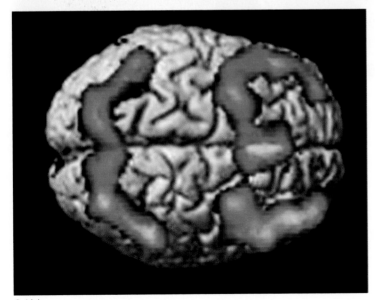

3.1(c)

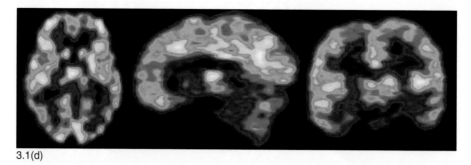

3.1(d)

Figure 3.1. Neuroimaging methods relevant to cognitive changes. (a) Structural MRI (gray and white matter atrophy); (b) diffusion tensor imaging (white matter connectivity); (c) functional MRI (brain activity), and (d) PET (brain metabolism). Reprinted with permission from Ahles and Saykin (2007)

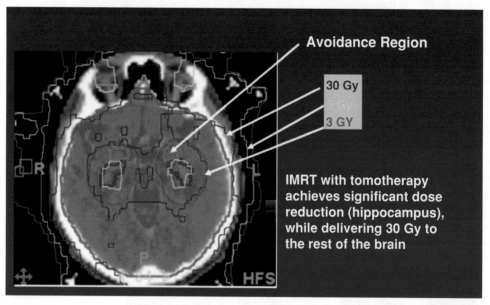

Figure 12.2. Hippocampus avoidance with intensity modulated radiotherapy (provided by Drs. Hazim Jaradat and Wolfgang Tome, University of Wisconsin)

4

Role of neuropsychological assessment in cancer patients

Elana Farace

Neurocognitive function is a very important issue in cancer survivorship. When present, neurocognitive deficits explain the lion's share of cancer survivors' reported decreased quality of life. However, scientific study of the neuropsychological sequelae of cancer is just beginning to be undertaken. A Medline search for 1996–2006 of "neuropsychology or neurocognitive" and "cancer" results in only 86 articles. Once those are selected to include only those that include information on cancer in adults (as opposed to pediatric cancer or adult survivors of pediatric cancers), written in English, only 34 papers remain. However, the relative paucity of research is in contrast to the recent attention given to this important topic, most recently in the Institute of Medicine Report *From Cancer Patient to Cancer Survivor*, in which cognitive dysfunction is listed as one of the important concerns of cancer survivors after treatment (Hewitt *et al.*, 2006).

Neurocognitive deficits in cancer patients are variable. When patients report having neuropsychological impairments, they may note them as being very minor (e.g., "I'm in a fog" or "I have a lot of 'senior moments'") or patients may have significant neurocognitive deficits that impair their ability to speak, remember, or act appropriately. Some patients are not aware of their own deficits and only caregivers have noticed the changes. A cancer patient with neurocognitive dysfunction may decline during some periods, such as during active treatment, and improve during inter-treatment intervals; however, often the opposite pattern can be seen. Patients will also differ from one another in terms of their objective deficits at any given time, and in terms of the impact of those deficits on their overall quality of life (QOL).

The neuropsychology of cancer is particularly complex due to the numerous mediators that affect an individual's abilities. For example, instead of a deficit occurring from a one-time injury, such as in a traumatic brain injury, the injury to the brain can come from a solid brain tumor (either a primary brain tumor or a metastasis), which then varies over time with tumor growth and treatment. Neurocognitive change may also result from changes in structure and function through radiation, chemotherapy, changes in hormonal status, and other factors that less directly affect brain function. Neurocognitive impairment can be masked or mimicked by psychological phenomena such as depression, anxiety, and somatization. Although cancer patients' neurocognitive ability typically declines at some point in the cancer trajectory, the pattern of decline is variable. Other patient-oriented factors, such as baseline intelligence, education level, mood, coping skills, and social support, are also likely mediators of neurocognitive ability.

Thus, the purpose of this chapter is to familiarize the reader with the importance of careful neuropsychological assessment throughout cancer survivorship. Neuropsychological assessment helps clinicians, patients, and family caregivers understand cancer disease, treatment, and survivorship sequelae. Neuropsychological assessment is also extremely useful in research, whether in determining the side-effects of an experimental treatment, as a primary focus of research aimed to improve QOL, or in determining future directions in the field. Each of these areas will be discussed in turn. Ideally, elucidation of these factors will improve decision-making by patients, families, and the clinicians who care for them. The ultimate goal is to maximize both survival and QOL, that is, to help patients live a longer life *and* a better life.

Benefit of neuropsychological assessment for clinical medical management of the cancer patient

Neuropsychological changes are very common presenting symptoms of a new brain tumor in a cancer patient, whether it is a primary brain tumor or a primary cancer elsewhere that has metastasized to the brain. The most frequent cause of new neuropsychological impairment in cancer survivors is metastatic brain tumors, the most common form of intracranial tumors in adults (Patchell, 1995). A complete review of brain metastases can be found in Chapter 12 in this volume. As treatment of the primary cancer improves and length of survival after diagnosis increases, the risk of metastases to the brain also increases (Carney, 1999; Chidel *et al.*, 2000; Vermeulen, 1998). Up to 170 000 new patients are diagnosed each year in the USA with brain metastases (Packer *et al.*, 1998). One-half of all invasive cancers will disseminate to the brain (Vermeulen, 1998) as shown on autopsy (Cairncross *et al.*, 1980) and 150 000–170 000 cancer patients develop symptomatic brain metastases annually (Chidel *et al.*, 2000; Vermeulen, 1998). Approximately 90% of patients with a history of cancer who present with a solitary brain lesion on magnetic resonance imaging (MRI) have a brain metastasis (Patchell & Tibbs, 1990). Between 21% and 86% of

patients with metastases to the brain either have or will develop multiple lesions (Sawaya *et al.*, 1995).

Neurological and neurocognitive impairment resulting from a metastatic lesion is very similar to the signs and symptoms of primary brain tumors (Cairncross *et al.*, 1980; Hirsch *et al.*, 1982). Mental status changes are one of the most frequent symptoms of a primary brain tumor (Klein *et al.*, 2001; Packer *et al.*, 1998). Neurocognitive impairment in primary brain tumor patients at baseline is very frequent, with 91% of patients having at least one area of deficit compared to the normal population, and 71% demonstrating at least three deficits (Tucha *et al.*, 2000). The following sections will detail the importance of neuropsychological evaluation in the multidisciplinary care of a cancer patient. More complete reviews of low-grade and high-grade gliomas can be found in Chapters 10 and 11, respectively.

Neuropsychological dysfunction at presentation

The presenting neurocognitive symptoms typically depend on where the new tumor or tumors are located (Farace *et al.*, 1995; Meyers, 2000; Meyers *et al.*, 2000b, Scheibel *et al.*, 1996). For example, left hemisphere lesions tend to produce changes in language (Hahn *et al.*, 2003) and lesions on the motor strip tend to cause seizures and/or paresis. Third ventricle tumors tend to cause impairments in memory, executive function, and manual dexterity (interestingly, independent of the effects of surgery or hydrocephalus) (Friedman *et al.*, 2003). Therefore, the onset of a new neuropsychological symptom can be a very important sign of new brain disease, which should encourage clinicians to investigate further.

The size and location of the brain tumor can also impact neurocognitive impairment, given that healthy brain tissue near the tumor may also be impacted by surgery and treatment. For example, in tumors that arise in areas with a difficult surgical approach (e.g., deep tumors) or tumors in "eloquent cortex" that are not very amenable to surgical resection (Laws *et al.*, 2003; Packer *et al.*, 1998), there is a risk for the surgical approach damaging healthy brain tissue, and the location of any bleeding will affect future neurocognitive status in a similar way to bleeding following a stroke (Meyers, 2000). Radiation fields may adversely influence normal brain tissue and corresponding neurocognitive function; even if brain tumors are treated with focused radiation such as radiosurgery, the adjacent normal tissue still receives a significant dose of radiation. Finally, the radiation field directed to structures adjacent to the brain, as is common in head and neck cancer, may overlap parts of the brain and cause neurocognitive impairment (Meyers *et al.*, 2000a). The biological bases of radiation-induced brain injury can be found in Chapter 7.

Tumor location is not the only predictor of neurocognitive deficit. Rate of tumor growth is a predictor of the degree of neurocognitive impairment – slow tumor growth may displace normal tissue slowly enough so as not to displace function too drastically (Anderson *et al.*, 1990) whereas rapid tumor growth will cause more severe deficits (Hom & Reitan, 1984). In a comparison of neuropsychological deficits between patients with brain tumors and patients with strokes, matched for lesion location, stroke patients were shown to have more severe neurocognitive deficits (Anderson *et al.*, 1990). Often a patient with a new brain tumor will develop brain edema, which is typically treated with glucocorticoids (Routh *et al.*, 1994; Vecht *et al.*, 1994). However, steroid therapy has been associated with neurobehavioral changes such as depression, hypomania, mood swings, anxiety, acute psychotic reactions, and even a case of obsessive-compulsive behavior disorder (Bick, 1983). Thus, the benefit from glucocorticoids can sometimes be offset by their side-effects.

For any new neuropsychological symptom in a cancer patient, neuropsychological assessment can help the medical clinician by diagnosing and quantifying the new deficit, and can help to distinguish the cause of the deficit from any mediators. A discussion of the utility of neuropsychological assessment beyond initial diagnosis will be explored next.

Cancer surveillance using neuropsychological assessment

Collecting "baseline" neuropsychological information from patients either before treatment or very early in their treatment course can provide an excellent benchmark for later analysis. There is evidence that neurocognitive decline may precede a change in the neuroimaging of the tumor, suggesting that neuropsychological surveillance may be more sensitive to tumor progression than traditional neuroimaging. In a landmark study, Meyers and Hess (2003) performed a baseline neuropsychological assessment on 80 patients with recurrent glioblastoma or anaplastic astrocytoma prior to beginning a clinical trial for recurrent/relapsed tumor. The patients were then assessed prior to each cycle of chemotherapy and an MRI was obtained at the same time. The median time for patients to deteriorate cognitively on any of the nine assessments was 7.4 weeks (95% confidence interval, 5.0–9.6); 61% of patients declined neurocognitively prior to radiographic progression and 25% declined at the same time as radiographic progression (4% declined after progression and 11% did not change neurocognitively). Figure 4.1 shows the time to neurocognitive progression versus neuroimaging progression for each individual patient (Meyers & Hess, 2003).

Neurocognitive decline has also been shown to predict MRI evidence of tumor progression in low-grade (Armstrong *et al.*, 2003) along with high-grade (Meyers, 2000; Meyers & Hess, 2003) gliomas and patients with brain metastases (Meyers *et al.*, 2004). Thus, neuropsychological surveillance can help clinicians to determine when their index of suspicion for radiographic change should occur (and concomitant changes in treatment be considered).

Neuropsychological side-effects of cancer treatment

Neuropsychological assessment can also help the oncologist to assess side-effects of treatment and to monitor for toxicity. Standard chemotherapies

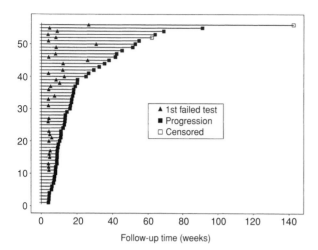

Figure 4.1. Event chart comparing time to neurocognitive failure on any of the tests (▲) and radiographic tumor progression (■) for each subject (*y* axis). "Censored" (□) indicates that the individual had not yet progressed. From Meyers and Hess (2003), with permission

for a number of different types of cancer have been related to neuropsychological deficits. For example, cytokines, interleukin-2, and corticosteroids have all been suggested to be agents that decrease neurocognitive function (Baile, 1996). Potential complications of chemotherapy include acute and chronic encephalopathy, cerebellar syndrome, and neuropathy. Chapter 8 of this volume discusses the effects of systemic treatment on neurocognitive function, and Chapter 9 describes the effects of hormonal treatment on neurocognitive function.

Conventional chemotherapy for breast cancer has been the most highly studied primary cancer in regards to the potential neurocognitive sequelae of treatment, colloquially referred to as "chemobrain." Several forms of adjuvant chemotherapy and secondary prevention such as tamoxifen have been shown to cause neurocognitive impairment, although there is some debate as to the degree of baseline neurocognitive impairment in this group (Bender *et al.*, 2001; Brezden *et al.*, 2000; Ganz, 1998; Olin, 2001; Paganini-Hill & Clark, 2000; Schagen *et al.*, 1999; van Dam *et al.*, 1998). One study revealed

worse neurocognitive impairment in breast cancer patients receiving adjuvant chemotherapy compared to controls (Brezden *et al.*, 2000) even after controlling for patient age, education level, and menopausal status. Long-term negative neurocognitive effects of standard chemotherapy for breast cancer and lymphoma have also been shown (Ahles *et al.*, 2002). An article by Ganz and colleagues (Ganz *et al.*, 2002) found that the only predictor of poor QOL 5–10 years after breast cancer diagnosis was having had past systemic adjuvant chemotherapy, suggesting possible long-term effects of neurocognitive impairment on QOL.

Radiation also may induce neurocognitive impairment, whether directed at the brain as in the case of primary or metastatic brain tumors, or when a radiation field overlaps the brain (e.g., head and neck cancers, lymphomas, etc.) (Meyers *et al.*, 2000a). Patients with small cell lung carcinoma (SCLC) may receive prophylactic cranial irradiation (PCI) to prevent the development of brain metastases. The use of PCI continues to be debated, as it has been shown to be associated with neurocognitive impairment, particularly in the neuropsychological domain of attention, within 2 years of diagnosis of SCLC (van De Pol *et al.*, 1997; Van Oosterhout *et al.*, 1996), and, in the presence of concurrent chemotherapy, SCLC patients showed significant neurocognitive impairment within 4 months of PCI (Ahles *et al.*, 1998).

Neurocognitive impairment following radiation therapy (RT) is likely to be dose dependent, and may appear immediately or as much as 30 years after completion of treatment (Keime-Guibert *et al.*, 1998). Radiation-induced progressive neurocognitive dysfunction, dementia, ataxia, and death in the absence of tumor recurrence have all been described (DeAngelis, 1994; DeAngelis *et al.*, 1989; Sheline *et al.*, 1980; Sundaresan *et al.*, 1981). Neurocognitive impairment caused by RT is typified by the well-defined profile of subcortical white matter dysfunction similar to that seen in the subcortical dementias (Cummings, 1990; Roman *et al.*, 1993) with deficits in the areas of information processing, executive functioning, memory, attention, and motor co-ordination (Archibald *et al.*, 1994; Hochberg & Slotnick, 1980; Imperato *et al.*, 1990; Lieberman *et al.*, 1982; Salander *et al.*, 1995; Scheibel *et al.*, 1996; Surma-Aho *et al.*, 2001; Taphoorn *et al.*, 1994). Radiation necrosis may also result in a focal lesion, which results in neurocognitive decline (although necrosis can often be temporarily alleviated with steroids) (Packer *et al.*, 1998). Treatment-related neurocognitive impairment can be discriminated from deficits caused by the tumor itself using standardized neuropsychological testing, with comparison of the pattern of deficits to the normal population and pre-radiation treatment patterns of neurocognitive impairment (Cummings, 1990; Meyers *et al.*, 2000b).

Discrimination of neurocognitive from psychological sequelae

Depression is extremely common in cancer survivors. Often cancer patients with metastatic or primary brain tumors develop *de novo* psychiatric symptoms (Lezak *et al.*, 2004). A significant number of patients with low-grade infiltrating tumors and meningiomas are referred for psychiatric consultation before the initial diagnosis or even imaging of the tumor (Packer *et al.*, 1998). Depression is a risk factor for treatment non-compliance (DiMatteo *et al.*, 2000) for which various psychoneuroendocrinological explanations have been proposed (Capuron *et al.*, 2001; Spiegel, 1996; Tashiro *et al.*, 2001). Depression has even been suggested to predict response to chemotherapy in breast cancer (Walker *et al.*, 1999).

Depression in cancer patients has been shown to predict shortened length of survival (Litofsky *et al.*, 2004; Spiegel, 1996). For example, one study of depression following stem-cell transplantation for malignancies found that depressed patients had a threefold greater risk of dying than non-depressed patients, adjusting for other prognostic factors (Loberiza *et al.*, 2002). A significant relationship between depression at 3 months post-surgery and length of survival has also been shown in a population of patients with malignant gliomas (Litofsky *et al.*, 2004).

When cancer patients have a structural brain lesion, psychiatric symptoms may depend on the location of the tumor (Irle *et al.*, 1994; Lezak & O'Brien, 1988). Hecaen (1962) found that 67% of patients with frontal lobe tumors exhibited confused states and dementia as would be expected. Patients with temporal lobe tumors have been shown to have personality changes and mood swings (Heilman *et al.*, 1993) and patients with right hemisphere tumors may also show paranoia, hallucinations, and agitation (Price & Mesulam, 1985). If the hypothalamic circuitry is disrupted, whether from the tumor, surgery, or treatment, there can be striking dysregulated behavior such as anxiety, depression, emotional lability, hypersexuality, reduced attention, memory loss, and impaired reasoning ability (Mechanick *et al.*, 1986).

Depression is thought to negatively impact patients' scores on neuropsychological assessment (Lezak & O'Brien, 1988), although recently this has been debated (Arfken *et al.*, 1999; Rohling *et al.*, 2002). It is not uncommon for patients to change clinically and appear to neurocognitively worsen, but on assessment it is determined that the only change was an increase in depression. Tumor-related neurocognitive impairment can be discriminated from depression using standardized neuropsychological testing, with comparison of the pattern of deficits to the normal population and pre-treatment patterns of neurocognitive impairment and mood (Meyers *et al.*, 2000b). A careful neuropsychological examiner can differentiate between neurocognitive impairment and depression, and make suggestions as to the best way to treat the depression.

Prognostic value of neuropsychological assessment

There is increasing evidence that baseline neuropsychological function is a significant predictor of length of survival in a number of patient populations including those with multiple sclerosis (Peyser *et al.*, 1990), dementia (Jelic *et al.*, 2000), and medically ill older adults (Arfken *et al.*, 1999). Meyers and colleagues (2000b) have shown that neurocognitive status (verbal memory performance) was strongly and independently related to length of survival in patients with recurrent glioma even after accounting for age, Karnofsky Performance Scale (KPS), and time since diagnosis. An analysis of 445 cancer patients with brain metastases also found that baseline Mini-Mental Status Exam (MMSE) scores were a significant predictor of length of survival, in a Cox proportional hazards model adjusting for age, gender and Karnofsky Performance Scale (KPS) (Murray *et al.*, 2000). The benefit of neurocognitive information added to a prognostic model has been shown in patients with leptomeningeal or parenchymal brain lesions (Meyers *et al.*, 2002). Another study found that baseline neurological deficits were an independent predictor of survival in patients with low-grade glioma (Pignatti *et al.*, 2002) although neuropsychological deficits were not directly tested. Therefore, as clinicians are called upon to discuss individual prognosis with the patient, information on baseline neurocognitive status may be helpful.

Benefit of neuropsychological assessment to the clinician

Thus, information on neurocognitive function from a neuropsychological assessment of the cancer patient can be beneficial to the clinician because:

- *De novo* neuropsychological symptoms in cancer patients help alert clinicians to the possibility of new brain disease.
- Neuropsychological surveillance can be useful to help predict brain tumor growth, and may be more sensitive to changes in tumor size than standard neuroimaging.
- Neurocognitive changes are measurable side-effects of treatments such as chemotherapy and radiation which significantly impact patients' QOL.
- A neuropsychological assessment can help distinguish brain disease from other neuropsycholo-

gical phenomena (e.g., undiagnosed depression causing a "pseudo-dementia").

Neuropsychological assessment should be performed in the case of any new neuropsychological symptom in a cancer patient, to help diagnose and quantify the new deficits, and to help distinguish the cause of the deficit from other mediators. Indeed, some major brain tumor centers are now moving toward having a baseline neuropsychological evaluation with neurocognitive surveillance as standard practice for all cancer patients with brain tumors.

Benefit of neuropsychological assessment for the patient and family caregivers

Neuropsychological assessment is performed with cancer patients to help determine the differential contributions of neurological and psychological factors to the patient's function. From a patient and family perspective, neurocognitive impairment has a significant negative impact on QOL. This phenomenon has most often been shown in cancer patients with malignant brain tumors, but the construct is very likely similar in other types of cancer when significant neurocognitive impairment is present.

We performed a study to better detail the relationships between cognitive impairment and QOL outcomes in a population of patients with malignant brain tumor (Farace & Shaffrey, 2000). Neuropsychological and QOL measures known to be sensitive to the neurocognitive effects of brain tumors were given to 30 patients with malignant brain tumors, and patients' caregivers were simultaneously given measures of QOL and caregiver burden. Patients' QOL was measured using the EORTC QLQ-C30 with Brain Cancer module BCM29 (Aaronson *et al.*, 1993) and caregivers were given the Family QOL Tool, a 20-item measure of caregiver QOL (Ferrell *et al.*, 1993), and Caregiver Strain, which measures perceived burden by caregivers (Robinson, 1983). The neuropsychological battery included measures of pre-morbid IQ, divided attention, problem-solving ability and cognitive flexibility, language, verbal

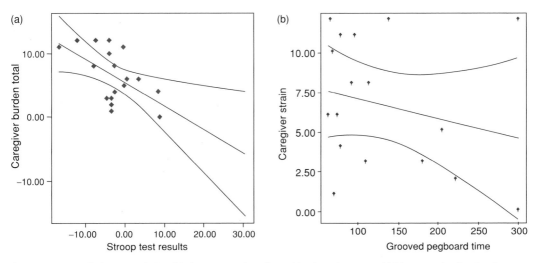

Figure 4.2. **a** Graph showing relationship between patients' cognitive impairment and higher caregiver burden (strong correlations with a test of divided attention; Stroop; $r = -0.56$). **b** Graph showing the lack of a relationship between patients' physical ability and caregiver burden, indicating that neurocognitive rather than physical impairment is a greater burden on caregivers

memory, visual memory, fine motor skills, psychomotor speed, and psychological distress. Patients included 14 men, 16 women; mean age was 49.5 years (range 20–77); mean years of education was 13 (range 6–18); 24/30 were right-handed; 28 were Caucasian, 2 African-American; mean estimated pre-morbid IQ was 105 (85–117) (Barona *et al.*, 1984); and median time since diagnosis was 8 months. Patients' cognitive impairment was significantly related to poor patient QOL. Patients' cognitive impairment was also strongly and negatively related to caregiver QOL and caregiver burden, particularly when the patient's impairment was in language and executive function. Patient and caregiver QOL was *not* correlated to measures of physical function, such as the Barthel Index (a measure of activities of daily living), or the grooved pegboard (a test of fine motor skill). The strong relationship between cognitive impairment and QOL suggests that neurocognitive outcome is an important component of overall QOL.

Figure 4.2a shows the significant relationship between patients' cognitive impairment and higher caregiver burden (strong correlations with a test of

divided attention; Stroop; $r = -0.56$). In Figure 4.2b, the *lack* of a relationship between patients' physical ability and caregiver burden can be seen, indicating that neurocognitive rather than physical impairment is a greater burden on caregivers.

In addition to the direct benefit to the medical clinicians detailed above, the benefit of neuropsychological assessment is clear because the patient and the family caregivers can receive individualized feedback on the assessment from the neuropsychologist, in order to help each patient best determine how to maximize QOL during survivorship. The assessment will help to elucidate the patient's psychological strengths and weaknesses related to neurological dysfunction, and the patient, family, and neuropsychologist work together to understand the results in an ecologically valid "real-world" perspective. This feedback session may be as short as a few minutes for an intact patient with few questions, or it may be as long as 1–2 h in situations where the patient's neuropsychological deficits are contributing to causing significant strain on the family system. Therefore, as a result of undergoing a neuropsychological evaluation, information is provided to the patient and caregivers regarding the patient's:

- Neurocognitive profile – to detail a profile of strengths and weaknesses and clarify what compensatory strategies ("work-around solutions") might help (e.g., memory aids, changes to home environment, counseling).
- Differential diagnosis – distinguishing between different conditions that have similar symptoms, such as depression versus memory problems versus tumor progression.
- Prognosis – how much will the patient improve or decline over time? What to expect, what to be looking for, why changes occur, and how to deal with changes.
- Ability to function independently – how can we maximize patients' independence?
- Rehabilitation potential – will the patient benefit from a referral to rehabilitation services (e.g., speech therapy, physical therapy, occupational therapy, vocational therapy, etc.)?
- Ability to return to work or school – what changes need to be made to get the patient back to work or school and what should be changed in those environments?
- Need for specialized school services – does the student need referrals to special education, or adaptations such as unlimited time on tests?
- Ability to drive a car or operate other vehicles or machinery (farm equipment, power tools, woodstove, oven, microwave, etc.).
- Legal issues – is the patient legally competent? Are they accurately representing their function? Might they benefit from an advanced directive and/or power of attorney?
- Disability – does the patient qualify for disability services? Referrals to social work to aid in application.
- Safety – for example is the patient safe to stay alone at home, or to care for small children, or to live by themselves?
- Psychological follow-up – could the patient benefit from counseling or psychotherapy or support groups? Referrals to physicians for a trial of an antidepressant or other medications.

- Caregiver support – does the caregiver need to have more assistance (e.g., other family, hired housecleaners, home nurse aid, support groups, etc.)?
- Any other questions about patient functioning.

Essentially, the neurocognitive assessment, to the patient and family caregiver, is a major part of helping cancer patients determine how to live their lives so as to maximize QOL, rather than how to fight the cancer per se.

Benefit of neuropsychological information to clinical cancer and survivorship research

A thorough review of the use of neurocognitive testing in clinical trials can be found in Chapter 23. A survey of academically based Canadian oncologists found that the majority identified QOL as a more appropriate endpoint than survival for future randomized controlled trials in cancer (Bezjak et al., 1998). The Food and Drug Administration (FDA) will also consider neurocognitive endpoints in clinical trials. As part of the FDA Project on Cancer Drug Approval Endpoints, there was a meeting on January 20, 2006, on Primary Brain Tumor Endpoints wherein public discussion and testimony was given on alternative endpoints in registration trials. The message of the presentation was that response, freedom from radiological progression and other imaging-based endpoints may not adequately reflect QOL in brain tumor patients. As a result, neurocognitive outcomes, and to a lesser extent patient-reported outcomes, are increasingly being included in clinical trials (Meyers & Brown, 2006). This serves to broaden the scope of approvable endpoints and adds valuable information regarding the clinical benefit of new agents.

REFERENCES

Aaronson N, Ahmedzai S, Bergman V, et al. (1993). The European Organization for Research and Treatment of Cancer QLQ-C30: a quality of life instrument for use in international trials in oncology. *J Natl Cancer Inst* **85**: 365–376.

Ahles TA, Silberfarb PM, Herndon J, 2nd, *et al.* (1998). Psychologic and neuropsychologic functioning of patients with limited small-cell lung cancer treated with chemotherapy and radiation therapy with or without warfarin: a study by the Cancer and Leukemia Group B. *J Clin Oncol* **16**: 1954–1960.

Ahles TA, Saykin AJ, Furstenberg CT, *et al.* (2002). Neuropsychologic impact of standard-dose systemic chemotherapy in long-term survivors of breast cancer and lymphoma. *J Clin Oncol* **20**: 485–493.

Anderson SW, Damasio H, Tranel D (1990). Neuropsychological impairments associated with lesions caused by tumor or stroke. *Arch Neurol* **47**: 397–405.

Archibald YM, Lunn D, Ruttan LA, *et al.* (1994). Cognitive functioning in long-term survivors of high-grade glioma. *J Neurosurg* **80**: 247–253.

Arfken CL, Lichtenberg PA, Tancer ME (1999). Cognitive impairment and depression predict mortality in medically ill older adults. *J Gerontol Series A-Biol Sci Med Sci* **54**: M152–M156.

Armstrong CL, Goldstein B, Shera D, *et al.* (2003). The predictive value of longitudinal neuropsychologic assessment in the early detection of brain tumor recurrence. *Cancer* **97**: 649–656.

Baile WF (1996). Neuropsychiatric disorders in cancer patients. *Curr Opin Oncol* **8**: 182–187.

Barona A, Reynolds CR, Chastain R (1984). A demographically based index of premorbid intelligence for the WAIS-R. *J Consult Clin Psychol* **52**: 885–887.

Bender CM, Paraska KK, Sereika SM, Ryan CM, Berga SL (2001). Cognitive function and reproductive hormones in adjuvant therapy for breast cancer: a critical review. *J Pain Symptom Manage* **21**: 407–424.

Bezjak A, Taylor KM, Ng P, *et al.* (1998). Quality-of-life information and clinical practice: the oncologist's perspective. *Cancer Prevent Control* **2**: 230–235.

Bick PA (1983). Obsessive-compulsive behavior associated with dexamethasone treatment. *J Nerv Mental Dis* **171**: 253–254.

Brezden CB, Phillips, KA, Abdolell M, *et al.* (2000). Cognitive function in breast cancer patients receiving adjuvant chemotherapy. *J Clin Oncol* **18**: 2695–2701.

Cairncross JG, Kim JH, Posner JB (1980). Radiation therapy for brain metastases. *Ann Neurol* **7**: 529–541.

Capuron L, Ravaud A, Gualde N, *et al.* (2001). Association between immune activation and early depressive symptoms in cancer patients treated with interleukin-2-based therapy. *Psychoneuroendocrinology* **26**: 797–808.

Carney DN (1999). Prophylactic cranial irradiation and small-cell lung cancer [editorial; comment]. *New Engl J Med* **341**: 524–526.

Chidel MA, Suh JH, Barnett GH (2000). Brain metastases: presentation, evaluation, and management. *Clevel Clin J Med* **67**: 120–127.

Cummings J (1990). Introduction. In: Cummings J (ed.) *Subcortical Dementia*. New York, Oxford University Press.

DeAngelis LM (1994). Management of brain metastases. *Cancer Invest* **12**: 156–165.

DeAngelis LM, Delattre JY, Posner JB (1989). Radiation-induced dementia in patients cured of brain metastases. *Neurology* **39**: 789–796.

DiMatteo MR, Lepper HS, Croghan TW (2000). Depression is a risk factor for noncompliance with medical treatment: meta-analysis of the effects of anxiety and depression on patient adherence. *Arch Intern Med* **160**: 2101–2107.

Farace E, Shaffrey ME (2000). Relationship of neurocognitive impairment to QOL in malignant brain tumor patients [abstract]. *J Neuropsychiatry Clin Neurosci* **13**: 1.

Farace E, Turkheimer E, Wilkniss S (1995). Utility of analyzing lesion location in an outcome study of traumatic brain injury [abstract]. International Neuropsychological Society. Seattle, WA. *J Int Neuropsychol Soc* **1**.

Ferrell B, Rhiner M, Rivera LM (1993). Development and evaluation of the family pain questionnaire. *J Psychosocial Oncol* **10**: 21–35.

Friedman MA, Meyers CA, Sawaya R (2003). Neuropsychological effects of third ventricle tumor surgery. *Neurosurgery* **52**: 791–798; discussion 798.

Ganz PA (1998). Cognitive dysfunction following adjuvant treatment of breast cancer: a new dose-limiting toxic effect? [letter; comment]. *J Natl Cancer Inst* **90**: 182–183.

Ganz PA, Desmond KA, Leedham B, *et al.* (2002). Quality of life in long-term, disease-free survivors of breast cancer: a follow-up study. *J Natl Cancer Inst* **94**: 39–49 [erratum in: *J Natl Cancer Inst* **94**:463].

Hahn CA, Dunn RH, Logue PE, *et al.* (2003). Prospective study of neuropsychologic testing and quality-of-life assessment of adults with primary malignant brain tumors. *Int J Radiat Oncol Biol Phys* **55**: 992–999.

Hecaen H (1962). Clinical symptomatology in right and left hemisphere lesions. In Mountcastle VB (ed.)

Interhemispheric Relations and Cerebral Dominance in Man: Baltimore, MD: Johns Hopkins University Press.

Heilman KM, Bowers D, Valenstein E (1993). Emotional disorders associated with neurological diseases. In Heilman KM, Valenstein E (eds.) *Clinical Neuropsychology*, 3rd edn. New York: Oxford University Press.

Hewitt M, Greenfield S, Stovall E (eds.) (2006). *From Cancer Patient to Cancer Survivor: Lost in Transition*. Washington DC: National Academies Press.

Hirsch FR, Paulson OB, Hansen HH, *et al.* (1982). Intracranial metastases in small cell carcinoma of the lung: correlation of clinical and autopsy findings. *Cancer* 50: 2433–2437.

Hochberg FH, Slotnick B (1980). Neuropsychologic impairment in astrocytoma survivors. *Neurology* 30: 172–177.

Hom J, Reitan RM (1984). Neuropsychological correlates of rapidly vs. slowly growing intrinsic cerebral neoplasms. *J Clin Neuropsychol* 6: 309–324.

Imperato JP, Paleologos NA, Vick NA (1990). Effects of treatment on long-term survivors with malignant astrocytomas. *Ann Neurol* 28: 818–822.

Irle E, Peper M, Wowra B, *et al.* (1994). Mood changes after surgery for tumors of the cerebral cortex. *Arch Neurol* 51: 164–174.

Jelic V, Johansson SE, Almkvist O, *et al.* (2000). Quantitative electroencephalography in mild cognitive impairment: longitudinal changes and possible prediction of Alzheimer's disease. *Neurobiol Aging* 21: 533–540.

Keime-Guibert F, Napolitano M, Delattre JY (1998). Neurological complications of radiotherapy and chemotherapy. *J Neurol* 245: 695–708.

Klein M, Taphoorn MJB, Heimans JJ, *et al.* (2001). Neurobehavioral status and health-related quality of life in newly diagnosed high-grade glioma patients. *J Clin Oncol* 19: 4037–4047.

Laws ER, Shaffrey ME, Morris A, *et al.* (2003). Surgical management of intracranial gliomas – does radical resection improve outcome? *Acta Neurochir Suppl* 85: 47–53.

Lezak MD, O'Brien KP (1988). Longitudinal study of emotional, social, and physical changes after traumatic brain injury. *J Learn Disabil* 21:456–463.

Lezak MD, Howieson DB, Loring DW (2004). *Neuropsychological Assessment* (4th edn.). New York: Oxford University Press.

Lieberman AN, Foo SH, Ransohoff J, *et al.* (1982). Long term survival among patients with malignant brain tumors. *Neurosurgery* 10: 450–453.

Litofsky NS, Farace E, Anderson F Jr., *et al.* (2004). Depression in patients with high-grade glioma: results of the Glioma Outcomes Project. *Neurosurgery* 54: 358–366; discussion 366–367.

Loberiza FR Jr., Rizzo JD, Bredeson CN, *et al.* (2002). Association of depressive syndrome and early deaths among patients after stem-cell transplantation for malignant diseases. *J Clin Oncol* 20: 2118–2126.

Mechanick JI, Hochberg FH, Larocque A (1986). Hypothalamic dysfunction following whole-brain irradiation. *J Neurosurg*, 65: 490–494.

Meyers CA (2000). Quality of life of brain tumor patients. In Bernstein M, Berger, MS (eds.) *Neuro-Oncology: The Essentials*. New York: Thieme Medical Publishers.

Meyers CA, Brown PD (2006). The role and relevance of neurocognitive assessment in clinical trials of patients with central nervous system tumors. *J Clin Oncol* 24: 1305–1309.

Meyers CA, Hess KR (2003). Multifaceted end points in brain tumor clinical trials: cognitive deterioration precedes MRI progression. *Neurooncology* 5: 89–95.

Meyers CA, Geara F, Wong PF, *et al.* (2000a). Neurocognitive effects of therapeutic irradiation for base of skull tumors. *Int J Radiat Oncol Biol Phys* 46: 51–55.

Meyers CA, Hess KR, Yung WKA, *et al.* (2000b). Cognitive function as a predictor of survival in patients with recurrent malignant glioma. *J Clin Oncol* 18: 646–650.

Meyers CA, Mehta MP, Rodrigus P, *et al.* (2002). Motexafin gadolinium (MGD) delays neurocognitive progression in patients with brain metastases from lung cancer: results of a randomized phase III trial. *Neurooncology* 4: 372.

Meyers CA, Smith JA, Bezjak A, *et al.* (2004). Neurocognitive function and progression in patients with brain metastases treated with whole-brain radiation and motexafin gadolinium: results of a randomized phase III trial. *J Clin Oncol* 22: 157–165.

Murray KJ, Scott C, Zachariah B, *et al.* (2000). Importance of the mini-mental status examination in the treatment of patients with brain metastases: a report from the Radiation Therapy Oncology Group protocol 91–04. *Int J Radiat Oncol Biol Phys* 48: 59–64.

Olin JJ (2001). Cognitive function after systemic therapy for breast cancer. *Oncology (Williston Park)* 15: 613–618; discussion 618: 621–624.

Packer RJ, Miller DC, Shaffrey MS, *et al.* (1998). Intracranial neoplasms. In Rosenberg RN, Pleasure DE (eds.) *Comprehensive Neurology* (2nd edn.) New York: John Wiley & Sons.

Paganini-Hill A, Clark LJ (2000). Preliminary assessment of cognitive function in breast cancer patients treated with tamoxifen. *Breast Cancer Res Treat* 64: 165–176.

Patchell RA (1995). Metastatic brain tumors. *Neurol Clin* 13: 915–925.

Patchell R, Tibbs P (1990). A randomised trial of surgery in the treatment of single metastases to the brain. *New Engl J Med* 22: 494–500.

Peyser JM, Rao SM, Larocca NG, *et al.* (1990). Guidelines for neuropsychological research in multiple sclerosis. *Arch Neurol* 47: 94–97.

Pignatti F, Van Den Bent M, Curran D, *et al.* (2002). Prognostic factors for survival in adult patients with cerebral low-grade glioma. *J Clin Oncol* 20: 2076–2084.

Price BH, Mesulam M (1985). Psychiatric manifestations of right hemisphere infarctions. *J Nerv Mental Dis* 173: 610–614.

Robinson B (1983). Validation of a caregiver strain index. *J Gerontol* 38: 344–388.

Rohling ML, Green P, Allen LM, *et al.* (2002). Depressive symptoms and neurocognitive test scores in patients passing symptoms validity tests. *Arch Clin Neuropsychol* 17: 205–222.

Roman GC, Tatemichi TK, Erkinjuntti T, *et al.* (1993). Vascular dementia: diagnostic criteria for research studies. Report of the NINDS-AIREN International Workshop. *Neurology* 43: 250–260.

Routh A, Khansur T, Hickman BT, *et al.* (1994). Management of brain metastases: past, present, and future. *Southern Med J* 87: 1218–1226.

Salander P, Karlsson T, Bergenheim T, *et al.* (1995). Long-term memory deficits in patients with malignant gliomas. *J Neurooncol* 25: 227–238.

Sawaya R, Rambo WM Jr., Hammoud MA, *et al.* (1995). Advances in surgery for brain tumors. *Neurol Clin* 13: 757–771.

Schagen SB, Van Dam FS, Muller MJ, *et al.* (1999). Cognitive deficits after postoperative adjuvant chemotherapy for breast carcinoma. *Cancer* 85: 640–650.

Scheibel RS, Meyers CA, Levin VA (1996). Cognitive dysfunction following surgery for intracerebral glioma: influence of histopathology, lesion location, and treatment. *J Neurooncol* 30: 61–69.

Sheline GE, Wara WM, Smith V (1980). Therapeutic irradiation and brain injury. *Int J Radiat Oncol Biol Phy* 6: 1215–1228.

Spiegel D (1996). Cancer and depression. *Br J Psychiatry Suppl* 30: 109–116.

Sundaresan N, Galicich JH, Deck MD, *et al.* (1981). Radiation necrosis after treatment of solitary intracranial metastases. *Neurosurgery* 8: 329–333.

Surma-Aho O, Niemela M, Vilkki J, *et al.* (2001). Adverse long-term effects of brain radiotherapy in adult low-grade glioma patients. *Neurology* 56: 1285–1290.

Taphoorn MJ, Schiphorst AK, Snoek FJ, *et al.* (1994). Cognitive functions and quality of life in patients with low-grade gliomas: the impact of radiotherapy. *Ann Neurol* 36: 48–54.

Tashiro M, Itoh M, Kubota K, *et al.* (2001). Relationship between trait anxiety, brain activity and natural killer cell activity in cancer patients: a preliminary PET study. *Psychooncology* 10: 541–546.

Tucha O, Smely C, Preier M, *et al.* (2000). Cognitive deficits before treatment among patients with brain tumors. *Neurosurgery* 47: 324–333; discussion 333–334.

Van Dam FS, Schagen SB, Muller MJ, *et al.* (1998). Impairment of cognitive function in women receiving adjuvant treatment for high-risk breast cancer: high-dose versus standard-dose chemotherapy. *J Natl Cancer Inst* 90: 210–218.

Van De Pol M, Ten Velde GP, Wilmink JT, *et al.* (1997). Efficacy and safety of prophylactic cranial irradiation in patients with small cell lung cancer. *J Neurooncol* 35: 153–160.

Van Oosterhout AG, Ganzevles PG, Wilmink JT, *et al.* (1996). Sequelae in long-term survivors of small cell lung cancer. *Int J Radiat Oncol Biol Phys* 34: 1037–1044.

Vecht CJ, Hovestadt A, Verbiest HB, *et al.* (1994). Dose-effect relationship of dexamethasone on Karnofsky performance in metastatic brain tumors: a randomized study of doses of 4, 8, and 16 mg per day. *Neurology* 44: 675–680.

Vermeulen SS (1998). Whole brain radiotherapy in the treatment of metastatic brain tumors. *Sem in Surg Oncol* 14: 64–69.

Walker LG, Heys SD, Walker MB, *et al.* (1999). Psychological factors can predict the response to primary chemotherapy in patients with locally advanced breast cancer. *Eur J Cancer* 35: 1783–1788.

5

Neuropsychological assessment of adults with cancer

Anne E. Kayl, Robert Collins, and Jeffrey S. Wefel

Introduction

The survival rate for patients diagnosed with some types of cancers has increased with advances in surgical techniques, radiotherapy, and the development of new chemotherapeutic agents. Although most patients continue to face aggressive multi-modality and multi-agent treatment to control or eradicate disease, cancer is not always regarded as the "terminal" disease of past decades. In fact, some types of cancer are best conceptualized as a chronic illness, more akin to diabetes, and are amenable to long-term management. It continues to be the case, however, that the majority of cancer patients will require treatment with therapies that are rarely specific to malignancy and often place normal tissues at risk. The central nervous system (CNS) appears particularly vulnerable to therapy-related changes, and there is ample evidence to suggest that many treatments are capable of producing cognitive dysfunction that can persist well after cessation of treatment. While it is easy to associate such cognitive changes to observable CNS tissue damage (e.g., post-surgical changes seen on imaging), many current treatments act at a molecular level of observation and the mechanism that links those various treatments to putative changes in a patient's cognitive functioning has not been fully elucidated. Neuropsychological assessment is well suited to quantify such cognitive impairments, which may bear directly on a person's ability to function in their environment; it also offers a methodology to evaluate the effectiveness and neurotoxic limitations of therapies at a level not typically accounted for in most clinical trials.

Neuropsychological assessment

There has been much written about neuropsychological assessment and the reader is referred to Chapter 2 in this book and elsewhere for a more in-depth review of this topic (see Lezak *et al.*, 2004). Briefly, neuropsychology is the study of brain–behavior relationships. Through individualized assessment, practitioners study the impact of injury or disease on brain function (Vanderploeg, 2000). Neuropsychological testing involves the administration of standardized psychometric instruments that comprehensively evaluate cognitive aspects of cerebral functioning to include attention, the ability to acquire new memories, the recall of stored memories, expressive speech, language comprehension, visual perception, executive functions, and mood. The assessment process includes the integration of test results with observations of the patient's behavior, patient report, and reports of family members and/or caregivers. Neuropsychological evaluations have traditionally been utilized to evaluate patients with known CNS injury or disease

Cognition and Cancer, eds. Christina A. Meyers and James R. Perry. Published by Cambridge University Press.

such as head injury, dementia, or stroke but this method has more recently been applied to a wider spectrum of medical disorders (see Tarter *et al.*, 2001).

Although recognition of the utility of cognitive assessment for persons with cancer has increased since the early 1990s, the focus of many clinicians, especially in cases with difficult-to-treat malignancies, remains on the achievement of disease control and/or symptom management. However, patients' cognitive and behavioral functioning, which is also more loosely studied under the rubric "quality of life," must be given consideration, especially when in the course of extending life expectancy there exists the possibility that added neurotoxicity will compromise a person's ability to function in their daily environment at a level that is individually satisfying. Even subtle cognitive deficits can significantly limit a patient's ability to perform their usual activities, but they may not be evident on casual observation or detectable via routine medical examinations. If unrecognized, these cognitive deficits can lead to inaccurate judgment on the part of the medical team regarding the patient's ability for self-care, requirements for supervision or special safety measures, and reliability in following his/her therapeutic regimen. Neuropsychological assessment in the cancer population provides quantitative, objective measurement of potentially subtle changes in a patient's cognitive function, allows for careful evaluation of the costs and benefits of a given treatment regimen or supportive therapy, has been shown to predict progression of disease prior to progression on imaging (Meyers & Hess, 2003), and can differentiate cancer-related impairment from stroke, dementia, or mood disturbance. The results of an appropriate cognitive assessment may also be used to guide interventions including compensatory strategy training (cognitive rehabilitation), pharmacotherapy (i.e., psychostimulants, antidepressants, or anxiolytics), or psychotherapy. In fact, improvement in cognitive function and delayed cognitive progression are now recognized as important study endpoints by the Food and Drug Administration (FDA).

The importance of cognitive evaluations in patient care and in clinical cancer trials is receiving greater recognition than previously, but assessment methods remain less than optimal in most cases. Cognitive assessment is a complex, multifaceted undertaking that requires specialized training. Although administration of tests is relatively simple, selection of appropriate measures and interpretation of results draws on a diverse set of skills requiring specialized, advanced training in the field of neuropsychology, as well as knowledge of the patient population under study. Case conceptualization relies on information obtained during clinical interviews with patients and caregivers, an understanding of the patient's sociocultural milieu, recognition of the idiosyncrasies of test construction and psychometrics, and knowledge of the human nervous system (Wefel *et al.*, 2004b). Finally, the literature is replete with studies inadequately assessing "cognitive functioning" in the cancer population. This suggests a limited appreciation of the underlying science that makes cognitive assessment a useful, complementary tool in the medical research setting.

Principles of neuropsychological assessment in the cancer population

There are both general testing and cancer-treatment-specific factors that should be given consideration in neuropsychological assessment, and these are not always independent of one another. General testing factors refer to broader principles of assessment that should be considered across all cancer populations, whereas cancer/treatment factors are more specifically concerned with putative mechanisms by which cognitive dysfunction might be induced. The following sections are divided into general and specific considerations but the type of questions being asked (e.g., research versus clinical) will also bear directly on testing issues. In theory and in practice, we advocate a purpose-driven approach, geared toward the goal of obtaining maximally relevant data with minimal patient burden.

Test selection

Test selection is crucial in both clinical and research settings and will necessarily vary given the hypotheses being evaluated. Standard assessments of performance status such as the Karnofsky Performance Status Scale (KPS) (Karnofsky & Burchenal, 1949) globally measure the patient's symptoms or ability for self-care and ambulation, but do not reliably or validly assess cognition (Hutchinson *et al.*, 1979). For example, a patient who is able to walk and perform basic activities of daily living may be rated as having a good performance status, but on more careful evaluation there may be clear evidence of unreliable memory, poor judgment, difficulty managing routine work, or significant personality change. Brief mental status evaluations such as the Mini-Mental State Examination (MMSE) (Folstein *et al.*, 1975) may superficially evaluate aphasia, apraxia, orientation, and attention, but neglect those functions most susceptible to chemotherapy-related change (learning and memory, processing speed, executive function, and fine motor control) (Meyers & Wefel, 2003).

The instruments used in the neuropsychological evaluation of persons with cancer should be sensitive to subtle changes in the aforementioned areas. They should be psychometrically sound, with established reliability and validity, and appropriate normative studies. As previously noted, the breadth of the assessment and the choice of instruments will necessarily vary with the purpose of the assessment, be it a clinical referral for diagnosis/documentation of impairment, a standardized research protocol, a capacity assessment, or to assist with transitions back to work or a return to school.

Although the specific measures selected will vary given the referral question, the patient's complaints, and the patient's estimated baseline level of functioning, most patients referred to the Neuropsychology Service at The University of Texas M. D.

Anderson Cancer Center receive measures tapping multiple cognitive domains (i.e., general intellectual skills, learning and memory, language, attention, visuospatial/visuoperceptual skills, processing speed, executive functions), motor functions, and mood. In this setting, the evaluation is typically completed in 1 day and lasts from 1 h to 4+ h depending on the purpose and goals of the assessment. For example, our service is involved in a variety of clinical trials evaluating the efficacy of novel and innovative treatments. The clinical trial battery is briefer than a typical neuropsychological assessment and is able to be completed by most patients in 60 min or less. The clinical trial battery includes measures that have alternative forms that allow for serial testing and are sensitive to changes in learning and memory processes, attention, processing speed, executive function, and fine motor co-ordination. In addition to the aforementioned domains, a patient referred prior to a planned return to educational pursuits will require a more thorough assessment of intellectual ability and academic achievement. Information gleaned from the assessment may be used to develop an individualized education plan, ensuring supports that will facilitate a successful transition. An evaluation to assist in the process of returning to competitive employment will certainly include an assessment of those domains sensitive to cancer-related and treatment-related cognitive changes, but should also include measures thought to be ecologically valid. That is, measures that may predict the patient's success in their chosen vocation. An evaluation requested to assist in ruling out dementia should include a thorough assessment of verbal and non-verbal learning and memory processes, as well as supporting cognitive domains that are known to be affected across different stages of various dementing disorders. Appropriate measures should, on interpretation, enable the neuropsychologist to differentiate between failures of learning, retrieval and/or consolidation processes. The evaluation should also include an assessment of apraxia, language (e.g., naming, lexical fluency, semantic fluency, auditory comprehension), agnosia, executive function, orientation, and visuoconstruction/visuoperception skills. To summarize, the selection of neuropsychological instruments cannot be a "one-size-fits-all" proposition. Although many patients diagnosed with and treated for cancer will evidence cognitive dysfunction, the measures chosen must take into account the purpose and goals of the assessment.

Assessment process

Once again, the reader is referred to Chapter 2 and other sources (Lezak *et al.*, 2004; Vanderploeg, 2000) for comprehensive discussions of the assessment procedure.

In general, the neuropsychological assessment should begin with a general introduction explaining why the patient was referred, as well as the nature of the evaluation. The clinical interview that typically precedes test administration may include family members and/or caregivers as well as the patient, but the testing portion of the examination should be completed in a quiet, distraction-free environment, with only the patient and examiner being present.

Establishing a good working relationship with the patient is crucial to the success of the evaluation. Practitioners must be sensitive to the many potential factors (demographic, psychological, sociocultural, medical, etc.) that may affect the patient's willingness or ability to actively participate in the assessment. Tasks included in the assessment should vary in difficulty, be sensitive to potential deficits, and should be administered in a standardized fashion. "Testing the limits" is a process that can provide valuable clinical information, but should be attempted only after a measure has been completed in the standardized format (Lezak *et al.*, 2004).

Timing of assessment(s)

The timing of the assessment is an important consideration for both general clinical and research purposes and, again, is in many ways dictated by the hypotheses being evaluated. In most clinical settings, a patient will be referred when there is impairment obvious to their treatment provider or caregiver. The timing of the assessment is, therefore, dictated by the referral. These assessments, however, often occur in the context of on going treatments and the impact of this should be accounted for. In clinical trials assessing the effect of a particular treatment, pre-treatment assessments are imperative to adequately discern change over time. From a methodological standpoint, the need for pre-treatment assessments has been undervalued in the cancer literature. In more recent studies pre-treatment cognitive dysfunction has been reported in patients with CNS disease (Fleissbach *et al.*, 2003; Tucha *et al.*, 2000), lung cancer (Meyers *et al.*, 1995), and breast cancer (Wefel *et al.*, 2004a). Often a patient may undergo several assessments over time and in this case it is important to employ measures with alternative forms, which are relatively resistant to practice effects (Wefel *et al.*, 2004b). When interpreting data from repeated assessments it is also imperative to determine if the magnitude of change across individual, and multiple measures, is clinically meaningful. We utilize a reliable change index (Jacobson & Truax, 1991), but there several ways to account for clinical change over time and there is no consensus in the field.

Cognitive domains of interest

In clinical referral cases, the neuropsychologist should select tests appropriate to answer the referral question (e.g., aphasia evaluation) for that particular patient. For patients with focal CNS disease, knowledge of brain–behavior relationships should guide initial test selection. As a general rule, the neuropsychological assessment of persons with cancer should also include measures of learning and memory, processing speed, executive function, and fine motor control, since these are the domains that have been found to be sensitive to disease-related and treatment-related change across disease groups.

The neuropsychological assessment of patients with cancer should include an evaluation of mood. In one study, nearly 50% of cancer patients interviewed had some type of psychiatric disorder; the majority of these were classified as adjustment disorders with features of anxiety and/or depression or major depression (Derogatis *et al.*, 1983). Unfortunately, mood remains under-assessed in the clinical care and research setting. Analysis of data from 598 patients enrolled in the Glioma Outcomes Project revealed a remarkable discordance, with physicians reporting depression in 15% of patients with high-grade gliomas, but depressive symptomology was reported by 93% of patients in the early post-operative period. Patient-reported depression increased throughout the 6-month period after surgery, but remained underdiagnosed and under-treated by physicians (Litofsky *et al.*, 2004).

Patient-reported outcomes

Though the importance of patient perceptions and experience in the clinical management of disease has long been recognized, the term "quality of life" has been criticized as being too broad and non-specific to be of scientific value. An FDA work group concurred and adopted the term "patient-reported outcomes" (PROs) to include any disease- or treatment-related study endpoint subjectively reported by the patient (Acquadro *et al.*, 2003). Health-related quality of life (HRQOL) measures are a subset of PROs, remaining subjective, but also providing patient evaluations of the impact of disease or treatment on their well-being.

Patient-reported outcomes are now commonly used in clinical trials since they provide a unique understanding of treatment outcome from the patient's perspective. In one recent review, PROs were reported in 30% of 215 FDA-approved product labels reviewed, and were the only type of endpoint used for 23 products (Willke *et al.*, 2004). Patient-reported outcomes complement clinical endpoints and factor into the evaluation of a treatment's impact. Cancer therapy may be associated with significant adverse side-effects, so it is important to weigh the impact of these effects against potentially small gains in survival (Osoba *et al.*, 2000; Wiklund, 2004).

There are numerous PROs available and critical review of a measure's development, psychometric properties, and generalizability is necessary to determine its appropriateness for use in a particular setting and with a particular patient population (Meyers, 1997). The Functional Assessment of Cancer Therapy (FACT) (Cella *et al.*, 1993) and the European Organization for Research and Treatment of Cancer QLQ-C30 (EORTC QLQ-C30) (Aaronson *et al.*, 1993) are two commonly referenced PROs in the cancer–cognition literature. Each includes functional scales (physical, emotional, social, functional) and symptom scales, with diagnosis-specific modules. Although they provide some insight into patient concerns and perceptions, PRO ratings do not reliably correlate with clinical/functional outcomes (Huang *et al.*, 2001) or cognitive status as evaluated by objective neuropsychological assessment (Taphoorn *et al.*, 1992).

Disease- and treatment-specific considerations

The assessment of patients with CNS disease

Whether primary or metastatic, CNS tumors nearly always cause cognitive dysfunction. The nature of the neuropsychological impairment observed in the individual patient is in part related to the site of the lesion. For example, tumors located in the left hemisphere of the brain may be associated with expressive and/or receptive language problems that impede communication, while right hemisphere tumors may be associated with perception problems, visual-spatial disturbances, or attention deficits. In cancer patients, deficiencies in learning efficiency and memory retrieval are common and prevalent among patients with right, as well as left hemisphere disease. Impairments of frontal lobe function (executive deficits manifested by impairments of cognitive flexibility, abstraction, motivation, planning and organizational skills, ability to benefit from experience, personality changes, etc.) are also prevalent and may occur in patients without clear evidence of frontal lobe involvement. Disruption of afferent and efferent frontal lobe connections has been suggested as a putative mechanism.

Although research on the neurobehavioral and cognitive changes associated with metastatic disease is not that voluminous, some data are available for review. In contrast to the neuropsychological profiles of patients with local CNS disease, individuals with metastatic brain involvement frequently present with more diffuse cognitive dysfunction. For example, we completed neuropsychological assessments on 55 patients with brain metastases (Kayl et al., 2001). The majority of these patients carried a primary diagnosis of lung cancer, melanoma, renal cancer, or breast cancer. In most cases, patients had a single metastatic lesion, but those with multiple metastases were not excluded. Impaired cognitive performance (defined as a score greater than 1 standard deviation from the normative mean) was demonstrated on measures of fine motor co-ordination speed (42% of patients), memory (free recall: 29%), and verbal fluency (20%) prior to treatment for their brain disease. In this group of patients, as in others with metastatic brain disease, the etiology of these impairments is unclear, but microscopic tumor infiltration, diaschisis, and treatment-related changes may be influencing their functioning.

The impact of radiation on cognitive function

Radiation therapy remains an important therapeutic tool in the care and management of patients with CNS disease. A comprehensive review is beyond the scope of this chapter, but the interested reader is referred to Chapter 7 in this volume, as well as those articles cited in the paragraphs that follow, for additional information. Risk factors for developing cognitive dysfunction and radiation necrosis include patient age >60 years, scheduled dosing >2 Gy per fraction, total dose, volume of brain irradiated, hyperfractionated schedules, shorter overall treatment time, concomitant or subsequent use of chemotherapy, and presence

of co-morbid vascular risk factors (e.g., diabetes) (Crossen et al., 1994; Gregor et al., 1996; Lee et al., 2002). Most studies that include neuropsychological assessment of patients before and following radiation therapy reveal significant impairments of information-processing speed, executive functions, memory, sustained attention, and motor co-ordination in those with no evidence of disease recurrence (Archibald et al., 1994; Helfre & Pierga, 1999; Hochberg & Slotnick, 1980; Imperato et al., 1990; Lang et al., 2000; Lieberman et al., 1982; Salander et al., 1995; Scheibel et al., 1996; Taphoorn et al., 1994). Even radiation not directed at the brain can cause cognitive impairment. For example, a substantial percentage of patients who receive therapeutic radiation for tumors of the anterior skull base have cognitive deficits. Memory impairment was detected in 80% of patients with paranasal sinus tumors, even though the brain was not the target of radiation (Meyers et al., 2000).

Impact of chemotherapy on cognitive function

Chemotherapy remains a useful weapon in the management of cancer, and has improved survival for patients with some types of disease. Potential CNS side-effects vary across agents but may appear as peripheral neuropathy, acute and reversible encephalopathy, cerebellar syndrome, or persistent cognitive dysfunction (Keime-Guibert et al., 1998). Cognitive and emotional changes reported during and after chemotherapy include memory loss, decreased information-processing speed, reduced attention, anxiety, and depression (Meyers & Abbruzzese, 1992). It has been estimated that as many as one-third of patients undergoing systemic chemotherapy evidence declines in cognitive function that interfere with their quality of life (Ferguson & Ahles, 2003).

Among patients treated for cancer, the term "chemobrain" is being used with increasing frequency to describe perceived cognitive declines. In a recently published prospective, randomized, longitudinal trial, Wefel et al. (2004a) found an association between cognitive dysfunction and chemotherapy in a subgroup of women with non-metastatic breast carcinoma. Patients received a baseline assessment prior to the initiation of chemotherapy with 5-fluorouracil, doxorubicin, and cyclophosphamide (FAC), approximately 3 weeks following chemotherapy, and again at 1 year post-treatment. Surprisingly, 33% of these women had evidence of cognitive dysfunction prior to the initiation of treatment. Within-subject analyses revealed that 61% of patients evidenced a decline in cognitive function between the baseline assessment and just after the cessation of chemotherapy. Cognitive decline occurred most often in the domains of attention, learning and memory, and processing speed. Of this subset of patients, 45% remained impaired, 45% improved, and 10% had a mixed pattern of improvement and persistent symptoms 1 year post-chemotherapy.

In some cases, chemotherapeutic agents have a mechanism of action that is expected to affect focal brain regions (Meyers *et al.*, 1997). Other potential mechanisms include direct neurotoxic effects of treatment leading to cortical atrophy or demyelination and microvascular changes (Saykin *et al.*, 2003). Certain chemotherapeutic agents are known to be especially neurotoxic. The incidence and severity of the neurotoxicities vary between agents and between individual patients, but cognitive changes have been associated with methotrexate (Madhyastha *et al.*, 2002; Mulhern *et al.*, 1988; Ochs *et al.*, 1991; Taphoorn & Klein, 2004), etoposide (Castello *et al.*, 1990; Chamberlain, 1997; Chamberlain & Kormanik, 1997), high-dose cytarabine (Geller *et al.*, 2001; Hwang *et al.*, 1985; Salinsky *et al.*, 1983; Schwartz *et al.*, 2000), 5-fluorouracil (Lipp, 1999), TNP-470 (Logothetis *et al.*, 2001), CI-980 (Meyers *et al.*, 1997), ifosfamide (Lipp, 1999), and cisplatin (Troy *et al.*, 2000). Please refer to Chapter 8 in this volume for a more detailed discussion of chemotherapy-related cognitive dysfunction.

Impact of immunotherapy and hormonal therapies on cognitive function

Cytokines such as interferon alpha (IFN-α) and interleukin-2 (IL-2) have been used in a number of therapeutic trials for primary brain tumors and leptomeningeal disease (LMD) (Meyers *et al.*, 1991a). These agents are known to have both acute and persistent neurotoxic side-effects. Acute toxicity is characterized by fever, headache, and myalgia, which generally resolves over several days. Subacute neurotoxicity, evident within a week of starting therapy, is characterized by inattention, slowed thinking, and lack of motivation. Patients may develop difficulty with memory, frontal lobe executive functions (e.g., problem-solving, planning, sequencing), motor co-ordination, and mood as treatment continues (Pavol *et al.*, 1995). These neurotoxic side-effects are not always reversible following treatment cessation (Meyers *et al.*, 1991b). Please refer to Chapter 8 in this volume for a more detailed discussion of biological response modifier-related cognitive dysfunction.

The brain may also be sensitive to changes in its hormonal milieu (Yaffe *et al.*, 1998). Tamoxifen (TAM) is a widely used selective estrogen receptor modulator for the treatment of breast cancer. In a prospective, longitudinal trial (Wefel & Meyers, 2004) completed at The University of Texas M. D. Anderson Cancer Center, adjuvant TAM therapy was found to be associated with significant neurotoxicity in a subgroup of women. This subgroup experienced significant dysfunction in the domains of memory, executive, and motor function, as well as increased emotional distress, decreased quality of life, and diminished ability to maintain productive activities. Hormonal therapies are also among the treatment options available to men diagnosed with prostate carcinoma. One type of hormonal therapy involves treatment with luteinizing-hormone-releasing hormone (LHRH) agonists, such as leuprolide (Lupron®) and goserelin (Zoladex®). This treatment prevents the testicles from producing testosterone, and also lowers estradiol levels (Dawson-Hughes, 2001). There is growing evidence that certain brain structures are susceptible to declines in hormone levels associated with LHRH therapy, but the mechanisms of these changes are not fully understood. The cognitive effects of hormonal agents are reviewed in Chapter 9 of this volume.

Fatigue

Fatigue is a common symptom of patients with cancer and may be related to anemia, insomnia, poor nutrition, proinflammatory cytokine activation, or metabolic disturbance. Cancer-related fatigue is not responsive to increased rest or sleep and can contribute to cognitive decline (Iop *et al.*, 2004; Nerenz *et al.*, 1982; Tierney *et al.*, 1991). An assessment of fatigue should include an assessment of severity and its functional impact on the patient's daily activities and perceived quality of life. In one study of older patients (over 60 years), fatigue was nearly universal, significantly interfered with subjects' general activity level, and was positively correlated with severity of depression (Respini *et al.*, 2003). Potential treatment avenues might include correction of underlying metabolic or endocrine disorders, addressing depression or insomnia, institution of light/moderate exercise, cognitive therapy, or pharmacotherapy with steroids, stimulants, or epoetin alfa to correct anemia (Iop *et al.*, 2004; Lesage & Portenoy, 2002).

Anemia

The majority of chemotherapy patients experience mild anemia (Hb <12 g/dl) and severe anemia may affect up to 80% of patients (Groopman & Itri, 1999). The causes of cancer-related anemia include infiltration of bone marrow by malignant cells, decreased hemoglobin (Hb) production secondary to treatment, iron deficiency, or low erythropoietin (EPO) levels. Anemia levels below 12 g/dl in patients undergoing chemotherapy have been associated with both fatigue and declines on measures of attention, speed of cognitive processing, verbal fluency, and verbal memory (Brown *et al.*, 1991; Jacobsen *et al.*, 2004; Marsh *et al.*, 1991; Temple *et al.*, 1995). Treatment of anemia results in improved cognitive function (Grimm *et al.*, 1990; Littlewood *et al.*, 2002; Straus, 2002).

Adjunctive medications

Interpretation of the results of a neuropsychological assessment may be complicated by the confounding effects of medications. Depending on the clinical situation, steroids may have positive or negative effects on neurocognitive function (Lewis & Smith, 1983; Martignoni *et al.*, 1992; Stoudemire *et al.*, 1996; Varney *et al.*, 1984; Wolkowitz *et al.*, 1990). Antiepileptic medications have also been associated with cognitive dysfunction (Taphoorn & Klein, 2004), the severity of which tends to increase with the use of multiple agents and with elevated serum levels (Ortinski & Meador, 2004). With the exception of topiramate, the newer antiepileptic agents (including lamotrigine, oxcarbazepine, and gabapentin) seem to have more favorable side-effect profiles, with less impact on cognition (Beyenburg *et al.*, 2004; Loring & Meador, 2004; Meador & Baker, 1997).

Affective distress

Depression and anxiety may also affect cognitive performance. While depression and anxiety are not uncommon in the cancer population, the diagnosis of depression in cancer patients is complicated by the difficulty in distinguishing vegetative symptoms attributable to a mood disorder from symptoms caused by the primary disease or its treatment (Valentine *et al.*, 2002). Assessment and diagnosis are important however, as depression has been shown to affect cognitive function, causing impairments in attention and other cognitive skills, including memory (Christensen *et al.*, 1997; Tarbuck & Paykel, 1995). Interestingly, cognitive impairment may vary as a function of the depressive disorders. In a 2004 study, Airaksinen *et al.* found that severely depressed individuals and patients with mixed anxiety-depression evidenced significant memory dysfunction, while dysthymic patients tended to show impairments of mental flexibility. In a 1996 study, Cull *et al.* failed to detect differences in cognitive test performance between patients complaining of concentration and memory difficulties and non-complainers. However, those reporting cognitive difficulties had significantly high scores on measures of anxiety, depression, and fatigue. Anxiety has been associated with reduced cognitive efficiency, memory problems, and distractibility.

Neurobiological evidence suggests that anxiety can affect medial temporal lobe structures, including the hippocampus, amygdala, and frontal-subcortical circuits, subserving some memory functions. In some cases, imaging studies have found associations between depression and decreased hippocampal volume (Bremner *et al.*, 2000; Steffens *et al.*, 2000; Videbech & Ravnkilde, 2004). Relative to normal, healthy controls, persons diagnosed with anxiety disorders evidence impairment on measures of memory and executive function, but verbal fluency and processing speed were statistically unaffected (Airaksinen *et al.*, 2005).

Conclusion

Neuropsychological *testing* (the act of test administration) is a relatively simple procedure, but neuropsychological assessment is a *process* requiring an understanding of test construction and psychometrics, functional neuroanatomy, behavioral neurology, and the patient's sociocultural milieu, and should only be undertaken by professionals with training in these domains.

The utility and value of neuropsychological assessment in the clinical management of cancer patients and in the evaluation of new treatments are becoming better recognized, but the quality of the research that has been published to date is less than optimal. The contemporary scientific literature is cluttered with poorly designed studies that may lead investigators and the readership to incorrect conclusions. Clinicians and researchers must keep a few basic principles in mind when developing a plan for assessment. First, test selection will vary depending on the question under consideration. Second, the measures chosen should have alternative forms or be relatively resistant to practice effects, characteristics that are especially important if one plans to test patients repeatedly. Third, selected measures should be psychometrically sound, with established reliability and validity, and appropriate normative studies. Finally, it is important to select measures that are sensitive to subtle changes in cognitive function often experienced by patients with cancer. Attention, processing speed, learning/memory functions, executive function, and motor skills are particularly vulnerable and should be carefully evaluated for signs of dysfunction. These are areas of cognition that cannot be adequately assessed using screening measures such as the oft-employed MMSE.

REFERENCES

Aaronson NK, Ahmedzai S, Bergman B *et al.* (1993). The European Organization for Research and Treatment of Cancer QLQ-C30: a quality-of-life instrument for use in international cancer trials in oncology. *J Natl Cancer Inst* **85**(5): 365–376.

Acquadro C, Berzon R, Dubois D *et al.* for the PRO Harmonization Group. (2003). Incorporating the patient's perspective into drug development and communication: an ad hoc force report of the Patient-reported Outcomes (PRO) Harmonization Group meeting at the Food and Drug Administration, February 16, 2001. *Value Health* **6**(5): 522–531.

Airaksinen E, Larsson M, Lundberg I *et al.* (2004). Cognitive functions in depressive disorders: evidence from a population-based study. *Psychol Med* **34**(1): 83–91.

Airaksinen E, Larsson M, Forsell Y (2005). Neuropsychological functions in anxiety disorders in population-based samples: evidence of episodic memory dysfunction. *J Psychiatr Res* **39**(2): 207–214.

Archibald YM, Lunn D, Ruttan LA *et al.* (1994). Cognitive functioning in long-term survivors of high-grade glioma. *J Neurosurg* **80**: 247–253.

Beyenburg S, Bauer J, Reuber M (2004). New drugs for the treatment of epilepsy: a practical approach. *Postgrad Med J* **80**: 581–587.

Bremner JD, Narayan M, Anderson ER *et al.* (2000). Hippocampal volume reduction in major depression. *Am J Psychiatry* **157**: 115–117.

Brown WE, Marsh J, Wolcott D *et al.* (1991). Cognitive function, mood and P3 latency: effects of the amelioration of anemia in dialysis patients. *Neuropsychologia* **29**: 35–45.

Castello MA, Clerico A, Deb G *et al.* (1990). High-dose carboplatin in combination with etoposide (JET regimen) for childhood brain tumors. *Am J Pediatr Hematol Oncol* **12**(3): 297–300.

Cella DF, Tulsky DS, Gray G *et al.* (1993). The Functional Assessment of Cancer Therapy Scale: development and validation of the general measure. *J Clin Oncol* **11**: 570–579.

Chamberlain MC (1997). Recurrent supratentorial malignant gliomas in children. Long-term salvage therapy with oral etoposide. *Arch Neurol* **54**(5): 554–558.

Chamberlain MC, Kormanik PA (1997). Chronic oral VP-16 for recurrent medulloblastoma. *Pediatr Neurol* **17**(3): 230–234.

Christensen H, Griffiths K, MacKinnon A *et al.* (1997). A quantitative review of cognitive deficits in depression and Alzheimer-type dementia. *J Int Neuropsychol Soc* **3**: 631–651.

Crossen JR, Garwood D, Glatstein E *et al.* (1994). Neurobehavioral sequelae of cranial irradiation in adults: a review of radiation-induced encephalopathy. *J Clin Oncol* **12**: 627–642.

Cull A, Hay C, Love SB *et al.* (1996). What do cancer patients mean when they complain of memory problems? *Br J Cancer* **74**(10): 1674–1679.

Dawson-Hughes B (2001). Bone loss accompanying medical therapies. *N Engl J Med* **354**(13): 989–991.

Derogatis LR, Morrow GR, Fetting J *et al.* (1983). The prevalence of psychiatric disorders among cancer patients. *J Am Med Assoc* **249**: 751–757.

Ferguson RJ, Ahles TA (2003). Low neuropsychologic performance among adult cancer survivors treated with chemotherapy. *Curr Neurol Neurosci Rep* **3**(3): 215–222.

Fliessbach K, Urbach H, Helmstaedter C *et al.* (2003). Cognitive performance and magnetic resonance imaging findings after high-dose systemic and intraventricular chemotherapy for primary central nervous system lymphoma. *Arch Neurol* **60**: 563–568.

Folstein MF, Folstein SE, McHugh PR (1975). A mini mental state: a practical method for grading the cognitive status of patients for the clinician. *J Psychiatr Res* **12**: 189–198.

Geller HM, Cheng KY, Goldsmith NK *et al.* (2001). Oxidative stress mediates neuronal DNA damage and apoptosis in response to cytosine arabinoside. *J Neurochem* **78**(2): 265–275.

Gregor A, Cull A, Traynor E *et al.* (1996). Neuropsychometric evaluation of long-term survivors of adult brain tumours: relationship with tumour and treatment parameters. *Radiother Oncol* **41**: 55–59.

Grimm G, Stockenhuber F, Schneeweiss B *et al.* (1990). Improvement in brain function in hemodialysis patients treated with erythropoietin. *Kidney Int* **38**: 480–486.

Groopman JE, Itri LM (1999). Chemotherapy-induced anemia in adults: incidence and treatment. *J Natl Cancer Inst* **91**: 1616–1634.

Helfre S, Pierga J (1999). Cerebral metastases: radiotherapy and chemotherapy. *Neuro-Chirurgie* **45**(5): 382–392.

Hochberg FH, Slotnick B (1980). Neuropsychologic impairment in astrocytoma survivors. *Neurology* **30**: 172–177.

Huang ME, Wartella JE, Kreutzer JS (2001). Functional outcomes and quality of life in patients with brain tumors: a preliminary report. *Arch Phys Med Rehabil* **82**: 1540–1546.

Hutchinson TA, Boyd NF, Feinstein AR *et al.* (1979). Scientific problems in clinical scales, as demonstrated in the Karnofsky Index of performance status. *J Chronic Dis* **32**(9–10): 661–666.

Hwang TL, Yung WK, Estey EH *et al.* (1985). Central nervous system toxicity with high dose Ara-C. *Neurology* **35**: 1475–1479.

Imperato JP, Paleologos NE, Vich NA (1990). Effects of treatment on long-term survivors with malignant astrocytomas. *Ann Neurol* **28**: 818–822.

Iop A, Manfredi AM, Bonura S (2004). Fatigue in cancer patients receiving chemotherapy: an analysis of published studies. *Ann Oncol* **15**: 712–720.

Jacobsen L, Garland M, Booth-Jones K *et al.* (2004). Relationship of hemoglobin levels to fatigue and cognitive functioning among cancer patients receiving chemotherapy. *J Pain Symptom Manage* **28**(1): 7–18 P.

Jacobson NS, Truax P (1991). Clinical significance: a statistical approach to defining meaningful change in psychotherapy research. *J Consult Clin Psychol* **59**(1): 12–19.

Karnofsky DA, Burchenal JH (1949). The clinical evaluation of chemotherapeutic agents in cancer. In Macleod CM (ed.) *Evaluation of Chemotherapeutic Agents* (pp. 191–205). New York: Columbia University Press.

Kayl AE, Seabrooke LF, Meyers CA (2001). Neurobehavioral changes due to metastatic brain tumors [abstract]. *Neurooncology* **3**(4): 339.

Keime-Guibert F, Napolitano M, Delattre J-Y (1998). Neurological complications of radiotherapy and chemotherapy. *J Neurol* **245**: 695–708.

Lang FF, Wildrick DM, Sawaya R (2000). Metastatic brain tumors. In Bernstein M, Berger MS (eds.) *Neuro-Oncology: The Essentials* (pp. 329–337). New York: Thieme Medical Publishers.

Lee AW, Kwong DLW, Leung S-F *et al.* (2002). Factors affecting risk of symptomatic temporal lobe necrosis: Significance of fractional dose and treatment time. *Int J Radiat Oncol Biol Phys* **53**: 75–82.

Lesage P, Portenoy RK (2002). Management of fatigue in the cancer patient. *Oncology* **16**(3): 373–378.

Lewis DA, Smith RE (1983). Steroid induced psychiatric syndromes. *J Affect Disord* **5**: 319.

Lezak MD, Howieson DB, Loring DW (2004). *Neuropsychological Assessment*, (4th edn.). New York: Oxford University Press.

Lieberman AN, Foo SH, Ransohoff J *et al.* (1982). Long term survival among patients with malignant brain tumors. *Neurosurgery* **10**: 450–453.

Lipp HP (1999). Neurotoxicity (including sensory toxicity) induced by cytostatics. In Lipp HP (ed.) *Anticancer Drug-Toxicity. Prevention, Management, and Clinical Pharmacokinetics* (pp. 431–454). New York: Marcel Dekker Inc.

Litofsky NS, Farace E, Anderson F, Meyers CA, Huang W, Laws ER (2004). Depression in patients with high-grade glioma: results of the Glioma Outcomes Project. *Neurosurgery* **54**(2): 358–366.

Littlewood TJ, Bajetta E, Nrtier JWR *et al.* (2002). Effects of epoetin alfa on hematologic parameters and quality of life in cancer patients receiving nonplatinum chemotherapy: results of a randomized, double-blind, placebo-controlled trial. *J Clin Oncol* **19**: 2865–2874.

Logothetis CJ, Wu KK, Finn LD *et al.* (2001). Phase I trial of the angiogenesis inhibitor TNP-470 for progressive androgen-independent prostate cancer. *Clin Cancer Res* **7**: 1198–1203.

Loring DW, Meador KJ (2004). Cognitive side effects of antiepileptic drugs in children. *Neurology* **62**: 872–877.

Madhyastha S, Somayaji SN, Raoe MS *et al.* (2002). Hippocampal brain amines in methotrexate-induced learning and memory deficit. *Can J Physiol Pharmacol* **80**(11): 1076–1084.

Marsh J, Brown WE, Wolcott D *et al.* (1991). RhuEPO treatment improves brain and cognitive function of anemic dialysis patients. *Kidney Int* **39**: 155–163.

Martignoni E, Costa A, Sinforiani E *et al.* (1992). The brain as a target for adrenocortical steroids: cognitive implications. *Psychoneuroendocrinology* **17**: 343.

Meador KJ, Baker GA (1997). Behavioral and cognitive effects of lamotrigine. *J Child Neurol* **12** [Suppl 1]: S44–47.

Meyers CA (1997). Issues of quality of life in neuro-oncology. In Vecht CJ (ed.) *Handbook of Clinical Neurology, Neuro-Oncology* (Part 1) (pp. 389–409). New York: Elsevier Science.

Meyers CA, Abbruzzese JL (1992). Cognitive functioning in cancer patients: effect of previous treatment. *Neurology* **42**: 434–436.

Meyers CA, Hess KR (2003). Multifaceted end points in brain tumor clinical trials: cognitive deterioration precedes MRI progression. *Neurooncology* **5**(2): 89–95.

Meyers CA, Wefel JS (2003). The use of the Mini-Mental State Examination to assess cognitive functioning in cancer trials: no ifs ands, buts, or sensitivity. *J Clin Oncol* **21**(19): 3557–3558.

Meyers CA, Obbens EAMT, Scheibel RS *et al.* (1991a). Neurotoxicity of intraventricularly administered alpha-interferon for leptomeningeal disease. *Cancer* **68**: 88–92.

Meyers CA, Scheibel RS, Forman AD (1991b). Persistent neurotoxicity of systemically administered interferon-alpha. *Neurology* **41**: 672–676.

Meyers CA, Byrne KS, Komaki R (1995). Cognitive deficits in patients with small cell lung cancer before and after chemotherapy. *Lung Cancer* **12**: 231–235.

Meyers CA, Kudelka AP, Conrad CA *et al.* (1997). Neurotoxicity of CI-980, a novel mitotic inhibitor. *Clin Cancer Res* **3**: 419–422.

Meyers CA, Geara F, Wong P-F *et al.* (2000). Neurocognitive effects of therapeutic irradiation for base of skull tumors. *Int J Radiat Oncol Biol Phys* **46**: 51–55.

Mulhern RK, Wasserman Al, Fairclough D *et al.* (1988). Memory function in disease-free survivors of childhood acute lymphoblastic leukemia given central nervous system prophylaxis with or without 1800 cGy cranial irradiation. *J Clin Oncol* **6**: 315–320.

Nerenz DR, Leventhal H, Love RR (1982). Factors contributing to emotional distress during chemotherapy. *Cancer* **50**: 1020–1027.

Ochs J, Mulhern RK, Fairclough D *et al.* (1991). Comparison of neuropsychologic functioning and clinical indicators of neurotoxicity in long-term survivors of childhood leukemia given cranial irradiation or parenteral methotrexate: a prospective study. *J Clin Oncol* **9**(1): 145–151.

Ortinski P, Meador KL (2004). Cognitive side effects of antiepileptic drugs. *Epilepsy Behav* **5**: S60–S65.

Osoba D, Brada M, Yung WKA *et al.* (2000). Health-related quality of life patients treated with temozolomide versus procarbazine for recurrent glioblastoma multiforme. *J Clin Oncol* **18**(7): 1481–1491.

Pavol MA, Meyers CA, Rexer JL *et al.* (1995). Pattern of neurobehavioral deficits associated with interferon-alfa therapy for leukemia. *Neurology* **45**: 947–950.

Respini D, Jacobsen PB, Thors C *et al.* (2003). The prevalence and correlates of fatigue in older cancer patients. *Crit Rev Oncol Hematol* **47**: 273–279.

Salander P, Karlsson T, Bergenheim T *et al.* (1995). Long-term memory deficits in patients with malignant gliomas. *J Neurooncol* **25**: 227–238.

Salinsky MC, Levine RL, Aubuchon JP *et al.* (1983). Acute cerebellar dysfunction with high-dose Ara-C therapy. *Cancer* **51**: 426–429.

Saykin AJ, Ahles TA, McDonald BC (2003). Mechanisms of chemotherapy-induced cognitive disorders: neuropsychological, pathophysiological, and neuroimaging perspectives. *Semin Clin Neuropsychiatry* **8**(4): 201–216.

Scheibel RS, Meyers CA, Levin VA (1996). Cognitive dysfunction following surgery for intracerebral glioma: influence of histopathology, lesion location, and treatment. *J Neurooncol* **30**: 61–69.

Schwartz J, Alster Y, Ben-Tal O *et al.* (2000). Visual loss following high-dose cytosine-arabinoside (ARA-C). *Eur J Haematol* **64**(3): 208–209.

Steffens DC, Byrum CE, McQuoid DR *et al.* (2000). Hippocampal volume in geriatric depression. *Biol Psychiatry* **48**: 301–309.

Stoudemire A, Anfinson T, Edwards J (1996). Corticosteroid-induced delirium and dependency. *Gen Hosp Psychiatry* **18**: 196–202.

Straus DJ (2002). Epoetin alfa as a supportive measure in hematologic malignancies. *Semin Hematol* **39** [4 Suppl 3]: 25–31.

Taphoorn MJB, Klein M (2004). Cognitive deficits in adult patients with brain tumors. *Lancet* **3**: 159–168.

Taphoorn MJB, Heimans JJ, Snoek FJ *et al.* (1992). Assessment of quality of life in patients treated for low grade glioma: a preliminary report. *J Neurol Neurosurg Psychiatry* **55**: 372–376.

Taphoorn MJB, Schiphorst CP, Snoek JF *et al.* (1994). Cognitive functions and quality of life in patients with low-grade gliomas: the impact of radiotherapy. *Ann Neurol* **36**: 48–54.

Tarbuck AF, Paykel ES (1995). Effects of major depression on the cognitive function of younger and older patients. *Psychol Med* **25**: 285–296.

Tarter RE, Butters M, Beers SR (2001). *Medical Neuropsychology* (2nd edn.). New York: Kluwer Academic/Plenum Publishers.

Temple RM, Deary IJ, Winney RJ (1995). Recombinant erythropoietin improves cognitive function in patients maintained on chronic ambulatory peritoneal dialysis. *Nephrol Dial Transplant* **10**: 1733–1738.

Tierney A, Leonard R, Taylor J *et al.* (1991). Side effects expected and experienced by women receiving chemotherapy for breast cancer. *Br Med J* **302**:272.

Troy L, McFarland K, Littman-Power S *et al.* (2000). Cisplatin-based therapy: a neurological and neuropsychological review. *Psychooncology* **9**: 29–39.

Tucha O, Smely C, Preier M *et al.* (2000). Cognitive deficits before treatment among patients with brain tumors. *Neurosurgery* **47**: 324–333.

Valentine AD, Passik SD, Massie MJ (2002). Psychiatric and psychosocial issues. In Levin VA (ed.) *Cancer in the Nervous System* (2nd edn.) (pp. 572–589). New York: Oxford University Press.

Vanderploeg RD (2000). Interview and testing: the data collection phase of neuropsychological evaluations. In Vanderploeg RD (ed.) *Clinician's Guide to Neuropsychological Assessment* (2nd edn.) (pp. 3–38). New Jersey: Lawrence Erlbaum Associates.

Varney NR, Alexander B, Macindoe JH (1984). Reversible steroid dementia in patients without steroid psychosis. *Am J Psychiatry* **141**: 369–372.

Videbech P, Ravnkilde B (2004). Hippocampal volume and depression: a meta-analysis of MRI studies. *Am J Psychiatry* **161**(11): 1957–1966.

Wefel JS, Lenzi R, Theriault RL *et al.* (2004a). The cognitive sequelae of standard-dose adjuvant chemotherapy in women with breast carcinoma. Results of a prospective, randomized, longitudinal trial. *Cancer* **100**(11): 2292–2299.

Wefel JS, Kayl AE, Meyers CA (2004b). Neuropsychological dysfunction associated with cancer and cancer therapies: a conceptual review of an emerging target. *Br J Cancer* **90**(9): 1691–1696.

Wefel JS, Meyers CA (2004). Tamoxifen associated neurotoxicity in women with breast cancer [abstract]. Final program 32nd Annual International Neuropsychological Society Conference: 185–186.

Wiklund I (2004). Assessment of patient-reported outcomes in clinical trials: the example of health-related quality of life. *Fundam Clin Pharmacol* **18**: 351–363.

Willke RJ, Burke LB, Erickson P (2004). Measuring treatment impact: a review of patient-reported outcomes and other efficacy endpoints in approved product labels. *Control Clin Trials* **25**: 535–552.

Wolkowitz OM, Reus VI, Weingartner H *et al.* (1990). Cognitive effects of corticosteroids. *Am J Psychiatry* **147**: 1297–1303.

Yaffe K, Grady D, Pressman A *et al.* (1998). Serum estrogen levels, cognitive performance, and risk of cognitive decline in older community women. *J Am Geriatr Soc* **46**(7): 918–920.

6

Neuropsychological assessment of children with cancer

Louise Penkman Fennell and Robert W. Butler

Introduction

Neuropsychology, broadly defined, is the study of brain–behavior relationships. The term was coined by William Osler in the early 1900s and gained wider appeal in the 1960s. The field was influenced by pioneers in neuroanatomy, neurology, and physiology, who began to explore the brain's functionality (Broca, 1865; Hughlings-Jackson, 1931; Lashley, 1950; Wernicke, 1874). Modern neuropsychology represents a blend of careful clinical observation grounded in the pioneering work of Alexandr Luria (1973), and a more actuarial approach that utilizes psychometric instruments to describe and quantify an individual's functioning (Halstead, 1947; Reitan, 1974). Neuropsychology has become a science of human behavior as it is influenced by brain functioning and by social, psychological, and cultural contexts.

Pediatric neuropsychologists are concerned with developmental issues and take into account the genetic, medical, environmental, behavioral, and sociocultural influences that impact the maturation of a child (Baron, 2004). The human nervous system is never static and development occurs across the lifespan. However, the rapidity of development in childhood and adolescence calls for a specific developmental focus when conducting evaluations with this age group.

At birth, infants have more than 100 billion neurons (Berger, 2005). In the first 2 years of life the brain undergoes a period termed transient exuberance when as many as 15 000 new connections are established per neuron (Thompson, 2000). Following this period of rapid growth, there is a period of rapid elimination of synapses called "pruning" that peaks in adolescence and is variable across different brain regions (Kolb & Wishaw, 2003). Frequently used synaptic connections are strengthened and unused connections are pruned. It is through this process of pruning that distributed neural networks that subserve functions such as language are developed. There are certain critical periods during development when the brain "expects" certain experiences from the environment (e.g., language stimulation) in order to develop. Studies of children who were deprived of appropriate environmental stimulation showed that they failed to develop expected skills (Ames, 1997; Gunnar, 2001; Rutter, 1998). However, it appears that these children can demonstrate accelerated development and the brain can recover to reach age-appropriate levels if the deprivation is brief in duration (Rutter, 1998). This supports the concept of critical periods for development.

In addition to synaptogenesis, dendritic arborization, and pruning, myelination is an important neurodevelopmental process that occurs across the

Cognition and Cancer, eds. Christina A. Meyers and James R. Perry. Published by Cambridge University Press.

lifespan to varying degrees. Myelin is the fatty sheath that surrounds the axon and is made from oligodendrocytes. It serves to insulate the axon and to prevent leakage of the electrical potential, and is responsible for speeded conduction of neural impulses. Myelination begins in the pre-natal period and continues into the adult years. Like synaptogenesis and pruning, myelination occurs in different cortical regions at different rates and is considered a gross index of cerebral maturation (Anderson, 2001; Kolb & Wishaw, 2003).

It is important to understand the dynamic nature of the child's nervous system in order to adequately understand how development may be interrupted or changed by an illness, injury, or toxic exposure. The plasticity of the child's nervous system may be most dramatically illustrated in cases of hemispherectomy. When one hemisphere is removed (e.g., to control refractory epilepsy), if the child is young enough some of the functions of the resected hemisphere can be taken over by the remaining, healthy hemisphere. In contrast, the mature nervous system is based on well-established connections and is less malleable. Although the adult nervous system does retain some degree of plasticity, it is not likely to reorganize in response to a catastrophic neurological event (e.g., stroke or severe traumatic brain injury) in the same way that a developing nervous system may.

Having said this, it is now understood that suffering brain damage early in life does not always result in fewer deficits. The premise that brain damage early in life is associated with a better outcome than brain damage later in life is known as the Kennard Principle (Finger, 1999; Finger & Wolf, 1988). This is a general statement and does not apply in many cases. The type and extent of injury determine whether a mature or developing nervous system is more resilient: greater recovery of function is typically seen following focal rather than diffuse injuries and many childhood injuries are diffuse in nature. Although compared to adults a child's nervous system may show more plasticity, defined as the capacity of the brain to continuously change its structure and ultimately its function (Kolb, 1995), children possess less well-established, acquired knowledge than adults. Also, their foundational skill base is less. So when an injury disrupts the ability to acquire new information, a child will be more compromised than an adult whose lifetime of education has created a broad base of knowledge and skills.

Childhood cancer

Dramatic progress in pediatric oncology has resulted in increased survival rates for certain types of cancer since the late 1980s to the time of writing. In the 1960s fewer than 5% of children diagnosed with acute lymphoblastic leukemia (ALL) survived for more than 5 years. In 2004 the 5-year survival rate for children with standard-risk ALL was approximately 85% (Ries *et al.*, 2005). Likewise, children with medulloblastoma were almost certain to die in the mid 1990s. In 2005, medulloblastomas had a 5-year survival rate of 70% (Reddick *et al.*, 2005). These dramatic increases in cure rates are attributable in great part to large-scale, well co-ordinated clinical trials carried out by groups such as Children's Oncology Group (COG) and its predecessors Pediatric Oncology Group (POG) and Children's Cancer Group (CCG). However, these medical advances have yielded a cohort of childhood cancer survivors with mild to severe neuropsychological impairments that are the result of life-saving treatments.

Acute lymphoblastic leukemia is the most common form of childhood malignancy. There are approximately 2400 individuals under the age of 20 diagnosed with ALL each year in the United States (Smith *et al.*, 1999). The peak incidence is during the pre-school years. Brain tumors are the second most common neoplasm of childhood (Ries *et al.*, 2005). Of these tumors, approximately 60% occur in the posterior fossa. The most common are gliomas such as astrocytoma, followed by medulloblastoma and ependymoma. Less commonly diagnosed are high-grade supratentorial gliomas and pineal tumors (Strother *et al.*, 2002). Although ALL and brain tumors are very different diseases, they have both been recognized as posing significant risks to neurodevelopment and ultimately academic and vocational functioning.

Brain tumors

The diagnosis of a brain tumor carries with it a risk to neuropsychological functioning. A tumor is a space-occupying lesion that can cause deficits through compression of brain structures. An obstructive brain tumor can cause hydrocephalus and an increase in intracranial pressure, which can ultimately be fatal if brainstem structures are compressed. Deficits can be focal or more diffuse depending upon tumor location and associated complications (Ris & Noll, 1994).

Surgery is an important component of both diagnosis and treatment unless the tumor is deemed inoperable. Medulloblastomas are the most common malignant brain tumor of childhood and most cases are diagnosed in the first decade of life (Strother *et al.*, 2002). They are aggressive tumors and treatment usually includes surgery, chemotherapy, and cranial-spinal radiation therapy (CRT) with a boost of focal radiation to the posterior fossa. Ependymomas are also treated with surgery, cranial-spinal or focal radiation, and chemotherapy. Low-grade gliomas are generally treated with surgery alone. See Chapter 14 for a more complete review of childhood brain tumors.

Acute lymphoblastic leukemia

Children with ALL are also at risk for neuropsychological dysfunction related to their treatment. Currently, standard treatment for ALL does not include CRT. However, children who present with ALL that has spread to the central nervous system (CNS) or whose disease relapses in the CNS do receive CRT at a lower dose than that typically administered for treatment of a malignant brain tumor. Because the CNS is a site of recurrence for this disease, intrathecal (IT) chemotherapy is used

for prophylaxis and has contributed to the high cure rate. Intrathecal chemotherapy consists of methotrexate (MTX) delivered in combination with other agents or alone, administered directly into the cerebrospinal fluid via lumbar puncture. When CRT and IT-MTX are administered concurrently, the risk for neuropsychological dysfunction increases (Bleyer *et al.*, 1990).

Young children are at the highest risk for neuropsychological dysfunction and subsequent academic difficulties due to radiation and/or chemotherapy treatment (Hopewell, 1998; Mulhern *et al.*, 1998; Ris *et al.*, 2001; Walter *et al.*, 1999). The immature brain is highly vulnerable to the diffuse effects of radiation and IT chemotherapy: young children have fewer well-established skills than older children when they receive treatment with its potentially disruptive influence on their development. It is generally thought that skills that are in a critical stage of development when a neurological insult occurs may be most susceptible to disruption (Dennis *et al.*, 1998). The rapid growth of the nervous system during early childhood is the reason for its significant vulnerability to treatment-related brain injury. It is important to also note that research indicates that treatment-related brain injury is progressive and that cognitive and academic deficits may not become evident until 12 months to several years post-treatment (Hoppe-Hirsch *et al.*, 1995; Langer *et al.*, 2002; Moleski, 2000).

Pattern of neuropsychological deficits

As stated, children treated with IT chemotherapy and/or CRT are at risk for neurodevelopmental delay and subsequent neuropsychological deficits. These deficits can lead to academic struggles and ultimately lower vocational success and health-related quality of life (HRQOL). Research examining the HRQOL of childhood cancer survivors documents the lowest level for children with CNS tumors. Children with leukemia and lymphoma have the next poorest HRQOL (Speechley *et al.*, 2002). For a discussion of the pattern of neuropsychological deficits observed following treatment for a brain tumor in childhood, please refer to Chapter 14 of this text.

The neuropsychological outcome of CRT was first studied in survivors of childhood ALL (Rowland *et al.*, 1984). Similar to brain tumor survivors, intellectual functioning has been shown to be compromised in children with ALL treated with CRT (Cousens *et al.*, 1988; Fletcher & Copeland, 1988; Rowland *et al.*, 1984; Spiegler *et al.*, 2006). However, IQ scores have also been shown to remain within the normal range (Langer *et al.*, 2002). In general, the level of global impairment tends not to be as severe as in the brain tumor population. These children are treated with a relatively low dose of CRT and a high dosage has been shown to be a risk factor for poor intellectual outcome (Picard & Rourke, 1995).

The pattern of deficits documented for children treated for ALL is similar to those seen in childhood brain tumors. Mulhern and Butler (2005) reviewed this literature and underscored the fact that non-dominant hemisphere functions seem to be differentially impacted. This includes non-verbal memory, visual motor integration, visual spatial reasoning, and visual perceptual abilities. Similarly, in an earlier comprehensive review Moleski (2000) documented attention and non-verbal memory problems as the most robust findings. In addition, these children show difficulties with fine motor and tactile-perceptual functioning due to the use of vincristine as a chemotherapy agent (Moleski, 2000). Lehtinen and colleagues (2002) studied motor-evoked potentials in children treated for ALL. Their findings support the persistence of peripheral, but not central, motor abnormalities in children up to 5 years post-treatment. These difficulties manifest themselves as gross and fine motor problems and children struggle with co-ordination for playing sports and with handwriting. In general, ALL survivors demonstrate more difficulties with arithmetic than with language based academic skills (Moleski, 2000).

The literature is mixed with respect to neuropsychological outcome in children treated with IT-MTX and not CRT. Mulhern and Butler (2004) estimate

the prevalence of some degree of neuropsychological impairment in this group of children to be at least 30%. In a number of studies examining children treated for ALL with CNS-directed chemotherapy only, Brown and colleagues showed that children who received CNS prophylactic chemotherapy were more impaired than their sibling controls on measures of dominant hemisphere skills (Brown & Maden-Swain, 1993; Brown *et al.*, 1992, 1998). Other authors have shown negligible impact on overall intellectual functioning when children with ALL are treated with IT chemotherapy alone (Langer *et al.*, 2002; Von der Weid *et al.*, 2003). Spiegler and colleagues (2006) assessed neurocognitive outcome in survivors of early childhood ALL 5–20 years post-treatment. They compared children treated with high-dose and very high-dose intravenous MTX and IT-MTX to a group of children treated with CRT and the same chemotherapy backbone. Their results showed no difference from population norms for the chemotherapy group, with survivors treated with CRT showing deficits. However, Moleski (2000) cautions that IT-MTX cannot be considered a benign agent. In her comprehensive review, she summarizes the mixed research findings available. Her overview indicated that in all studies using sibling controls instead of the general norms, there was a significant difference in overall intellectual functioning for patients treated with IT chemotherapy. In addition, children treated with CRT alone fare better than children treated with IT-MTX in combination with CRT, suggesting a possible synergistic neurotoxic effect (Bleyer *et al.*, 1990).

Researchers interested in the neuropsychological impact of treatment for ALL are focused on investigating core cognitive processes such as attention, processing speed, and working memory. Deficits in these core processes are seen as underlying the overall intellectual deterioration and academic difficulty that has been observed. Processing speed, working memory, vigilance, and cognitive flexibility deficits have been reported in ALL survivors (Butler & Copeland, 2002; Langer *et al.*, 2002; Schatz *et al.*, 2000). Buzier and colleagues (2005) showed that IT chemotherapy alone has been associated with attention dysfunction. They identified intensified treatment and young age as being associated with worse performance.

In sum, deficits have been reported in a number of different areas. However, attention, processing speed, executive functioning, non-verbal problem solving, and non-verbal memory appear to be most impacted for children with brain tumors and ALL. Verbal skills tend to be better preserved except in very young children. However, the presentation of each individual child will be mediated by both risk and protective factors such as gender (see Moore, 2005 for a brief overview), age, treatment, pre-existing complications, and parental social class (see Moleski, 2000, for a brief discussion).

Implications for neuropsychological assessment

Children treated with CRT and/or IT chemotherapy with MTX are at substantial risk of neuropsychological dysfunction with implications for academic, vocational and social functioning, and, ultimately, quality of life. Neuropsychological follow-up of these survivors is now described as standard care (Children's Oncology Group, 2004; Duffner, 2004).

Serial assessments

Children treated for brain tumors or ALL evidence a delayed onset of neuropsychological deficits that may progress over time. As such, it is important to take a serial approach to testing this group of children. It does not suffice to test a child once at the end of treatment. Serial assessment presents particular challenges in the selection of instruments, detection of meaningful change, and determining when and how often to test. More often now, serial testing is built into treatment protocols. However, for many children, planning when testing should take place is left up to the neuropsychologist.

Depending upon the age of the child and treatment protocol, it may be helpful to conduct a neu-

ropsychological assessment when treatment ends. This provides information for the school about any special accommodations that need to be made to optimize a child's re-integration into school. For children with ALL, treatment duration is approximately 30 months and many children are able to continue at school during treatment. For these children, it may be necessary to conduct a neuropsychological assessment during treatment, particularly if teachers are noticing changes in the child's performance at school.

Re-testing should not be carried out excessively. Children can be "over-tested." Some children remember the test materials and this can contribute to significant practice effects. Sometimes neuropsychologists will use alternative test forms or different tests to attempt to control for this problem. However, only a handful of tests are available in alternative forms. In addition, this is not a perfect solution since alternative forms have been shown to evidence practice effects when administered serially (Beglinger *et al.*, 2005; Franzen *et al.*, 1996). When different tests are used, it is sometimes difficult to compare scores for the purposes of evaluating the child's progression of learning because the test norms may be very different. In an optimal situation a child should be administered the same measures when possible, at an appropriate inter-test interval. A general practice of clinicians is to use 6–12 months as the minimum inter-test interval. However, test manuals provide reliability estimates for much shorter durations of time. Currently, data are lacking for inter-test intervals that more closely approximate clinical practice. For a thorough discussion of approaches to detecting clinically significant change over time in children the reader is referred to Baron (2004).

Decisions made about when to test a child may be dependent on the child's age when the first assessment is conducted. Obviously, younger children will need to be seen more often. Some neuropsychologists make it their practice to leave it up to families and educators to contact them if the child encounters more problems over time. This can be a way to manage heavy demands on one's time.

However, some parents find it more difficult to be proactive than others, and some children risk not receiving adequate follow-up if educators or parents do not initiate the assessment. Other practitioners set up a more structured plan where children are booked in advance to come back for a re-assessment in 12–36 months following the first assessment. The time interval may depend on the age and grade placement of the child and the severity of neuropsychological dysfunction. It may be helpful to see children at important educational transition points. For example, a child who is assessed in the third grade (at about 9 years of age) may receive a follow-up neuropsychological assessment when he or she transitions to junior high school (sixth or seventh grade, i.e., aged 12–14 years) and then a final assessment at the beginning of high school. This updated assessment information can be taken with the child into their new educational setting so that educators can make the most well-informed decisions about appropriate placement and educational focus.

Liaison with the school

Unfortunately, most very busy educators and school psychologists do not have the time or the resources to be particularly well informed about the issues facing child cancer survivors when they return to school. Educators may assume that once the cancer treatment is over that the child should return to their pre-morbid level of functioning. Similarly, they may assume that an end-of-treatment neuropsychological assessment that revealed no areas of concern may signal a positive educational future for a child. However, this is clearly not always the case because these children often sustain a progressive injury with deficits that manifest over time. Many times a neuropsychologist is not available to evaluate child cancer survivors and they are seen by a school psychologist who is not trained in brain development issues or the underlying neuropathology of brain injury acquired through cancer treatment. When a neuropsychologist is available, it is important that their involvement with

the child cancer survivor continues beyond the testing office, and that communication is established between the neuropsychologist and the educational professionals at the child's school. The neuropsychologist's role is to teach these individuals about the nature of the child's injury and subsequent deficits and how they translate into practical challenges to learning and social development in the classroom. Furthermore, the neuropsychologist is instrumental in ensuring that the child receives adequate follow-up over time and that new teachers each year are educated about the child's specific needs.

Approaches to assessment

Neuropsychological assessments for child cancer survivors should be comprehensive because a multitude of deficits have been described. Similarly, research studies reflect information about groups of children whereas neuropsychological assessments in clinical settings are carried out within the idiographic context, and generalized statements drawn from research findings may or may not apply. Research findings serve as a guideline to suggest which areas of cognitive function are likely to be impacted and help to direct clinical assessment planning.

Traditionally, neuropsychological assessment has been a fairly lengthy process. This is due to the number of areas of cognitive function that are evaluated and the need for rest breaks to ensure adequate effort on the part of the examinee. However, in more recent years various pressures have forced neuropsychologists to find ways to work more quickly yet still provide a comprehensive description of the strengths and weaknesses of their patient and provide relevant, useful recommendations.

We present an overview of a thorough neuropsychological assessment that addresses the areas of deficit experienced by child cancer survivors (see Table 6.1 for a discussion of individual tests). The approach to assessment considered here is in the spirit of the flexible battery. With the fixed battery

Table 6.1. Areas to evaluate in a comprehensive neuropsychological assessment and sample measures for school-age child cancer survivors: neurocognitive measures

Area of function	Sample tests[a]	Comments
Overall intellectual functioning	Wechsler tests (Wechsler, 2003, 2002, 1999, 1997), i.e.: – Wechsler Preschool and Primary Intelligence Scale (3rd edn.) (WPPSI-III) – Wechsler Intelligence Scale for Children (4th edn.) (WISC-IV) – Wechsler Adult Intelligence Scale (3rd edn.) (WAIS-III) – Wechsler Abbreviated Scale of Intelligence (WASI)	The Wechsler tests are the most widely used of the intelligence scales in North America and have strong psychometric properties.
	Differential Ability Scales (DAS) (Elliott, 1990)	The DAS is an alternative to the Wechsler tests and provides a General Cognitive Ability (CGA) score. It has a good normative base and strong psychometric properties. However, the DAS lacks a comparable battery across the age ranges because subtests change as do the factors that subtests load on
	Stanford-Binet Intelligence Scale (5th edn.) (SB5) (Roid, 2003)	The Stanford-Binet Scales provide large ceilings and floors and may provide better coverage when evaluating individuals at the extreme ends of the distribution
Learning and memory	California Verbal Learning Test for Children (CVLT-C) (Delis *et al.*, 1994)	The CVLT-C provides numerous useful indices including learning slope which can be compared against normative data
	Children's Memory Scale (CMS) (Cohen, 1997) Faces Picture memory Stories	Story recall tests such as those on the Wide Range Assessment of Memory and Learning (WRAML) and the CMS provide useful complementary information about the ability to learn and remember meaningful information. Used together, a comprehensive picture of verbal memory abilities can be obtained
	Wide Range Assessment of Memory and Learning (2nd edn.) (WRAML-II) (Sheslow & Adams, 2004) Story Memory Verbal Learning Picture Memory	Both the WRAML and the CMS provide tests of visual memory that do not require a motor response. This can be very useful when evaluating children who may not be able to demonstrate what they remember because of problems with visual motor output

Table 6.1. (*cont.*)

Area of function	Sample tests	Comments
Design memory	Rey–Osterrieth Complex Figure Test (RCFT) (Corwin & Bylsma, 1993)	The RCFT has a number of administration and scoring systems. It provides considerable information and is used as an indicator of visual spatial abilities, executive functions (particularly planning and organizational abilities), and visual motor integration in additional to incidental visual memory
Attention and working memory	Freedom from Distractibility Index (FDI) of the WISC-IV	FDI provides information about a child's short-term attention and working memory abilities. Other widely available batteries contain subtests sensitive to working memory dysfunction [e.g., WRAML-II, CMS, Woodcock–Johnson Tests of Cognitive Ability – (3rd edn., TEA-Ch)]
	Test of Everyday Attention for Children (TEA-Ch) (Manly *et al.*, 1999)	The TEA-Ch is a unique test battery designed to comprehensively evaluate attention. It is very long when given in its entirety, but it does not provide a global score so giving the subtests individually does not violate the psychometrics of the test. It provides measures of sustained attention in the auditory modality. Children enjoy the interesting activities and materials and it is available in alternative forms
	Continuous Performance Tasks (CPTs) (various)	CPTs evaluate sustained attention or vigilance. They provide numerous indices such as omission and commission errors and response speed. They are not specific enough to be diagnostic of attention deficit hyperactivity disorder alone but provide useful information about inattentiveness and impulsivity. They are tedious and children tend to dislike them and compliance can be an issue
	Rating scales – e.g., Child Behavior Checklist (CBCL) (Achenbach, 2001); Behavior Assessment Scale for Children (BASC) (Reynolds & Kamphaus, 2004); Conners' Rating Scales – Revised (Conners, 2001)	Parent, teacher and self-rating scales are helpful to obtain information about attention performance in real-world settings. Rating scales such as the CBCL and BASC provide coverage of a wide range of problem areas but do not examine attention functioning. A measure such as the Conner's is more specific to attention and behavioral regulation difficulties
Processing speed	WISC-IV Processing Speed Index (PSI)	The Perceptual Organization factor of the WISC-IV is influenced by processing speed but PSI provides a more direct measure. Care must be taken to rule out confounds of slow processing speed such as fine motor or visual tracking difficulties
	Academic fluency measures from the Woodcock–Johnson (3rd edn.) Tests of Achievement (WJ3) (McGrew *et al.*, 2001)	Academic fluency measures provide estimates of processing speed in a relevant context that is applicable to school functioning

(*cont.*)

Table 6.1. (*cont.*)

Area of function	Sample tests	Comments
Executive function	Wisconsin Card Sorting Test (WCST) (Heaton, 1981) Category Test (CT) (Knights & Tymchuk, 1968)	The WCST and CT are less sensitive to anterior lesions than originally believed but they remain useful measures of planning, shifting, flexible thinking, and concept formation. Both demonstrate significant practice effects because of the novel learning component and their use in serial assessments should be carefully considered
	Delis-Kaplan Tests of Executive Function (D-KEFS) (Delis *et al.*, 2001)	The D-KEFS provides a compilation of executive function measures that are normed on the same national sample
	Tower of London (Shallice, 1982) Tower of Hanoi (Simon, 1975)	Tower tasks have grown in popularity and may be less sensitive to practice effects than the WCST or CT. For a thorough review of the strengths and weaknesses and psychometric properties of Tower tasks see Baron (2004)
	Behavior Rating Inventory of Executive Function (BRIEF) (Gioia *et al.*, 2000)	The BRIEF was developed in an effort to address issues of ecological validity and the insensitivity of laboratory-based measures of EF. The BRIEF is a parent and teacher report instrument with a large normative database. There is now a pre-school version. A strength of this measure is that it is a measure of EF developed specifically for children and is not a downward extension of an adult measure
Language	Comprehensive Test of Phonological Processing (CTOPP) (Wagner *et al.*, 1999)	The CTOPP may be used as a follow-up measure for in-depth assessment when a child shows difficulties with the development of language-based skills, particularly reading
	Receptive One-Word Picture Vocabulary Test (ROWPVT) (Brownell, 2000) Expressive One-Word Picture Vocabulary Test (EOWPVT) (Gardner, 2000)	The other measures listed will provide estimates of expressive and receptive vocabulary development as well as language comprehension skills. Taken together with the verbal subtests of the overall intellectual measures, a screening of language function can be accomplished
	Peabody Picture Vocabulary Test (PPVT) (Dunn & Dunn, 1997) Token Test (De Renzi & Faglioni, 1978)	
Visual perceptual, motor, spatial, and constructional abilities	Beery Developmental Test of Visual Motor Integration (VMI) (Beery & Beery, 2004)	Screening for adequate visual perceptual and visuomotor abilities using tasks such as the VMI can help in the interpretation of more complex tasks such as the RCFT
	Block Design, Matrices subtests of the Wechsler tests Judge of line orientation (Benton *et al.*, 1983)	

Table 6.1. (*cont.*)

Area of function	Sample tests	Comments
	Rey–Osterreith Complex Figure Test (RCFT)	
Motor and sensory perceptual	Grooved Pegboard (Klove, 1963) Purdue Pegboard (Tiffin & Asher, 1948) Astereognosis (Benton *et al.*, 1994) Finger Tapping (Halstead, 1947)	Tests listed represent commonly used measures of fine motor skills, motor speed, and sensory perceptual ability
Academic achievement	Wechsler Individual Achievement Test (2nd edn.) (WIAT-II) (Wechsler, 2001) Woodcock–Johnson (3rd edn.) Tests of Achievement (WJ3) Wide Range Achievement Test (3rd edn.) (WRAT-3) (Wilkinson, 1993)	The WIAT-II or WJ3 are preferred measures when in-depth information about a child's academic functioning is required. The various subtests can help to pinpoint which specific academic areas are problematic for a particular child. The WRAT-3 is a screener only and should be used as such
Psychosocial functioning	BASC-II; CBCL Adaptive Behavior Assessment System (2nd edn.) (ABAS-II) (Harrison & Oakland, 2003)	Rating scales that provide coverage of a range of both problem and adaptive behaviors are good starting points to screen for psychological and social issues that may impact a child's functioning. These may be followed up with a more in-depth assessment of a child's psychological functioning if necessary The ABAS-II is a measure of adaptive functioning. It is useful for determining how a child may be functioning in their home, school and community settings

[a]Complete references for all tests are found in the test list at the end of the chapter.

approach, a pre-determined battery of tests is given to every child. The battery is generally designed to evaluate all necessary areas. With the flexible battery approach, a core battery of tests is given in order to generate hypotheses about a child's areas of strengths and weakness. These hypotheses are followed-up by the selection of additional tests based on the child's performance on the core battery. This approach is also influenced by the process approach (Kaplan, 1988), which underscores the importance of attending to the individual's process or test-taking style to guide the neuropsychological exploration. The end result is that the assessment is tailored to the individual child and more tests are given in an area where a child is having difficulty to further tease out the nature of that difficulty.

It may be helpful to think of a neuropsychological assessment as a challenge to the functioning of the CNS. The child's performance will be influenced by the degree of impairment of the CNS and by the complexity of the task. It is an evaluation of a child's ability to take in or receive information through their senses, to integrate and process this information, and to interact with their environment through the production of a response. Cognitive processes impacting a child's ability to adequately take in information in addition to basic sensation and perceptual ability include attention, processing speed, and working memory. Memory abilities also impact the ability to process information. Higher level processing of information includes visual spatial reasoning, language processing and problem solving, and the integration of information across modalities in association areas of the brain. Skills impacting a child's ability to produce meaningful output in order to interact with his or her environment

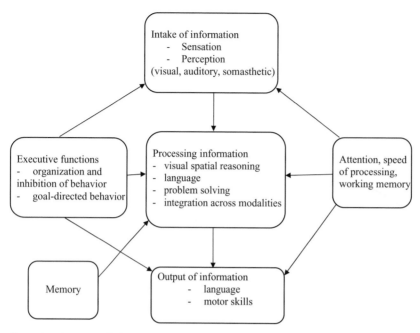

Figure 6.1. Neuropsychological Assessment Heuristic

include fine and gross motor skills and language. A child's ability to produce meaningful output is moderated by executive functions, which help to organize responses and inhibit behavior when necessary. The dynamic interplay of input-processing/integration-output is a useful heuristic to consider when trying to ensure that there is adequate coverage of domains of cognitive function in a comprehensive neuropsychological assessment of the child cancer patient or survivor (see Figure 6.1). In addition, psychological functioning is a key part of the neuropsychological assessment and will be discussed further at a later point in this chapter.

Following our overview of the key areas to evaluate, we will present two approaches to neuropsychological assessment of the child cancer patient that represent attempts to provide rich, meaningful information in a short period of time through the use of a streamlined core battery of tests. These assessments might best be thought of as screening assessments. In particular situations, neuropsychologists may need to follow-up with more inten-sive assessment of specific areas of weakness in order to make useful recommendations for home and school.

Areas to evaluate

Overall intellectual functioning

Both research and clinical reports typically use overall intellectual level as a global index of a child's functioning. The subtest scores for each individual are compared to each other (ipsative comparison), as well as to population norms, thus discerning areas of relative strength and weakness within an individual child's neuropsychological pro-file. The IQ score will place the child in perspective relative to others of similar age within the general population (Baron, 2004) and it is a good predictor of school performance (see Sternberg *et al.*, 2001, for an overview of the predictive value of the IQ score). It is extremely important to measure this domain of functioning in more severely compromised children. Intellectual functioning is one of the diagnostic criteria, together with adaptive functioning deficits, for a diagnosis of mental retardation. Some children treated for malignant brain tumors with CRT at a young age meet criteria for this diagnosis. In addition, some of the more commonly used intellectual tests provide a large normative base and opportunities for detailed statistical analysis of strengths and weaknesses. Another benefit of using a well-known and well-normed instrument such as the Wechsler scales is that it is possible to track rate of learning over time by examining normative and raw scores in an individual child over different assessments. This is not always possible with other instruments where ceiling effects, learning effects, small normative samples or changes in items across age ranges can limit the ability to track learning rates over time.

The IQ tests are global instruments and should be interpreted as such. Oftentimes, detailed conclusions about brain function are generated based on poor performance on one subtest of a broader intellectual measure by inexperienced clinicians. According to Baron (2004) specific neuropsychological instruments are much better suited to making detailed inferences about brain function. Oftentimes the instrument used will be dictated by the school board or institution in which an individual psychologist works.

In a different viewpoint, Lezak *et al.* (2004) advocate strongly against the use of overall IQ indices. An in-depth discussion of the argument is beyond the scope of this chapter. Briefly, they caution that with any derived score, important information is lost and the overall score is not always representative or meaningful. They also describe unfortunate uses of an IQ "cut off" score that limits access to services for individuals. It is important to consider these issues and the well-trained clinician should examine test scores from every vantage point before making inferences about brain function. We believe that an overall IQ score can be useful to neuropsychological assessment. However, a complete understanding of the limitations of this overall score is crucial.

Learning and memory

The assessment of learning and memory is necessary to the comprehensive neuropsychological assessment and nowhere is it more important than in the assessment of children and adolescents. Failures to learn and remember new information and to retrieve information at a later time will ultimately lead to impaired functioning because of the importance of acquiring new knowledge to future learning and development. The assessment of learning and memory can be conceptualized by modality (visual and auditory-verbal), as well as within an information-processing model of memory functioning (i.e., encoding, consolidation, storage, retrieval, and recognition). A thorough discussion of the many models of memory functioning is beyond the scope of this chapter. The interested reader is referred to Lezak *et al.* (2004) for a review of memory models.

Memory batteries are often lengthy and time consuming and contain a number of subtests that may or may not add useful clinical information. For this reason, Baron (2004) recommends a needs-based selection of individual subtests. This may compromise the statistical properties of the test to some degree, but the experienced clinician can remain cognizant of these limitations and integrate the information in a meaningful way.

A child's capacity and motivation to adequately attend to information should be sufficiently screened because of the importance of intact attention to support memory functioning. The ability to retain information over the short term needs to be evaluated by tests of immediate memory. The duration for "long-term" memory assessment in a day-long neuropsychological assessment is obviously limited and most memory tests include a delay that is about 20 min in duration. More information about a child's ability to learn, retain, and retrieve information over the long term can be gleaned from background information about the child's functioning in their home and school environment. This contextual information should be considered together with the results of memory testing to develop an overall conceptualization of a child's memory abilities.

Learning should be assessed by both repeated and one-time exposure to determine a child's capacity for single trial learning as well as their rate of learning (e.g., learning curve) over time. Memory for rote information (e.g., a list of words), as well as memory for information with more salience (e.g., stories) should be assessed. When assessing for new learning, both free recall and recognition formats should be used. This allows for delineation of whether difficulties in remembering are related to problems with encoding or retrieval.

Non-verbal memory has been implicated as an area of deficit in child cancer survivors. Therefore, it is an area that should not be omitted. Non-verbal memory is usually evaluated through a reproduction format (e.g., drawing) or through a recognition format (e.g., pointing). Obviously, these two formats are not equivalent and may provide additive information. This is particularly true in the case where a child has visuomotor difficulty and is challenged by drawing. It will be difficult for the clinician to ascribe failure on a test of non-verbal memory to memory dysfunction if the child is poor at drawing. In this case, a task without visuomotor demands may be helpful.

Apparent problems in memory can be produced by a variety of other difficulties such as problems with attention, motivation, working memory, executive functions, and impaired language comprehension. As well, emotional dysfunction can disrupt learning and memory. It is important to carefully evaluate for the presence of difficulties in these areas before determining that a child has memory dysfunction.

Core cognitive processes: attention, processing speed, working memory

Assessment of what are now commonly referred to as "core" cognitive processes is critical to any neuropsychological assessment. Intact neuropsychological functioning is dependent on adequate performance of these important processes as they support the "taking in" of information. If a child cannot attend to information, or processes information extremely slowly, he or she will have limited opportunity to optimally utilize cognitive resources. The neuropsychological late-effects research base has pointed to deficits in these areas as driving many of the observed declines in other areas of functioning and subsequent academic failure.

Attention

Attention is not a unitary construct, despite common reference to a general skill called "attention." There are several models of attention that influence clinicians' approaches to its evaluation and a thorough discussion is beyond the scope of this chapter (e.g., Mirsky *et al.*, 1991; Posner & Petersen, 1990; Sohlberg & Mateer, 1987). Drawing from these models, the subset of skills that fall under the overall rubric of attention is broad and includes: sustained, focused, selective, divided, alternating, shifting, and resistance to distraction. Sohlberg and Mateer's (1987) model is helpful in a clinical setting because it conceptualizes attention in a hierarchical manner going from the most basic form of attention, arousal and responding to the environment, to higher levels of attentional complexity that demand more cognitive capacity (such as alternating attention). It is helpful for the comprehensive neuropsychological assessment to attempt to evaluate attentional functioning in as many of these domains as possible. At a minimum, clinicians should evaluate span of attention, sustained attention, and more complex attention such as the divided or alternating types. Visual scanning is also important to assess because of its relevance to schoolwork (particularly reading and test taking). Attention is demanded by many different tasks and conclusions about attention functioning can be drawn from subtests of various test batteries.

It is important to remain aware that attention is closely related to motivation (Baron, 2004) and can fluctuate widely over the course of a day. Test order and breaks should be considered in order to manage fatigue and motivation, which can impact performance on tests of attention. For this reason, it is also important to obtain estimates of attention functioning in daily life through the use of parent and teacher report measures. These estimates can be obtained through relatively broad parent and teacher report instruments such as the Behavior Assessment Scale for Children – 2nd Edition (BASC-II; Reynolds & Kamphaus, 2004) or through the use of specific attention rating scales such as the Conners' Rating Scales – Revised (Conners, 2001).

Working memory

Working memory is considered by many to fall under the broad rubric of executive functions. In fact, Baddeley and Hitch's model (1974) conceptualizes working memory as being comprised of a Central Executive which manages two slave systems: the visual spatial scratchpad and the phonological or articulatory loop. In addition, working memory tasks have been shown to activate the prefrontal cortex (Goldman-Rakic, 1992). Working memory is also considered a form of attention. In fact, Baddeley himself has written a chapter entitled "Working memory or working attention?" (Baddeley 1993) which captures the difficulty in differentiating between the two concepts. Some may think of it as a form of memory given its label. However it is conceptualized or labeled, working memory is considered a core cognitive process and is closely related to attentional ability because of its role in supporting both the input and processing of information. As discussed above, this is a potential area of deficit for the child cancer survivor.

Working memory is the attentional store that we use to hold information in mind for short periods of time while we do something with it. For example, while making a phone call the number is held in working memory until dialing is finished. Simple span tasks such as Digit Span, which is a subtest of the Wechsler tests of intelligence from ages 6 and up, are one way of assessing working memory; however, more complex tasks with greater demands on working memory are more sensitive.

Processing speed

Given the importance of myelin in the speeded conduction of neural impulses, it is not surprising that processing speed deficits have been noted in child cancer survivors with CNS impact. The importance of adequate processing speed to success at school is evident. If a child cannot keep up with the pace of presentation of information or is unable to demonstrate knowledge because testing time frames are too short, he or she will struggle academically.

Executive function

The construct of executive function (EF) is very broad. It has been described as an umbrella term encompassing a number of subdomains (Baron, 2004). Several useful models of EFs have been developed (Fuster, 1980; Shallice, 1988; Stuss & Alexander, 2000; Stuss & Anderson, 2004). Executive functions have been conceptualized as encompassing the skills required for purposeful, goal-directed behavior (Anderson, 2001). For this reason, EF skills can be considered to play a very important role in the quality of an individual's output and therefore their interaction with the environment. The assessment of EF in the pediatric oncology population will be discussed here in general terms, recognizing that considerable discussion could be devoted to the assessment of individual areas of EF alone, such as planning or response inhibition. For a more thorough discussion of the assessment of EF in children the interested reader is referred to Anderson *et al.* (2001) and Baron (2004).

There has been some debate about whether it is appropriate to assess executive functioning in children. Given that the prefrontal cortex is the putative seat of EF, that this cortical area is the last to reach maturation (Fuster, 1993), and the finding that children do not perform as well as adults on tests of executive functioning (Chelune & Baer, 1986), it may seem inappropriate to assess for this domain in young children. Recently, research has provided evidence for EF skill development in children (Levin *et al.*, 1991; Passler *et al.*, 1985; Welsh *et al.*, 1991) and for deficits in these areas following brain injury relative to normally developing children (Anderson & Moore, 1995). However, behavioral descriptors of executive dysfunction in adults such as poor self-control, impulsivity, and poor planning may not be warranted for children, given the developmental appropriateness of children being unable to plan and organize a busy day or demonstrate adequate self-control in some situations. An example of the complexity of assessing EFs in children and adolescents is provided by Todd *et al.*, (1996). They found evidence of planning difficulties in both brain-injured and normally developing adolescents. This underscores the importance of basing our assessment of EF in children within a developmental context and using instruments that provide an adequate normative database reflecting the normal development of EF in childhood and adolescence.

An additional challenge in the assessment of EFs in any age group is the lack of sensitivity of many laboratory-based tasks to deficits in these areas. Deficits in these skills are often difficult to detect in structured clinical settings with structured assessment instruments. Therefore, clinicians often rely on anecdotal evidence from the patient or from family members. Because EF is such a broad term, many tests are needed to assess for deficits in each of its subdomains. In her review, Anderson (2001) noted that most test batteries designed for children do not include measures of EF. Despite these challenges it is important to include the assessment of EF when evaluating the child cancer survivor. Deficits in this area will manifest in daily life as problems with organization, time management, behavioral control, and will negatively impact not only learning but also social development.

Language

According to Baron (2004), the speech and language portion of a neuropsychological assessment should include screening of: conversational fluency, phonological processing, generative fluency, comprehension, repetition, naming, reading, writing, spelling, and praxis. To this list we would add both receptive and expressive vocabulary development. Basic language skills develop relatively early in life. Therefore, they are usually intact in children treated for malignant brain tumors and ALL unless they have intense neurotoxic treatment delivered in infancy, prior to language development. However, more subtle difficulties with language may be evident. It is important to be aware that children treated with cisplatin for a brain tumor may suffer hearing loss. This may have an obvious impact on language development.

When children evidence language difficulties it is helpful to utilize the specialized expertise of our speech and language colleagues. However, neuropsychological assessment should include measures of language functioning to put the entire assessment in context and to document areas requiring further follow-up by a speech and language pathologist.

Non-verbal skills: visual perceptual, visual motor, visual spatial, and visual constructional abilities

The non-verbal domain of cognitive functioning is probably one of the most complex areas to evaluate. A wide array of skills comprise this domain. It may be helpful to think of visually mediated skills for the input (i.e., visual perceptual functioning) and for the output (i.e., visual motor) of information, as well as skills for higher level processing of visual information (e.g., mental rotation and spatial reasoning), and complex integrative skills such as the recognition of facial expression and object recognition. One of the reasons why this is such a difficult area to assess adequately is that it is extremely difficult to create tests that measure discrete areas of functioning within this domain. Difficulties in other areas such as visual acuity, speed, or constructional problems may inadvertently lead a clinician to conclude that a child has difficulties with non-verbal reasoning. It is very important to rule out deficits in other domains that contribute to task performance.

Deficits in non-verbal skills can contribute to academic struggles. For example, a child with spatial difficulties may struggle with arithmetic because he or she cannot line up numbers for mathematical operations. Spatial difficulties can also contribute to difficulties with writing. As the research reviewed earlier indicates, this functional domain is impacted by CRT and IT chemotherapy.

Tests of visual recognition, discrimination and matching can aid in the evaluation of visual perceptual abilities. More complex perceptual tasks of mental rotation and the understanding of spatial relationships can tap into more integrative, higher-level non-verbal reasoning. Difficulties with earlier levels of perception must be ruled out before it can be discerned that a child has a higher-level deficit in visual reasoning.

Motor and sensory perceptual function

Assessment of basic motor and sensory function is important to rule out deficits in these input/output pathways, which may confound assessment findings. Childhood cancer survivors often have difficulties with movement and basic sensation related to their treatment. Vincristine is known to cause peripheral neuropathy. Children who undergo surgery for brain tumors may have cranial nerve deficits that interfere with their sensory and motor functioning. Children with tumors of the posterior fossa may have problems with movement related to cerebellar involvement and this should be carefully observed and considered in the interpretation of test findings.

Academic achievement

Performance on standardized measures of academic achievement is often included as part of a neuropsychological assessment although this does not fall uniquely within the realm of the neuropsychologist. The referral question may dictate whether academic achievement is included in the assessment. It may not be necessary when evaluating a child for a baseline prior to beginning CRT because pertinent and up-to-date school information may be available. However, it can be very useful when determining where a child is functioning academically when planning for return to school after a long absence. Tests that provide a more in-depth analysis of a child's academic strengths and weaknesses are preferred over a screener when the goal is to make relevant recommendations for school planning.

Psychosocial and adaptive functioning

The terms neurocognitive and neuropsychological have been used interchangeably in the literature in recent years. However, we would like to propose an important distinction. The term "neurocognitive" implies the assessment of cognition or thinking skills and of the integrity of underlying neurological substrates. The term "neuropsychological" implies assessment of an individual's brain functioning, and therefore their various thinking skills or cognition, within the context of their psychological functioning. To return to our earlier definition, neuropsychology is a science of human behavior as it is influenced by brain functioning and by social, psychological, and cultural context. The brain should not be assessed in isolation but must be considered within the various contexts of the individual person. The impact of anxiety and depression on neuropsychological test performance is well documented (see Lezak et al., 2004, for an overview) and therefore should be considered in a neuropsychological evaluation.

For this reason we do not feel that a neuropsychological assessment is complete without taking into account emotional or intrapsychic and social factors that may impact test performance. The clinical interview is a rich source of information about a child's emotional functioning. Furthermore, this information can be quantified and compared to normative data through the use of parent- and teacher-reported behavior-rating scales. Older children can report on their own experience. Specific instruments may be warranted for exploration of specific concerns about depression or anxiety. This is not to say that a neuropsychological assessment can take the place of a comprehensive and thorough evaluation by a clinical psychologist specializing in children's emotional disorders. However, the "psychology" in neuropsychology should not be forgotten and a child's emotional state should be screened as part of the neuropsychological evaluation. Emotional status may impact test interpretation and the creation of relevant and useful recommendations.

The Children's Oncology Group (COG) neuropsychology test battery

The development of the COG test battery represents a major accomplishment and should streamline the collection of data for multisite COG clinical trials. It was put together by members of the neuropsychology subcommittee of COG in an effort to standardize neuropsychological data collection being conducted within the various COG treatment studies. It was difficult to draw robust conclusions from the data generated because different measures were used across sites and within the same patient over time. A further challenge was the time needed to complete these often lengthy batteries. In times of cost containment and managed care, neuropsychological assessments cannot always be completed, particularly for research purposes.

The goals of the core battery are to assess the key domains of neurocognitive functioning that are sensitive to the presence of a brain tumor and/or the treatment effects of cancer, and to do so in a time-efficient manner (Moore, 2005; P. Brouwers, personal communication, 2005). The test battery was designed to represent the minimum standard of care and other tests can be added for a particular study protocol if necessary. The choice of instruments was driven by a need to select tests that cover the full age range (from infancy to adulthood), are psychometrically sound, and are commonly available and widely used by psychologists in practice (see Tables 6.2 and 6.3 for a list of the core neuropsychological test battery). The battery illustrated covers the age range of 6–16 years only. Modified batteries were also developed to cover the 1–5 years age

Table 6.2. COG Neuropsychology Test Battery for the 6- to 16-year-old age group. Neurocognitive measures. *WASI* Wechlser Abbreviated Scale of Intelligence, *WRAT-3* Wide Range Assessment Test (3rd edn.), *CVLT-C* California Verbal Learning Test for Children, *CPT-II* Continuous Performance Test (2nd edn.), *D-KEFS* Delis–Kaplan Executive Function System, *BRIEF* Behavior Rating Inventory of Executive Function, *EOWPVT* Expressive One-Word Picture Vocabulary Test, *ROWPVT* Receptive One-Word Picture Vocabulary Test

Area of function	Measure[a]
Overall intellectual functioning	WASI
Academic achievement	WRAT-3
Memory	CVLT-C
	Children's Memory Scale – selected subtests
Attention	CPT-II
Executive function	NEPSY – verbal fluency
	Contingency Naming Test
	D-KEFS – Tower of London
Language	BRIEF – parent report
	EOWPVT
	ROWPVT

[a]Complete references for all tests are found in the test list at the end of the chapter.

range and the 16 years to adult age range, but these are not shown.

Although the COG battery represents a major effort toward standardized assessment for research purposes, some challenges remain. Processing speed and visuomotor functioning are not well represented in this battery and problems with both are frequently observed in survivors of ALL and brain tumors. A further challenge has been the need to satisfy research and clinical demands with the same test battery. The COG battery was clearly created as a research instrument. However, because of the comprehensiveness of the assessment, many of the measures may also need to be administered for clinical purposes. In some settings

Table 6.3. Measures of psychosocial, adaptive functioning and quality of life. *PedsQL* Varni Pediatric Quality of Life Inventory, *BASC-II* Behavior Assessment System for Children (2nd edn.), *ABAS-II* Adaptive Behavior Assessment Scale (2nd edn.)

Areas assessed	Measure[a]
Quality of life	PedsQL 4.0 Generic Version – parent report (Varni *et al.*, 1999)
Psychosocial functioning including parent report of attention function	BASC-II
Adaptive functioning	ABAS-II

[a]Complete references for all tests found in the test list at the end of the chapter.

the child's health insurance pays for the assessment or the child is already scheduled to be seen for a clinical assessment. In these situations it is often advantageous for the assessment data to be used for both research and clinical purposes, which can create some conflicts. This is an ongoing challenge that the COG neuropsychology subcommittee will address.

Oregon Health Sciences University test battery

This test battery was assembled by the second author to provide a brief, yet comprehensive, core screening battery of tests providing information that is very relevant to the school setting. Like the COG test battery, it has been designed to cover the full age range from 1 year of age through to adulthood. The battery used with the age range 6–16 years is displayed in Tables 6.4 and 6.5. The test battery is streamlined in that it can be completed in only 2–3 h, and it is comprehensive, covering the major areas of cognitive function discussed above, cor-responding with areas of cortical and subcortical brain function. Because the tests comprising the battery were selected on the basis of their good psychometric properties and sensitivity, they represent a wide variety of normative data. This is a drawback of this battery and psychometric knowledge and clinical expertise are essential to inferring appropriate interpretations.

Future directions in pediatric oncology and neuropsychology

The most important future direction in pediatric oncology in addition to increasing cure rates is to provide a cure at a smaller price, without such detriment to neurodevelopment. Medical researchers are investigating ways to provide a high chance of cure with lower radiation dosage (Packer *et al.*, 1999), and investigations of neuroprotective agents are also underway (Drachtman *et al.*, 2002).

In concert with medical attempts to reduce the neurotoxicity of treatment, neuropsychologists are turning their focus from assessment to treatment. Treatment may include educational strategies and compensations that can be implemented once children return to school, or specific targeted intervention strategies that may be delivered prophylactically while a child is on treatment.

The Cognitive Remediation Program (CRP) (Butler, 1998; Butler & Copeland, 2002) is an approach to the treatment of acquired brain injury in child cancer survivors, and has received the most systematic study. This is a tripartite model and draws from the fields of special education/educational psychology, clinical psychology, and brain injury rehabilitation. Children meet individually with a therapist for 2-h sessions for 20 weeks. Massed practice activities are administered using the Attention Process Training (APT) techniques developed by Sohlberg and Mateer (1987). These activities focus on exercising attentional processes and are alternated with more

Table 6.4. Oregon Health Sciences University Test Battery for the 6- to 16-year-old age group: neurocognitive measures. *WASI* Wechlser Abbreviated Scale of Intelligence, *WISC-III* Wechsler Intelligence Scale for Children (3rd edn.), *WRAT-3* Wide Range Assessment Test (3rd edn.), *WRAML* Wide Range Assessment of Memory and Learning, *CMS* Children's Memory Scale, *CPT-II* Continuous Performance Test (2nd edn.), *WCST* Wisconsin Card Sorting Test, *BRIEF* = Behavior Rating Inventory of Executive Function

Area of function	Measure[a]
Overall intellectual functioning	WASI
Academic achievement	WRAT-3
Memory	Figural Memory (Wechsler, 1945)
	Memory Cards (Keller *et al.*, 1999)
	Sentence Memory from the WRAML
	Story Memory from the CMS
Attention and working memory	Digit Span from the WISC-III
	CPT-II (Conners and Staff of Multi-Health Systems, 2000)
Processing speed	Coding from the WISC-III (Wechsler, 1991)
Executive function	Color-Word Test (Golden, 1978)
	WCST
	Tower of London (Keller *et al.*, 1999)
	BRIEF – parent report
Non-dominant hemisphere function (visual spatial processing)	Line Orientation (Benton *et al.*, 1983)
	Facial Recognition (Benton *et al.*, 1983)
	Visual Orientation Test (Hooper, 1983)
Language	Boston Naming Test (Kaplan *et al.*, 1983)
	Token Test Short Form (De Renzi & Faglioni, 1978)

[a]Complete references for all tests are found in the test list at the end of the chapter.

intrinsically interesting computer games that also exercise attention and problem-solving abilities. The participants are also provided instruction in metacognitive strategies designed to help them with preparing to complete a task, improve their on-task performance, and post-task strategies. This is all conducted within the context of psychotherapeutic support, drawing from clinical psychology. A cognitive-behavioral approach is used to assist the participant in re-framing challenges, acknowledging strengths, monitoring internal dialogue, stress inoculation, and the development of positive self-statements.

Results published thus far are promising using CRP methods to improve attentional functioning in childhood cancer survivors. Mulhern and Butler (2004) described a recently completed Phase III clin-ical trial of the CRP program involving seven institutions across the United States of America. Although there are no published findings available yet, it is extremely exciting to see such a large-scale study of a behavioral intervention. For a review of the published literature in this area, the interested reader is referred to Penkman (2004).

There is nothing in the literature to date looking at the efficacy or feasibility of prophylactic interventions (i.e., remediation programs or academic interventions delivered while a child is still on medical treatment and prior to the documentation of neuropsychological dysfunction). However, Penkman and Scott-Lane (2007) report a case study where an academic intervention was delivered prophylactically to a child treated for medulloblastoma. Some improvement and maintenance of reading skills in

Table 6.5. Measures of psychosocial functioning. *BASC* Behavior Assessment System for Children, *PSI-3* Parenting Stress Index (3rd edn.), *SIPA* Stress Index for Parents of Adolescents

Areas assessed	Measure[a]
Psychosocial functioning	BASC – parent report
	PSI-3/SIPA (Abidin, 1995)

[a]Complete references for all tests are found in the test list at the end of the chapter.

the context of decline in most other areas was documented. Mulhern and Butler (2004) underscore the potential usefulness of early, prophylactic interventions for children known to be at increased risk.

With survival as a reasonably expected outcome now in childhood cancer and knowledge amassed regarding the potential cost of treatment, it is imperative that clinicians make more concerted efforts to communicate with parents about realistic expectations. Not telling parents that their child may experience learning disabilities following CRT is no longer defensible given the large research base that is now available to guide the provision of information. Parents should be given information about research findings and how these findings may relate to their child. There is still much unknown about why certain children experience considerable deficits and others exposed to the same treatment do not. Further delineation of both the treatment and patient characteristics related to higher risk is necessary.

Although neuropsychology has moved in the direction of providing behavioral treatments for acquired brain injury, neuropsychological assessment remains the primary task and there is much work to be done to improve upon current assessment techniques. The approaches to assessment discussed in this chapter represent movements toward streamlining the neuropsychological assessment process without losing crucial information about a child's strengths and weaknesses. Given the economic conditions of most hospital and clinic environments this has been an important focus.

However, it is time to begin thinking creatively about our approach to neuropsychological assessment and to move beyond the drive for efficiency.

Ecological validity is a key issue for neuropsychology. What use are our tests if they are not meaningful in the real world? Parent, teacher, and self-report measures have been developed in recent years to attempt to garner some glimpse into a child's day-to-day real-world functioning. These represent an important first step, however it is our belief that as a profession we need to take a further step forward and create assessment techniques that are more behaviorally oriented in addition to our laboratory based tests. The creation of virtual reality technology represents an effort to link testing more closely to a classroom environment. The ecological validity of our assessment techniques will be further supported through the completion of validity studies that examine the meaning of our test findings in the classroom environment.

In summary, an exciting future awaits neuropsychologists working with child cancer survivors. It is an area filled with hope for greater chance of cure at a smaller price. There remains a vast territory of unexplored possibilities in both the treatment and assessment domains.

REFERENCES

Ames E (1997). *The Development of Romanian Orphanage Children Adopted to Canada* [Final Report to the National Welfare Grants Program: Human Resources Development Canada]. Burnaby, British Columbia: Simon Fraser University.

Anderson DM, Rennier KM, Ziegler RS *et al.* (2001). Medical and neurocognitive late effects among survivors of childhood central nervous system tumors. *Cancer* **92**: 2709–2719.

Anderson V (2001). Assessing executive functions in children: biological, psychological, and developmental considerations. *Pediatr Rehabil* **4**: 119–136.

Anderson V, Moore C (1995). Age at injury as a predictor of outcome following pediatric head injury. *Child Neuropsychol* **1**: 187–202.

Baddeley A (1993). Working memory or working attention? In: Baddeley A, Weiskrantz L (eds.) *Attention: Selection, Awareness, and Control* (pp. 152–170). New York: Oxford University Press.

Baddeley AD, Hitch G (1974). Working memory. In Bower GA (ed.) *The Psychology of Learning and Motivation*. New York: Academic Press.

Baron IS (2004). *Neuropsychological Evaluation of the Child*. Oxford: Oxford University Press.

Beglinger LJ, Gaydos B, Tangphao-Daniels O *et al.* (2005). Practice effects and the use of alternate forms in serial neuropsychological testing. *Arch Clin Neuropsychol* **20**: 517–529.

Berger K (2005). *The Developing Person Through the Lifespan* (6th edn.). New York: Worth Publishers.

Bleyer WA, Fallavollita J, Robison L *et al.* (1990). Influence of age, sex, and concurrent intrathecal methotrexate therapy on intellectual function after cranial irradiation during childhood: a report from Children's Cancer Study Group. *Pediatric Hematol Oncol* **7**: 329–338.

Broca P (1865). Sur le siege de la faculte du langage articule. *Bull Soc Anthropol* **6**: 377–396.

Brown RT, Maden-Swain A (1993). Cognitive, neuropsychological, and academic sequelae in children with leukemia. *J Learn Disabil* **26**: 74–90.

Brown RT, Maden-Swain A, Pais R *et al.* (1992). Chemotherapy for acute lymphocytic leukemia: cognitive and academic sequelae. *J Pediatr* **121**: 885–889.

Brown RT, Maden-Swain A, Walco GA *et al.* (1998). Cognitive and academic late effects among children previously treated for acute lymphocytic leukemia receiving chemotherapy as CNS prophylaxis. *J Pediatr Psychol* **23**: 333–340.

Butler RW (1998). Attentional processes and their remediation in childhood cancer. *Pediatr Oncol Suppl* **1**: 75–78.

Butler RW, Copeland DR (2002). Attentional processes and their remediation in children treated for cancer: a literature review and the development of a therapeutic approach. *J Int Neuropsychol Soc* **8**: 115–124.

Buzier AI, de Sonneville LMJ, Van Den Heuvel-Eibrink MM *et al.* (2005). Chemotherapy and attentional dysfunction in survivors of childhood acute lymphoblastic leukemia: effect of treatment intensity. *Pediatr Blood Cancer* **45**: 281–290.

Chelune GJ, Baer RA (1986). Developmental norms for the Wisconsin Card Sorting Test. *J Clin Exp Neuropsychol* **8**: 219–228.

Children's Oncology Group (2004). *Long-Term Follow-up Guidelines for Survivors of Childhood, Adolescent, and Young Adult Cancers*, version 1.2. Retrieved March 20, 2008, from http://www.survivorshipguidelines.org.

Conners CK (2001). *Conners' Rating Scales – Revised (CRS-R)*. Toronto, ON: Multi-Health Systems, Inc.

Cousens P, Waters F, Said J *et al.* (1988). Cognitive effects of cranial irradiation in leukemia: a survey and meta-analysis. *J Child Psychol Psychiatry* **29**: 839–852.

Dennis M, Hetherington R, Spiegler B (1998). Memory and attention after childhood brain tumors. *Med Pediatr Oncol Suppl* **1**: 25–33.

Drachtman RA, Cole PD, Golden CB *et al.* (2002). Dextromethorphan is effective in the treatment of subacute methotrexate toxicity. *Pediatr Hematol Oncol* **19**: 319–327.

Duffner PK (2004). Long-term effects of radiation therapy on cognitive and endocrine function in children with leukemia and brain tumors. *Neurologist* **10**: 293–310.

Finger S (1999). Margaret Kennard on sparing and recovery of function: a tribute on the 100th anniversary of her birth. *J Historical Neurosci* **8**: 269–285.

Finger S, Wolf C (1988). The "Kennard effect" before Kennard. The early history of age and brain lesions. *Arch Neurol* **45**: 1136–1142.

Fletcher JM, Copeland DR (1988). Neurobehavioral effects of central nervous system prophylactic treatment of cancer in children. *J Clin Exp Neuropsychol* **10**: 495–538.

Franzen MD, Paul D, Iverson GL (1996). Reliability of alternate forms of the Trail Making Test. *Clin Neuropsychol* **10**: 125–129.

Fuster JM (1980). *The Prefrontal Cortex*. New York: Raven Press.

Fuster JM (1993). Frontal lobes. *Curr Opin Neurobiol* **3**: 160–165.

Goldman-Rakic PS (1992). Working memory and the mind. *Sci Am* **267**: 111–117.

Gunnar ME (2001). Effects of early deprivation: findings from orphanage reared-infants and children. In Nelson CA, Luciana M (eds.) *Developmental Cognitive Neuroscience* (pp. 617–629). Cambridge, MA: MIT Press.

Halstead WC (1947). *Brain and Intelligence: A Quantitative Study of the Frontal Lobes*. Chicago, IL: University of Chicago Press.

Hopewell JW (1998). Radiation injury to the central nervous system. *Med Pediatr Oncol Suppl* **1**: 1–9.

Hoppe-Hirsch E, Brunet L, Laroussinie F *et al.* (1995). Intellectual outcome in children with malignant tumors of the posterior fossa: influence of the field of irradiation and quality of surgery. *Childs Nerv Syst* **11**: 340–346.

Hughlings-Jackson J (1931). In Taylor J (ed.) *Selected Writings of John Hughlings-Jackson*. London: Hodder.

Kaplan E (1988). A process approach to neuropsychological assessment. In Boll T, Bryant BK (eds.) *Clinical Neuropsychology and Brain Function: Research, Measurement, and Practice* (pp. 143–155). Washington DC: American Psychological Association.

Kolb B (1995). *Brain Plasticity and Behavior*. New Jersey: Lawrence Erlbaum Associates.

Kolb B, Wishaw IQ (2003). *Fundamentals of Human Neuropsychology* (5th edn.). New York: Worth Publishers.

Langer T, Martus P, Ottensmeier H *et al.* (2002). CNS late-effects after ALL therapy in childhood. Part III. Neuropsychological performance in long-term survivors of childhood ALL: impairments in concentration, attention, and memory. *Med Pediatr Oncol* **38**: 320–328.

Lashley KD (1950). In search of the engram. *Symp Soc Exp Biol* **4**: 454–482.

Lehtinen SS, Huuskonen UE, Harila-Saari AH *et al.* (2002). Motor nervous system impairment persists in long-term survivors of childhood acute lymphoblastic leukemia. *Cancer* **94**: 2466–2473.

Levin HS, Culhane KA, Hartmann J *et al.* (1991). Developmental changes in performance on tests of purported frontal lobe functioning. *Dev Neuropsychol* **7**: 377–395.

Lezak M, Howieson DB, Loring DW (2004). *Neuropsychological Assessment* (4th edn.). New York: Oxford University Press.

Luria AR (1973). *The Working Brain*. New York: Basic Books.

Mirsky AF, Anthony BJ, Duncan CC *et al.* (1991). Analysis of the elements of attention: a neuropsychological approach. *Neuropsychol Rev* **2**: 109–145.

Moleski M (2000). Neuropsychological, neuroanatomical and neurophysiological consequences of CNS chemotherapy for acute lymphoblastic leukemia. *Arch Clin Neuropsychol* **15**: 603–630.

Moore BD (2005). Neurocognitive outcomes in survivors of childhood cancer. *J Pediatr Psychol* **30**: 51–63.

Mulhern RK, Butler RW (2004). Neurocognitive sequelae of childhood cancers and their treatment. *Pediatr Rehabil* **7**: 1–14.

Mulhern RK, Butler RW (2005). Neuropsychological late effects. In Brown RT (ed.) *Pediatric Hematology/ Oncology: A Biopsychosocial Approach*. New York: Oxford University Press.

Mulhern RK, Kepner JL, Thomas PR *et al.* (1998). Neuropsychologic functioning of survivors of childhood medulloblastoma randomized to receive conventional or reduced-dose craniospinal irradiation: a pediatric oncology group study. *J Clin Oncol* **16**: 1723–1728.

Packer RJ, Goldwein J, Nicholson HS *et al.* (1999). Treatment of children with medulloblastoma with reduced-dose cranial spinal radiation and adjuvant chemotherapy: A Children's Cancer Group Study. *J Clin Oncol* **17**: 2127–2136.

Passler MA, Isaac W, Hynd GW (1985). Neuropsychological development of behavior attributed to frontal lobe functioning in children. *Dev Neuropsychol* **1**: 349–370.

Penkman LC (2004). Remediation of attention deficits in children: a focus on childhood cancer, traumatic brain injury and attention deficit disorder. *Pediatr Rehabil* **7**: 111–123.

Penkman LC, Scott-Lane L (2007). Prophylactic academic intervention for children treated with cranial radiation therapy. *Dev Neurorehabil* **10**: 19–26.

Picard EM, Rourke BP (1995). Neuropsychological consequences of prophylactic treatment for acute lymphocytic leukemia. In Rourke BP (ed.). *Syndrome of Nonverbal Learning Disabilities* (pp. 282–330). New York: Guilford Press.

Posner MI, Petersen SE (1990). The attention system of the brain. *Annu Rev Neurosci* **13**: 25–42.

Reddick WE, Glass JO, Palmer SL *et al.* (2005). Atypical white matter volume development in children following craniospinal irradiation. *Neurooncology* **7**: 12–19.

Reitan RM (1974). Methodological problems in clinical neuropsychology. In Reitan RM, Davison LA (eds.) *Clinical Neuropsychology: Current Status and Applications* (pp. 19–46). Washington, DC: Hemisphere Publishing Corporation.

Reynolds CR, Kamphaus RW (2004). *Behavior Assessment System for Children* (2nd edn.). Circle Pines, MN: AGS Publishing.

Ries LAG, Eisner MP, Kosary CL *et al.* (eds.) (2005). SEER Cancer Statistics Review, 1975–2002, NCI. Bethesda, MD, http://seer.cancer.gov/csr/1975˙2002/, based on November 2004 SEER data submission, posted to SEER website 2005.

Ris MD, Noll RB (1994). Long-term neurobehavioral outcome in pediatric brain tumor patients: review and methodological critique. *J Clin Exp Neuropsychol* **16**: 21–42.

Ris MD, Packer R, Goldwein J *et al.* (2001). Intellectual outcome after reduced-dose radiation therapy plus adjuvant chemotherapy for medulloblastoma: a children's cancer group study. *J Clin Oncol* **19**: 3470–3476.

Rowland JH, Glidewell OJ, Sibley RF *et al.* (1984). Effects of different forms of central nervous system prophylaxis on neuropsychologic function in childhood leukemia. *J Clin Oncol* **12**: 1327–1355.

Rutter M (1998). Developmental catch up, and deficit, following adoption after severe global early privation. *J Child Psychol Psychiatry* **39**: 465–476.

Schatz J, Kramer JH, Ablin A *et al.* (2000). Processing speed, working memory, and IQ: a developmental model of cognitive deficits following cranial radiation therapy. *Neuropsychology* **14**: 189–200.

Shallice T (1988). *From Neuropsychology to Mental Structure*. Cambridge, UK: Cambridge University Press.

Smith MA, Ries LA, Gurney JG *et al.* (eds.) (1999). *SEER Cancer Statistics Review, 1973–1995. Cancer Incidence and Survival among Children and Adolescents: United States SEER Program 1975–1995*. NCI. Bethesda, MD: National Institutes of Health NIH Pub. No. 99–4649.

Sohlberg M, Mateer C (1987). *Attention Process Training (APT)*. Washington, DC: Association for Neuropsychological Research and Development.

Speechley KN, Barrera ME, Shaw A *et al.* (2002). Health related quality of life (HRQL) in childhood cancer survivors (<17): survivor-control comparisons and impact of age, gender and cancer type. Poster presented at the sixth World Congress of Psycho-Oncology; 2002; Banff, Alberta.

Spiegler BJ, Kennedy K, Maze R *et al.* (2006). Comparison of long-term neurocognitive outcomes in young children with acute lymphoblastic leukemia treated with cranial radiation or high-dose or very high-dose intravenous methotrexate. *J Clin Oncol* **24**: 3858–3864.

Sternberg RJ, Grigorenko EL, Bundy DA (2001). The predictive value of IQ. *Merrill Palmer Q* **47**: 1–41.

Strother D, Pollack I, Fisher PG *et al.* (2002). Tumors of the central nervous system. In Pizzo PA, Poplack DG (eds.) *Principles and Practice of Pediatric Oncology* (4th edn.) (pp. 751–824). Philadelphia, PA: Lippincott Williams & Wilkins.

Stuss DT, Alexander MP (2000). Executive functions and the frontal lobes: a conceptual review. *Psychol Res* **63**: 289–298.

Stuss DT, Anderson V (2004). The frontal lobes and theory of mind: developmental concepts from adult focal lesion research. *Brain Cogn* **55**: 69–83.

Thompson RF (2000). *The Brain* (3rd edn.). New York: Worth Publishers.

Todd JA, Anderson VA, Lawrence J (1996). Planning skills in head injured adolescents and their peers. *Neuropsychol Rehabil* **6**: 81–99.

Von der Weid N, Mosimann I, Hirt A *et al.* (2003). Intellectual outcome in children and adolescents with acute lymphoblastic leukemia treated with chemotherapy alone: Age and sex-related differences. *Eur J Cancer* **39**: 353–365.

Walter AW, Mulhern RK, Gajjar A *et al.* (1999). Survival and neurodevelopmental outcome of young children with medulloblastoma at St. Jude Children's Research Hospital. *J Clin Oncol* **17**: 3720–3728.

Welsh MC, Pennington BF, Grossier DB (1991). A normative-developmental study of executive function: a window on prefrontal function in children. *Dev Neuropsychol* **7**: 131–149.

Wernicke C (1874). *Der aphasische Symptomenkomplex*. Breslau, Poland: M. Cohn and Weigert.

LIST OF TESTS

Abidin RR (1995). *Parent Stress Index* (3rd edn.). Odessa, FL: Psychological Assessment Resources.

Achenbach T (2001). *Child Behavior Checklist (CBCL)*. Burlington, VT: ASEBA.

Beery KE, Beery NA (2004). *The Beery-Buktenica Developmental Test of Visual-Motor Integration*. Minneapolis, MN: NCS Pearson, Inc.

Benton AL, Hamsher KD, Vanery NR, Spreen O (1983). *Contributions to Neuropsychological Assessment: A Clinical Manual*. New York: Oxford University Press.

Benton AL, Sivan AB, Hamsher KD, Vanery NR, Spreen O (1994). *Contributions to Neuropsychological Assessment: A Clinical Manual* (2nd edn.). New York: Oxford University Press.

Brownell R (2000). *Receptive One-Word Picture Vocabulary Test–2000 Edition*. Novato, CA: Academic Therapy Publications.

Cohen MJ (1997). *Children's Memory Scale (CMS)*. New York: The Psychological Corporation.

Conners CK (2001). *Conners' Rating Scales – Revised (CRS-R)*. Toronto, ON: Multi-Health Systems, Inc.

Conners CK, Staff of Multi-Health Systems (2000). *Conners' Continuous Performance Test (CPT-II)*. North Tonawanda, NY: Multi-Health Systems, Inc.

Corwin J, Bylsma FW (1993). Translations of excerpts from Andre Rey's *Psychological Examination of Traumatic Encephalopathy* and PA Osterreith's *The Complex Figure Copy Test. Clin Neuropsychol* **7**: 3–21.

De Renzi E, Faglioni P (1978). Development of a shortened version of the Token Test. *Cortex* **14**: 42–49.

Delis D, Kramer JH, Kaplan E, Ober BA (1994). *California Verbal Learning Test – Children's Version (CVLT-C)*. San Antonio, TX: The Psychological Corporation.

Delis D, Kaplan E, Kramer J (2001). *Delis-Kaplan Executive Function System (D-KEFS)*. San Antonio, TX: The Psychological Corporation.

Dunn LM, Dunn LM (1997). *Examiner's Manual for the Peabody Picture Vocabulary Test* (3rd edn.) *(PPVT-III)*. Circle Pines, MN: American Guidance Service.

Elliott CD (1990). *Differential Ability Scales (DAS)*. San Antonio, TX: The Psychological Corporation.

Gardner MF (2000). *Expressive One-Word Picture Vocabulary Test–2000 Edition*. Novato, CA: Academic Therapy Publications.

Gioia G, Isquith PK, Guy SC, Kenworthy L (2000). *Behavior Rating Inventory of Executive Function*. Odessa, FL: Psychological Assessment Resources.

Golden JC (1978). *Stroop Color and Word Test*. Chicago, IL: Stoelting Co.

Halstead WC (1947). *Brain and Intelligence: A Quantitative Study of the Frontal Lobes*. Chicago, IL: University of Chicago Press.

Harrison PL, Oakland T (2003). *Adaptive Behavior Assessment System* (2nd edn.) *(ABAS-II)*. San Antonio, TX: Harcourt Assessment, Inc.

Heaton RK (1981). *Wisconsin Card Sorting Test (WCST)*. Odessa, FL: Psychological Assessment Resources.

Hooper HE (1983). *Hooper Visual Orientation Test*. Los Angeles, CA: Western Psychological Services.

Kaplan EF, Goodglass H, Weintraub S (1983). *The Boston Naming Test*. Philadelphia, PA: Lea & Febiger.

Keller FR, Davis CM, Davis HP (1999). *Memory Cards Test*. Colorado Springs, CO: Colorado Assessment Tests.

Klove H (1963). Clinical neuropsychology. In Foster FM (ed.) *The Medical Clinics of North America*. New York: Saunders.

Knights RM, Tymchuk AJ (1968). An evaluation of the Halstead-Reitan Category Test for children. *Cortex* **4**: 403–414.

Korkman M, Kirk U, Kemp S (1997). *NEPSY: A Developmental Neuropsychological Assessment*. San Antonio, TX: The Psychological Corporation.

Manly T, Robertson IH, Anderson V, Nimmo-Smith I (1999). *The Test of Everyday Attention for Children: Manual (TEA-Ch)*. Bury St. Edmunds: Thames Valley Test Company, Ltd.

McGrew KS, Woodcock RW, Maher N (2001). *The Woodcock-Johnson III Tests of Achievement (WJ3)*. Itsaca, IL: Riverside Publishing.

Reynolds CR, Kamphaus RW (2004). *Behavior Assessment System for Children* (2nd edn.) *(BASC-II)*. Circle Pines, MN: AGS Publishing.

Roid GH (2003). *Stanford-Binet Intelligence Scales* (5th edn.) *(SB5)*. Itsaca, IL: Riverside Publishing.

Shallice T (1982). Specific impairments of planning. *Philos Trans R Soc Lond* **298**: 199–209.

Sheslow D, Adams W (2004). *Wide Range Assessment of Memory and Learning* (2nd edn.) *(WRAML-II)*. Lutz, FL: Psychological Assessment Resources.

Simon HA (1975). The functional equivalence of problem solving skills. *Cogn Psychol* **7**: 268–288.

Tiffin J, Asher EJ (1948). The Purdue Pegboard: norms and studies of reliability and validity. *J Appl Psychol* **32**: 234–247.

Varni JW, Seid M, Rode CA (1999). The PedsQL: measurement model for the pediatric quality of life inventory. *Med Care* **37**(2): 126–139.

Wagner RK, Toregensen JK, Rashotte CA (1999). *Examiner's Manual: The Comprehensive Test of Phonological Processing*. Austin, TX: PRO-ED, Inc.

Wechsler D (1945). A standardized memory scale for clinical use. *J Psychol* **19**: 87–95.

Wechsler D (1991). *Wechsler Intelligence Scale for Children* (3rd edn.) *(WISC-III)*. San Antonio, TX: The Psychological Corporation.

Wechsler D (1997). *Wechsler Adult Intelligence Scale* (3rd edn.) *(WAIS-III)*. San Antonio, TX: The Psychological Corporation.

Wechsler D (1999). *Wechsler Abbreviated Scale of Intelligence (WASI)*. San Antonio, TX: The Psychological Corporation.

Wechsler D (2001). *Wechsler Individual Achievement Test* (2nd edn.) *(WIAT-II)*. San Antonio, TX: Harcourt Assessment, Inc.

Wechsler D (2002). *Wechsler Preschool and Primary Scale of Intelligence* (3rd edn.) *(WPPSI-III)*. San Antonio, TX: The Psychological Corporation.

Wechsler D (2003). *Wechsler Intelligence Scale for Children* (4th edn.) *(WISC-IV)*. San Antonio, TX: The Psychological Corporation.

Wilkinson GS (1993). *WRAT-3: The Wide Range Achievement Test Administration Manual* (3rd edn.). Wilmington, DE: Wide Range.

Effects of cancer and cancer treatment on cognition

7

Biological bases of radiation injury to the brain

Edward G. Shaw and Mike E. Robbins

Introduction

Neoplasms of the central nervous system (CNS) are a pathologically diverse group of benign and malignant tumors for which a variety of management strategies, including observation, surgery, radiation therapy, and/or chemotherapy, are employed. Regardless of the type of CNS tumor treated, what usually limits the dose of radiation that can be utilized, and therefore what typically determines the local control and cure rate of that tumor, are the tolerance doses of the adjacent or underlying normal tissues in and around the CNS. This chapter will outline the biological principles of CNS radiation tolerance and radiation-induced CNS injury, with an emphasis on the brain.

Pathogenesis of radiation-induced CNS injury

Classical model of parenchymal or vascular target cells

Vascular abnormalities and demyelination are the predominant histological changes seen in radiation-induced CNS injury. Classically, late delayed injury was viewed as due solely to a reduction in the number of surviving clonogens of either parenchymal, i.e., oligodendrocyte (Van den Maazen et al., 1993), or vascular, i.e., endothelial

(Calvo et al., 1988), target cell populations leading to white matter necrosis.

Vascular hypothesis

Proponents of the vascular hypothesis argue that vascular damage leads to ischemia with secondary white matter necrosis. In support of this hypothesis is the large amount of data describing radiation-induced vascular changes including blood vessel (primarily arterial) wall thickening, vessel dilation, and endothelial cell nuclear enlargement (Calvo et al., 1988; Reinhold et al., 1990; Schultheiss & Stephens, 1992). Quantitative studies in the irradiated rat brain have noted time- and dose-related reductions in the number of endothelial cell nuclei and blood vessels prior to the development of necrosis (Reinhold et al., 1990). Further, recent boron neutron capture studies, in which radiation was delivered essentially to the vasculature alone, still led to the development of white matter necrosis (Morris et al., 1996). In contrast, radiation-induced white matter necrosis has been reported in the absence of vascular changes (Schultheiss & Stephens, 1992). Moreover, while the vascular hypothesis argues that ischemia is responsible for white matter necrosis, the most sensitive component of the CNS to oxygen deprivation, the neuron, is located in the gray matter, a relatively radioresistant region. Thus, it seems unlikely that radiation injury is due to damage to the vasculature alone.

Cognition and Cancer, eds. Christina A. Meyers and James R. Perry. Published by Cambridge University Press.
© Cambridge University Press 2008.

Parenchymal hypothesis

The parenchymal hypothesis for radiation-induced CNS injury focuses on the oligodendrocyte, required for the formation of myelin sheaths. The key cell for the generation of mature oligodendrocytes is the oligodendrocyte type 2 astrocyte (O-2A) progenitor cell (Raff et al., 1983). Ionizing radiation results in the loss of the reproductive capacity of the O-2A progenitor cells in the rat CNS (van der Maazen et al., 1991a, 1991b). It is hypothesized that radiation-induced loss of O-2A progenitor cells leads to a failure to replace oligodendrocytes resulting in demyelination. However, a mechanistic link between loss of oligodendrocytes and demyelination has yet to be established. Further, while the kinetics of oligodendrocytes is consistent with the early transient demyelination seen in so-called early delayed reactions (discussed later in chapter), it is inconsistent with the late onset of white matter necrosis (Hornsey et al., 1981). Thus, it is unlikely that loss of O-2A progenitor cells and oligodendrocytes alone can lead to late radiation-induced CNS injury.

Recent findings suggest that the classic model of parenchymal or vascular target cells is oversimplistic. Pathophysiological data from a variety of late responding tissues, including the brain and spinal cord, indicate that the expression of radiation-induced normal tissue injury involves complex and dynamic interactions between several cell types within the particular organ (Jaenke et al., 1993; Moulder et al., 1998; Schultheiss & Stephens, 1992). In the brain, these include not only the oligodendrocytes and endothelial cells, but also the astrocytes, microglia, and neurons. These now are viewed not as *passive* bystanders, merely dying as they attempt to divide, but as *active* participants in an orchestrated response to injury (Tofilon & Fike, 2000). This new paradigm offers the exciting possibility that radiation-induced CNS injury can be modulated by the application of therapies directed that alter the steps in the chain of events leading to the clinical expression of damage. Since the cascade of events does not occur in tumors, where direct clonogenic cell kill predominates, such treatments should not negatively impact antitumor efficacy.

Astrocytes

Once considered to be the "brain glue," providing a supportive role for neuronal distribution and interactions in the normal CNS, astrocytes are now recognized as a heterogeneous class of cells with many important and diverse functions (Volterra & Meldelosi, 2005). Astrocytes secrete a variety of cytokines, proteases, and growth factors that regulate the response of the vasculature, neurons, and oligodendrocyte lineage (Horner & Palmer, 2003). Recent data suggest that hippocampal astrocytes are capable of regulating neurogenesis by instructing the stem cells to adopt a neuronal fate (Muller et al., 1995). In addition, astrocytes assume a critical role in the reaction of the CNS to various forms of injury, including ionizing radiation, and are vital for the protection of endothelial cells, oligodendrocytes, and neurons from oxidative stress (Song et al., 2002). In response to injury, astrocytes exhibit two common reactions: a relatively acute cellular swelling and a more chronic reactive gliosis (Pekny & Nilsson, 2005). Of note, time- and dose-dependent increases in astrocyte number have been observed in the irradiated rat and mouse brain (Calvo et al., 1988; Chiang et al., 1993; Reinhold et al., 1990). In addition to increased cell number, an increase in glial fibrillary acidic protein (GFAP) staining intensity indicative of reactive astrocytes has been observed (Chiang et al., 1993). However, the precise pathogenic mechanism(s) impacted by the astrocyte in radiation-induced CNS injury remains unknown.

Microglia

Microglia form approximately 10% of the total glial cell population in the adult CNS (Vaughan & Peters, 1974) and are considered the main mediators of neuroinflammation (Van Rossum & Hanisch, 2004). Microglia respond to virtually all pathological events in the CNS, and in most pathological settings are assisted by infiltrating macrophages. Upon activation, they can proliferate, phagocytose, and enhance or exacerbate injury through the production of reactive oxygen species (ROS), lipid metabolites, and hydrolytic enzymes (Stoll & Jander, 1999). Irradiation of the rat spinal cord results in a progressive increase in the number of microglial cells 4 and 6 months post-irradiation (Siegal *et al.*, 1996). Similar increases in activated microglia have been observed in the irradiated rat (Mildenberger *et al.*, 1990) and dog (Nakagawa *et al.*, 1996) brain. In addition, cranial irradiation studies suggest that radiation-induced microglial activation leads to decreased neurogenesis in the rat dentate subgranular zone (DSZ) of the hippocampus and is associated with spatial memory retention memory deficits (Monje *et al.*, 2002; Rola *et al.*, 2004). Thus, microglia may play a role in determining the severity of radiation-induced injury in the CNS.

Neurons

In view of the classic model of radiation-induced normal tissue injury, where DNA damage and loss of slow-turnover stem-cell populations leads to late effects, the non-proliferating neuron was thought to be radioresistant and a non-participant in radiation-induced CNS injury. Recent reviews of the clinical aspects of radiation-induced brain injury (Armstrong *et al.*, 2004; Crossen *et al.*, 1994; Mulhern *et al.*, 2004; Sarkissian, 2005) describe chronic and progressive cognitive dysfunction both in children (Anderson *et al.*, 2000; Roman & Sperduto, 1995) and adults (Abayomi, 1996; Moore *et al.*, 1992) following whole-brain or large-field irradiation, suggesting that neurons are indeed sensitive to radiation. Moreover, *in vivo* and *in vitro* experimental studies have shown radiation-induced changes in hippocampal cellular activity, synaptic efficiency, and spike generation (Bassant & Court, 1978; Surma-aho *et al.*, 2001), and in neuronal gene expression (Pellmar & Lepinski, 1993). Thus, it seems likely that radiation-induced alterations in neuron function play a role in the development and progression of radiation-induced CNS injury. An additional and important component of radiation injury is the relatively recent observation that ionizing radiation can inhibit hippocampal neurogenesis.

Neural stem cells and neurogenesis

The hippocampus is central to short-term declarative memory and spatial information processing. It consists of the dentate gyrus, CA3 and CA1 regions. The dentate gyrus represents a highly dynamic structure and a major site of postnatal and adult neurogenesis. Resident in the hippocampus are neural stem cells, self-renewing cells capable of generating neurons, astrocytes, and oligodendrocytes (Gage *et al.*, 1998; Noel *et al.*, 1998). Neurogenesis depends on the presence of a specific neurogenic microenvironment; both endothelial cells and astrocytes can promote/regulate neurogenesis (Palmer *et al.*, 1997; Song *et al.*, 2002). Experimental studies have indicated that brain radiation results in increased apoptosis and neuron loss (Nakaya *et al.*, 2005; Palmer *et al.*, 2000), with neonatal mice being more susceptible than postnatal animals (Nakaya *et al.*, 2005), decreased cell proliferation, and a decreased stem/precursor cell differentiation into neurons within the neurogenic region of the hippocampus (Bellinzona *et al.*, 1996; Monje *et al.*, 2002; Snyder *et al.*, 2003). Rats irradiated with a single dose of 10 Gy produce only 3% of the new hippocampal neurons formed in control animals (Snyder *et al.*, 2003). Of note, these changes were observed after doses of radiation that failed to produce demyelination and/or white matter necrosis in the rat brain.

Further evidence demonstrating the importance of the microenvironment for successful neurogenesis comes from studies showing that non-irradiated stem cells transplanted into the irradiated hippocampus failed to generate neurons; this may reflect a pronounced microglial inflammatory response, since neuroinflammation is a strong inhibitor of neurogenesis (Mizumatsu *et al.*, 2003; Nakaya *et al.*, 2005). In contrast to the reduction in neurogenesis, gliogenesis appears to be enhanced after irradiation: microglia and immature oligodendrocytes increase in total and relative number in both *in vitro* and *in vivo* conditions (Monje *et al.*, 2002). These results suggest that brain irradiation does not eradicate hippocampal progenitor cells or even alter their intrinsic capability to produce new neurons, but radiation induces currently undefined signals that regulate the proliferation, differentiation, and survival of these cells.

Contemporary view on the pathogenesis of radiation-induced CNS injury

Based on the assumption that the CNS has a limited repertoire of responses to injury, the response of the CNS to other forms of insult has been used by Tofilon and Fike (2000) to model a more contemporary view of the pathogenesis of radiation-induced CNS damage. In this model, radiation not only causes acute cell death, but also induces an intrinsic recovery/repair response in the form of specific cytokines and may initiate secondary reactive processes that result in the generation of a persistent oxidative stress and/or chronic inflammation (Robbins & Zhao, 2004).

Data published in the last several years suggest a primary role for chronic oxidative stress and reactive oxygen/nitrogen oxide species (ROS/RNOS) in radiation-induced brain injury. Initial indirect evidence showed that irradiation of the rat brain inhibited hippocampal neurogenesis, associated with a marked increase in the number and activation status of microglia in the neurogenic zone (Monje *et al.*, 2002). Subsequent studies showed that inhibiting microglial activation using indomethacin restored hippocampal neurogenesis (Monje *et al.*, 2003).

Direct experimental evidence for radiation-induced oxidative/nitrosative stress has been obtained from studies using neonatal and adult rats and mice. Fukuda *et al.* (2004) treated one hemisphere of postnatal-day-8 rats or postnatal-day-10 mice with a single dose of 4–12 Gy of 4-MV X-rays. Time-dependent increases in nitrosative stress, assessed in terms of nitrotyrosine formation, were observed in the subventricular zone and the granular cell layer of the dentate gyrus 2–12 h post-irradiation. An oxidative stress, evidenced as a significant increase in lipid peroxidation measured using malondialdehyde, was noted in the adult male mouse hippocampus 2 weeks after brain irradiation with a single dose of 10 Gy (Limoli *et al.*, 2004). In accompanying *in vitro* studies using isolated multipotent neural precursor cells derived from the rat hippocampus, Limoli *et al.* (2004) showed that the levels of ROS were significantly elevated when the cells were cultured at low cell density and were associated with elevated proliferation and increased metabolic, primarily mitochondrial, activity. The ROS appeared to result from altered mitochondrial function that ultimately compromised the growth rate of the neural precursor cells. At high cell densities, intracellular ROS and oxidative damage were reduced; this was associated with a concomitant increase in manganese superoxide dismutase (MnSOD) expression. Irradiation-induced depletion of neural precursor cells assessed in the subgranular zone also led to increased ROS and altered proliferation, confirming the *in vitro* studies. To further test the role of ROS, mice were treated with the antioxidant α-lipoic acid (LA). The administration of LA *in vivo* reduced cell proliferation in both unirradiated and irradiated mice. Indeed, the effect of LA was less marked due to the pronounced reduction of precursor cell numbers observed after irradiation. Of note, LA treatment in irradiated mice lowered malondialdehyde levels in hippocampal tissue, supporting the active role of radiation-induced oxidative stress in radiation-induced brain injury. More recently, Rola *et al.* (2005) reported a chronic inflammatory response in the mouse DSZ 9 months following high-LET (linear energy transfer) brain irradiation; expression of the CCR2 receptor, important in neuroinflammation (Banisadr *et al.*, 2002), increased in the irradiated brains as compared to the sham-irradiated control brains. In addition, *in vitro* irradiation of rat neural precursor cells subjected to chronic exogenous oxidative stress showed increased radiosensitivity (Limoli *et al.*, 2006).

Laboratory studies of therapeutic interventions for radiation-induced CNS injury

As noted earlier, radiation-induced CNS injury has been well characterized in terms of histological criteria as well as radiobiological parameters. In contrast, details of the molecular, cellular, and biochemical processes responsible for the expression and progression of radiation-induced CNS injury currently remain limited. Thus, the rational application of interventional procedures directed at reducing the severity of late radiation injury has been problematical. Several pragmatic but unspecific approaches have been used.

Intrathecal administration of the classic radioprotector WR-2721 (amifostine) before spinal cord irradiation resulted in a dose-modifying factor of 1.3 and a prolongation of median latency to myelopathy by 63% at the effective dose in 50% of subjects (ED_{50}) (Monje *et al.*, 2003). Fike *et al.* (1994) observed that the polyamine synthesis inhibitor α-difluoromethylornithine reduced the volume of radionecrosis and contrast enhancement in the irradiated dog brain; a delayed increase in microglia was also noted (Nakagawa *et al.*, 1996). Hornsey *et al.* (1990) hypothesized that treating rats with the iron-chelating agent desferrioxamine would reduce hydroxyl-mediated reperfusion-related injury in the irradiated spinal cord. Rats were fed a low-iron diet from 85 days after local spinal cord irradiation and received desferrioxamine (30 mg in 0.3 ml, s.c., 3 times per week) from day 120, the time at which changes in vascular permeability were noted. The onset of ataxia due to white matter necrosis was delayed and the incidence of lesions was reduced after single doses of 25 and 27 Gy. The steroid dexamethasone also delayed the development of radiation-induced ataxia along with a reduction in regional capillary permeability. In contrast, indomethacin did not appear to affect any of these endpoints. In the pig, administration of the polyunsaturated fatty acids γ-linolenic acid (GLA; 18C:3n-6) and eicosapentaenoic acid (EPA; 20C:5n-3), starting the day after spinal cord irradiation, was associated with a reduced incidence of paralysis,

from 80% down to 20% (Hopewell *et al.*, 1993). More recently, El-Agamawi *et al.* (1996) reported that GLA significantly reduced the onset of paralysis following spinal cord irradiation in 5-week-old rats. Prophylactic hyperbaric oxygen (HBO) has also been used to try to prevent radiation-induced myelopathy in a rat model. Using a dose of 65 Gy in 10 fractions with or without 30 HBO treatments following the irradiation, Sminia *et al.* (2003) did not demonstrate any preventive value to HBO. In fact, there was a "tendency towards radiosensitization" in the HBO-treated rats (Sminia *et al.*, 2003). Administration of ramipril, an angiotensin converting enzyme inhibitor, from 2 weeks to 6 months after stereotactic irradiation with a single dose of 30 Gy was associated with a reduction in the severity of optic neuropathy (Kim *et al.*, 2004).

Attempts have been made to rectify the radiation-induced decrease in neurogenesis. Rezvani *et al.* (2002) transplanted neural stem cells 90 days after irradiation of the rat spinal cord with a single dose of 22 Gy. While 100% of irradiated rats treated with saline exhibited paralysis within 167 days of irradiation, the paralysis-free survival rate of rats treated with neural stem cells was approximately 34% at 183 days. Conversely, non-irradiated stem cells transplanted into the irradiated rat hippocampus failed to generate neurons, although gliogenesis was spared (Rezvani *et al.*, 2002). Preliminary data suggest that insulin-like growth factor-1 (IGF-1) may show efficacy in not only preventing radiation myelopathy in adults (Nieder *et al.*, 2000) but also in ameliorating the radiation-induced cognitive dysfunction observed in the rat following whole-brain irradiation (Lynch *et al.*, 2002). Other growth factors besides IGF-1, such as platelet-derived growth factor, vascular endothelial growth factor, and beta fibroblast growth factor, may also play a role in modulating radiation-induced CNS tissue injury (Andratschke *et al.*, 2005).

As discussed above, recent data suggest a role for chronic inflammation in the development and progression of radiation-induced late effects, and provide a rationale for the application of anti-inflammatory interventions to mitigate

Table 7.1. Factors associated with radiation tolerance of the normal central nervous system (CNS) tissues (modified from Leibel & Sheline, 1991; Schultheiss et al., 1995; Sheline et al., 1980)

Factor[a]	Factors for increased risk of CNS injury	CNS tolerance increased by:
Total dose	Higher total dose	Decreasing total dose
Fractionation	Hypofractionation	Hyperfractionation[b]
Radiation dose	Radiosensitizers	Radioprotectors
Dose per fraction	Dose per fraction >180–200 cGy	Dose/fraction to ≤180–200 cGy
Volume	Increased volume, e.g., whole-organ radiation	Decreasing volume, e.g., partial organ radiation
Host factors	Medical illness, e.g., hypertension, diabetes	Unknown
Beam quality	High-LET radiation beams, e.g., neutrons	Low-LET beams, e.g., photons
Adjunctive therapy	Concomitant use of CNS toxic drugs, e.g., methotrexate	Avoid concomitant use drugs, or use sequentially

[a]Total time is not a major determinant of normal CNS tissue tolerance.
[b]Defined as multiple daily fractions, usually two with doses per fraction of 180–200 cGy, usually 100–120 cGy, separated by 4–8 h, to total doses higher than those given with "standard" fractionation.

radiation-induced brain injury (Robbins & Zhao, 2004). Given the anti-inflammatory properties of the peroxisomal proliferator-activated receptor (PPAR)γ agonists in neurological disease (Feinstein, 2003), Zhao et al. (2007) investigated the ability of the PPARγ agonist pioglitazone (Pio) to modulate radiation-induced cognitive impairment using a well-characterized rat model (Brown et al., 2005). Young adult male F344 rats received one of the following: (1) fractionated whole-brain irradiation (WBI); 40 or 45 Gy γ rays in 4 or 4.5 weeks, respectively, 2 fractions/week, and normal diet; (2) sham irradiation and normal diet; (3) WBI plus Pio (120 ppm) prior, during, and for 4 or 54 weeks post-irradiation; (4) sham irradiation plus Pio; and (5) WBI plus Pio starting 24 h after completion of WBI. Administration of Pio prior to, during, and for 4 or 54 weeks after WBI prevented the radiation-induced cognitive impairment. Of interest, administration of Pio for 54 weeks starting after completion of fractionated WBI substantially, but not significantly, reduced the radiation-induced cognitive impairment (Zhao et al., 2007). The ability of Pio to modulate experimental radiation-induced cognitive impairment is very significant; Pio (Actos) has been prescribed for several years as an anti-diabetic agent, and thiazolidinedione drugs (TZDs)

appear to be effective in the treatment of a variety of brain disorders (Bordet et al., 2006). Further, PPARγ agonists induce antineoplastic signaling pathways in a variety of cancer cell lines, animal models, and humans, including gliomas (Grommes et al., 2004). Translating these findings to the clinic offers the promise of not only improving the quality of life for long-term brain tumor survivors, but also increasing their therapeutic window.

Clinical aspects of CNS radiation tolerance

The radiation tolerance of the CNS is dependent on a number of factors, including total dose, dose per fraction, total time, volume, host factors, radiation quality (linear energy transfer), and adjunctive therapies. Table 7.1 defines the role of these factors in radiation tolerance and injury to the brain, as well as ways in which they might be modified to increase tolerance (i.e., reduce injury) (Leibel & Sheline, 1991; Schultheiss et al., 1995).

Table 7.2 shows partial and whole-organ tolerance doses for the brain and spinal cord, and includes doses predicted to result in a 5% and 50% probability of injury 5 years following treatment with radiation ($TD_{5/5}$ and $TD_{50/5}$, respectively) (Emami

Table 7.2. Tolerance doses for normal central nervous system tissues[a] (modified from Emami et al., 1991; Rubin & Casarett, 1968)

CNS tissue	$TD_{5/5}$ (Gy)	$TD_{50/5}$ (Gy)	Endpoint
Rubin and Casarett (1968)			
Brain			Infarction, necrosis
Whole	60	70	
Partial (25%)	70	80	
Spinal cord			Infarction, necrosis
Partial (10-cm length)	45	55	
Emami et al. (1991)			
Brain			Infarction, necrosis
One-third	60	75	
Two-thirds	50	65	
Whole	40	60	
Brainstem			Infarction, necrosis
One-third	60	–	
Two-thirds	53	–	
Whole	50	65	
Spinal cord			Myelitis, necrosis
5 cm	50	70	
10 cm	50	70	
20 cm	47	–	
Cauda equina	60	75	Clinically apparent nerve damage
Brachial plexus			Clinically apparent nerve damage
One-third	62	77	
Two-thirds	61	76	
Whole	60	75	

[a] Assumes 2 Gy per fraction, 5 days per week.

et al., 1991; Rubin & Casarett, 1968). These values are derived from mathematical models of brain and spinal cord tolerance based on clinical data describing instances of radiation injury and the total doses and fraction sizes at which they occurred.

None of the mathematical models account for the factors listed in Table 7.1, nor do they adequately predict radiation tolerance or injury. The power-law model described by Sheline et al. (1980) represents a modification of the Ellis Nominal Standard Dose formula (Ellis, 1969):

$$Neuret = (D)(N^{-0.41})(T^{-0.03})$$

where D = total dose, N = number of fractions, and T = time.

The linear quadratic model links the response to fractionated irradiation to the fractional reproductive survival of clonogenic target cells. Fractionation data can be analyzed using the formula shown below:

$$E = n(\alpha d + \beta d^2)$$

where the effect (E) is a linear and quadratic function of the dose per fraction (d) and a function of the fraction number (n). This equation allows determination of the α/β ratio, a measure of the "bendiness" of the underlying putative target cell survival curve. For brain and spinal cord, an average α/β ratio of 2 Gy appears appropriate (Fowler, 1992).

Based on these various models, the $TD_{5/5}$ for the whole brain and for part of the brain is 50 ± 10 Gy and 60 ± 10 Gy, respectively. For a 10-cm segment of spinal cord the $TD_{5/5}$ is 45–50 Gy (Table 7.2). Although the $TD_{50/5}$ value for spinal cord is lower than that for brain, there are no robust data to support this difference. Rather, the sequelae of spinal cord radiation injury are perceived as greater than those of brain injury; therefore, tolerance doses have been lowered arbitrarily. In clinical practice, $TD_{5/5}$ and $TD_{1/5}$ values of 60–65 Gy and 50–55 Gy for partial brain irradiation and $TD_{5/5}$ and $TD_{1/5}$ values of 55–60 Gy and 45–50 Gy for a limited segment of spinal cord are commonly used. Clinical data have borne out these somewhat empiric dose ranges. In a study of 203 adults with supratentorial low-grade glioma, patients were randomized to partial brain treatment fields with either 50.4 Gy in 28 fractions of 1.8 Gy each or 64.8 Gy in 36 fractions of 1.8 Gy (Shaw *et al.*, 2002). Radiation necrosis developed in 1% of patients who received 50.4 Gy and 5% of those who had 64.8 Gy. In a retrospective study of 53 head and neck cancer patients undergoing typical posterior cervical treatment in fields including the cervical spinal cord to doses greater than 56 Gy in fraction sizes of ≤2 Gy, the incidence of radiation myelopathy was 1.9% (McCunniff & Liang, 1989). In a subsequent study of 1048 lung cancer patients treated with thoracic radiation on three Medical Research Council Lung Cancer Working Party clinical trials, the only patients who developed radiation myelopathy were those treated with 3 Gy fractions or larger. The 2-year risk of radiation myelopathy was 2.2%–2.5% among patients receiving thoracic spinal cord doses of 17 Gy in 2 fractions or 39 Gy in 13 fractions. The authors concluded that a total cord dose of 48 Gy given in 2-Gy fractions was safe (Macbeth *et al.*, 1996). These data emphasize the importance of both total dose and dose per fraction in determining CNS tolerance to radiation. These concepts are implied in the neuret model of brain tolerance, in which fraction size, which is related to "N" (number of fractions), is far more important than "T" (time), given that the exponent for N is much larger than that for T. The $TD_{5/5}$ values given

Table 7.3. Tolerance doses for miscellaneous normal tissues of the cranium (modified from Cooper *et al.*, 1995; Emami *et al.*, 1991; Gordon *et al.*, 1995; Sklar & Constine, 1995)

Normal tissue	$TD_{5/5}$ (Gy)	$TD_{50/5}$ (Gy)	Manifestations of severe injury
Ear (middle/ external)	30–55	40–65	Acute or chronic serous otitis
Eye			
Retina	45	65	Blindness
Lens	10	18	Cataract formation
Optic nerve or chiasm	50	65	Blindness

for brain and spinal cord tolerance assume a fraction size of 180–200 cGy per day. For primary CNS tumor patients being treated with curative intent, fraction size should rarely exceed 200 cGy daily, and, in most situations, should be 180–200 cGy (including areas or volumes of "hot spots"). Fraction sizes greater than 200 cGy daily (usually 250–300 cGy) are commonly used for palliation of brain metastases and spinal cord compression, but only because such patients are not expected to live long enough to manifest late radiation-induced brain or spinal cord injury.

Tables 7.2 and 7.3 show the tolerance doses for other normal tissues of the CNS, including the brainstem, eye, ear, optic chiasm, optic nerve, and pituitary gland. The clinical manifestations of severe injury to these structures are listed in the table (Cooper *et al.*, 1995; Gordon *et al.*, 1995; Sklar & Constine, 1995).

Quantitative scoring of CNS toxicity

Radiation injury is usually described in terms of its time course and severity. Acute injury occurs during the course of brain and spinal cord irradiation, and is extremely uncommon, although acute side-effects of radiation do occur, such as fatigue, hair loss, and skin erythema. More common are the early delayed reactions, which occur several weeks

Table 7.4. RTOG and EORTC central nervous system toxicity tables[a] (modified from Cox *et al.*, 1995)

Acute toxicity grade, brain			
1 Fully functional status (i.e., able to work) with minor neurological findings; no medication needed	2 Neurological findings sufficient to require home care; nursing assistance may be required; medications including steroids and anti-seizure agents may be required	3 Neurological findings requiring hospitalization for initial management	4 Serious neurological impairment that includes paralysis, coma, or seizures >3 per week despite medication and/or hospitalization required
Chronic toxicity grade, brain			
1 Mild headache; slight lethargy	2 Moderate headache; great lethargy	3 Severe headaches; severe CNS dysfunction (partial loss of power or dyskinesia)	4 Seizure or paralysis; coma
Chronic toxicity grade, spinal cord			
1 Mild Lhermitte's syndrome	2 Severe Lhermitte's syndrome	3 Objective neurological findings at or below cord level treated	4 Monoplegia, paraplegia, or quadriplegia

[a] Grade 0 toxicity, none; grade 1, mild; grade 2, moderate; grade 3, severe; grade 4, life threatening; grade 5, fatal.

to months after radiation has been completed, and the late delayed reactions, which occur beyond several months (and usually between 1 and 2 years) following treatment.

Clinically, radiation-induced toxicities are usually graded as mild, moderate, severe, life-threatening, or fatal, and are defined in an organ-specific manner. Table 7.4 shows the toxicity tables used for brain tumor clinical research protocols by the Radiation Therapy Oncology Group (RTOG) and its European counterpart, the European Organisation for the Research and Treatment of Cancer (EORTC) (Cox *et al.*, 1995). Alternatively, the National Cancer Institute (NCI) Common Terminology Criteria for Adverse Events version 3.0 can be used (http://ctep.cancer.gov/reporting/ctc.html). To measure quality of life in brain tumor patients undergoing combined modality therapy including brain radiation, a commonly used and validated assessment tool is the Functional Assessment of Cancer Therapy (FACT) that includes the brain subscale (Weitzner *et al.*, 1995).

Early delayed reactions are thought to occur, at least in part, due to the effects of radiation on the oligodendroglial or myelin-producing cells, resulting in an interruption of myelin synthesis. Myelin forms a concentric sheath that surrounds the axons or nerve fibers. In the brain, this is clinically manifest as somnolence, increased irritability, loss of appetite, and sometimes an exacerbation of underlying tumor-associated symptoms or signs. When this symptom complex occurs in children following whole brain radiation, it is called the "somnolence syndrome." In the spinal cord, symptoms of demyelination include electric-shock-like paresthesias radiating into the arms that occur with flexion of the neck, or Lhermitte's syndrome. Early delayed reactions are nearly always transient, lasting several weeks to months, and do not predict for subsequent injury (Esik *et al.*, 2003). Late delayed reactions, in contrast, are usually irreversible. The underlying mechanisms of late delayed reactions are thought to include (but are not limited to) injury to the capillary endothelium leading to narrowing or obliteration of the arteries supplying blood to the brain or spinal cord, and direct damage to all the cells in the CNS. For both early and late delayed reactions, the result is radiation necrosis, which is tissue damage

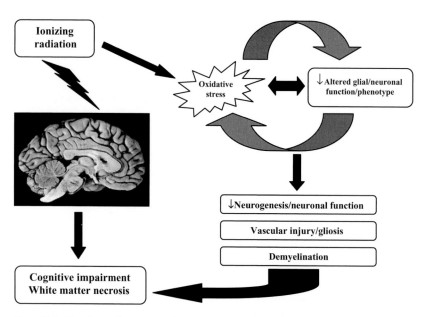

Figure 7.1. Putative pathogenic mechanisms involved in the development and progression of radiation-induced late effects in the brain. Brain irradiation is hypothesized to lead to both acute and chronic oxidative stress/inflammation, with resultant alterations in glial and neuronal phenotype that lead to additional and persistent oxidative stress. Accompanying these changes in brain cell phenotype are decreased neurogenesis and neuronal function, vascular injury, gliosis and changes in myelin composition/demyelination. The functional consequence of radiation-induced brain injury is cognitive impairment that may or may not be accompanied by white matter necrosis

to the substance or white matter of the brain and/or spinal cord. The clinical symptoms and signs of radiation necrosis are either the direct result of tissue damage, or indirectly result from swelling of the adjacent normal tissues in response to the necrotic material. Brain necrosis may be asymptomatic if it occurs in non-critical areas, e.g., anterior frontal and temporal lobes, but usually is associated with symptoms that are location specific (e.g., necrosis in the motor gyrus would result in a contralateral hemiparesis). Spinal cord necrosis is usually symptomatic, and may include sensory and motor loss in the legs or arms and legs, depending on the spinal cord level of the injury, as well as sphincter impairment of the bowel and bladder.

Conclusions

Radiation-induced injury to the CNS, including both the brain and spinal cord, is a complex pro-cess resulting from acute cell death as well as an intrinsic recovery/repair response inducing specific cytokines and secondary reactive processes that result in persistent oxidative stress and/or chronic inflammation (Figure 7.1).

There is evidence that multiple cells are involved, including the endothelium, oligodendrocytes, astrocytes, microglia, neurons, and neural stem cells. Neuroprotective and neurotherapeutic approaches have been utilized both in the laboratory and clinical settings (Table 7.5) with variable degrees of success. Laboratory research focused on the pathobiology of radiation-induced CNS injury as well as the development of effective preventive and therapeutic approaches remain areas of active investigation.

ACKNOWLEDGMENTS

Supported by NCI grants CA112593, CA122318, and by an unrestricted educational grant from Elekta Instruments Inc., Norcross, GA.

Table 7.5. Possible preventive and therapeutic interventions for radiation-induced brain injury. (*bFGF* Basic fibroblast growth factor, *IGF-1* insulin-like growth factor-1, *PDGF* platelet derived growth factor, *PPARγ* peroxisomal proliferator-activated receptor, gamma, *VEGF* vascular endothelial growth factor)

Intervention	Reference
Amifostine (WR-2721)	Spence *et al.*, 1986
α-difluoromethylornithine	Fike *et al.*, 1994; Nakagawa *et al.*, 1996
Desferrioxamine	Hornsey *et al.*, 1990
Polyunsaturated fatty acids	Hopewell *et al.*, 1993; El-Agamawi *et al.*, 1996
Hyperbaric oxygen	Sminia *et al.*, 2003
Angiotensin-converting enzyme inhibitors	Kim *et al.*, 2004
Indomethacin	Monje *et al.*, 2003
Neural stem cells	Rezvani *et al.*, 2002
PDGF, IGF-1, VEGF, bFGF	Andratschke *et al.*, 2005
PPARγ agonists	Zhao *et al.*, 2007

REFERENCES

Abayomi OK (1996). Pathogenesis of irradiation-induced cognitive dysfunction. *Acta Oncol* **35**: 659–663.

Anderson VA, Godber T, Smibert E *et al.* (2000). Cognitive and academic outcome following cranial irradiation and chemotherapy in children: a longitudinal study. *Br J Cancer* **82**: 255–262.

Andratschke NH, Nieder C, Price RE *et al.* (2005). Potential role of growth factors in diminishing radiation therapy neural tissue injury. *Semin Oncol* **32** [2 Suppl. 3]: S67–70.

Armstrong CL, Gyato K, Awadalla AW *et al.* (2004). A critical review of the clinical effects of therapeutic irradiation damage to the brain: the roots of the controversy. *Neuropsychol Rev* **14**: 65–86.

Banisadr G, Quéraud-Lesaux F, Boutterin MC *et al.* (2002). Distribution, cellular localization and functional role of CCR2 chemokine receptors in adult rat brain. *J Neurochem* **81**: 257–269.

Bassant MH, Court L (1978). Effect of whole-body gamma irradiation on the activity of rabbit hippocampal neurons. *Radiat Res* **75**: 595–606.

Bellinzona M, Gobbel GT, Shinohara C *et al.* (1996). Apoptosis is induced in the subependyma of young adult rats by ionizing irradiation. *Neurosci Lett* **208**: 163–166.

Bordet R, Gelé P, Duriez P *et al.* (2006). PPARs: a new target for neuroprotection. *J Neurol Neurosurg Psychiatry* **77**: 285–287.

Brown WR, Thore CR, Moody DM *et al.* (2005). Vascular damage after fractionated whole-brain irradiation in rats. *Radiat Res* **164**: 662–668.

Calvo W, Hopewell JW, Reinhold HS *et al.* (1988). Time- and dose-related changes in the white matter of the rat brain after single doses of X rays. *Br J Radiol* **61**: 1043–1052.

Chiang C-S, McBride WH, Withers HR (1993). Radiation-induced astrocytic and microglial cellular hyperplasia. *Radiother Oncol* **29**: 60–68.

Cooper JS, Fu K, Marks J *et al.* (1995). Late effects of radiation in the head and neck region. *Int J Radiat Oncol Biol Phys* **31**: 1141–1164.

Cox JD, Stetz J, Pajak TF (1995). Toxicity criteria of the Radiation Therapy Oncology Group and the European Organization for Research and Treatment of Cancer. *Int J Radiat Oncol Biol Phys* **31**: 1341–1346.

Crossen JR, Garwood D, Glatstein E *et al.* (1994). Neurobehavioral sequelae of cranial irradiation in adults: a review of radiation-induced encephalopathy. *J Clin Oncol* **12**: 627–642.

El-Agamawi AY, Hopewell JW, Plowman PN *et al.* (1996). Modulation of normal tissue responses to radiation. *Br J Radiol* **69**: 374–375.

Ellis F (1969). Dose, time fractionation: a clinical hypothesis. *Clin Radiol* **20**: 1–7.

Emami B, Lyman J, Brown A *et al.* (1991). Tolerance of normal tissue to therapeutic irradiation. *Int J Radiat Oncol Biol Phys* **21**: 109–122.

Esik O, Csere T, Stefantis K *et al.* (2003). A review on radiogenic Lhermitte's sign. *Pathol Oncol Res* **9**: 115–120.

Feinstein DL (2003). Therapeutic potential of peroxisomal proliferator-activated receptor agonists for neurological disease. *Diabetes Technol Ther* **5**: 67–73.

Fike JR, Goebbel GT, Martob J *et al.* (1994). Radiation brain injury is reduced by the polyamine inhibitor alpha-difluoromethylornithine. *Radiat Res* **138**: 99–106.

Fowler JF (1992). Brief summary of radiobiological principles in fractionated radiotherapy. *Semin Radiat Oncol* **2**: 16–21.

Fukuda H, Fukuda A, Zhu C *et al.* (2004). Irradiation-induced progenitor cell death in the developing brain is resistant to erythropoietin treatment and caspase inhibition. *Cell Death Differ* **11**: 1166–1178.

Gage FH, Kempermann G, Palmer TD *et al.* (1998). Multi-potent progenitor cells in the adult dentate gyrus. *J Neurobiol* **36**: 249–266.

Gordon KB, Char DH, Sagerman RH (1995). Late effects of radiation on the eye and ocular adnexa. *Int J Radiat Oncol Biol Phys* **31**: 1123–1140.

Grommes C, Landreth GE, Heneka MT (2004). Antineoplastic effects of peroxisome proliferator-activated receptor γ agonists. *Lancet Oncol* **5**: 419–429.

Hopewell JW, Van Den Aardweg GJMJ, Morris GM *et al.* (1993). Unsaturated lipids as modulators of radiation damage in normal tissues. In Horrobin DF (ed.). *New Approaches to Cancer Treatment* (pp. 88–106). London: Churchill Communications Europe.

Horner PJ, Palmer TD (2003). New roles for astrocytes: the nightlife of an "astrocyte". La vida loca! *Trends Neurosci* **26**: 597–603.

Hornsey S, Myers R, Coultas PG *et al.* (1981). Turnover of proliferative cells in the spinal cord after X irradiation and its relation to time-dependent repair of radiation damage. *Br J Radiol* **54**: 1081–1085.

Hornsey S, Myers R, Jenkinson T (1990). The reduction of radiation damage to the spinal cord by postirradiation administration of vasoactive drugs. *Int J Radiat Oncol Biol Phys* **18**: 1437–1442.

Jaenke RS, Robbins MEC, Bywaters T *et al.* (1993). Capillary endothelium: target site of renal radiation injury. *Lab Invest* **57**: 551–565.

Kim JH, Brown SL, Kolozsvary A *et al.* (2004). Modification of radiation injury by Ramipril, inhibitor of the angiotensin-converting enzyme, on optic neuropathy in the rat. *Radiat Res* **161**: 137–142.

Leibel SA, Sheline GE (1991). Tolerance of the brain and spinal cord to conventional irradiation. In Gutin P, Liebel SA, Sheline GE (eds.) *Radiation Injury to the Nervous System* (1st edn.) (pp. 211–238). New York: Raven Press.

Limoli CL, Rola R, Giedzinski E *et al.* (2004). Cell-density-dependent regulation of neural precursor cells function. *Proc Natl Acad Sci USA* **101**: 16052–16057.

Limoli CL, Giedzinski E, Baure J *et al.* (2006). Altered growth and radiosensitivity in neural precursor cells subjected to oxidative stress. *Int J Radiat Biol* **82**: 640–647.

Lynch CD, Sonntag WE, Wheeler KT (2002). Radiation-induced dementia in aged rats: effects of growth hormone and insulin-like growth factor 1 [Abstract]. *Neuro-Oncology* **4**: 354.

Macbeth FR, Wheldon TE, Girling DJ *et al.* (1996). Radiation myelopathy: estimates of risk in 1048 patients in three randomized trials of palliative radiotherapy for non-small cell lung cancer. The Medical Research Council Lung Cancer Working Party. *Clin Oncol (R Coll Radiol)* **8**: 176–181.

McCunniff AJ, Liang AJ (1989). Radiation tolerance of the cervical spinal cord. *Int J Radiat Oncol Biol Phys* **16**: 675–678.

Mildenberger M, Beach TG, McGeer EG *et al.* (1990). An animal model of prophylactic cranial irradiation: histologic effects at acute, early and delayed stages. *Int J Radiat Oncol Biol Phys* **18**: 1051–1060.

Mizumatsu S, Monje ML, Morhardt DR *et al.* (2003). Extreme sensitivity of adult neurogenesis to low doses of X-irradiation. *Cancer Res* **63**: 4021–4027.

Monje ML, Mizumatsu S, Fike JR *et al.* (2002). Irradiation induced neural precursor-cell dysfunction. *Nature Med* **8**: 955–961.

Monje ML, Toda H, Palmer TD (2003). Inflammatory blockade restores adult hippocampal neurogenesis. *Science* **302**: 1760–1764.

Moore BD, Copeland DR, Ried H *et al.* (1992). Neurophysiological basis of cognitive deficits in long-term survivors of childhood cancer. *Arch Neurol* **49**: 809–817.

Morris GM, Coderre JA, Bywaters A *et al.* (1996). Boron neutron capture irradiation of the rat spinal cord: histopathological evidence of a vascular-mediated pathogenesis. *Radiat Res* **146**: 313–320.

Moulder J, Robbins MEC, Cohen EP *et al.* (1998). Pharmacologic modification of radiation-induced late normal tissue injury. In Mittal BB, Purdy JA, Ang KK (eds.) *Radiation Therapy* (pp. 129–151). Norwell, MA: Kluwer.

Mulhern RK, Merchant TE, Gajjar A *et al.* (2004). Late neurocognitive sequelae in survivors of brain tumours in childhood. *Lancet Oncol* **5**: 399–408.

Muller HW, Junghans U, Kappler J (1995). Astroglial neurotrophic and neurite-promoting factors. *Pharmacol Ther* **65**: 1–18.

Nakagawa M, Bellinzona M, Seilhan TM *et al.* (1996). Microglial responses after focal radiation-induced injury are affected by alpha-difluoromethylornithine. *Int J Radiat Oncol Biol Phys* **36**: 113–123.

Nakaya K, Hasegawa T, Flickinger JC *et al.* (2005). Sensitivity to radiation-induced apoptosis and neuron loss declines rapidly in the postnatal mouse neocortex. *Int J Radiat Biol* **81**: 545–554.

Nieder C, Price RE, Rivera B *et al.* (2000). Both early and delayed treatment with growth factors can modulate the development of radiation myelopathy (RM) in rats [Abstract]. *Radiother Oncol* **56** [Suppl. 1]: S15.

Noel F, Gumin GJ, Raju U *et al.* (1998). Increased expression of prohormone convertase-2 in the irradiated rat brain. *FASEB J* **12**: 1725–1730.

Palmer TD, Takahashi J, Gage FH (1997). The adult rat hippocampus contains primordial neural stem cells. *Mol Cell Neurosci* **8**: 389–404.

Palmer TD, Willhoite AR, Gage FH (2000). Vascular niche for adult hippocampal neurogenesis. *J Comp Neurol* **425**: 479–494.

Pekny M, Nilsson M (2005). Astrocyte activation and reactive gliosis. *Glia* **50**: 427–434.

Pellmar TC, Lepinski DL (1993). Gamma radiation (5–10 Gy) impairs neuronal function in the guinea pig hippocampus. *Radiat Res* **136**: 255–261.

Raff MC, Miller RH, Noble M (1983). A glial progenitor cell that develops in vitro into an astrocyte or an oligodendrocyte depending on culture medium. *Nature* **303**: 390–396.

Reinhold HS, Calvo W, Hopewell JW *et al.* (1990). Development of blood vessel-related radiation damage in the fimbria of the central nervous system. *Int J Radiat Oncol Biol Phys* **18**: 37–42.

Rezvani M, Birds DA, Hodges H *et al.* (2002). Modification of radiation myelopathy by the transplantation of neural stem cells in the rat. *Radiat Res* **156**: 408–412.

Robbins MEC, Zhao W (2004). Chronic oxidative stress and radiation-induced late normal tissue injury: a review. *Int J Radiat Biol* **80**: 251–259.

Rola R, Raber J, Rizk A *et al.* (2004). Radiation-induced impairment of hippocampal neurogenesis is associated with cognitive deficits in young mice. *Exp Neurol* **188**: 316–330.

Rola R, Sarkissian V, Obenaus A *et al.* (2005). High-LET radiation induces inflammation and persistent changes in markers of hippocampal neurogenesis. *Radiat Res* **164**: 556–560.

Roman DD, Sperduto PW (1995). Neuropsychological effects of cranial radiation: current knowledge and future directions. *Int J Radiat Oncol Biol Phys* **31**: 983–998.

Rubin P, Casarett GW (1968). *Clinical Radiation Pathology* (Vols 1 and 2). Philadelphia, PA: WB Saunders.

Sarkissian V (2005). The sequelae of cranial irradiation on human cognition. *Neurosci Lett* **382**: 118–123.

Schultheiss TE, Stephens LC (1992). Permanent radiation myelopathy. *Br J Radiol* **65**: 737–753.

Schultheiss TE, Kun LE, Ang KK *et al.* (1995). Radiation response of the central nervous system. *Int J Radiat Oncol Biol Phys* **31**: 1093–1112.

Shaw E, Arusell R, Scheithauer B *et al.* (2002). A prospective randomized trial of low-versus high-dose radiation therapy in adults with supratentorial low-grade glioma: initial report of a NCCTG-RTOG-ECOG Study. *J Clin Oncol* **20**: 2267–2276.

Sheline GE, Wara WM, Smith V (1980). Therapeutic irradiation and brain injury. *Int J Radiat Oncol Biol Phys* **6**: 1215–1218.

Siegal T, Pfeffer MR, Meltzer A *et al.* (1996). Cellular and secretory mechanisms related to delayed radiation-induced microvessel dysfunction in the spinal cord of rats. *Int J Radiat Oncol Biol Phys* **36**: 649–659.

Sklar CA, Constine LS (1995). Chronic neuroendocrinological sequelae of radiation therapy. *Int J Radiat Oncol Biol Phys* **31**: 1113–1122.

Sminia P, Van Der Kleij AJ, Carl UM *et al.* (2003). Prophylactic hyperbaric oxygen treatment and rat spinal cord irradiation. *Cancer Lett* **191**: 59–65.

Snyder JS, Kee N, Wojtowicz JM (2003). Effects of adult neurogenesis on synaptic plasticity in the rat dentate gyrus. *J Neurophysiol* **85**: 2423–2431.

Song H, Stevens CF, Gage FH (2002). Astroglia induce neurogenesis from adult neural stem cells. *Nature* **417**: 39–44.

Spence AM, Krohn KA, Edmonson SW *et al.* (1986). Radioprotection in rat spinal cord with WR-2721 following cerebral lateral intraventricular injection. *Int J Radiat Oncol Biol Phys* **12**: 1479–1482.

Stoll G, Jander S (1999). The role of microglia and macrophages in the pathophysiology of the CNS. *Prog Neurobiol* **58**: 233–247.

Surma-aho O, Niemalä M, Vilkki J *et al.* (2001). Adverse long-term effects of brain radiotherapy in adult low-grade glioma patients. *Neurology* **56**: 1285–1290.

Tofilon PJ, Fike JR (2000). The radioresponse of the central nervous system: a dynamic process. *Radiat Res* **153**: 357–370.

Van Der Maazen RWM, Kleiboer BJ, Verhagen I *et al.* (1991a). Irradiation in vitro discriminates between different O-2A progenitor cell subpopulations in the perinatal central nervous system of rats. *Radiat Res* **128**: 64–72.

Van Der Maazen RWM, Verhagen I, Kleiboer BJ *et al.* (1991b). Radiosensitivity of glial progenitor cells of the prenatal and adult rat optic nerve studies by an in vitro clonogenic assay. *Radiother Oncol* **20**: 258–264.

Van Den Maazen RWM, Kleiboer BJ, Berhagen I *et al.* (1993). Repair capacity of adult rat glial progenitor cells determined by an in vitro clonogenic assay after in vitro or in vivo fractionated irradiation. *Int J Radiat Biol* **63**: 661–666.

Van Rossum D, Hanisch UK (2004). Microglia. *Metab Brain Dis* **19**: 393–411.

Vaughan DW, Peters A (1974). Neuroglial cells in the cerebral cortex of rats from young adulthood to old age: an electron microscopic study. *J Neurocytol* **3**: 405–429.

Volterra A, Meldelosi J (2005). Astrocytes from brain glue to communication elements: the revolution continues. *Nat Rev Neurosci* **6**: 626–640.

Weitzner MA, Meyers CA, Gelke CK *et al.* (1995). The Functional Assessment of Cancer Therapy (FACT) scale: development of a brain subscale and revalidation of the general version (FACT-G) in patients with primary brain tumors. *Cancer* **75**: 1151–1161.

Zhao W, Payne V, Tommasi E *et al.* (2007). Administration of the peroxisomal proliferator-activated receptor γ agonist pioglitazone during fractionated brain irradiation prevents radiation-induced cognitive impairment. *Int J Radiat Oncol Biol Phys* **67**: 6–9.

8

Cognitive dysfunction related to chemotherapy and biological response modifiers

Jeffrey S. Wefel, Robert Collins, and Anne E. Kayl

Chemotherapy-related cognitive dysfunction

The successful management of many cancers has been achieved largely through aggressive use of therapy, which now generally combines surgery, radiation, chemotherapy, and immunotherapy. Many of these treatment strategies, including chemotherapy, are not highly specific and therefore place normal tissues and organs at risk. While the brain is afforded some protection from systemic treatments via the blood–brain barrier, it is increasingly recognized that many agents gain access to this environment via direct and/or indirect mechanisms, potentially contributing to central nervous system (CNS) toxicity. Furthermore, treatment strategies designed to disrupt or penetrate the blood–brain barrier are being explored as treatment options for a number of cancers including primary CNS lymphoma and brain metastases (Doolittle *et al.*, 2006). Evidence will be presented supporting the existence of both chemotherapy-related cognitive dysfunction and unique neurobehavioral/psychiatric manifestations associated with biological response modifiers generally, and interferon alpha in particular.

Incidence and nature of chemotherapy-related cognitive dysfunction

Adult patients presenting with complaints of "chemobrain" or "chemofog" typically report cognitive symptoms arising soon after initiating treatment. For many patients, these symptoms persist even after therapy is complete. It is not uncommon for many patients and providers to treat these symptoms as an expected, albeit unfortunate, side-effect of treatment. Persistent symptoms are also a cause of considerable distress for individuals who are unable to return to their previous scholastic, occupational, or social activities (or are able to do so only with significant additional mental effort). There has been additional concern that cancer and cancer therapies may increase an individual's susceptibility to late emerging cognitive dysfunction (Heflin *et al.*, 2005); however, this has yet to be conclusively established (Roe *et al.*, 2005; Wefel & Meyers, 2005).

The most commonly described cognitive problems include difficulties with memory, attention, information-processing speed, and organization (i.e., executive dysfunction). In patients with chemotherapy-related cognitive dysfunction, the

Cognition and Cancer, eds. Christina A. Meyers and James R. Perry. Published by Cambridge University Press.

neuropsychological evaluation frequently uncovers difficulties in sustaining focused attention that parallel patient reports of episodes during which they "space out" and lose their concentration. Deficits in working memory and executive function are also common and may correspond to patient reports of disorganization and difficulty multi-tasking. Measures of information-processing speed and fine motor function suggest further inefficiencies in cognitive and motor functions. Memory testing is generally consistent with reduced learning efficiency and memory-retrieval deficits in the context of relatively better memory consolidation processes. This reflects patient reports of forgetfulness for recent events and details of conversations, misplacing items, and repeating themselves in conversations. Notably, it is rare to see syndromes of aphasia, agnosia or apraxia that suggest disturbance in cortical brain areas. This pattern of cognitive performance is suggestive of preferential dysfunction of frontal subcortical networks (Kayl et al., 2006).

While there is rich anecdotal and clinical evidence for the existence of "chemobrain" (Staat & Segatore, 2005), the cognitive and neurobehavioral sequelae associated with chemotherapeutic agents have rarely been systematically studied. An emerging body of literature is beginning to characterize the cognitive and neurobehavioral sequelae of chemotherapeutic agents with chemotherapy-related cognitive dysfunction occurring in 15%–70% of patients (Bender et al., 2006; Moleski, 2000; Shilling et al., 2005; Wefel et al., 2004b). However, few methodologically rigorous studies exist to guide clinical practice. Most studies are retrospective, fail to incorporate assessments of pre-treatment cognitive and neurobehavioral function, consist of small and heterogeneous samples of patients who often received heterogeneous chemotherapeutic regimens, lack appropriate control groups, and suffer from poor measurement selection. Further studies are clearly warranted to address both the possible acute sequelae and the long-term effects of these treatments. A recently published meta-analysis (Anderson-Hanley et al., 2003) summarizing the cognitive sequelae of chemotherapy based on heterogeneous studies in adult cancer patients treated with chemotherapy reported statistically significant deficits in memory, executive, and motor function compared to normative expectations. However, when studies without a pre-treatment baseline evaluation were excluded, there was no evidence of a statistically significant effect on domains of cognitive function. This may reflect: (1) that the disease itself contributes to the cognitive dysfunction experienced by patients even before they receive potentially neurotoxic therapies (Wefel et al., 2004a); (2) that a subgroup of patients generally appear to develop these neurotoxicities suggesting pharmacogenetic vulnerabilities; and (3) that there is variability across different chemotherapeutic agents in their degree of neurotoxicity. For example, CI-980 was studied in a Phase II trial as a potential therapy for individuals with ovarian and colorectal cancer. This agent is a synthetic mitotic inhibitor that shares structural and functional similarities with colchicine, crosses the blood–brain barrier, and binds to tubulin at the colchicine-binding site. Cognitive testing including monitoring of memory function was a component of this protocol due to colchicine's ability to selectively damage cholinergic neurons in and around the hippocampus and basal forebrain, structures critical to learning and memory functions. Serial testing demonstrated declines in memory function using standardized neuropsychological measures (Meyers et al., 1997).

In the pediatric literature, there is mixed evidence for chemotherapy-related cognitive and neurobehavioral dysfunction. The majority of these studies were completed in patients diagnosed with acute lymphocytic leukemia (ALL) or brain tumors, and were frequently complicated by the administration of cerebral radiation. However, after multi-agent chemotherapy for ALL there are reports of deficits in attention, memory, visuoconstruction, visuomotor and tactile-perceptual skills, as well as achievement in arithmetic and, less frequently, spelling and reading skills (Moleski, 2000; Moor, 2005). Please refer to Chapters 6 and 14 for a more detailed review of the cognitive and neurobehavioral sequelae of cancer and cancer therapy in children.

Patients may also report symptoms of depression, anxiety, and fatigue. While there are many studies demonstrating the relationship between alterations in mood and cognitive dysfunction in other populations, studies of chemotherapy-related cognitive dysfunction have consistently failed to demonstrate such a link. Moreover, patient-reported cognitive dysfunction does not correlate with objective evidence of cognitive dysfunction (as assessed through formal, standardized neuropsychological testing). Rather, mood disturbance is positively correlated with self-reported cognitive dysfunction (Castellon et al., 2004; Jenkins et al., 2006; Schagen et al., 2002). Thus, comprehensive neuropsychological assessments are necessary to assist in the differential diagnosis of cognitive dysfunction and/or mood disorder.

Common neurologic toxicities have been characterized for a host of chemotherapeutic agents (see Table 8.1) and include a variety of non-specific neurologic syndromes including: *acute encephalopathy* characterized by a confusional state, insomnia, and often agitation; *chronic encephalopathy* characterized by cognitive dysfunction consistent with a "subcortical dementia," incontinence, and gait disturbance; *leukoencephalopathy*; a *cerebellar syndrome* with symptoms ranging from ataxia to a pancerebellar syndrome; and a variety of *peripheral neuropathies*. Unfortunately, it is often difficult to discern the specific effect attributable to individual agents as they are commonly administered in multi-agent combinations.

Risk factors and mechanisms underlying cognitive and neurobehavioral toxicity

Although the relationship between chemotherapy and cognitive dysfunction has not been fully elucidated, there is agreement that cognitive dysfunction associated with chemotherapy is a measurable toxicity. Several risk factors have been identified that appear to increase the risk of developing neurotoxicity associated with chemotherapy, including: (1) exposure to higher doses due to planned use of high-dose regimens or high concentrations of the parent drug and/or its metabolite due to impaired

systemic clearance and/or pharmacogenetic modulation of drug pharmacokinetics (Shah, 2005); (2) additive or synergistic effects of multi-agent chemotherapy; (3) additive or synergistic effects of multi-modality therapy that includes administration of chemotherapy either concurrently with or subsequent to cerebral radiation (Sheline et al., 1980; Sul & DeAngelis, 2006); (4) intra-arterial administration with blood–brain barrier disruption; and (5) intrathecal administration (Delattre & Posner, 1995; Jansen et al., 2005; Keime-Guibert et al., 1998; Sul & DeAngelis, 2006; Taphoorn & Klein, 2004; Weiss & Vogelzang, 1993).

The mechanisms by which these agents impact CNS function have been reported to occur through both direct and indirect pathways. It is also likely that the influence of specific mechanisms varies at different time points in the course of an emerging neurotoxicity. Though not exhaustive, Table 8.2 provides an overview of the mechanisms that may be involved in the development of cognitive and neurobehavioral toxicities.

Metabolic abnormalities can be induced by various chemotherapeutic agents and may be responsible for alterations in cognitive and neurobehavioral function. Both high and intermediate doses of 5-fluorouracil (5-FU) have been reported to cause encephalopathy in association with hyperammonemia. With normalization of ammonia levels, the encephalopathy resolved (Kim et al., 2006). Methotrexate, a folate antagonist, has been reported to decrease dihydrofolate reductase leading to deficiencies in *S*-adenosylmethionine (SAM). A deficiency of SAM has been associated with demyelination (Shuper et al., 2000), and polymorphisms of genes involved in methionine metabolism appear to place individuals at greater risk for this neurotoxicity (Linnebank et al., 2005). Methotrexate has also been reported to lead to hyperhomocysteinemia, high levels of neurotransmitters including homocysteic acid, cysteine sulfinic acid, and homocysteine sulfonic acid, and toxic levels of adenosine. These abnormalities may lead to *mineralizing microangiopathy* in the white matter, *NMDA-mediated excitotoxicity*, and *alterations in brain monoamines* (i.e., norepinephrine, dopamine,

Table 8.1. Primary neurotoxicities associated with chemotherapeutic agents. (*BCNU* Bischloroethyl nitrosurea, carmustine, *CHOP* cyclophosphamide, adriamycin, vincristine and prednisone, *5-FU* 5-fluorouracil, *SERMs* selective estrogen receptor inhibitors, *VM-26* teniposide, *VP-16* etoposide)

Syndrome/mechanism	Chemotherapy
Acute encephalopathy[e]	Ara-C
	L-Asparaginase
	Cisplatin
	5-FU
	Fludarabine[a]
	Thalidomide
	Pentostatin[a]
	Ifosfamide
	Interferon alpha
	Interleukin-1 and -2
	Methotrexate[a,b,c]
	Nitrosureas[a,d]
	Procarbazine
	Vincristine
	Tamoxifen
	VP-16[a]
Leukoencephalopathy[e]	Ara-C
	L-Asparaginase
	BCNU[a,d]
	Cisplatin
	Cyclophosphamide
	5-FU
	Fludarabine[a]
	Ifosfamide
	Methotrexate[a]
	Nitrosureas
	Paclitaxel
	Vincristine
Reversible posterior leukoencephalopathy	Ara-C
	Cisplatin
	Multi-agent chemo such as CHOP and other combinations (including the following agents: adriamycin, cyclophosphamide, vincristine, ifosfamide, etoposide, and Ara-C)
	Fludarabine[a]
	Ciclosporin
	Tacrolimus
Seizures	Ara-C
	L-Asparaginase
	BCNU[a,d]
	Busulfan[a]

Table 8.1. (*cont.*)

Syndrome/mechanism	Chemotherapy
	Cisplatin
	Cyclophosphamide[a]
	5-FU
	Fludarabine[a]
	Ifosfamide
	Interferon alpha[a]
	Interleukin-2
	Methotrexate[a]
	Vincristine
	VP-16[a]
Chronic encephalopathy[e]	Ara-C[b,c]
	BCNU[a,c]
	Carmofur
	Fludarabine[a]
	5-FU (± levamisole)
	Ifosfamide
	Methotrexate[a,b,c]
Cerebellar syndrome	Ara-C
	Cytosine arabinoside[a]
	5-FU (± levamisole)
	Methotrexate
	Procarbazine
Peripheral neuropathy	Ara-C
	Cisplatin
	Carboplatin
	Oxaliplatin
	Procarbazine
	Suramin
	Taxanes (paclitaxel, docetaxel)
	Thalidomide
	Vinca alkaloids (vincristine, vinorelbine)
	VM-26
	VP-16
Cardiotoxicity	Anthracyclines (adriamycin, epirubicin)
Ototoxicity[e]	Carboplatin
	Cisplatin
Chemotherapy-related alterations in hormonal function	Alkylating agents
	Carboplatin
	Cisplatin
	Doxorubicin
	5-FU
	Methotrexate

(*cont.*)

Table 8.1. (*cont.*)

Syndrome/mechanism	Chemotherapy
	SERMs
	Aromatase inhibitors
	Estrogen antagonists
	Androgen deprivation therapy
Chemotherapy-related anemia	Myelosuppressive chemotherapies[f]

Note: Adapted from: Delattre & Posner, 1995; Jansen *et al.*, 2005; Keime-Guibert *et al.*, 1998; Rottenberg, 1991; Sul & DeAngelis, 2006; Weiss & Vogelzang, 1993.
[a] Especially if given in high doses.
[b] Especially if administered intrathecally.
[c] Especially if administered intravenously.
[d] Especially if administered intra-arterially.
[e] Especially if therapy includes both chemotherapy and radiation therapy.
[f] See review article by Groopman and Itri (1999).

serotonin) (Haykin *et al.*, 2006; Madhyastha *et al.*, 2002; Quinn & Kamen, 1996). Encephalopathy has also been reported in association with the syndrome of inappropriate antidiuretic hormone secretion (SIADH) secondary to intravenous vincrisitine or cyclophosphamide treatment (Lipp, 1999), hyperglycemia secondary to L-asparaginase, streptozocin or corticosteroid use, and salt-wasting nephropathy due to cisplatin (Gilbert & Armstrong, 1996).

Across all classes of chemotherapeutic agents, *anemia* has been estimated to occur in up to 80% of patients (Cunningham, 2003) and is a well known side-effect of myelosuppressive chemotherapies. Anemia may cause cerebral hypoxia due to diminished circulating erythrocyte levels and hemoglobin concentration (Birgegård *et al.*, 2005) and is associated with patient reports of reduced quality of life, as well as *fatigue* and cognitive dysfunction (Groopman & Itri, 1999; O'Shaughnessy *et al.*, 2005; Wagner *et al.*, 2005).

Chemotherapy-induced menopause (Knobf, 2006; Molina *et al.*, 2005) and treatments targeting sex-hormone systems in both women (Eberling *et al.*, 2004; Jenkins *et al.*, 2004) and men (Green *et al.*, 2002; Jenkins *et al.*, 2005; Mottet *et al.*, 2006) have been implicated in the development of cog-

nitive dysfunction. In women, the incidence of ovarian failure due to chemotherapy is variable (20%–100%) and depends on the patient's age, the

Table 8.2. Potential mechanisms of chemotherapy-associated cognitive and neurobehavioral dysfunction

Acute/subacute	
∨	Metabolic abnormalities
∨	Alterations in excitatory neurotransmitters
∨	Anemia
∨	Fatigue
∨	Hormonal dysfunction
∨	Secondary inflammatory response
∨	Indirect chemical toxicity and oxidative stress
∨	Myeloencephalopathy
∨	Demyelination
∨	Leukoencephalopathy
∨	Microvascular injury
∨	Direct neurotoxic injury to cerebral parenchyma
∨	Cerebral atrophy
∨	Non-CNS organ toxicity (e.g., cardiotoxicity)
Late/delayed	Secondary malignancies

dose and regimen of chemotherapy, and prior or concurrent use of radiation therapy (Molina *et al.*, 2005). Estrogen receptors have been found in the hypothalamus, anterior pituitary, amygdala, and CA1 of the hippocampus (McEwen & Alves, 1999). The mechanisms by which estrogen benefits cognitive function include: (1) increasing cholinergic activity through its actions on choline acetyl-transferase; (2) maintenance of dendritic spine density on CA1 pyramidal cells of the hippocampus; (3) facilitating induction of long-term potentiation in the hippocampus; (4) increasing serotonergic and cholinergic activity; (5) altering lipoprotein; and (6) decreasing the risk of cerebral ischemia (Yaffe *et al.*, 1998). It remains unclear whether the cognitive and neurobehavioral effects of hormonal manipulations arise through the estrogen receptors (including aromatization of androgens to estradiol in men) or via androgen receptors. Please refer to Chapter 9 for a more comprehensive review of this literature.

Pro-inflammatory cytokine activation may contribute to the cognitive and neurobehavioral sequelae associated with chemotherapy. Several studies have reported increases in interleukins IL-1β, -6, -8, -10, IFN-γ, tumor necrosis factor alpha (TNF-α), and granulocyte monocyte colony stimulating factor associated with different schedules of paclitaxel, docetaxel, etoposide and carboplatin (Penson *et al.*, 2000; Pusztai *et al.*, 2004; Tsavaris *et al.*, 2002). The ability of distinct chemotherapeutic agents to induce similar pro-inflammatory cytokine activity has been hypothesized to occur through the common activation of p38 mitogen-activated protein kinase (Wood *et al.*, 2006). Alternatively, the appearance of cancer-related symptom clusters after exposure to different cytokines has been attributed to activation of nuclear factor-kappa B (Lee *et al.*, 2004). Similarly, adriamycin has been demonstrated to increase *oxidative stress* in the brain, which may lead to cell dysfunction or cell death and thus contribute to the symptoms of chemobrain (Joshi *et al.*, 2005).

Myeloencephalopathy may develop after intrathecal administration of vincristine (Alcaraz *et al.*, 2002) or methotrexate (Garcia-Tena *et al.*, 1995) with devastating adverse effects. This subacute process typically occurs within days to weeks after treatment and can involve progressive limb weakness, cranial nerve palsies, seizures, visual disturbance, coma, and even death (Moleski, 2000). Methotrexate, especially when accompanied by radiation therapy, has also been reported to cause *microvascular injury* including mineralizing microangiopathy, vasodilatation, endothelial damage, and stroke-like *leukoencephalopathy* (Moleski, 2000). Whether this represents ischemic events, *demyelination* or edema within the cerebral white matter is a matter of ongoing research (Brown *et al.*, 1998; Haykin *et al.*, 2006).

Gray and white matter volume loss as well as hippocampal atrophy have been described in association with some chemotherapeutic treatments (Madhyastha *et al.*, 2002; Saykin *et al.*, 2003; Schneiderman, 2004). However, these findings have not always been replicated (Yoshikawa *et al.*, 2005) suggesting the need for further investigation. Appreciation of the ability of the adult brain to generate new neurons has stimulated investigation into questions regarding the impact of chemotherapies on neurogenesis. Crandall *et al.* (2004) reported that long-term exposure to 13-*cis*-retinoic acid was associated with decreased hippocampal neurogenesis and cell proliferation in the hippocampus and subventricular zone as well as impaired spatial learning and memory in young adult mice. Other late emerging side-effects that may be associated with cognitive and neurobehavioral dysfunction include the development of *cardiotoxicity* (e.g., myopericarditis, arrhythmia, pericardial effusion, cardiomyopathy, congestive heart failure) (Jensen, 2006; Johnson, 2006; Lipshultz, 2006; Steinherz & Yahalom, 1993) and secondary malignancies (e.g., leukemia and myelodysplastic syndrome) (Shapiro & Recht, 2001).

Neuroimaging and neurophysiologic correlates of chemotherapy-related cognitive dysfunction

Chemotherapy-related structural imaging changes, primarily involving the white matter, have been frequently identified as possible manifestations of a neurotoxic syndrome. However, recent high-dose chemotherapeutic protocols used in the management of primary CNS lymphoma have demonstrated a dissociation between imaging findings and cognitive outcomes with patients developing treatment-related white matter pathology in the context of stable cognitive function (Fliessbach *et al.*, 2003).

Functional neuroimaging techniques are beginning to be utilized to help understand the appearance of cognitive dysfunction, the underlying mechanisms of that dysfunction, and the potential for recovery of cognitive processes (see Chapter 3). Silverman *et al.* (2007) compared female breast cancer survivors who had been treated with chemotherapy 5–10 years previously and breast cancer survivors and non-breast cancer survivors with no history of chemotherapy exposure. During a memory-related cognitive activation paradigm, [^{15}O] water positron emission tomography (PET) revealed increased activation in the left inferior frontal gyrus and posterior cerebellum near the midline for chemotherapy-treated survivors and in the left parietal region for untreated survivors. Resting metabolism, as evaluated by [^{18}F]-fluorodeoxyglucose PET, did not differ significantly between the groups. However, survivors treated with both chemotherapy and tamoxifen showed decreased metabolism in the lentiform nucleus compared to survivors treated with chemotherapy alone.

Electroencephalography (EEG) with event-related potentials has also been employed to study aspects of information processing in female breast cancer survivors who had been treated with chemotherapy 2–5 years earlier and with tamoxifen (Kreukels *et al.*, 2006). Survivors who received high-dose therapy demonstrated decreased P3 amplitude relative to untreated controls, but were not significantly different from survivors treated with standard-dose chemotherapy.

A variety of metabolic and evoked potential techniques have been used to evaluate brain function in pediatric ALL survivors treated with methotrexate (Moleski, 2000). Abnormalities of cerebral glucose

metabolism rate have been detected, with evidence suggesting a relationship between lower IQ and lower thalamus-to-cortex ratio. Cortical hypoperfusion has been demonstrated using single photon emission computed tomography (SPECT). In addition, EEG studies have documented increased P300 latency and slowed reaction times after treatment, with significant correlations between P300 latencies and IQ and achievement test scores.

Pharmacogenetic modulation of chemotherapy-related cognitive dysfunction

Clinically, and in most studies to date, cognitive and neurobehavioral dysfunction has been found to occur only in a subgroup of patients. This finding has provoked interest in clarifying the pharmacogenetic differences that may underlie an individual's vulnerability to these side-effects. Polymorphisms that alter the pharmacodynamics of chemotherapeutic agents may place individuals at greater risk through increased exposure to potentially toxic agents secondary to reduced detoxification and/or increased permeability of agents across the blood–brain barrier (Largillier *et al.*, 2006; McAllister *et al.*, 2004; Okcu *et al.*, 2004). In children with leukemia treated with methotrexate-containing regimens with or without cranial radiation, polymorphisms of genes modulating the folate pathway have been associated with diminished IQ (Krajinovic *et al.*, 2005). The relationships between polymorphisms in genes responsible for various repair processes (e.g., apolipoprotein E) and the development of cognitive dysfunction are receiving increased attention (Ahles *et al.*, 2003; Chen *et al.*, 1997). Recent studies have also examined the relationship between brain-derived neurotrophic factor and memory (Egan *et al.*, 2003), and catechol-O-methyl transferase and executive function (Egan *et al.*, 2001). There is evidence that polymorphisms in these genes are related to differences in cognitive function amongst healthy individuals. It is unknown whether these same polymorphisms confer an additional risk to an individual exposed to a potentially neurotoxic treatment.

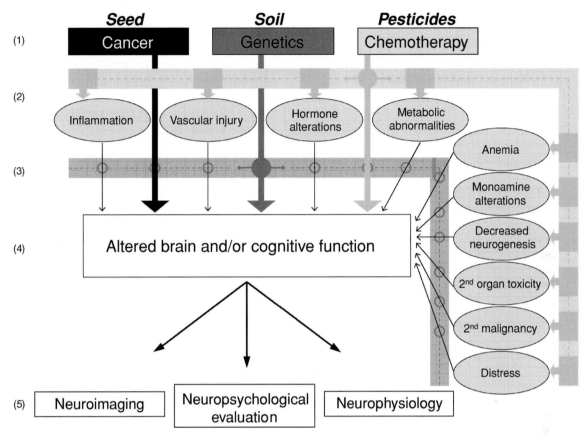

Figure 8.1. A conceptual model of the relationship between cancer, chemotherapy, and genetics in the development of abnormalities in brain and/or cognitive function

Figure 8.1 provides a model by which disease ("seed"), genetics ("soil"), and therapies ("pesticides") may impact on brain structure and function. For ease of discussion this model has been organized into 5 layers. Layer 1 lists three primary potential contributing factors to altered brain and/or cognitive function (layer 4). There are likely direct effects of the disease, the therapy, and host genetics on brain and/or cognitive function, which are represented by the large arrows. Layer 2 shows the mechanisms by which chemotherapy is believed to affect brain and/or cognitive function and is represented by the light gray ovals. The dark gray bar in layer 3 demonstrates the modulatory effect that host genetic characteristics are believed to exert on the expression of altered brain and/or cognitive func-

tion. Layer 5 represents the methods that have been employed to measure and characterize the alterations in brain and/or cognitive function including structural and functional neuroimaging techniques, neurophysiologic studies, and neuropsychological evaluations. Importantly, the mechanisms represented in layer 2 are not believed to be mutually exclusive and it is likely that a number of these mechanisms directly and indirectly influence the expression of one other. For example, inflammatory processes such as cytokine activation may directly affect brain and/or cognitive function and also contribute to vascular injury, which itself can lead to altered brain and/or cognitive function. Additionally, cancer may invoke a variety of the mechanisms associated with chemotherapy (i.e., inflammation, metabolic abnormalities) and thereby contribute to alterations in brain and/or cognitive function.

Biological response modifiers

Modification of the cancer patient's immune response, such that a therapeutic advantage is subsequently conferred, is the underlying principle of treating with biological response modifiers (BRMs; also referred to as immunotherapy) (National Institutes of Health, 2003). Given the various means by which a person's immune system can respond to foreign substances, BRMs represent a wide range of treatments that often differ fundamentally in their mechanisms. Cytokines, vaccines, monoclonal antibodies, thymic factors, and colony stimulating factors are all examples of BRMs (Clark, 1996). Biological response modifiers can: (1) directly or indirectly augment the patient's immunological defenses; (2) modify tumor cells such that the patient's immunological response is increased; or (3) bolster the patient's ability to manage toxicities secondary to other cancer treatments (Mihich, 2000). It should also be noted that some chemotherapy drugs (e.g., adriamycin, vincristine, cyclophosphamide), which are typically thought to be *immunosuppressive*, can produce *immunoaugmentative* effects (depending on dosing and regimen) and under certain circumstances convey a therapeutic benefit through augmentation of a patient's antitumor host defense (Mihich, 2000).

The impact of treatment with BRMs on cognition is complex, in part due to the wide ranging mechanisms by which these agents act. Monoclonal antibodies, which recognize specific antigens, are generally not thought to produce neurotoxic effects or secondary cognitive impairment. Colony stimulating factors, such as hematopoietic growth factors, may improve overall quality of life and ameliorate cognitive impairment that occurs secondary to treatment-related anemia (Brown *et al.*, 1991; Massa *et al.*, 2006). Other BRMs (e.g., interleukins), like many chemotherapy agents, have

been associated with the development of cognitive dysfunction. Some BRMs may also cause psychiatric symptoms such as depression or hallucinations that may require additional treatment. The remainder of this chapter will focus on the cytokine interferon alpha (IFN-α), which demonstrates the potential neurotoxic effects of these agents in terms of both producing cognitive dysfunction and inducing affective distress. As with the literature examining the effects of chemotherapy on cognition, there are few well-designed studies in the cancer population that fully elucidate the effects of IFN-α, and even fewer that assess the association of other BRMs (e.g., IFN-β, interleukins, TNF-α, etc.) with cognitive dysfunction. While it is beyond the scope of this chapter to review the putative mechanisms for all of the BRMs, the reader is encouraged to use the existing literature on IFN-α as a model.

Interferon alpha

Interferon alpha prevents carcinogenesis by inducing an innate immunological response from the patient. While the exact mechanism through which IFN works has not been fully elucidated, the downstream effects are natural killer and T cell responsiveness driving an immunological response, which, in turn, exerts an effect on cellular proliferation and differentiation (Krause *et al.*, 2003; Meyers & Whiteside, 1996; Tompkins, 1999). That IFN induces a natural immunological response explains its use in the treatment of a variety of medical conditions, including malignancies, infectious diseases, and neurodegenerative diseases (Cirelly & Tyring, 1995; Meyers & Valentine, 1995). For example, IFN has demonstrated effectiveness, and is approved by the Food and Drug Administration (FDA), for the treatment of chronic myelogenous leukemia, hepatitis C, and melanoma. Interferon has also been used for the treatment of multiple sclerosis, amytrophic lateral sclerosis, and HIV-1, with limited success. In combination with chemotherapy (i.e., 13-*cis*-retinoic acid, CRA), IFN has received recent attention as a viable component in the preventative treatment of advanced squamous cell carcinoma of the head and neck (Büntzel & Küttner, 1998; Shin *et al.*, 2001), although the benefit of CRA and IFN may be most robust for locally advanced disease rather than metastatic disease (Shin *et al.*, 2002).

Interferon-related side-effects

The side-effect profile for IFN is an important consideration, as neurotoxicity may prohibit patients from gaining maximum benefit from the therapy (Valentine *et al.*, 1998). Approximately 11% of patients treated with IFN elect to discontinue treatment because of adverse effects (Spiegel, 1989). Negative effects are seen immediately after initial treatment, as many patients experience flu-like symptoms (e.g., fever, chills, body aches, etc.). In most cases this is transient and responsive to non-steroidal anti-inflammatory agents (Meyers & Valentine, 1995). In normal, healthy controls, a single dose of 1.5 million international units (MIU) has been shown to decrease reaction time 6 h and 10 h after injection (Smith *et al.*, 1988). (As a reference, most cancer patients receive much higher doses for longer periods of time.) Fatigue tends to be the most serious side-effect, often persisting for the duration of treatment, and is most frequently reported across trials. It is estimated that between 70% and 100% of patients undergoing IFN treatment experience fatigue, with 10%–40% requiring dose reduction (Malik *et al.*, 2001). Psychiatric symptoms, usually increased depression, are also reported in 15%–50% of patients receiving IFN treatment (Dieperink *et al.*, 2000; Meyers *et al.*, 1991; Valentine & Meyers, 2005), although the clinical picture may vary to include mania.

Increased depression has been observed within the first month of treatment and has been linked to neurovegetative, emotional/affective, and cognitive symptoms (Capuron *et al.*, 2004). Consistent with this, the effects of IFN for the treatment of chronic myelogenous leukemia (IFN alone and in combination with chemotherapy) were shown to increase depressive symptoms independent of fatigue (Scheibel *et al.*, 2004). Both fatigue and mood alterations tend to remit following cessation

of treatment, although persisting effects of each have been noted (Malik *et al.*, 2001; Meyers *et al.*, 1991; Strite *et al.*, 1997). Antidepressant pharmacotherapies have been found to be effective in a number of trials (Goldman, 1994; Malek-Ahmadi & Ghandour, 2004; Musselman *et al.*, 2001; Valentine & Meyers, 2005). Many argue that pre-treatment screening coupled with close serial monitoring of a patient's mood is an appropriate strategy to balance the risks of this neurotoxicity against the potential adverse side effects of pharmacotherapies used prophylactically for symptom prevention (Valentine & Meyers, 2005).

Nature and course of interferon-related cognitive dysfunction

In addition to fatigue and increased depression, IFN has been associated with cognitive impairment. However, findings across studies have not been consistent, and there has been criticism with regard to methodological limitations and/or qualitative differences in the assessment of cognitive functioning. For example, Pavol *et al.* (1995) retrospectively assessed the cognitive functioning of 25 patients with chronic myelogenous leukemia undergoing treatment with IFN. There was variability with regard to IFN dosage and chronicity of treatment, with an average weekly dose of 51 MIU (range: 17–77) for 26 months (range: 1 week to 84 months). Patients evidenced impairments in verbal memory, visual motor scanning, and executive functioning, suggesting frontal subcortical network dysfunction. Given the nature of the design (i.e., no pre-treatment data available), however, it was not possible to conclude if the pattern of cognitive deficits was related to pre-existing depression or disease-related cognitive dysfunction. In contrast, Mayr *et al.* (1999) found improvements on four tasks (e.g., measure of attention, recall of a 10-digit number, three simple multiplication problems, and tapping a pencil for 30 s) in 14 patients with myeloproliferative disorders. All patients received IFN treatment for a year, with assessments at 3-month intervals post-baseline, with an average weekly dose of 25 MIU (range: 10–35). However, interpretation of their findings is limited by their selection of tasks, which have not been validated and may be susceptible to large uncontrolled practice effects. Bender *et al.* (2000) assessed information-processing speed and vigilance in 18 patients with melanoma randomized to high-dose IFN (100 MIU per week), low-dose IFN (9 MIU per week), or observation control (6 per arm) and reported no changes in cognitive functioning after a 3-month interval (between-group analyses were not made). Unfortunately, the design itself was likely underpowered ($n = 16$ and 13 at 3 and 6 months, respectively) and demographic and group data were not presented to facilitate more detailed analysis (Bender *et al.*, 2000).

To date, few methodologically rigorous studies have assessed the cognitive effects associated with IFN treatment. Caraceni *et al.* (1998) assessed focused attention, short-term memory, executive function, and mood in 64 patients randomized to IFN (dose = 9 MIU per week) or observation for the treatment of malignant melanoma. Patients were assessed at baseline, 1, 3, 6, and 12 months. For each patient, the largest negative change on each measure from any one of the assessments relative to baseline was determined and these were collapsed across groups to form outcome measures. Relative to baseline, IFN patients evidenced no changes on measures of cognition or mood. Group means and effect sizes were not reported. A significant selection bias appears possible, as the 64 patients agreeing to participate were a subset of the 113 enrolled in the actual clinical trial. More recently, Scheibel *et al.* (2004) assessed the cognitive effects of IFN for the treatment of chronic myelogenous leukemia. In all, 30 patients on protocols receiving IFN ($n = 13$, average weekly dose = 40 MIU) or IFN in combination with chemotherapy ($n = 17$, average weekly dose = 52 MIU) were assessed across domains of verbal memory, verbal fluency, graphomotor speed, visual motor scanning and sequencing, and mood. Evidence for cognitive dysfunction was found in both groups, as over half of the patients in the study evidenced a decline of at least 1.5 SD on at least one or more of the cognitive measures. Increases in depressive symptoms across groups

were also noted, independent of cognitive dysfunction. Declines over time on measures of divided attention and graphomotor speed were demonstrated for both treatment groups, whereas the combination therapy additionally produced declines on measures of verbal learning and verbal fluency. The authors suggest the findings are not inconsistent with frontal-subcortical dysfunction (i.e., impaired information processing and executive functioning) but their data appear to more reliably support frontal subcortical dysfunction in the combination group alone, rather than both IFN and combination treatments. There is, however, some evidence supporting IFN-related frontal subcortical dysfunction, as patients exhibiting neurotoxic effects from IFN demonstrated reversible diffuse EEG abnormalities with intermittent delta activity (e.g., slowing) in the frontal lobes (Farkkila *et al.*, 1984; Honigsberger *et al.*, 1983; Smedley *et al.*, 1983). Additionally, hypometabolism in the prefrontal cortex has been reported following low-dose treatment with IFN (Juengling *et al.*, 2000).

Mechanisms underlying cognitive and neurobehavioral toxicity

The mechanisms by which IFN causes cognitive effects, including possible alteration of frontal circuitry, are not fully understood (Malik *et al.*, 2001; Schaefer *et al.*, 2002; Valentine *et al.*, 1998). Numerous studies suggest: (1) changes in the endocrine system, (2) dysregulation of neurotransmitter systems, and (3) activation of secondary cytokine pathways as possible mechanisms (Schaefer *et al.*, 2002; Valentine *et al.*, 1998).

Interferon is structurally and functionally similar to adrenocorticotropic hormone (Blalock & Smith, 1980; Blalock & Stanton, 1980) and is known to stimulate cortisol release into the human bloodstream (Menzies *et al.*, 1996). Increased cortisol levels have been associated with mood disorders through perturbations of the hypothalamic–pituitary–adrenal axis (HPA) (Nemeroff *et al.*, 1992). Endocrinologic disturbance including disruption of the hypothalamic–pituitary–thyroid axis (HPT) resulting in thyroid abnormalities may also contribute to the mood and cognitive dysfunction associated with IFN therapy (Valentine *et al.*, 1998).

Interferon interacts directly with the opioid receptor system, as it is structurally similar to endogenous opioids (Blalock & Smith, 1980), and some of the clinical manifestations of IFN treatment are similar to opioid-like effects (e.g., catatonia and analgesia). Moreover, IFN may indirectly modulate other neurotransmitter systems (e.g., dopamine, serotonin), through either opioidergic or secondary cytokine mechanisms (Schaefer *et al.*, 2003).

Though not well studied, IFN influences other cytokines, specifically inducing the production of interleukins IL-1, IL-2, IL-6 and TNF (Taylor & Grossberg, 1998). These particular cytokines are known to play a central role in stimulation of the HPA and suppression of the HPT (Zaloga *et al.*, 2001). As previously noted, HPA and HPT alterations may explain mood and cognitive changes during treatment. Moreover, animal models suggest that cytokines (e.g., IL-2) modulate serotonin levels in the prefrontal cortex (Lacosta *et al.*, 2000).

Intervention strategies to prevent or manage cognitive and neurobehavioral dysfunction

Chemotherapy and immunotherapy are necessary components of the management and eradication of many types of cancer. Although not all patients will experience treatment-related neurotoxicity, for a subpopulation of patients cognitive and/or behavioral symptoms are distressing and disruptive. Clearly, there is an opportunity and a very real need to explore therapies that may prevent negative side-effects or minimize the impact and extent of symptoms that are already present. Ideally, these interventions should be tailored to the symptom (e.g., anemia, durable fatigue, memory-retrieval deficit) and be based on the hypothesized mechanism. While determining the nature of the symptom is often feasible, our understanding of the etiologic mechanisms underlying these symptoms is limited in most cases.

Clinical experience and research has informed clinicians about the risks involved with certain regimens (e.g., high dose or intrathecal treatment) and administration schedules (e.g., concomitant use of radiation therapy and chemotherapy) such that many neurotoxicities have been reduced while continuing to achieve adequate cancer control (Keime-Guibert *et al.*, 1998; Lipp, 1999). In cases where a specific mechanism underlying the neurotoxicity has been characterized, targeted treatment strategies have been explored. For example, treatment with naltrexone (i.e., a μ-opioid receptor antagonist) was effective in relieving neurotoxic side-effects in seven of nine patients undergoing IFN treatment for hematological malignancies (Valentine *et al.*, 1995). Musselman *et al.* (2001) demonstrated the benefit of pre-treatment with paroxetine (selective serotonin reuptake inhibitor) in minimizing depression in melanoma patients receiving IFN treatment.

However, empirically supported therapies for persistent cognitive and neurobehavioral dysfunction are limited. Stimulant therapies have proven effective in treating the cognitive dysfunction that is common in cancer patients (Meyers *et al.*, 1998). Other pharmacologic interventions commonly used to treat other diseases affecting cognitive function are currently being explored (Barton & Loprinzi, 2002; see Chapter 22). Cognitive and behavioral intervention strategies that have been studied in the traditional rehabilitation literature with stroke and traumatic brain injury survivors may also be employed. These interventions often focus on compensatory strategy training, stress management, energy conservation and psycho-education (see Chapters 20, 21).

REFERENCES

Ahles TA, Saykin AJ, Noll WW *et al.* (2003). The relationship of APOE genotype to neuropsychological performance in long-term cancer survivors treated with standard dose chemotherapy. *Psychooncology* **12**: 612–619.

Alcaraz A, Rey C, Concha A *et al.* (2002). Intrathecal vincristine: fatal myeloencephalopathy despite cerebrospinal fluid perfusion. *J Toxicol Clin Toxicol* **40**: 557–561.

Anderson-Hanley C, Sherman ML, Riggs R *et al.* (2003). Neuropsychological effects of treatments for adults with cancer: a meta-analysis and review of the literature. *J Int Neuropsychol Soc* **9**: 967–982.

Barton D, Loprinzi C (2002). Novel approaches to preventing chemotherapy-induced cognitive dysfunction in breast cancer: the art of the possible. *Clin Breast Cancer* **3** [Suppl. 3]: S121–S127.

Bender CM, Yasko JM, Kirkwood JM *et al.* (2000). Cognitive function and quality of life in interferon therapy for melanoma. *Clin Nurs Res* **9**: 352–363.

Bender CM, Sereika SM, Berga SL *et al.* (2006). Cognitive impairment associated with adjuvant therapy in breast cancer. *Psychooncology* **15**: 422–430.

Birgegård G, Aapro MS, Bokemeyer C *et al.* (2005). Cancer-related anemia: pathogenesis, prevalence, and treatment. *Oncology* **68** [Suppl. 1], 3–11.

Blalock JE, Smith EM (1980). Human leukocyte interferon: structural and biological relatedness to adrenocorticotropic hormones and endorphins. *Proc Natl Acad Sci USA* **77**: 5972–5974.

Blalock JE, Stanton JD (1980). Common pathways of interferon and hormonal action. *Nature* **283**: 406–408.

Brown MS, Stemmer SM, Simon JH *et al.* (1998). White matter disease induced by high-dose chemotherapy: longitudinal study with MR imaging and proton spectroscopy. *Am J Neuroradiol* **19**: 217–221.

Brown WS, Marsh JT, Wolcott D *et al.* (1991). Cognitive function, mood and p3 latency: effects of the amelioration of anemia in dialysis patients. *Neuropsychologia* **29**: 35–45.

Büntzel J, Küttner K (1998). Chemoprevention with interferon alfa and 13-*cis* retinoic acid in the adjunctive treatment of head and neck cancer. *Auris Nasus Larynx* **25**: 413–418.

Capuron L, Ravaud A, Miller AH *et al.* (2004). Baseline mood and psychosocial characteristics of patients developing depressive symptoms during interleukin-2 and/or interferon-alpha cancer therapy. *Brain Behav Immun* **18**: 205–213.

Caraceni A, Gangeri L, Martini C *et al.* (1998). Neurotoxicity of interferon-α in melanoma therapy: results from a randomized clinical trial. *Cancer* **83**: 482–489.

Castellon SA, Ganz PA, Bower JE *et al.* (2004). Neurocognitive performance in breast cancer survivors exposed to adjuvant chemotherapy and tamoxifen. *J Clin Exp Neuropsychol* **26**: 955–969.

Chen Y, Lomnitski L, Michaelson DM *et al.* (1997). Motor and cognitive deficits in apolipoprotein E-deficient mice after closed head injury. *Neuroscience* **80**: 1255–1262.

Cirelly R, Tyring SK (1995). Major therapeutic uses of interferons. *Clin Immunother* **3**: 27–87.

Clark JW (1996). Biological response modifiers. *Cancer Chemother Biol Response Modif* **16**: 239–273.

Crandall J, Sakai Y, Zhang J *et al.* (2004). 13-*cis*-Retinoic acid suppresses hippocampal cell division and hippocampal-dependent learning in mice. *Proc Natl Acad Sci USA* **101**: 5111–5116.

Cunningham RS (2003). Anemia in the oncology patient: cognitive function and cancer. *Cancer Nurs* **26**: 38S–42S.

Delattre JY, Posner JB (1995). Neurological complications of chemotherapy and radiation therapy. In Aminoff MJ (ed.). *Neurology and General Medicine* (2nd edn.) (pp. 421–445). New York: Churchill Livingstone.

Dieperink E, Willenbring M, Ho SB (2000). Neuropsychiatric symptoms associated with hepatitis C and interferon alpha: a review. *Am J Psychiatry* **157**: 867–876.

Doolittle ND, Peereboom DM, Christoforidis GA *et al.* (2006). Delivery of chemotherapy and antibodies across the blood-brain barrier and the role of chemoprotection, in primary and metastatic brain tumors: report of the Eleventh Annual Blood-Brain Barrier Consortium meeting. *J Neurooncol* **81**: 81–91.

Eberling JL, Wu C, Tong-Turnbeaugh R *et al.* (2004). Estrogen- and tamoxifen-associated effects on brain structure and function. *Neuroimage* **21**: 364–371.

Egan MF, Goldberg TE, Kolachana BS *et al.* (2001). Effect of COMT Val108/158 met genotype on frontal lobe function and risk for schizophrenia. *Proc Natl Acad Sci USA* **98**: 6917–6922.

Egan MF, Kojima M, Callicott JH *et al.* (2003). The BDNF val66met polymorphism affects activity-dependent secretion of BDNF and human memory and hippocampal function. *Cell* **112**: 257–269.

Farkkila M, Iivanainen M, Roine R *et al.* (1984). Neurotoxic and other side effects of high dose interferon in amyotrophic lateral sclerosis. *Acta Neurol Scand* **70**: 42–46.

Fliessbach K, Urbach H, Helmstaedter C *et al.* (2003). Cognitive performance and magnetic resonance imaging findings after high-dose systemic and intraventricular chemotherapy for primary central nervous system lymphoma. *Arch Neurol* **60**: 563–568.

Garcia-Tena J, Lopez-Andreu JA, Ferris J *et al.* (1995). Intrathecal chemotherapy related myeloencephalopathy in a young child with acute lymphoblastic leukemia. *Pediatr Hematol Oncol* **12**: 377–385.

Gilbert MR, Armstrong TS (1996). Neurotoxicities. In Kirkwood J, Lotze M, Yasko J (eds.) *Current Cancer Therapeutics* (2nd edn.) (pp. 364–371). Philadelphia, PA: Current Medicine.

Goldman LS (1994). Successful treatment of interferon alfa-induced mood disorder with nortriptyline. *Psychosomatics* **35**: 412–413.

Green HJ, Pakenham KI, Headley BC *et al.* (2002). Altered cognitive function in men treated for prostate cancer with luteinizing hormone-releasing hormone analogues and cyproterone acetate: a randomized controlled trial. *BJU Int* **90**: 427–432.

Groopman JE, Itri LM (1999). Chemotherapy-induced anemia in adults: incidence and treatment. *J Natl Cancer Inst* **91**: 1616–1634.

Haykin ME, Gorman M, van Hoff J *et al.* (2006). Diffusion-weighted MRI correlates of subacute methotrexate-related neurotoxicity. *J Neurooncol* **76**: 153–157.

Heflin LH, Meyerowitz BE, Hall P *et al.* (2005). Cancer as a risk factor for long-term cognitive deficits and dementia. *J Natl Cancer Inst* **97**: 854–856.

Honigsberger L, Fielding JW, Priestman TJ (1983). Neurological effects of recombinant human interferon. *Br J Med* **286**: 719.

Jansen C, Miakowski C, Dodd M *et al.* (2005). Potential mechanisms for chemotherapy-induced impairments in cognitive function. *Oncol Nurs Forum* **32**: 1151–1163.

Jenkins VA, Shilling V, Fallowfield L *et al.* (2004). Does hormone therapy for the treatment of breast cancer have a detrimental effect on memory and cognition? A pilot study. *Psychooncology* **13**: 61–66.

Jenkins VA, Bloomfield DJ, Shilling VM *et al.* (2005). Does neoadjuvant hormone therapy for early prostate cancer affect cognition? Results from a pilot study. *BJU Int* **96**: 48–53.

Jenkins V, Shilling V, Deutsch G *et al.* (2006). A 3-year prospective study of the effects of adjuvant treatments on cognition in women with early stage breast cancer. *Br J Cancer* **94**: 828–834.

Jensen BV (2006). Cardiotoxic consequences of anthracycline-containing therapy in patients with breast cancer. *Semin Oncol* **33** [Suppl. 8]: S15–S21.

Johnson SA (2006). Anthracycline-induced cardiotoxicity in adult hematologic malignancies. *Semin Oncol* **33** [Suppl. 8]: S22–S27.

Joshi G, Sultana R, Tangpong J *et al.* (2005). Free radical mediated oxidative stress and toxic side effects in brain induced by the anti cancer drug adriamycin: insight into chemobrain. *Free Radic Res* **39**: 1147–1154.

Juengling FD, Ebert D, Gut O *et al.* (2000). Prefrontal cortical hypometabolism during low-dose interferon alpha treatment. *Psychopharmacology* **152**: 383–389.

Kayl AE, Wefel JS, Meyers CA (2006). Chemotherapy and cognition: effects, potential mechanisms and management. *Am J Ther* **13**: 362–369.

Keime-Guibert F, Napolitano M, Delattre JY (1998). Neurological complications of radiotherapy and chemotherapy. *J Neurol* **245**: 695–708.

Kim YA, Chung HC, Choi HJ *et al.* (2006). Intermediate dose 5-fluorouracil-induced encephalopathy. *Jpn J Clin Oncol* **36**: 55–59.

Knobf MT (2006). Reproductive and hormonal sequelae of chemotherapy in women. *Am J Nurs* **106** [Suppl. 3]: 60–65.

Krajinovic M, Robaey P, Chiasson S *et al.* (2005). Polymorphisms of genes controlling homocysteine levels and IQ score following treatment for childhood ALL. *Pharmacogenomics* **6**: 293–302.

Krause I, Valesini G, Scrivo R *et al.* (2003). Autoimmune aspects of cytokine and anticytokine therapies. *Am J Med* **115**: 390–397.

Kreukels BPC, Schagen SB, Ridderinkhof KR *et al.* (2006). Effects of high-dose and conventional-dose adjuvant chemotherapy in patients with breast cancer: an electrophysiologic study. *Clin Breast Cancer* **7**: 67–78.

Lacosta S, Merali Z, Anisman H (2000). Central monoamine activity following acute and repeated systemic interleukin-2 administration. *Neuroimmunomodulation* **8**: 83–90.

Largillier R, Etienne-Grimaldi MC, Formento JL *et al.* (2006). Pharmacogenetics of capecitabine in advanced breast cancer patients. *Clin Cancer Res* **12**: 5496–5502.

Lee BN, Dantzer R, Langley KE *et al.* (2004). A cytokine-based neuroimmunologic mechanism of cancer-related symptoms. *Neuroimmunomodulation* **11**: 279–292.

Linnebank M, Pels H, Klecza N *et al.* (2005). MTX-induced white matter changes are associated with polymorphisms of methionine metabolism. *Neurology* **64**: 912–913.

Lipp HP (1999). Neurotoxicity (including sensory toxicity) induced by cytostatics. In Lipp HP (ed.). *Anticancer Drug Toxicity: Prevention, Management, and Clinical Pharmacokinetics* (pp. 431–453). New York: Marcel Dekker, Inc.

Lipshultz SE (2006). Exposure to anthracyclines during childhood causes cardiac injury. *Semin Oncol* **33** [Suppl. 8]: 8–14.

Madhyastha S, Somayaji SN, Rao MS *et al.* (2002). Hippocampal brain amines in methotrexate-induced learning and memory deficit. *Can J Physiol Pharmacol* **80**: 1076–1084.

Malek-Ahmadi P, Ghandour E (2004). Bupropion for treatment of interferon-induced depression. *Ann Pharmacother* **38**: 1202–1205.

Malik UR, Makower DF, Wadler S (2001). Interferon-mediated fatigue. *Cancer* **92** [Suppl]: 1664–1668.

Massa E, Madeddu C, Lusso MR *et al.* (2006). Evaluation of the effectiveness of treatment with erythropoietin on anemia, cognitive functioning and functions studied by comprehensive geriatric assessment in elderly cancer patients with anemia related to cancer chemotherapy. *Crit Rev Oncol Hematol* **57**: 175–182.

Mayr N, Zeitlhofer J, Deecke L *et al.* (1999). Neurological function during long-term therapy with recombinant interferon alpha. *J Clin Neurosci* **11**: 343–348.

McAllister TW, Ahles TA, Saykin AJ *et al.* (2004). Cognitive effects of cytotoxic cancer chemotherapy: predisposing risk factors and potential treatments. *Curr Psychiatr Rep* **6**: 364–371.

McEwen BS, Alves SE (1999). Estrogen actions in the central nervous system. *Endocr Rev* **20**: 279–307.

Menzies R, Phelps C, Wiranowska M *et al.* (1996). The effect of interferon-alpha on the pituitary-adrenal axis. *J Interferon Cytokine Res* **16**: 619–629.

Meyers CA, Valentine AD (1995). Neurological and psychiatric effects of immunological therapy. *CNS Drugs* **3**: 56–68.

Meyers CA, Scheibel RS, Forman AD (1991). Persistent neurotoxicity of systemically administered interferon-alpha. *Neurology* **41**: 672–676.

Meyers CA, Kudelka AP, Conrad CA *et al.* (1997). Neurotoxicity of CI-980, a novel mitotic inhibitor. *Clin Cancer Res* **3**: 419–422.

Meyers CA, Weitzner MA, Valentine AD *et al.* (1998). Methylphenidate therapy improves cognition, mood, and function of brain tumor patients. *J Clin Oncol* **16**: 2522–2527.

Meyers JN, Whiteside TL (1996). Immunotherapy of squamous cell carcinoma of the head and neck. In Meyers EN, Suen JY (eds.). *Cancer of the Head and Neck* (pp. 805–817). Philadelphia, PA: WB Saunders Company.

Mihich E (2000). Historical overview of biologic response modifiers. *Cancer Invest* **18**: 456–466.

Moleski M (2000). Neuropsychological, neuroanatomical, and neurophysiological consequences of CNS chemotherapy for acute lymphoblastic leukemia. *Arch Clin Neuropsychol* **15**: 603–630.

Molina JR, Barton DL, Loprinzi CL (2005). Chemotherapy-induced ovarian failure. *Drug Safety* **28**: 401–416.

Moor BD (2005). Neurocognitive outcomes in survivors of childhood cancer. *J Pediatr Psychol* **30**: 51–63.

Mottet N, Prayer-Galetti T, Hammerer P *et al.* (2006). Optimizing outcomes and quality of life in the hormonal treatment of prostate cancer. *BJU Int* **98**: 20–27.

Musselman DL, Lawson DH, Gumnick JF *et al.* (2001). Paroxetine for the prevention of depression induced by high-dose interferon alpha. *N Engl J Med* **344**: 961–966.

National Institutes of Health (2003). *Biological Therapy. Treatments that use your Immune System to Fight Cancer.* [Brochure]. NIH Publication No. 03–5406.

Nemeroff CB, Krishnan KR, Reed D *et al.* (1992). Adrenal gland enlargement in major depression: a computed tomographic study. *Arch Gen Psychiatry* **49**: 384–387.

Okcu MF, Selvan M, Wang L *et al.* (2004). Glutathione *S*-transferase polymorphisms and survival in primary malignant glioma. *Clin Cancer Res* **10**: 2618–2625.

O'Shaughnessy JA, Svetislava JV, Holmes FA *et al.* (2005). Feasibility of quantifying the effects of epoetin alpha therapy on cognitive function in women with breast cancer undergoing adjuvant or neoadjuvant chemotherapy. *Clin Breast Cancer* **5**: 439–446.

Pavol MA, Meyers CA, Rexer JL *et al.* (1995). Pattern of neurobehavioral deficits associated with interferon alpha therapy for leukemia. *Neurology* **45**: 947–950.

Penson RT, Kronish K, Duan Z *et al.* (2000). Cytokines IL-1beta, IL-2, IL-6, IL-8, MCP-1, GM-CSF and TNF-alpha in patients with epithelial ovarian cancer and their relationship to treatment with paclitaxel. *Int J Gynecol Cancer* **1**: 33–41.

Pusztai L, Mendoza TR, Reuben JM *et al.* (2004). Changes in plasma level of inflammatory cytokines in response to paclitaxel chemotherapy. *Cytokine* **25**: 94–102.

Quinn CT, Kamen BA (1996). A biochemical perspective of methotrexate neurotoxicity with insight on nonfolate rescue modalities. *J Invest Med* **44**: 522–530.

Roe CM, Behrens MI, Xiong C *et al.* (2005). Alzheimer disease and cancer. *Neurology* **64**: 895–898.

Rottenberg DA (ed.) (1991). *Neurological Complications of Cancer Treatment*. Boston, MA: Butterworth-Heinemann.

Saykin AJ, Ahles TA, McDonald BC (2003). Mechanisms of chemotherapy-induced cognitive disorders: neuropsychological, pathophysiological, and neuroimaging perspectives. *Semin Clin Neuropsychiatry* **8**: 201–216.

Schaefer M, Engelbrecht MA, Gut O *et al.* (2002). Interferon alpha (IFN-α) and psychiatric syndromes: a review. *Prog Neuropsychopharmacol Biol Psychiatry* **26**: 731–746.

Schaefer M, Schwiger M, Pich M *et al.* (2003). Neurotransmitter changes by interferon-alpha and therapeutic implications. *Pharmacopsychiatry* **36** [Suppl. 3]: S203–S206.

Schagen SB, Muller MJ, Boogerd W *et al.* (2002). Cognitive dysfunction and chemotherapy: neuropsychological findings in perspective. *Clin Breast Cancer* **3** [Suppl]: S100–S108.

Scheibel RS, Valentine AD, O'Brien S *et al.* (2004). Cognitive dysfunction and depression during treatment with interferon alpha and chemotherapy. *J Neuropsychiatry Clin Neurosci* **16**: 1–7.

Schneiderman B (2004). Hippocampal volumes smaller in chemotherapy patients. *Lancet Oncol* **5**: 202.

Shah RR (2005). Mechanistic basis of adverse drug reactions: the perils of inappropriate dose schedules. *Expert Opinion Drug Safety* **4**: 103–128.

Shapiro CL, Recht A (2001). Drug therapy – side effects of adjuvant treatment of breast cancer. *New Engl J Med* **344**: 1997–2008.

Sheline GE, Wara WM, Smith V (1980). Therapeutic irradiation and brain injury. *Int J Radiat Oncol Biol Phys* **6**: 1215–1228.

Shilling V, Jenkins V, Morris R *et al.* (2005). The effects of adjuvant chemotherapy on cognition in women with breast cancer – preliminary results of an observational longitudinal study. *Breast* **14**: 142–150.

Shin DM, Khuri FR, Murphy B *et al.* (2001). Combined interferon-alpha, 13-*cis*-retinoic acid, and alpha tocopherol in locally advanced head and neck squamous cell carcinoma: novel bioadjuvant phase II trial. *J Clin Oncol* **19**: 3010–3017.

Shin DM, Glisson BS, Khuri FR *et al.* (2002). Phase II and biological study of interferon alpha, retinoic acid, and cisplatin in advanced squamous cell skin cancer. *J Clin Oncol* **20**: 364–370.

Shuper A, Stark B, Kornreich L *et al.* (2000). Methotrexate treatment protocols and the central nervous system: significant cure with significant neurotoxicity. *J Child Neurol* **15**: 573–580.

Silverman DH, Dy CJ, Castellon SA *et al.* (2007). Altered frontocortical, cerebellar, and basal ganglia activity in adjuvant-treated breast cancer survivors 5–10 years after chemotherapy. *Breast Cancer Res Treat* **103**(3): 303–311.

Smedley H, Katrak M, Sikora K *et al.* (1983). Neurological effects of recombinant interferon alpha. *Br Med J* **286**: 262–264.

Smith A, Tyrrell D, Coyle K *et al.* (1988). Effects of interferon alpha on performance in man: a preliminary report. *Psychopharmacology* **96**: 414–416.

Spiegel RJ (1989). The alpha interferons: clinical overview. *Urology* **34**: 75–79.

Staat K, Segatore M (2005). The phenomenon of chemo brain. *Clin J Oncol Nurs* **9**: 713–721.

Steinherz LJ, Yahalom J (1993). Cardiac complications of cancer therapy. In DeVita VT, Jr., Hellman S, Rosenberg SA (eds.) *Cancer Principles and Practice of Oncology* (4th edn.) (pp. 2370–2385). Philadephia, PA: J.B. Lippincott Company.

Strite D, Valentine AD, Meyers CA (1997). Manic episodes in two patients treated with interferon alpha. *J Neuropsychiatry* **9**: 273–276.

Sul JK, DeAngelis LM (2006). Neurologic complications of cancer chemotherapy. *Semin Oncol* **33**: 324–332.

Taphoorn MJB, Klein M (2004). Cognitive deficits in adult patients with brain tumors. *Lancet Neurol* **3**: 159–168.

Taylor JL, Grossberg SE (1998). The effects of interferon-α on the production and action of other cytokines. *Semin Oncol* **25** [Suppl. 1]: S3–S29.

Tompkins WA (1999). Immunomodulation and therapeutic effects of the oral use of interferon-α: mechanism of action. *J Interferon Cytokine Res* **19**: 817–828.

Tsavaris N, Kosmas C, Vadiaka M *et al.* (2002). Immune changes in patients with advanced breast cancer undergoing chemotherapy with taxanes. *Br J Cancer* **87**: 21–27.

Valentine AD, Meyers CA (2005). Neurobehavioral effects of interferon therapy. *Curr Psychiatry Rep* **7**: 391–395.

Valentine AD, Meyers CA, Talpaz M (1995). Treatment of neurotoxic side effects of interferon-alpha with naltrexone. *Cancer Invest* **13**: 561–566.

Valentine AD, Meyers CA, Kling MA *et al.* (1998). Mood and cognitive side effects of interferon-α therapy. *Semin Oncol* **25**: 39–47.

Wagner LI, Sweet JJ, Desa J *et al.* (2005). Prechemotherapy hemoglobin (Hgb) and cognitive impairment among breast cancer patients. *J Clin Oncol* **23**: 760S.

Wefel JS, Meyers CA (2005). Cancer as a risk factor for dementia: a house built on shifting sand. *J Natl Cancer Inst* **97**: 788–789.

Wefel JS, Lenzi R, Theriault R *et al.* (2004a). "Chemobrain" in breast cancer? A prologue. *Cancer* **101**: 466–475.

Wefel JS, Lenzi R, Theriault R *et al.* (2004b). The cognitive sequelae of standard dose adjuvant chemotherapy in women with breast cancer: results of a prospective, randomized, longitudinal trial. *Cancer* **100**: 2292–2299.

Weiss RB, Vogelzang NJ (1993). Miscellaneous toxicities. In DeVita VT, Jr., Hellman S, Rosenberg SA (eds.) *Cancer Principles and Practice of Oncology* (4th edn.) (pp. 2349–2358). Philadelphia, PA: JB Lippincott Company.

Wood LJ, Nail LM, Gilster A *et al.* (2006). Cancer chemotherapy-related symptoms: evidence to suggest a role for proinflammatory cytokines. *Oncol Nurs Forum* **33**: 535–542.

Yaffe K, Sawaya G, Lieberburg I *et al.* (1998). Estrogen therapy in postmenopausal women effects of cognitive function and dementia. *J Am Med Assoc* **279**: 688–695.

Yoshikawa E, Matsuoka Y, Inagaki M *et al.* (2005). No adverse effects of adjuvant chemotherapy on hippocampal volume in Japanese breast cancer survivors. *Breast Cancer Res Treat* **92**: 81–84.

Zaloga GP, Bhatt B, Marik P (2001). Critical illness and systemic inflammation. In Becker KL (ed.) *Endocrinology and Metabolism* (3rd edn.) (pp. 2068–2076). Philadelphia, PA: Lippincott Williams & Wilkins.

9

Effect of hormones and hormonal treatment on cognition

Christien Schilder, Sanne Schagen, and Frits van Dam

Introduction

This chapter will address the possible influences of hormonal therapy on cognitive functioning. Hormonal therapy is an important treatment option for, among others, breast and prostate cancer. While there is increasing evidence that *chemotherapy* induces cognitive dysfunction in a subgroup of patients (Tannock *et al.*, 2004), the effects of *hormonal therapy* on cognitive functioning have not been investigated thoroughly. Actually, it is conceivable that hormonal therapy also influences cognitive performance. After all, hormonal therapies interfere with serum levels of reproductive hormones (particularly estrogens and androgens) or with hormonal actions. There are indications that reproductive hormones are important in cognitive functioning (Bender *et al.*, 2001). The mechanisms of action of reproductive hormones on brain structures are not entirely understood. One of the possibilities is that these hormones act through estrogen and androgen receptors that are present in those brain structures important for cognitive function, for example the hippocampi and the cerebral cortex (Norbury *et al.*, 2003). Furthermore, it has been suggested that reproductive hormones have a beneficial effect on neurotransmitters that are involved in cognitive processes (Cholerton *et al.*, 2002; Norbury *et al.*, 2003).

Hormonal therapy is increasingly used for breast and prostate cancer, often for long periods and by elderly patients. Because intact cognitive functioning is essential for independent living and activities of daily life, elucidation of the possible effects of the various hormonal agents and treatment regimens is becoming increasingly important. The first part of this chapter will provide an introduction to the influence of reproductive hormones on cognitive functions from a neuropsychological point of view. In the second part, the mechanisms of action of the different hormonal agents that are used in cancer treatment are described and the neuropsychological literature on the impact of hormonal therapy on cognitive functioning is critically reviewed. Finally, some methodological aspects of the investigation of the complex relations between hormone levels and neuropsychological test scores are addressed.

The role of reproductive hormones in cognitive function

The influence of hormones begins in the prenatal period of life. Prenatal reproductive hormones exert long-lasting organizational influences on brain and behavior. It is suggested that the early presence of androgens may organize the male brain to enhance certain spatial functions (Sanders *et al.*, 2002). In

Cognition and Cancer, eds. Christina A. Meyers and James R. Perry. Published by Cambridge University Press.
© Cambridge University Press 2008.

adulthood, fluctuations in reproductive hormone levels (ranging from daily to monthly to seasonally) may cause small fluctuations in cognitive functioning. Later in life, levels of most reproductive hormones decline with age, and it is hypothesized that this decline is associated with age-related decline in cognitive functioning. Androgens and estrogens are present at different levels in men and women. In men, androgens, in particular testosterone, predominate. In women, estrogens are the predominating reproductive hormones (Green *et al.*, 2000).

The influence of reproductive hormones on cognition in healthy women

In premenopausal women, the levels of estrogen fluctuate during the menstrual cycle. Neuropsychological studies suggest that these fluctuations have an influence on cognitive performance. In general, it is found that high levels of estrogens are beneficial to performance on tasks at which women as a group excel (particularly tasks on verbal memory, verbal fluency, and some fine motor skills), but detrimental to tasks in which men as a group excel (particularly tasks on mental rotation and spatial perception) (Hampson, 1990; Hausmann *et al.*, 2000; Maki *et al.*, 2002). Studies on the influence of testosterone on cognitive functioning in women suggest that daily fluctuations are associated with spatial performance: early in the morning, when testosterone levels are relatively high, spatial performance is better than later in the morning, when testosterone levels are relatively lower (Sanders *et al.*, 2002).

The declining levels of reproductive hormones during the menopausal transition give another opportunity to relate changes in hormone levels to cognitive functioning in women. During menopause, levels of estrogen decrease substantially but gradually. This gradual decline, however, does not result in clearly measurable declines in the performance on cognitive tests during the years of the menopausal transition (Henderson *et al.*, 2003; Meyer *et al.*, 2003). However, surgically induced menopause, in which estrogen levels drop abruptly, has been reported to induce a

clear acute change in cognitive performance, most prominently on aspects of short- and long-term verbal memory (Phillips & Sherwin, 1992; Sherwin, 1988; Verghese *et al.*, 2000). However, there are few data on the long-term effects of physiological or surgical menopause on cognitive functioning (Barrett-Connor & Kritz-Silverstein, 1993).

After the menopausal transition, estrogen levels are low, but in that low range individual hormone levels vary between women. Some authors have investigated the relationship between estrogen levels and cognitive performance in postmenopausal women. The most consistent finding is that higher endogenous estrogen levels are related to better scores on verbal memory tasks (Drake *et al.*, 2000; Hogervorst *et al.*, 2004; Wolf & Kirschbaum, 2002), indicating that even small variations in the low range of estrogen levels are related to cognitive performance.

In the last few decades, numerous studies have evaluated the possible influences of hormone replacement therapy (HRT, mostly prescribed for relieving menopausal symptoms) on cognitive functioning and the risk of developing dementia. Initially, observational studies showed a significantly reduced risk for developing dementia and Alzheimer's disease in HRT users (Yaffe *et al.*, 1998). However, there were concerns about attributing the reduced risk to the use of HRT, because HRT users tend to be healthier and better educated than non-users, factors that are in themselves protective against cognitive decline. To avoid this "healthy user bias," the effects of HRT were investigated in a large randomized, placebo-controlled study, the Women's Health Initiative Memory Study (WHIMS). In this study, the effects of estrogen with or without a progestin on probable dementia and, secondarily, mild cognitive impairment were examined. Contrary to the expectations, a significantly increased risk of "probable dementia" was found in the estrogen-plus-progestin group; the "estrogen alone" group showed a non-significant increase in probable dementia. Remarkably, the risk of mild cognitive impairment, thought to be a precursor to Alzheimer's disease, was not increased in either group (Espeland *et al.*, 2004; Rapp *et al.*, 2003; Shumaker *et al.*, 2003, 2004). After these surprising results were published, several authors tried to explain them. One possible explanation is that the women in the WHIMS were already too old at the time HRT was initiated for it to have any protective effect. It is hypothesized that there is a limited period of time after cessation of ovarian function over which HRT is likely to protect cognitive functioning. One possible explanation for such a "limited time window" is that the rather rapid depletion of estrogen at the time of menopause may have a particularly pronounced effect on neurons. Hormone replacement therapy could conceivably prevent that detrimental effect. It is also possible that, after a long period of depletion of estrogen, neurons become less sensitive to estrogen, or that older neurons have reduced responsivity to the hormone (Sherwin, 2005). Another possible explanation for the findings in WHIMS is the choice of HRT preparation. In that study, conjugated equine estrogen (with or without a progestin) was used, an agent that elevates steady-state levels of estrone (a less potent estrogen) instead of replicating premenopausal variations in hormone levels. It is possible that these particular HRT preparations fail to induce a positive effect on cognitive functions (Gleason *et al.*, 2005). Consequently, important questions about the impact of HRT on cognitive functioning and the risk on dementia remain. These questions center around issues such as the timing of initiation, duration of treatment and type of HRT regimen (Maki, 2004).

The influence of reproductive hormones on cognition in healthy men

In men, the influence of reproductive hormones on cognitive function has also been the subject of investigation. One way to study this is to use the natural fluctuations in testosterone levels. As in women, testosterone levels in men show daily fluctuations. It is found that young men score better on spatial tasks late in the morning, when testosterone levels are relatively low, than early in the morning,

when testosterone levels are higher (Sanders *et al.*, 2002). The correlations are in the opposite direction from the correlations found in women, indicating that there might be an optimum level of testosterone for the performance of spatial tasks that is situated in the "lower male range."

In men, testosterone levels decline modestly but consistently with age (Juul & Skakkebaek, 2002). Because circulating estrogens arise through aromatization of testosterone, estrogens decrease as well with increasing age. Ironically, because the testes never stop the secretion of testosterone entirely, elderly men have higher levels of both testosterone and estrogen than elderly women (Sherwin, 2003). It is hypothesized that because of this difference, men are less susceptible to Alzheimer's disease than women (Bowen *et al.*, 2005).

This age-related decline of reproductive hormones is used to investigate the impact of hormone levels on cognitive function in men. Unfortunately, studies that tried to find correlations between endogenous estrogen and testosterone levels and cognitive performance in aging men mainly show inconsistent results. In several studies, age seems to play a modifying role in the relationship between hormone levels and cognitive functions. For example, one study only found a positive correlation between estrogen levels and spatial span performance, and between testosterone levels and speed of information processing in the age range of 61–72 years (Hogervorst *et al.*, 2004). Another study found a positive relationship between testosterone levels and global cognitive performance as assessed by the Mini-Mental State Examination (MMSE) in their oldest age category, 70–80 years of age (Muller *et al.*, 2005). Other studies failed to find any significant relationship between circulating hormone levels and cognitive performance (Fonda *et al.*, 2005; Wolf & Kirschbaum, 2002), while one study only found a correlation between bioavailable testosterone (but not total testosterone) and cognitive performance (Yaffe *et al.*, 2002).

Apart from the possibility that estrogen may protect against cognitive decline and Alzheimer's disease, there are questions concerning the role of declining testosterone levels in the development of cognitive decline and Alzheimer's disease in aging men. This becomes even more important because of the finding that men with Alzheimer's disease show lower testosterone levels than men of the same age without Alzheimer's disease (Hogervorst *et al.*, 2001; Rosario *et al.*, 2004). These findings are ambiguous, however, because of the possibility that depleted testosterone levels in men with Alzheimer's disease may actually be a consequence of the disease rather than a cause. Research to resolve this ambiguity is ongoing. There are some preliminary results that indicate that a low free testosterone level occurs before the diagnosis of Alzheimer's disease and is possibly a risk factor (Moffat *et al.*, 2004), but more prospective longitudinal studies are needed to assess the impact of long-term testosterone levels on cognitive decline and Alzheimer's disease. In fact, if testosterone levels turn out to be a risk factor for cognitive decline and Alzheimer's disease, this will have important consequences for the role of androgen substitution therapy in prevention and treatment.

While the potential role of androgen substitution therapy for the prevention and treatment of Alzheimer's disease is unclear, the impact of short-term use of this therapy on cognitive functioning has in fact been investigated in several studies. Androgen substitution therapy is used by men of all ages who experience symptoms of hypogonadism, such as decreased muscle mass and bone density, fatigue, decreased energy levels and decreased libido (Juul & Skakkebaek, 2002). But studies of the impact of androgen substitution on cognitive functioning have also produced conflicting results. Some authors found a beneficial effect on measures of working memory (Janowsky *et al.*, 2000), spatial memory (Cherrier *et al.*, 2001), verbal memory (Cherrier *et al.*, 2001), and verbal fluency (O'Connor *et al.*, 2001), whereas other authors did not find any significant correlation with scores on cognitive tests (Haren *et al.*, 2005; Kenny *et al.*, 2002; Wolf *et al.*, 1997). Even within the cognitive domain of spatial abilities, the findings are contradictory: one study suggests a beneficial effect (Cherrier *et al.*, 2001),

while another study suggests a detrimental effect (O'Connor *et al.*, 2001).

Neuroimaging studies

To unravel the complex associations between levels of reproductive hormones and cognitive functioning, some authors used the assistance of neuroimaging techniques. These techniques are predominantly used in studies on supplementation of reproductive hormones. The results suggest that HRT in women is capable of altering brain structure and brain activation patterns, especially in brain regions that are important for memory (Cook *et al.*, 2002; Eberling *et al.*, 2000; Luoto *et al.*, 2000; Maki & Resnick, 2000; Resnick *et al.*, 1998; Schmidt *et al.*, 1996; Shaywitz *et al.*, 1999). Furthermore, testosterone treatment in hypogonadal men increases cerebral perfusion in various brain regions (Azad *et al.*, 2003). However, the clinical significance of these alterations is not clear and needs further investigation.

Conclusions

Although the relationships between reproductive hormones and cognitive functioning have been addressed in many different studies, they appear to be complex and, in many cases, unclear. There is increasing evidence that, in general, reproductive hormones play a modest role in cognitive functioning. For estrogen, the most consistent effects are found on verbal memory performance in women (Sherwin, 2000). The relationship between androgens and cognitive functioning seems to be a complex one. Androgens particularly appear to affect spatial abilities but in a complex way: it has been suggested that there might be an optimal testosterone level, situated in the "lower male range." Both lower and higher levels of testosterone may have a detrimental effect on spatial performance. Until now, many questions regarding the impact of substitution of hormones on cognitive functioning, and the relationship between reproductive hormone levels and the risk of dementia are still unanswered.

Hormonal therapy in breast and prostate cancer: is there an influence on cognitive function?

The section above shows that neuropsychological and neuroimaging studies provide evidence for a relationship between reproductive hormones and cognitive functions. In addition, reproductive hormones play a major role in the etiology and treatment in breast and prostate cancer. Hormonal therapy interferes with reproductive hormone levels or with the activity of reproductive hormones. Therefore, it has been suggested that hormonal therapies may have an effect on cognitive function as well. This section will point out the possible effects of hormonal therapy on cognitive function. After an introduction to the mechanisms of action of various hormonal therapies in the treatment of breast and prostate cancer, an overview will be given of the studies on the effects of hormonal therapies on cognitive function.

The role of hormonal therapies in cancer treatment

Hormonal therapy plays a prominent and increasing role in the treatment of breast and prostate cancer. The healthy breasts and prostate are dependent on reproductive hormones, as are a high percentage of the malignant tumors that originate from these organs. Interference with the hormonal milieu will slow down or stop the growth of the tumor in many cases. There are several methods to achieve this interference in the hormonal milieu (Tripathy & Benz, 2001).

Originally, deprivation of reproductive hormones was achieved by ovariectomy or irradiation of the ovaries in women and orchiectomy in men. Despite the efficacy of these methods, patient acceptance is usually poor because of the irreversibility of the intervention. In the 1980s, luteinizing-hormone-releasing hormone (LHRH) analogs were introduced. These drugs are used to produce "reversible" chemical castration in both sexes. In women, these drugs suppress ovarian production of estrogen, while in men the production of testosterone by the testes is reduced. The most used LHRH agonists are leuprolide and goserelin (Hellerstedt & Pienta, 2002; Miller, 1996).

In *breast cancer* treatment, tamoxifen is widely used in both pre- and postmenopausal patients. In the 1960s, when the drug was synthesized, it was demonstrated to have antiproliferating effects in the breast. The drug appeared to be capable of binding to the estrogen receptors in breast tissue, thereby preventing estrogen from initiating the estrogenic effects. Tamoxifen thus became widely known as an anti-estrogen. Since then, it has been discovered that it, paradoxically, has many estrogenic qualities, including agonist effects on bone, blood lipids, and the endometrium (Osborne *et al.*, 2000). This finding led to the development of new drugs with specific and selective effects on the estrogen receptor function. Currently, tamoxifen and related drugs are collectively known as selective estrogen receptor modulators (SERMs) (Goss & Strasser, 2001). SERMs such as tamoxifen are tolerated relatively well. However, their estrogenic as well as anti-estrogenic qualities can lead to a variety of side-effects, including thromboembolic events, hot flashes, and the risk of endometrial cancer with prolonged use.

The introduction of aromatase inhibitors as a new class of agents has extended the treatment options for breast cancer patients. The enzyme aromatase is required for the peripheral conversion of testosterone and androstenedione to estrogen, the final step in the estrogen biosynthesis pathway (Visvanathan & Davidson, 2003). Aromatase inhibitors almost completely inhibit the action of this enzyme. Consequently, aromatase inhibitors lower the level of circulating estrogen by almost 100% (Simpson & Dowsett, 2002).

In *prostate cancer*, hormonal therapy plays an important role, especially in metastatic disease, although in the adjuvant and neoadjuvant settings its role is increasing. The most frequently used option is androgen deprivation by means of LHRH agonists, such as leuprolide and goserelin. Treatment with LHRH agonists initially results in a rise in serum testosterone levels, potentially causing stimulation of tumor growth and accompanying side-effects, such as increased bone pain. To prevent this "tumor flare," LHRH treatment is often preceded by treatment with an "anti-androgen." Anti-androgens block the effect of the testosterone surge on androgen receptors, preventing testosterone from exerting its growth-promoting effect on the tumor. The most commonly used anti-androgens are flutamide and bicalutamide. The use of anti-androgens can be continued for 2–4 weeks. Another possibility is to combine LHRH agonist treatment with anti-androgen treatment for longer periods. Anti-androgens can also be used as monotherapy (Sharifi *et al.*, 2005). In order to optimize the treatment outcome and reduce long-term toxicities related to testosterone deficiency, "intermittent androgen suppression" (IAS) is introduced as a treatment option. In IAS, androgen suppression (6–9 months) is alternated with an off-treatment period in which testosterone levels return to physiologic levels. As the "prostate-specific androgen" (PSA) reaches a certain threshold, treatment is reinstated (Cherrier *et al.*, 2003).

Hormonal therapies in breast cancer: the influence on cognitive functioning

To date, there is only limited information about the impact of the different hormonal therapies for breast cancer on cognitive function. Much of the evidence for the impact of LHRH agonists on cognitive functioning comes from studies with young women who received those agents for benign gynecologic conditions. In one study, young female LHRH-agonist users (mean age 32.4 years) reported a decrease in memory function (Newton *et al.*, 1996). Studies that used neuropsychological tests show mixed results: one study showed a decrease in verbal memory function in young women (mean age 34.2 years) after 3 months of leuprolide treatment (Sherwin & Tulandi, 1996), while another

study in young women (mean age 27 years) did not find any effect on cognition after similar treatment (Owens *et al.*, 2002). For breast cancer patients, data on the impact of LHRH agonists on cognitive function are scarce. In one study on adjuvant tamoxifen and/or goserelin therapy, premenopausal breast cancer patients (mean age 45 years) reported on a questionnaire increased memory and concentration problems during the period of treatment. However, an increase was also found in the tamoxifen group and in an untreated control group (Nystedt *et al.*, 2000).

Data on the impact of tamoxifen on cognitive function are also preliminary. The finding that tamoxifen treatment often induced hot flashes led to the hypothesis that tamoxifen acts as an estrogen antagonist within the central nervous system and may in the long term lead to cognitive deficits (Benson, 2002). Experimental evidence for a detrimental effect on memory was found in two experiments with mice. The results suggest that tamoxifen impairs memory function (especially the retrieval of spatial information) in mice (Chen *et al.*, 2002a, 2002b).

In four studies with patients that made use of neuropsychological tests, tamoxifen users were included (see Table 9.1 for more detailed information).

Paganini-Hill and Clark (2000) were the first to investigate the impact of tamoxifen on cognitive functioning. They mailed a questionnaire, including three neuropsychological tests (clock drawing, copying a box drawing, narrative writing), to breast cancer patients. They analyzed data from 1163 women: 710 women had taken tamoxifen and 453 had never used it. The tamoxifen group was divided in two subgroups, past users ($n = 428$) and current users ($n = 241$). Using a cross-sectional design, they found few differences between test scores of women who had used tamoxifen for the standard 5 years and never-users. However, more women who had used tamoxifen for 5 years or longer reported seeing their physician for memory problems than non-users. Current users also had significantly lower mean complexity scores on the narrative writing

Table 9.1. Overview of the studies on the impact of hormonal therapy on cognitive functioning in breast cancer. (*ATAC* Anastrozole, tamoxifen and combined trial, *GHQ* General Health Questionnaire, *HRT* hormone replacement therapy, *MMSE* Mini-Mental State Examination, *MRI* magnetic resonance imaging, *NART* National Adult Reading Test, *PET* positron emission tomography, *WMS* Wechsler Memory Scale)

Study	Goal	Patients and comparisons	Cognitive measures	Biological measures	Design and statistical analysis
Paganini-Hill & Clark (2000). Preliminary assessment of cognitive function in breast cancer patients treated with tamoxifen. *Breast Cancer Res Treat* **64**: 165–176.	To assess the effect of tamoxifen on cognitive function	Breast cancer patients 1. Past tamoxifen users (short-term: <4 years; standard-term: 4–5 years; long-term: 6+years) (*n* = 428) 2. Current tamoxifen users (short-term: <4 years; standard-term: 4–5 years; long-term: 6+years) (*n* = 241) 3. Never users (*n* = 453)	Clock drawing task Copying a box drawing Narrative writing to describe a pictured scene Tests were mailed to the patients and completed at home		Cross-sectional design. Patients recruited from a population-based case-control study of women with primary breast cancer Group comparison, mean scores per test Group comparison of percentage patients with errors
		Affective measures Geriatric Depression Scale	*Cognitive complaints* Questions in questionnaire		
			Conclusion Little differences between test scores of women who had used tamoxifen for the standard 5 years and never users More women who had used tamoxifen for the standard term or longer reported seeing their physician for memory problems than non-users	*Remarks* Limitations of the study: • Current users had significantly lower mean complexity score on the narrative writing task • The battery of tests was small and didn't contain a test of verbal memory • Patients were not randomly assigned to receive tamoxifen • It was impossible to classify over 20% of the patients by their duration of use • Tests were mailed to the patients, it is not sure that they did them without guidance • Non-responders were more likely to be less educated, single and not Caucasian	

(*cont.*)

Table 9.1. (*cont.*)

Study	Goal	Patients and comparisons	Cognitive measures	Biological measures	Design and statistical analysis
Ernst *et al.* (2002). The effects of tamoxifen and estrogen on brain metabolism in elderly women. *J Natl Cancer Inst* 94(8): 592–597.	Assessment of the effects of tamoxifen and estrogen on the brain chemistry of elderly women	Three groups of age-matched women from local community 1. Breast cancer patients treated with tamoxifen 20 mg/day for at least 2 years (mean ± sd = 4.4 ± 1.7 years) (*n* = 16) 2. Healthy women using HRT for at least 2 years (mean ± sd = 20.8 ± 10.5 years) (*n* = 27) 3. Healthy controls (*n* = 33)	Modified MMSE Digit Symbol substitution test Trailmaking A	Four metabolites in the brain (*myo*-inositol; creatine; N-acetyl-containing compounds; choline-containing compounds) measured by proton magnetic resonance spectroscopy	Cross-sectional design; Mean scores per test/mean concentration per metabolite
		Affective measures	*Conclusion* No differences in scores on cognitive tests Lower *myo*-inositol concentration in HRT and tamoxifen group compared with controls, suggesting a similar, maybe neuroprotective effect of both agents	*Remarks* This article is criticized by other authors. It is stated that there are alternative explanations for the lower *myo*-inositol concentrations in the brain	
		Cognitive complaints			

Reference	Aims	Sample/Groups	Measures	Results	Design/Analysis
Eberling *et al.* (2004). Estrogen- and tamoxifen-associated effects on brain structure and function. *Neuroimage* **21**: 364–371.	To evaluate the effects of estrogen and tamoxifen on cognitive testing, on PET measures on brain metabolism and MRI measures of hippocampus atrophy	40 postmenopausal women, recruited by advertisement Three groups 1. Tamoxifen group: breast cancer patients using tamoxifen ($n = 10$) 2. Estrogen group: women currently taking unopposed estrogen ($n = 15$) 3. Women not taking tamoxifen or estrogen ($n = 15$)	MMSE Verbal episodic memory (VEM) Semantic memory (object naming) Verbal attention span (VAS) Pattern recognition (PR) *Affective measures* Center for Epidemiological Studies – Depression Scale (CES-D) *Cognitive complaints*	*Conclusion* The tamoxifen group showed significantly poorer performance on the semantic memory test than the other two groups PET measures: the tamoxifen group showed widespread areas of hypometabolism in some areas of the frontal lobe (inferior and dorsal lateral areas) relative to the other two groups MRI measures: the tamoxifen group had smaller right hippocampal volumes than the estrogen group (borderline significance) *Remarks* The authors state that the findings provide support for an antagonistic role of tamoxifen on certain brain areas that are related to cognitive function Limitations: • Relatively small sample sizes • Differences in estrogen or tamoxifen use with respect to dosage and duration could affect the results • Cognitive function of the tamoxifen group could be influenced by general anesthesia, stress or depression	Each subject underwent an MRI scan and a PET scan At the MRI scan, hippocampal volumes were rated Cross-sectional design For the cognitive scores: group means were calculated PET data: group comparisons of glucose metabolism MRI data: ratings of hippocampal volume were compared between groups

(cont.)

Table 9.1. (*cont.*)

Study	Goal	Patients and comparisons	Cognitive measures	Biological measures	Design and statistical analysis
Shilling V. *et al.* (2003). The effects of hormone therapy on cognition in breast cancer *J Steroid Biochem Mol Biol* **86**: 405–412.	To establish whether significant cognitive deficit exists in women receiving hormone therapy for breast cancer To develop a statistical package that is sensitive to the potential effects of estrogen deficiency on cognition	Breast cancer patients from the ATAC trial: 1. Patient group (n = 94) consisting of three subgroups: • Tamoxifen + anastrozole placebo • Anastrozole + tamoxifen placebo • Anastrozole + placebo 2. Healthy control group (n = 35) *Cognitive complaints* Broadbent Cognitive Failures Questionnaire (25 items) *Affective measures* Beck Depression Inventory GHQ-12	NART WMS III: logical memory I + II WMS III: faces I + II WMS III: spatial span WMS III: digit span WMS III: letter-number sequencing Kendrick digit copying task *Conclusion* The patient group did not differ from the control group on measures of working memory, attention and visual memory, but was significantly impaired on measures of verbal memory and processing speed. Cognitive performance was not significantly related to length of time on trial or psychological morbidity	*Remarks* The study was not designed or powered to investigate differences between treatment arms	Cross-sectional design Group comparisons Raw scores for each of the cognitive measures were converted to z-scores using the mean score of the control group as a reference Correlational analyses between cognitive measures and depression measures, and between length of treatment and cognitive performance

task. This study suggests that current use of tamoxifen may adversely affect cognition. However, the interpretation of the results is problematic because the cognitive assessments were sent by mail and, consequently, the data may be unreliable. Furthermore, the selected tests were insensitive and not adequate with regard to the expected cognitive functions affected by tamoxifen. For example, the assessment did not include a test of verbal memory.

Ernst *et al.* (2002) found more or less opposite results. They used proton magnetic resonance spectroscopy, a neuroimaging technique that measures concentrations of biochemical markers associated with brain injury, to study the impact of tamoxifen and HRT on brain function. They compared brain metabolism of women with breast cancer who received tamoxifen ($n = 16$) with healthy women who had received HRT ($n = 27$) and with healthy controls ($n = 33$). They looked at four biochemical markers. In addition, they used three neuropsychological tests (one screening instrument and two tests for psychomotor speed). In the neuropsychological part of the study, they found no differences in group means on the tests. In the spectroscopy part, they found reduced concentrations of *myo*-inositol in the brains of women treated with tamoxifen and in the women who used HRT, compared with control women. They suggested that patients might receive neuroprotective benefits both from HRT and from tamoxifen. However, this study has been highly critiqued, for both its design and its interpretation of the results, by Ganz *et al.* (2002), who state that alternative explanations for the lower *myo*-inositol concentrations in the brain in estrogen and tamoxifen users should be considered. The lower *myo*-inositol concentrations could, for example, reflect the lifelong exposure to endogenous and exogenous estrogen. After all, older women that develop breast cancer often have higher circulating levels of estrogen after menopause compared to women who do not develop breast cancer.

In a neuroimaging study, Eberling *et al.* (2004) evaluated the effects of tamoxifen and estrogen on positron emission tomography (PET) measures of brain glucose metabolism and magnetic resonance imaging (MRI) measures on hippocampal atrophy. In addition, five neuropsychological tests were used [MMSE, object naming, attention span (Digit Span), verbal memory, and pattern recognition]. Subjects were 40 postmenopausal women (10 tamoxifen users, 15 estrogen users and 15 controls). The tamoxifen group showed significantly poorer performance on the naming test than the other two groups. The other neuropsychological tests and the depression questionnaire showed no significant differences between groups. On the PET measures, the tamoxifen group showed widespread parts of hypometabolism in some parts of the frontal lobe (inferior and dorsal lateral areas) relative to the other groups. In comparison with women not taking estrogen or tamoxifen, the estrogen group showed higher rates of metabolism in the inferior frontal cortex and temporal cortex. On the MRI measures, the tamoxifen group had smaller right hippocampal volumes than the estrogen group, but this effect was of borderline significance. The authors concluded that their findings provide support for an anti-estrogenic role of tamoxifen in certain brain areas that are related to cognitive function.

Although data on tamoxifen are sparse, the cognitive effects of another SERM (raloxifene) are well documented. Tamoxifen and raloxifene differ in their profiles of estrogenic and anti-estrogenic qualities. Raloxifene is primarily used in treatment and prevention of osteoporosis. Two large randomized placebo-controlled studies of postmenopausal women with osteoporosis reported no significant detrimental effects of raloxifene on cognitive performance (Nickelsen *et al.*, 1999; Yaffe *et al.*, 2001). Moreover, raloxifene (120 mg/day) resulted in a reduced risk of cognitive impairment (Yaffe *et al.*, 2005). Even though raloxifene does not play an important role in the treatment of breast cancer, these results may be important for tamoxifen users because of similarities between the agents (both have estrogenic and anti-estrogenic properties). However, it is possible that differences in the profiles of estrogenic and anti-estrogenic properties result in distinctly different effects on cognitive functioning.

The impact of aromatase inhibitors on cognitive functioning remains virtually unknown. Because these agents induce a substantial drop in circulating estrogens, it is supposed that alterations in cognitive functions are associated with these treatments. After all, as stated earlier, variations in the low range of postmenopausal hormone levels are found to be associated with variations in cognitive functions. Beside tamoxifen users, Shilling *et al.* (2003) included patients treated with anastrozole (an aromatase inhibitor) in their study on the effects of hormone therapy on cognition. They tested, in a cross-sectional design, 94 breast cancer patients from the anastrozole, tamoxifen and combined (ATAC) trial and 35 non-cancer controls. Patients were randomized to receive tamoxifen, anastrozole or tamoxifen/anastrozole in combination. Cognitive assessments consisted of a range of memory and attention functions. The patient group (consisting of tamoxifen users, anastrozole users and users of the combination) did not differ from the control group on measures of working memory, attention, or visual memory, but had significantly impaired verbal memory and processing speed compared to the control group. Cognitive performance was not significantly related to the length of time in the trial or measures of psychological morbidity. The authors state that the study was not designed or able to investigate differences in effects between tamoxifen and anastrozole on cognitive function, and speculate that differences in test scores may reflect the different activities of tamoxifen and anastrozole. The overall conclusion from the study was that the adverse effect of hormone therapy on cognition seems to be specific (i.e., on verbal memory and processing speed) rather than widespread.

Hormonal therapies in prostate cancer: the influence on cognitive functioning

Just as in hormonal therapy in breast cancer, information about the impact of hormonal therapy for prostate cancer on cognitive functioning is limited (see Table 9.2 for a description of the conducted studies). The first authors to systematically investigate the impact of hormonal therapy in prostate cancer were Green *et al.* (2002). They tested 65 prostate cancer patients who were randomized between four treatment modalities: two types of LHRH agonists (leuprorelin and goserelin), anti-androgen monotherapy with cyproterone acetate and close clinical monitoring. They compared baseline scores with scores after 6 months of treatment. They found that goserelin users (one of the LHRH agonists) had improved their performance on a task for visual memory. In the domain of verbal memory, goserelin users had improved their score on one test of verbal memory (recalling prose passages) but worsened their score on another verbal memory task (list learning). Patients randomized to "close clinical monitoring" also improved on the prose verbal memory task. Besides comparing mean scores, the authors examined the differences between baseline and follow-up scores for each patient. They found that none of the "close monitoring" patients showed a significant change in cognitive variables over 6 months. For patients receiving active treatment, 24 out of 50 showed a decrease on at least one cognitive task and 7 out of 50 on two or more tasks.

Salminen *et al.* (2003, 2004, 2005) published three studies on the influence of androgen deprivation therapy on cognitive functioning. In the first study (Salminen *et al.*, 2003), they tested 25 prostate cancer patients at baseline (before starting therapy) and after 6 and 12 months of therapy. The therapy started with 250 mg flutamide (an anti-androgen) three times a day for 4 weeks. An LHRH agonist was added after 2 weeks and lasted 12 months. Patients acted as their own controls in the follow-up. The authors did not find any impairment in cognitive functioning during androgen deprivation therapy; on the contrary, they found an improvement in the scores of an object recall task and a semantic memory task. In two additional studies on an identical patient population, associations between estrogen and testosterone levels and scores on cognitive tasks were investigated (Salminen *et al.*, 2004, 2005). Serum samples of testosterone, free testosterone, and estradiol were taken at baseline

Table 9.2. Overview of the studies on the impact of hormonal therapy on cognitive functioning in prostate cancer. (*AVLT* Auditory Verbal Learning Test, *CAMCOG* cognitive and self-contained part of the Cambridge Examination for Mental Disorders of the Elderly, *CPA* cyproterone acetate, *PSA* prostate-specific antigen, *SHBG* sex hormone binding globulin, *SOP* subjected-ordered pointing, *WAIS* Wechsler Adult Intelligence Scale, *WMS-R* Wechsler Memory Scale, Revised)

Study	Goal	Patients and comparisons	Cognitive measures	Biological measures	Design and statistical analysis
Green *et al.* (2002). Altered cognitive function in men treated for prostate cancer with luteinizing hormone-releasing hormone (LHRH) analogues and cyproterone acetate: a randomized controlled trial. *BJU Int* **90**: 427–432.	To report the first systematic investigation of the cognitive effects of LHRH analogs on prostate cancer patients	65 prostate cancer patients, randomly assigned to four conditions: 1. Treatment with leuprorelin (LHRH analog); *n* = 19 2. Treatment with goserelin (LHRH analog); *n* = 20 3. Treatment with (steroidal anti-androgen); *n* = 11 4. Close monitoring; *n* = 15	WMS-R visual memory WMS-R verbal memory AVLT Rey complex figure; immediate and delayed recall WMS-R Attention and concentration index WAIS Digit Symbol Controlled Oral Word Association Test Trail Making Test A and B Stroop test Victoria version WAIS-R 4 subtests	Periodic serum assays of testosterone and PSA were collected to check patient compliance	Longitudinal design. Cognitive assessments at baseline and at 6 months. Group × time analyses were conducted for serum, cognitive and emotional measures. The "reliable change index" was used to more closely examine individual results and to identify clinically significant cognitive changes
	Affective measures Depression Anxiety Stress Scales (DASS-21)		*Conclusion* A significant decrease on ≥1 task was observed for 9 out of 19 patients on leuprorelin, 9 out of 20 patients on goserelin, 6 out of 11 patients on CPA and none out of 15 patients on close monitoring.	*Conclusion (continued)* Limitations of the study: • Small sample size • Control group had higher average intelligence and education than active treatment groups	*Remarks*
		Cognitive complaints The results suggest that patients treated with goserelin improved performance on WMS-R visual and verbal memory measures but decreased performance on the AVLT measure of verbal memory The close monitoring group increased their performance on the WMS verbal memory test			

(*cont.*)

Table 9.2. (cont.)

Study	Goal	Patients and comparisons	Cognitive measures	Biological measures	Design and statistical analysis
Cherrier et al. (2003). The effects of combined androgen blockade on cognitive function during the first cycle of intermittent androgen suppression in patients with prostate cancer. J Urol **170**: 1808–1811.	To evaluate the effects of androgen deprivation on cognitive function.	Two groups: 1. 19 patients with prostate cancer (52–76 years of age) receiving intermittent androgen suppression therapy 2. 15 healthy community dwelling control participants	Spatial memory: • Route test Spatial ability: • Block design test • Mental rotation test Verbal memory: • Proactive interference test • Story recall test Verbal ability: Letter fluency test Executive function: Stroop color word test • Visual working memory task	Serum total testosterone levels and free testerone levels were obtained from the patient group	Longitudinal design: cognitive testing occurred twice before the start of treatment, after 9 months of treatment, and after 3 months of treatment
	Affective measures	*Cognitive complaints*	*Conclusion* 9 months of combined androgen blockade resulted in: • A beneficial effect on verbal memory • A detrimental effect on one measure of spatial ability (mental rotation).	*Conclusion (continued)*	*Remarks* Preliminary results because of: • Small sample size
Salminen et al. (2003). Androgen deprivation and cognition in prostate cancer. Br J Cancer **89**: 971–976.	To assess whether cognitive functioning is impaired during 12 months of androgen deprivation therapy	Two groups: • 25 prostate cancer patients receiving neoadjuvant androgen depression therapy for 12 months in connection with radical radiotherapy	WAIS similarities WAIS Digit span WAIS Digit-symbol Substitution subtest WAIS block design Verbal fluency (animals) Picture naming task Naming time (immediate and delayed) Word list recall	Longitudinal design: • Patients were tested at baseline (before start of therapy); and at 6 and 12 months of therapy • Patients acted as their own controls in the follow-up • Healthy controls were tested once	

	Aim	Participants / Intervention	Measures	Conclusion	Remarks
		• 52 healthy control males (baseline measurement only)	*Affective measures* Beck Depression Inventory Quality of Life forms (EORTC QLQ-C30) with additional items on sexual functioning, physical and mental discomfort, worry, role functioning, limitations in daily activities and bother due to prostate cancer or treatments	*Cognitive complaints* No impairment in cognitive performances was found during androgen deprivation therapy	Benton Visual Recognition (form C) Wechsler Visual Memory Span MMSE CogniSpeed Reaction times (4 subtests) *Conclusion* Improvement was observed in object recall (naming time, immediate and delayed); and semantic memory (similarities). In QOL, impairment in physical functioning was observed.	*Conclusion (continued)* Limitations of the study: • Small sample size • The authors didn't control for practice effects • The healthy controls were only used for a comparison with the cognitive performances of the patient group at baseline, limiting the possibilities of interpretation
Salminen *et al.* (2004). Associations between serum testosterone fall and cognitive function in prostate cancer patients *Clin Cancer Res* **10**: 7575–7582.	To investigate the associations between serum testosterone decline and specific cognitive functions in newly diagnosed prostate cancer patients treated with androgen deprivation therapy	23 prostate cancer patients receiving androgen deprivation therapy for 12 months: • 250 mg of flutamide 3 times a day for 4 weeks • From week 2: 11.25 mg leuprolide every 3 months	WAIS similarities WAIS Digit Span WAIS Digit-Symbol Substitution subtest WAIS block design Verbal fluency (animals) Picture naming task Naming time (immediate and delayed) Word list recall Benton Visual Recognition (C)		Serum samples for hormone analysis were collected at baseline and at 6 and 12 months Serum testosterone, free testosterone and sexual hormone binding globulin were determined Longitudinal design. Changes in hormone levels and in cognitive performance from baseline to 6 and 12 months were calculated and compared Regression analysis and correlations were used to study the

Remarks

(cont.)

Table 9.2. (cont.)

Study	Goal	Patients and comparisons	Cognitive measures	Biological measures	Design and statistical analysis
			Wechsler Visual Memory Span MMSE CogniSpeed Reaction times (4 subtests)		associations between changes in hormone levels and cognitive performances
	Affective measures Beck Depression Inventory *Cognitive complaints*		*Conclusion* Testosterone decline was associated with visuo motor slowing, slowed reaction times in some attentional domains including working, memory and impaired hit-rate in a vigilance test, impaired delayed recall and recognition speed of letters. Improvement in object recall	*Conclusion (continued)* Limitations of the study: • Small sample size	*Remarks*
Salminen *et al.* (2005). Estradiol and cognition during androgen deprivation in men with prostate carcinoma. *Cancer* **103** (7): 1381–1387.	To investigate the association of androgen-deprivation-induced estradiol decline with cognition in prostate carcinoma	23 prostate cancer patients receiving androgen deprivation therapy for 12 months: • 250 mg of flutamide 3 times a day for 4 weeks • from week 2: 11.25 mg leuprolide every 3 months	WAIS similarities WAIS Digit Span WAIS Digit-Symbol Substitution subtest WAIS block design Verbal fluency (animals) Picture naming task Naming time (immediate and delayed) Word list recall Benton Visual Recognition (C) Wechsler Visual Memory Span MMSE CogniSpeed Reaction times (4 subtests)	Serum samples for hormone analysis were collected at baseline and at 6 and 12 months Serum testosterone and estradiol were determined	Longitudinal design. Changes in hormone levels and in cognitive performance from baseline to 6 and 12 months were calculated and compared Regression analysis and correlations were used to study the associations between changes in hormone levels and cognitive performances

	Affective measures	Cognitive complaints	Conclusion	Conclusion (continued)	Remarks
	Beck Depression Inventory		Estrogen decline during androgen deprivation therapy was associated with a decline in visual memory and recognition speed at 6 months and with an improvement of verbal fluency at 12 months		Limitations of the study: • Small sample size
Almeida *et al.* (2004). One year follow-up study of the association between chemical castration, sex hormones, beta-amyloid, memory and depression in men. *Psychoneuroendocrinology* **29**: 1071–1081.	To clarify whether testosterone depletion and receptor blockade are associated with changes in mood and cognitive functions in humans	Prostate cancer patients who were prescribed intermittent androgen deprivation treatment with leuprolide (an LHRH analog) every 3 months for 36 weeks and flutamide 250 mg (an anti-androgen) for 36 weeks. *n* = 40; mean age = 72.4)	CAMCOG WMS-III word list WMS-III verbal paired associates WMS-III visual reproduction WAIS-III block design	Blood was drawn every visit to monitor plasma levels of PSA estradiol, testosterone and beta-amyloid	Longitudinal design Naturalistic study Patients were tested 1 week prior to baseline, at baseline and after 4, 12, 24, 36 weeks of treatment. At 36 weeks, treatment was discontinued and patients were re-assessed at 42, 48 and 54 weeks after baseline Multivariate analysis of variance for repeated measures; correlations

(cont.)

Table 9.2. (cont.)

Study	Goal	Patients and comparisons	Cognitive measures	Biological measures	Design and statistical analysis
	Affective measures Beck Depression Inventory Beck Anxiety Inventory	*Cognitive complaints* Discontinuation of treatment was linked to an improvement on the CAMCOG, and on recall total scores on the word list test and the verbal paired associates test	*Conclusion* No effect on the block design test	*Conclusion (continued)* Limitations of the study: • Small sample size • The authors didn't control for practice effects due to repetitive testing	*Remarks*
Jenkins *et al.* (2005). Does neoadjuvant hormone therapy for early prostate cancer affect cognition? Results from a pilot study. *BJU Int* **96**: 48–53.	To examine, in a prospective study, the influence that temporary reversible medical castration for localized prostate cancer has on cognition, by assessing whether temporary (3–5 months) treatment with a LHRH agonist before radical radiotherapy had a short- or long-term effect on cognitive function *Affective/QOL measures* General Health Questionnaire Functional Assessment of Cancer Therapy – Prostate (FACT – P) Trial Outcome Index	32 patients with localized prostate cancer, treated in a neoadjuvant setting 18 healthy control subjects *Cognitive complaints* Semi-structured interview at the final assessment	Intelligence: • National Adult Reading Test Verbal ability: • Phonemic verbal fluency task Verbal memory: • Rey Auditory Verbal Learning Test Visual memory: • Complex Figure Task Working memory: • WMS III Digit Span • WMS III Spatial Span Processing Speed: • Kendrick Assessment of Cognitive Ageing battery *Conclusion* Short-term LHRH therapy for early-stage prostate cancer has modest consequences on cognitive functioning in some men. The most affected cognitive domain is spatial ability	At all three time points serum free and bound testosterone, beta-estradiol and sex-hormone binding globulin (SHBG) levels were determined *Conclusion (continued)* Limitations of the study: • Small sample size • The authors didn't control for practice effects due to repetitive testing	Longitudinal design Naturalistic study Cognitive assessments at baseline, at 3 months of therapy and 9 months later Group comparisons of test scores were made using one-way and repeated measures ANOVA or chi-squared tests *Remarks*

Beer *et al.* (2006). Testosterone loss and estradiol administration modify memory in men. *J Urol* **175**: 130–135.	To examine the impact of androgen deprivation and subsequent estradiol therapy on the long-term and working memory of patients with prostate cancer	18 patients with androgen-independent prostate cancer, starting second-line hormonal treatment with transdermal estradiol 18 prostate cancer patients on continuous androgen deprivation 17 community dwelling healthy control subjects	Verbal memory: • Paragraph recall immediate recall • Paragraph recall delayed recall Working memory: • SOP • Trail Making Test • MMSE • WAIS-R Vocabulary	At the two time points serum total and free testosterone, estradiol and SHBG levels were determined	Longitudinal design Naturalistic study Cognitive assessments at baseline and 4 weeks later Repeated measures ANOVA were used to compare performance across the two study visits. One-way ANOVA with Tukey-HSD post hoc corrections or paired *t*-tests with Bonferroni corrections were used to examine main effects *Remarks*
			Affective/QOL measures Geriatric Depression Scale POMS	*Cognitive complaints* Patients on hormonal therapy performed worse on verbal memory and information-processing speed. Performance on working memory measures do not differ between groups *Conclusion* Patients that received estradiol therapy improved their verbal memory performance compared to baseline *Conclusion (continued)* Limitations of the study: • Small sample size • Short study duration	

(cont.)

Table 9.2. (*cont.*)

Study	Goal	Patients and comparisons	Cognitive measures	Biological measures	Design and statistical analysis
Taxel *et al.* (2004). The effect of short-term estradiol therapy on cognitive function in older men receiving hormonal suppression therapy for prostate cancer. *J Am Geriatr Soc* **52**: 269–273.	To determine the effect of estrogen alone (without the influence of testosterone) on cognitive function in older prostate cancer patients	27 patients receiving treatment with LHRH agonists for localized prostate cancer after primary treatment, or planning to receive neoadjuvant treatment with LHRH agonists for stage B or C prostate cancer	Verbal memory: • Rey AVLT Visual memory: • Benton visual retention test Executive function: • Stroop color word test • Trail Making Test • Controlled oral word association test MMSE	At the two time points serum testosterone, estrogen and SHBG levels were determined	Longitudinal design Cognitive assessments at baseline and 9 weeks later Repeated measures ANOVA were used to examine changes in hormone levels over time. Cognitive function data were analyzed with repeated measures MANOVA
		Patients were randomized between 1 mg/day $17\text{-}\beta$ micronized estradiol versus placebo	*Conclusion* Short-term treatment with low-dose estrogen resulted in a improvement of 2 out of 17 test scores (information-processing speed, executive functioning)	*(Conclusion continued)* No differences between the groups in any other measure. No difference in self-reported cognitive deficits or depressive symptoms	
	Affective/	*Cognitive complaints* Cognitive failures questionnaire			*Remarks* Limitations of the study: • Small sample size • Short study duration
	QOL measures Beck Depression Inventory				

and at 6 and 12 months. Significant associations were found between testosterone decline and slowing on some cognitive tasks, mostly in the domain of attention. Testosterone decline was also associated with less careful performance on a vigilance task. Furthermore, an association was found between testosterone decline and improvement in object recall. Estradiol decline during androgen deprivation therapy was associated with a decline in visual memory and recognition speed at 6 months of therapy, and an improvement in verbal fluency after 12 months of therapy.

Two studies evaluated the influence of combined androgen deprivation therapy on cognitive functioning. Cherrier *et al.* (2003) investigated patients ($n = 19$) who received as initial therapy flutamide (an anti-androgen; 250 mg three times daily). After 2 weeks, monthly injections of 7.5 mg leuprolide (an LHRH agonist) were administered for 9 months in addition to flutamide. They used a healthy control ($n = 15$, mean age of patients and controls together: 65 years). After 9 months, the therapy was, depending on PSA levels, continued or discontinued and re-initiated later. Patients were tested twice before the start of treatment, after 9 months of treatment and 3 months after discontinuation of treatment. They concluded that 9 months of androgen deprivation therapy resulted in a detrimental effect on one measure of spatial ability (mental rotation test). Discontinuation of the therapy resulted in a beneficial effect on verbal memory. Almeida *et al.* (2004) assessed 40 patients (mean age 72.4 years) twice before the start of treatment and four times during combined androgen deprivation treatment. After discontinuation, of treatment, patients were re-assessed another three times. Their results suggest that not initiation, but discontinuation, of treatment was associated with significant improvements in cognitive performance, particularly on a cognitive screening test and a verbal memory test. Visuospatial abilities were not influenced by introduction or discontinuation of treatment.

Jenkins *et al.* (2005) studied the relationship between temporary hormonal therapy (3–5 months) and cognitive performance in a neoadjuvant setting. Patients with localized prostate cancer ($n = 32$, mean age 67.5 years) had cognitive assessments before the start of treatment with LHRH agonists, after 3 months of therapy and 9 months later. Eighteen healthy control men (mean age 65.4 years) completed the cognitive assessments at the same times. The tests covered a broad range of cognitive functions. The results did not show an overall group effect of the treatment, but revealed that 47% of the patients, versus 17% of the controls, showed cognitive decline in at least one task after 3 months of treatment. The decline was most often in the domains of spatial memory and spatial ability. Nine months later the proportions of subjects with cognitive decline did not differ between both groups (34% versus 28%).

Two studies evaluated the influence of estrogen on cognitive functioning in prostate cancer patients. Beer *et al.* (2006) analyzed working memory and long-term memory in patients with androgen independent prostate cancer ($n = 18$); assessments took place before the start of second-line hormonal therapy with transdermal estradiol and 4 weeks later. The same assessments were performed in an age-matched patient group undergoing continued androgen deprivation therapy ($n = 18$) and a control group consisting of age-matched healthy community dwelling men ($n = 17$). The authors concluded that patients on hormonal therapy performed worse on measures of verbal memory and information processing speed compared to healthy controls, but not on measures of working memory. Patients who received estradiol therapy improved their verbal memory performance compared to baseline. Taxel *et al.* (2004) examined the influence of estrogen on cognitive function in prostate cancer patients receiving LHRH agonists. Patients treated with LHRH agonists were randomized between additional estradiol treatment ($n = 13$) and placebo ($n = 10$). Cognitive assessments took place before the start of the estradiol therapy and 9 weeks later. In this study, no clear effect of the estrogen therapy on cognitive functioning was found: on only 2 out of 17 cognitive measures (on information-processing speed and executive function) did the estradiol-treated patients show a statistically significant increase in performance compared to placebo-treated patients.

Methodological aspects

Although the conducted studies give some evidence that hormonal therapy in the treatment of cancer impacts cognitive functioning, many questions about the character, extent, and reversibility of the effects remain. Furthermore, the mechanisms of action of hormones and hormonal therapy on brain structures are complex and have only been partially elucidated. In addition, the neuropsychological studies on this topic show methodological weaknesses that probably cause under- or overestimation of the reported effects. The following are several methodological issues.

Sample size

Most of the studies had small sample sizes. Of 11 studies, 9 had sample sizes of only 10–37 patients (Almeida *et al.*, 2004; Cherrier *et al.*, 2003; Eberling *et al.*, 2004; Ernst *et al.*, 2002; Green *et al.*, 2002; Jenkins *et al.*, 2005; Salminen *et al.*, 2003; Salminen *et al.*, 2004; Salminen *et al.*, 2005). If a healthy control group was used, sample sizes were also small (15–35 subjects), and sometimes the control subjects differed from the patient groups in terms of age and intelligence. It is likely that small study populations make it difficult to detect significant differences in test scores. However, several small but well-designed studies (for example Eberling *et al.*, 2004) found significant differences even in small groups of subjects, supporting the hypothesis that effects of hormonal therapy on cognitive function go beyond normal variations in test scores.

Cross-sectional versus prospective studies

Studies of breast cancer are all cross-sectional and lack a baseline measurement. As a consequence, the results of these studies do not reflect individual changes over time associated with a particular treatment. The studies on prostate cancer do not have this shortcoming: all include a baseline measurement. However, prospective studies contend with other methodological problems, such as (possibly selective) loss of subjects to follow-up. Furthermore, repeated administrations of neuropsychological tests can yield what appears to be improvement in cognitive function due to practice that is not a true change in cognitive status. In general, an adequate method to correct for practice effects was not used in the reviewed prospective studies. In fact, stable test scores in a patient group when improvement is to be expected could actually reflect a decrease in cognitive functioning. Please refer to Chapter 23 for a more extensive description of test characteristics that are important to consider in longitudinal trials. Finally, the value of the baseline measurement should not be overestimated: at the time of baseline measurement, patients often have to cope with the diagnosis of cancer and may undergo other treatments as well, such as surgery or radiotherapy. These factors themselves could influence cognitive performance.

Selection of cognitive measures

The neuropsychological tests and the number of tests used vary highly between the studies. One study only used three tests (Paganini-Hill & Clark, 2000), while others used an extensive battery of tests. Often no rationale for the test selection was given. Since little is known about the influence of hormonal treatments on cognitive functioning, it is important to use a battery of tests that cover a broad range of cognitive functions so as not to miss possible cognitive effects through shortcomings in test selection. From the literature, there is evidence that reproductive hormones have an impact on distinct cognitive domains; estrogens particularly impact verbal memory, while androgens possibly influence visuospatial functions in particular. Therefore, it is remarkable that in the studies with breast cancer patients only one out of four studies included a verbal memory test (Shilling *et al.*, 2003). Another problem arises when tests are categorized under different cognitive domains. A specific cognitive domain can be represented by a variety of tests that can vary highly in degree of complexity and that may not be assessing exactly the same cognitive ability. This leads to disparity in the findings and, as a consequence, confusion about the role of the hormonal therapy (Jenkins *et al.*, 2005).

Self-reported cognitive complaints

Neuropsychological test scores frequently lack a clear association with self-reported cognitive problems in daily life. Most of the studies described above lack data on self-reported cognitive problems. Therefore, the question arises as to the extent to which the neuropsychological test scores actually reflect cognitive problems that patients have to deal with in daily life.

Anxiety, depression, fatigue, and psychosocial distress

It is known that mood problems, anxiety, fatigue, and psychosocial distress can have detrimental effects on cognitive test performance. In addition, cancer patients are more likely to suffer from these symptoms than healthy controls. Moreover, hormonal therapy itself possibly influences mood, psychosocial distress, and fatigue (Almeida *et al.*, 2004; Herr & O'Sullivan, 2000). For a good understanding of associations between psychosocial factors, mood factors, and cognitive performance, a thorough assessment and description of these different factors and their mutual dependencies is required (Schagen, 2002).

Comparisons of group means versus analysis of test scores of individuals

In most studies, mean test scores of groups are compared (Almeida *et al.*, 2004; Cherrier *et al.*, 2003; Eberling *et al.*, 2004; Ernst *et al.*, 2002; Paganini-Hill & Clark, 2000; Salminen *et al.*, 2003; Shilling *et al.*, 2003). Comparing group means can obscure indi-

vidual variations in test scores. A subgroup of patients with deviant test scores, or a subgroup whose scores improve or decline more than those of others may not be detected by comparing means. Only two studies used a method of determining individual decline (Green *et al.*, 2002; Jenkins *et al.*, 2005), and showed clearly that more patients in the active treatment groups suffered from significant decreases on one or more test scores compared to a non-treatment patient group or a non-cancer control group.

Conclusions

Although many questions remain unanswered regarding the influence of reproductive hormones on cognitive functioning, there is increasing evidence that reproductive hormones, and therapies that act on these hormones, can have a rather modest effect on cognitive functioning. In healthy men and women, the most consistent results come from studies on natural fluctuations and, in addition, on surgically induced menopause in women. These studies suggest that higher estrogen levels are associated with better performance on verbal memory tasks. Testosterone levels are mostly found to influence visuospatial abilities, in a way that suggests an optimal testosterone level, situated in the "lower male range." In any case, the relationships between reproductive hormones and cognitive functioning are complex and, to date, only partially elucidated.

Although many neuropsychological studies have been conducted on hormone substitution in healthy persons, the results of these studies are far from conclusive. The results of these supplementation studies vary from a beneficial effect or no effect at all, to a detrimental effect on cognitive functioning. Neuroimaging studies show that estrogens and testosterone are capable of changing brain-activation patterns, but the clinical significance of these results is unknown.

Many questions remain unanswered about the possible influence of hormonal therapies in the treatment of cancer on cognitive functioning. In breast cancer studies, three out of four studies suggest a slightly detrimental effect on cognitive functioning. On the basis of these studies, it is impossible to draw conclusions about the cognitive domains that are most vulnerable to the effects of the hormonal agents. In prostate cancer studies, mixed results were found without a clear and understandable pattern. Detrimental as well as beneficial effects were found.

Most of the studies showed methodological shortcomings, among others small sample sizes, a lack of baseline measurements, a lack of control for practice effects, inadequate selection of cognitive tests, inadequate determination of cognitive decline, and a lack of data on mood, anxiety, fatigue, and psychosocial distress.

The role of hormonal therapy in cancer treatment is increasing, and the medical grounds for prescribing this kind of treatment are expanding. As a consequence, increasing numbers of, often elderly, patients use hormonal therapy. Because intact cognitive functioning is essential for independent living and activities in daily life, it is important that the effects on cognition of the various hormonal agents and treatment regimens are included in long-term safety and quality-of-life studies. Large-scale studies that use appropriate controls and that include measures of symptoms of depression, anxiety, psychosocial distress, and fatigue are needed. Such studies should, among others, include verbal memory and spatial ability tasks, because these cognitive domains are probably the most vulnerable to hormonal effects. Furthermore, research that addresses mechanisms that might explain the results from neuropsychological studies is needed. Finally, probably the most important issue that needs attention is the experience of patients who use the various hormonal agents. After all, little is known about their cognitive complaints during therapy or the relationship between their complaints and test scores, psychosocial features, and health characteristics. Information from these studies can be used to make patients and clinicians aware of any potentially harmful cognitive side-effects that have to be balanced against benefits of the hormonal treatments.

REFERENCES

Almeida OP, Waterreus A, Spry N *et al.* (2004). One year follow-up study of the association between chemical castration, sex hormones, beta-amyloid, memory and depression in men. *Psychoneuroendocrinology* **29**: 1071–1081.

Azad N, Pitale S, Barnes WE *et al.* (2003). Testosterone treatment enhances regional brain perfusion in hypogonadal men. *J Clin Endocrinol Metab* **88**: 3064–3068.

Barrett-Connor E, Kritz-Silverstein D (1993). Estrogen replacement therapy and cognitive function in older women. *J Am Med Assoc* **269**: 2637–2641.

Beer TM, Bland LB, Bussiere JR *et al.* (2006). Testosterone loss and estradiol administration modify memory in men. *J Urol* **175**: 130–135.

Bender CM, Paraska KK, Sereika SM *et al.* (2001). Cognitive function and reproductive hormones in adjuvant therapy for breast cancer: a critical review. *J Pain Symptom Manag* **21**: 407–424.

Benson JR (2002). Re: The effects of tamoxifen and estrogen on brain metabolism in elderly women. *J Natl Cancer Inst* **94**: 1336–1337.

Bowen RL, Martins RN, Gregory CW *et al.* (2005). Dementia and testosterone levels in men. *J Am Med Assoc* **293**: 551.

Chen D, Wu CF, Shi B *et al.* (2002a). Tamoxifen and toremifene cause impairment of learning and memory function in mice. *Pharmacol Biochem Behav* **71**: 269–276.

Chen D, Wu CF, Shi B *et al.* (2002b). Tamoxifen and toremifene impair retrieval, but not acquisition, of spatial information processing in mice. *Pharmacol Biochem Behav* **72**: 417–421.

Cherrier MM, Asthana S, Plymate S *et al.* (2001). Testosterone supplementation improves spatial and verbal memory in healthy older men. *Neurology* **57**: 80–88.

Cherrier MM, Rose AL, Higano C (2003). The effects of combined androgen blockade on cognitive function during the first cycle of intermittent androgen suppression in patients with prostate cancer. *J Urol* **170**: 1808–1811.

Cholerton B, Gleason CE, Baker LD *et al.* (2002). Estrogen and Alzheimer's disease: the story so far. *Drugs Aging* **19**: 405–427.

Cook IA, Morgan ML, Dunkin JJ *et al.* (2002). Estrogen replacement therapy is associated with less progression of subclinical structural brain disease in normal elderly women: a pilot study. *Int J Geriatr Psychiatry* **17**: 610–618.

Drake EB, Henderson VW, Stanczyk FZ *et al.* (2000). Associations between circulating sex steroid hormones and cognition in normal elderly women. *Neurology* **54**: 599–603.

Eberling JL, Reed BR, Coleman JE *et al.* (2000). Effect of estrogen on cerebral glucose metabolism in postmenopausal women. *Neurology* **55**: 875–877.

Eberling JL, Wu C, Tong-Turnbeaugh R *et al.* (2004). Estrogen- and tamoxifen-associated effects on brain structure and function. *Neuroimage* **21**: 364–371.

Ernst T, Chang L, Cooray D *et al.* (2002). The effects of tamoxifen and estrogen on brain metabolism in elderly women. *J Natl Cancer Inst* **94**: 592–597.

Espeland MA, Rapp SR, Shumaker SA *et al.* (2004). Conjugated equine estrogens and global cognitive function in postmenopausal women: Women's Health Initiative Memory Study. *J Am Med Assoc* **291**: 2959–2968.

Fonda SJ, Bertrand R, O'Donnell A *et al.* (2005). Age, hormones, and cognitive functioning among middle-aged and elderly men: cross-sectional evidence from the Massachusetts Male Aging Study. *J Gerontol A Biol Sci Med Sci* **60**: 385–390.

Ganz PA, Castellon SA, Silverman DH (2002). Estrogen, tamoxifen, and the brain. *J Natl Cancer Inst* **94**: 547–549.

Gleason CE, Cholerton B, Carlsson CM *et al.* (2005). Neuroprotective effects of female sex steroids in humans: current controversies and future directions. *Cell Mol Life Sci* **62**: 299–312.

Goss PE, Strasser K (2001). Aromatase inhibitors in the treatment and prevention of breast cancer. *J Clin Oncol* **19**: 881–894.

Green HJ, Pakenham KI, Gardiner RA (2000). Effects of luteinizing hormone releasing hormone analogs on cognition in women and men: a review. *Psychol Health Med* **5**: 407–418.

Green HJ, Pakenham KI, Headley BC *et al.* (2002). Altered cognitive function in men treated for prostate cancer with luteinizing hormone-releasing hormone analogues and cyproterone acetate: a randomized controlled trial. *BJU Int* **90**: 427–432.

Hampson E (1990). Variations in sex-related cognitive abilities across the menstrual cycle. *Brain Cogn* **14**: 26–43.

Haren MT, Wittert GA, Chapman IM *et al.* (2005). Effect of oral testosterone undecanoate on visuospatial cognition, mood and quality of life in elderly men with low-normal gonadal status. *Maturitas* **50**: 124–133.

Hausmann M, Slabbekoorn D, Van Goozen SH *et al.* (2000). Sex hormones affect spatial abilities during the menstrual cycle. *Behav Neurosci* **114**: 1245–1250.

Hellerstedt BA, Pienta KJ (2002). The current state of hormonal therapy for prostate cancer. *CA Cancer J Clin* **52**: 154–179.

Henderson VW, Guthrie JR, Dudley EC *et al.* (2003). Estrogen exposures and memory at midlife: a population-based study of women. *Neurology* **60**: 1369–1371.

Herr HW, O'Sullivan M (2000). Quality of life of asymptomatic men with nonmetastatic prostate cancer on androgen deprivation therapy. *J Urol* **163**: 1743–1746.

Hogervorst E, Williams J, Budge M *et al.* (2001). Serum total testosterone is lower in men with Alzheimer's disease. *Neuroendocrinol Lett* **22**: 163–168.

Hogervorst E, De Jager C, Budge M *et al.* (2004). Serum levels of estradiol and testosterone and performance in different cognitive domains in healthy elderly men and women. *Psychoneuroendocrinology* **29**: 405–421.

Janowsky JS, Chavez B, Orwoll E (2000). Sex steroids modify working memory. *J Cogn Neurosci* **12**: 407–414.

Jenkins VA, Bloomfield DJ, Shilling VM *et al.* (2005). Does neoadjuvant hormone therapy for early prostate cancer affect cognition? Results from a pilot study. *BJU Int* **96**: 48–53.

Juul A, Skakkebaek NE (2002). Androgens and the ageing male. *Hum Reprod Update* **8**: 423–433.

Kenny AM, Bellantonio S, Gruman CA *et al.* (2002). Effects of transdermal testosterone on cognitive function and health perception in older men with low bioavailable testosterone levels. *J Gerontol A Biol Sci Med Sci* **57**: M321–M325.

Luoto R, Manolio T, Meilahn E *et al.* (2000). Estrogen replacement therapy and MRI-demonstrated cerebral infarcts, white matter changes, and brain atrophy in older women: the Cardiovascular Health Study. *J Am Geriatr Soc* **48**: 467–472.

Maki PM (2004). Hormone therapy and risk for dementia: where do we go from here? *Gynecol Endocrinol* **19**: 354–359.

Maki PM, Resnick SM (2000). Longitudinal effects of estrogen replacement therapy on PET cerebral blood flow and cognition. *Neurobiol Aging* **21**: 373–383.

Maki PM, Rich JB, Rosenbaum RS (2002). Implicit memory varies across the menstrual cycle: estrogen effects in young women. *Neuropsychologia* **40**: 518–529.

Meyer PM, Powell LH, Wilson RS *et al.* (2003). A population-based longitudinal study of cognitive functioning in the menopausal transition. *Neurology* **61**: 801–806.

Miller WR (1996). *Estrogens and Endocrine Therapy for Breast Cancer. Estrogen and Breast Cancer.* Heidelberg: Springer Verlag.

Moffat SD, Zonderman AB, Metter EJ *et al.* (2004). Free testosterone and risk for Alzheimer disease in older men. *Neurology* 62: 188–193.

Muller M, Aleman A, Grobbee DE *et al.* (2005). Endogenous sex hormone levels and cognitive function in aging men: is there an optimal level? *Neurology* 64: 866–871.

Newton C, Slota D, Yuzpe AA *et al.* (1996). Memory complaints associated with the use of gonadotropin-releasing hormone agonists: a preliminary study. *Fertil Steril* 65: 1253–1255.

Nickelsen T, Lufkin EG, Riggs BL *et al.* (1999). Raloxifene hydrochloride, a selective estrogen receptor modulator: safety assessment of effects on cognitive function and mood in postmenopausal women. *Psychoneuroendocrinology* 24: 115–128.

Norbury R, Cutter WJ, Compton J *et al.* (2003). The neuroprotective effects of estrogen on the aging brain. *Exp Gerontol* 38: 109–117.

Nystedt M, Berglund G, Bolund C *et al.* (2000). Randomized trial of adjuvant tamoxifen and/or goserelin in premenopausal breast cancer – self-rated physiological effects and symptoms. *Acta Oncol* 39: 959–968.

O'Connor DB, Archer J, Hair WM *et al.* (2001). Activational effects of testosterone on cognitive function in men. *Neuropsychologia* 39: 1385–1394.

Osborne CK, Zhao H, Fuqua SA (2000). Selective estrogen receptor modulators: structure, function, and clinical use. *J Clin Oncol* 18: 3172–3186.

Owens JF, Matthews KA, Everson SA (2002). Cognitive function effects of suppressing ovarian hormones in young women. *Menopause* 9: 227–235.

Paganini-Hill A, Clark LJ (2000). Preliminary assessment of cognitive function in breast cancer patients treated with tamoxifen. *Breast Cancer Res Treat* 64: 165–176.

Phillips SM, Sherwin BB (1992). Effects of estrogen on memory function in surgically menopausal women. *Psychoneuroendocrinology* 17: 485–495.

Rapp SR, Espeland MA, Shumaker SA *et al.* (2003). Effect of estrogen plus progestin on global cognitive function in postmenopausal women: the Women's Health Initiative Memory Study: a randomized controlled trial. *J Am Med Assoc* 289: 2663–2672.

Resnick SM, Maki PM, Golski S *et al.* (1998). Effects of estrogen replacement therapy on PET cerebral blood flow and neuropsychological performance. *Horm Behav* 34: 171–182.

Rosario ER, Chang L, Stanczyk FZ *et al.* (2004). Age-related testosterone depletion and the development of Alzheimer disease. *J Am Med Assoc* 292: 1431–1432.

Salminen E, Portin R, Korpela J *et al.* (2003). Androgen deprivation and cognition in prostate cancer. *Br J Cancer* 89: 971–976.

Salminen EK, Portin RI, Koskinen A *et al.* (2004). Associations between serum testosterone fall and cognitive function in prostate cancer patients. *Clin Cancer Res* 10: 7575–7582.

Salminen EK, Portin RI, Koskinen AI *et al.* (2005). Estradiol and cognition during androgen deprivation in men with prostate carcinoma. *Cancer* 103: 1381–1387.

Sanders G, Sjodin M, de Chastelaine M (2002). On the elusive nature of sex differences in cognition: hormonal influences contributing to within-sex variation. *Arch Sex Behav* 31: 145–152.

Schagen SB (2002). Cognitive function following chemotherapy: a study in breast cancer patients. Ph.D Thesis. University of Amsterdam.

Schmidt R, Fazekas F, Reinhart B *et al.* (1996). Estrogen replacement therapy in older women: a neuropsychological and brain MRI study. *J Am Geriatr Soc* 44: 1307–1313.

Sharifi N, Gulley JL, Dahut WL (2005). Androgen deprivation therapy for prostate cancer. *J Am Med Assoc* 294: 238–244.

Shaywitz SE, Shaywitz BA, Pugh KR *et al.* (1999). Effect of estrogen on brain activation patterns in postmenopausal women during working memory tasks. *J Am Med Assoc* 281: 1197–1202.

Sherwin BB (1988). Estrogen and/or androgen replacement therapy and cognitive functioning in surgically menopausal women. *Psychoneuroendocrinology* 13: 345–357.

Sherwin BB (2000). Oestrogen and cognitive function throughout the female lifespan. *Novartis Found Symp* 230: 188–196.

Sherwin BB (2003). Steroid hormones and cognitive functioning in aging men: a mini-review. *J Mol Neurosci* 20: 385–393.

Sherwin BB (2005). Estrogen and memory in women: how can we reconcile the findings? *Horm Behav* 47: 371–375.

Sherwin BB, Tulandi T (1996). "Add-back" estrogen reverses cognitive deficits induced by a gonadotropin-releasing hormone agonist in women with leiomyomata uteri. *J Clin Endocrinol Metab* 81: 2545–2549.

Shilling V, Jenkins V, Fallowfield L *et al.* (2003). The effects of hormone therapy on cognition in breast cancer. *J Steroid Biochem Mol Biol* 86: 405–412.

Shumaker SA, Legault C, Rapp SR *et al.* (2003). Estrogen plus progestin and the incidence of dementia and mild cognitive impairment in postmenopausal women: the

Women's Health Initiative Memory Study: a randomized controlled trial. *J Am Med Assoc* **289**: 2651–2662.

Shumaker SA, Legault C, Kuller L *et al.* (2004). Conjugated equine estrogens and incidence of probable dementia and mild cognitive impairment in postmenopausal women: Women's Health Initiative Memory Study. *J Am Med Assoc* **291**: 2947–2958.

Simpson ER, Dowsett M (2002). Aromatase and its inhibitors: significance for breast cancer therapy. *Recent Prog Horm Res* **57**: 317–338.

Tannock IF, Ahles TA, Ganz PA *et al.* (2004). Cognitive impairment associated with chemotherapy for cancer: report of a workshop. *J Clin Oncol* **22**: 2233–2239.

Taxel P, Stevens MC, Trahiotis M *et al.* (2004). The effect of short-term estradiol therapy on cognitive function in older men receiving hormonal suppression therapy for prostate cancer. *J Am Geriatr Soc* **52**: 269–273.

Tripathy D, Benz CC (2001). Hormones and cancer. In Greenspan FS, Gardner DG (eds.) *Basic and Clinical Endocrinology*. New York: Lange Medical Books.

Verghese J, Kuslansky G, Katz MJ *et al.* (2000). Cognitive performance in surgically menopausal women on estrogen. *Neurology* **55**: 872–874.

Visvanathan K, Davidson NE (2003). Aromatase inhibitors as adjuvant therapy in breast cancer. *Oncology (Huntingt)* **17**: 335–342, 347.

Wolf OT, Kirschbaum C (2002). Endogenous estradiol and testosterone levels are associated with cognitive performance in older women and men. *Horm Behav* **41**: 259–266.

Wolf OT, Neumann O, Hellhammer DH *et al.* (1997). Effects of a two-week physiological dehydroepiandrosterone substitution on cognitive performance and well-being in healthy elderly women and men. *J Clin Endocrinol Metab* **82**: 2363–2367.

Yaffe K, Sawaya G, Lieberburg I *et al.* (1998). Estrogen therapy in postmenopausal women: effects on cognitive function and dementia. *J Am Med Assoc* **279**: 688–695.

Yaffe K, Krueger K, Sarkar S *et al.* (2001). Cognitive function in postmenopausal women treated with raloxifene. *N Engl J Med* **344**: 1207–1213.

Yaffe K, Lui LY, Zmuda J *et al.* (2002). Sex hormones and cognitive function in older men. *J Am Geriatr Soc* **50**: 707–712.

Yaffe K, Krueger K, Cummings SR *et al.* (2005). Effect of raloxifene on prevention of dementia and cognitive impairment in older women: the Multiple Outcomes of Raloxifene Evaluation (MORE) randomized trial. *Am J Psychiatry* **162**: 683–690.

10

Low-grade gliomas

Martin J. B. Taphoorn and Charles G. Niël

Introduction

Low-grade gliomas (LGG) are diffusely infiltrating primary tumors of the cerebral hemispheres, and originate from glial tissue (Kleihues & Cavanee, 2000). Patients with these tumors, like any patient with a brain disease, may experience cognitive complaints and have cognitive deficits on examination. In LGG patients, who usually have a paucity of neurological deficits, these cognitive complaints and deficits may be particularly prominent, in contrast to patients with high-grade gliomas (HGG). In HGG patients, the rapidly growing tumor typically gives rise to hemiparesis or increased intracranial pressure, which may overshadow more subtle cognitive deficits (Ashby & Shapiro, 2004; Rees, 2002). Moreover, LGG patients have a relatively good prognosis with median survival rates ranging from 5 to more than 15 years. Long-term-surviving LGG patients run the risk of late toxicity of treatment. Tumor and treatment effects may impair cognitive functioning in these patients during the course of their disease and have a deleterious impact on the quality of life of the patient and their family.

Epidemiology and biology, pathology and genetics, clinical and imaging features, prognostic factors in LGG

Epidemiology and biology

The percentage of low-grade tumors amongst gliomas, the most common primary brain tumor, ranges between 15% and 20% (Kleihues & Cavanee, 2000). The incidence of gliomas in adults is 5 to 7 per 100 000 (Bondy & Wrensch, 1996). This figure has remained stable for many years, unlike that of other brain tumors such as primary central nervous system (CNS) lymphoma, which is increasing in incidence. Low-grade glioma typically develops in young adults. There is a slight preponderance in men (male:female ratio 1.3:1). Only the diffusely growing LGG of the cerebral hemispheres in adults will be discussed here. The pilocytic astrocytoma (mainly occurring in children in the posterior fossa), and the optic nerve glioma, both regarded as LGG, should be treated differently from the hemispheric LGG in adults, and they have a different prognosis (Kleihues & Cavanee, 2000). Also, relatively rare tumors such as the gangliocytoma

Cognition and Cancer, eds. Christina A. Meyers and James R. Perry. Published by Cambridge University Press.
© Cambridge University Press 2008.

and the dysembryoplastic neuro-ectodermal tumor (DNET), considered as belonging to the group of LGG, will not be discussed here due to their different behavior and prognosis (Rees, 2002). The same holds true for brainstem astrocytomas and gliomatosis cerebri, which both may show low-grade features on histopathological examination (Ashby & Shapiro, 2004).

In contrast to HGG, which are rapidly growing tumors leading to neurological deficit and increased intracranial pressure, LGG in the adult may remain silent for a long time (Ashby & Shapiro, 2004; Rees, 2002). Still, LGG are not benign tumors; by far the majority of LGG patients will, in due time, die from progressive tumor growth after dedifferentiation to a high-grade tumor. Although there is increasing knowledge on molecular tumor biology in general and on genetic abnormalities in all kinds of tumors, including gliomas, the etiology of gliomas remains still unknown (Rasheed et al., 1999). Environmental factors, such as food substances, alcohol, coffee, smoking, and the use of cellular phones, have been studied, with no or only a minor increased risk for glioma revealed (Christensen et al., 2005; Efird et al., 2004; Hardell et al., 2007; Huncharek et al., 2003; Rasheed et al., 1999; Takebayashi et al., 2008). The only known risk factor for gliomas is radiation therapy in the past (Salvati et al., 1991). Many years following therapeutic irradiation of the head there is a small chance that a glioma may occur.

Gliomas are more likely to arise in patients with genetic tumor syndromes such as neurofibromatosis, and the rarely occurring Turcot syndrome and Li-Fraumeni syndrome (Kleihues & Cavanee, 2000). Also, siblings of glioma patients without any known genetic syndrome have an increased risk for gliomas (Hemminki & Li, 2003).

Pathology and genetics

Based on histopathological examination, which is the gold standard for the diagnosis of LGG (Kleihues & Cavanee, 2000), the diffusely growing gliomas are classified as astrocytomas, oligodendrogliomas or mixed gliomas. Astrocytomas account for about 80% of all gliomas. Histological variants of astrocytomas are the fibrillary astrocytoma, the gemistocytic astrocytoma, and the protoplasmatic astrocytoma. The gemistocytic variant is particularly prone to dedifferentiation into a HGG. Subsequently, a distinction is made between low-grade and high-grade tumors. The absence of high-grade features such as mitoses, necrosis, nuclear atypia, and microvascular proliferation implies a low-grade tumor. In the current World Health Organization (WHO) classification the formerly applied grading system (grades I–IV for astrocytic tumors and grades A–D for oligodendroglial tumors) has been abandoned. A LGG is thus denominated as "astrocytoma," "oligodendroglioma" or "oligo-astrocytoma" (Kleihues & Cavanee, 2000).

Although the histopathology of gliomas has prognostic significance, this analysis is by definition subjective because it is based on visual criteria. Moreover, due to the heterogeneous nature of gliomas, high-grade features may be missed on histopathological examination, especially in small (stereotactic) biopsy specimens ("sampling error") (Jackson et al., 2001). Therefore, the definite diagnosis should always be based on the combination of histopathological, clinical, and radiological features.

It is believed that genetic analysis of gliomas, next to histopathological examination, will play a major role in future neuro-oncology (Fuller et al., 2002; Godard et al., 2003; Idbaih et al., 2007; Iwadate et al., 2004). As we have not in the past been able to define subsets of (low-grade) gliomas that are responsive to specific treatments, the value of these therapies may have been underestimated.

In LGG, frequent mutations of the tumor suppression gene p53 have been known to exist for a long time and are found in approximately 75% of cases. Other genetic changes include a gain of chromosome 7q, amplification of 8q, loss of heterozygosity (LOH) on 10p and 22q, and overexpression of platelet-derived growth factor receptor (PDGFR) (Kleihues & Cavanee, 2000). As these tumors dedifferentiate to high-grade tumors many other mutations will occur, reflecting the aggressive behavior of these tumors (Rees, 2002). This genetic pathway is quite different from that of tumors that are high grade from the start, such as the de novo glioblastoma multiforme, in which p53 mutations are very rare, but where epidermal growth factor receptor (EGFR) overexpression and PTEN (phosphatase and tensin homolog deleted on chromosome 10) mutation is frequently observed (Kleihues & Cavanee, 2000). Only recently has a link been made between specific genetic abnormalities in anaplastic oligodendroglioma (allelic loss of chromosomes 1p and 19q), the response to chemotherapy, and survival (Cairncross *et al.*, 1998). Also in LGG, both astrocytoma and oligodendroglioma types, genetic aberrations of chromosomes 1p and 19q have been described (Hirose *et al.*, 2003; Kaloshi *et al.*, 2007; Smith *et al.*, 2000; Watanabe *et al.*, 2002).

Clinical and imaging features

The majority of LGG patients present with one or more (focal) seizures but have no other symptoms (Ashby & Shapiro, 2004; Rees, 2002). Typically, no abnormalities are found on neurological examination; the features of a rapidly growing tumor such as a HGG leading to neurological deficit and increased intracranial pressure are absent. Even so, many patients with LGG appear to have problems with cognitive functioning at presentation (Pahlson *et al.*, 2003; Taphoorn & Klein, 2004). In some patients the tumor may be detected by chance, as imaging was performed for other reasons (e.g., head trauma, tension headache, dizziness).

On imaging, LGG are hypodense lesions on computed tomography (CT) with relatively little mass effect and no contrast enhancement. On magnetic resonance imaging (MRI), T2-weighted sequences or fluid-attenuated inversion recovery (FLAIR) images demonstrate a diffusely infiltrating high-signal lesion with slight mass effect (Figure 10.1). There is no contrast enhancement of the low-signal lesion on T1-weighted sequences (Recht *et al.*, 1992). Compared with CT, MRI is more sensitive in detecting LGG. The presence of calcifications in the lesion suggests an oligodendroglioma rather than an astrocytoma. Both CT and MR imaging have their limitations in determining whether a lesion is an LGG. An arachnoid cyst or an infarction with atypical clinical presentation may be mistaken for an LGG. Also, a ganglioglioma and a DNET, which are rare tumors in adults and are most frequently located in the (medial) temporal lobe, may have features similar to LGG. Still, these tumors are more sharply demarcated from surrounding tissue than LGG and a ganglioglioma may enhance with contrast agent. More importantly, the distinction between a high-grade and a low-grade tumor may be difficult: histopathological examination of about 35% of "typical" LGG on imaging reveals high-grade features, with the highest probability in patients over age 40 (Ginsberg *et al.*, 1998; Scott *et al.*, 2002).

More recently developed imaging modalities such as diffusion-weighted imaging (DWI), MR spectroscopy (MRS), and functional positron emission tomography (PET) have been unable to clearly improve the specificity of standard MRI (Herholz *et al.*, 1998; Knopp *et al.*, 1999; Kono *et al.*, 2001; Vuori *et al.*, 2004), although perfusion-weighted MR imaging (PWI) might be of help in differentiating low-grade from high-grade tumors (Maia *et al.*, 2005).

Prognostic factors in LGG

The natural history of an LGG is unpredictable. Some patients may remain free from clinical and radiological signs of tumor progression for several decades, whereas in others progression and de-differentiation to a high-grade tumor occur within weeks to months from the initial presentation (Ashby & Shapiro, 2004; Rees, 2002). Tumor progression results in an increased incidence of epileptic seizures, neurological deficit, and/or increased intracranial pressure. The majority of LGG patients will die from their disease sooner or later, unless intercurrent diseases occur. The median survival of LGG patients ranges from 5 to 10 years according to a large number of studies (Ashby & Shapiro, 2004; Johannesen *et al.*, 2003; Rees, 2002). This wide range may be explained by the earlier diagnosis of LGG with MRI currently compared to CT.

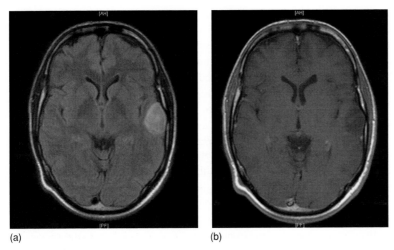

(a)   (b)

Figure 10.1. A 37-year-old male, presenting with focal seizures. (a) On MRI (FLAIR image): left temporal lesion, no surrounding edema, no mass effect; (b) T1-weighted image after gadolinium: no contrast enhancement

One study of oligodendroglioma even indicated a median survival of more than 15 years (Olson *et al.*, 2000).

Prognostic factors in LGG are age (patients over the age of 35–40 years have a worse prognosis than younger patients) and tumor histology (oligodendroglioma has a better prognosis compared to astrocytoma) (Leighton *et al.*, 1997; Vecht, 1993). Also, LGG patients who present solely with epilepsy have a better outlook than those who have neurological deficit on presentation. Next to these factors, tumor size and location (i.e., tumor extending into the other hemisphere) may have prognostic implications as well, according to the analysis of a large sample of LGG patients (Pignatti *et al.*, 2002). Sorting the patients from this sample according to five negative prognostic factors (age >40 years, neurological deficit, astrocytic histology, tumor size >6 cm, tumor crossing the midline) into a low-risk group (0–2 negative factors) and a high-risk group (3–5 factors) resulted in a median survival of 7.7 years in the favorable group versus 3.2 years in the unfavorable group.

More recently observed prognostic factors are cognitive function, the activity of the DNA repair enzyme *O*-6-methylguanine methyltransferase and

loss of chromosome 1p/19q (Brown *et al.*, 2004; Kaloshi *et al.*, 2007; Komine *et al.*, 2003; Levin *et al.*, 2006).

Therapeutic management

Surgery

Surgery in LGG may have two goals: a tissue biopsy is necessary to make the histopathological diagnosis (and to perform molecular genetics); and reduction of tumor mass may be intended to relieve neurological symptoms and signs and/or to enhance survival.

Surgery to reduce tumor mass is controversial in LGG (Ashby & Shapiro, 2004; Dropcho, 2004; Rees, 2002). This especially holds true for surgery to improve survival in cases without increased intracranial pressure. The majority of LGG patients do not have neurological symptoms and signs that may improve following reduction of tumor mass, but some do. Examples are patients with cystic tumors causing neurological deficit or patients with medication-resistant epilepsy that may be relieved by tumor resection ("epilepsy-surgery").

Despite technical developments in surgery, such as intraoperative-guided imaging and functional mapping, the infiltrative growth pattern of LGG prevents surgical cure. A review of the extent of resection as a factor influencing outcome in LGG suggested that there is no proof that surgery improves survival (Keles *et al.*, 2001) but a more recent review contested this (Sanai and Berger 2008). However, a recent retrospective study found that extent of resection was associated with significantly longer overall survival and minimal morbidity, suggesting improved patient outcome with maximal resection of hemispheric LGG (Smith *et al.*, 2008).

Using intraoperative-guided imaging and functional mapping in patients with LGG, surgery even in eloquent brain locations is feasible with very limited lasting neurological deficits due to the operation (Duffau, 2003a, 2003b, 2004).

Since neither radiation therapy nor chemotherapy following surgery has been demonstrated to improve survival in the majority of LGG patients, a so-called wait and see policy is often adopted in LGG patients with favorable prognostic factors (Ashby & Shapiro, 2004; Dropcho, 2004; Recht *et al.*, 1992; Rees, 2002). This conservative policy is in contrast to the earlier statement that LGG are not benign tumors, and that some are known to be responsive to treatment due to certain genetic features. A "wait and see" policy should only be advocated in patients under 40 years old who present with epilepsy and have no abnormalities on neurogical examination. Also, the typical features of an LGG should be found on imaging. In these cases, even a biopsy may be deferred (Reijneveld *et al.*, 2001). A second MRI should be performed after a 3-month interval to rule out the development of a high-grade tumor. In the case of a stable clinical situation and no signs of tumor progression on imaging, the "wait and see" approach may be continued with clinical and MRI follow-up once or twice a year, until progression occurs. A slow and slight increase in tumor size is normally observed over time in these patients on critical measurements of tumor volume (Mandonnet *et al.*, 2003). This, however, does not necessarily imply dedifferentiation of the tumor.

Radiotherapy

Based on several retrospective analyses in LGG patients, (focal) external radiotherapy resulted in improved survival (Cairncross, 2000; Shaw *et al.*, 1989). As other retrospective studies did not demonstrate a survival benefit of radiotherapy, selection bias was presumed to be a confounding factor (Cairncross, 2000). Adversaries of radiation therapy in LGG also point to irreversible long-term side-effects of radiation that may result in severe cognitive deterioration (Choucair *et al.*, 1997).

At present, the controversy on (early) radiation treatment in LGG has been ended to some extent by the results of prospective randomized trials in both Europe and the USA. Two trials comparing high-dose with low-dose radiation (59.4 versus 45 Gy; 64.8 versus 50.4 Gy) did not demonstrate a survival benefit for high-dose radiation (Karim *et al.*, 1996; Shaw *et al.*, 2002). Moreover, based on the results of the European trial (EORTC 22844) high-dose radiation resulted in a worse health-related quality of life (Kiebert *et al.*, 1998). Research on the dose dependency of neurotoxicity and of treatment is, however, hampered by the constant technical evolution in radiation oncology. The earlier-mentioned prospective randomized trials, one starting in 1984 (Karim *et al.*, 1996) and the other in 1986 (Shaw *et al.*, 2002), failed to demonstrate better results from a higher radiation dose. This might, in part, be caused by suboptimal dose definition compared to current standards: at the time these studies were performed, dose definition was merely an obligation to describe radiation dose in a uniform way, resulting in good inter-institutional dose comparability in multisite trials (ICRU report 29, 1979) rather than the clear and uniform individual dose description that is necessary to study dose-related clinical outcome. It was not until 1993 that the International Convention on Radiation Units (ICRU) defined radiation dose in an unequivocal way.

Of even more importance is the EORTC 22845 randomized trial of over 300 LGG patients, comparing early radiotherapy to observation only following surgery or biopsy. Progression-free survival was significantly longer in the radiotherapy group than in the observation group; however, overall survival was not different as reported in two interim analyses (Karim *et al.*, 2002; Van den Bent *et al.*, 2005). As quality of life was not studied, it is unknown whether clinical deterioration was postponed by early radiotherapy. Based on the results of these trials, early radiotherapy in LGG patients with favorable prognostic factors has been largely abandoned.

Patients with histologically proven LGG who are older than 40 and/or have (progressive) neurological deficit are likely to benefit from early radiation (Pignatti *et al.*, 2002). Focal radiation is currently applied with total doses ranging from 45 to 60 Gy in fractions of up to 2 Gy. Also, patients with medication-refractory epilepsy due to the tumor may benefit from radiation of their LGG (Rogers *et al.*, 1993).

Chemotherapy

Systemic chemotherapy is not a primary treatment for LGG patients currently. In line with the effective chemotherapeutic treatment of high-grade oligodendroglioma and high-grade oligoastrocytoma with PCV chemotherapy (procarbazine, lomustine, also known as CCNU®, and vincristine) or temozolomide, these agents have also been applied to low-grade oligodendroglial tumors in several phase II studies (Buckner *et al.*, 2003; Hoang-Xuan *et al.*, 2004; Kaloshi *et al.*, 2007; Levin *et al.*, 2006; Pace *et al.*, 2003; Quinn *et al.*, 2003; Stege *et al.*, 2005; Van den Bent *et al.*, 1998, 2003). Objective responses on imaging have been reported but may be difficult to appreciate due to the absence of contrast enhancement of LGG. MR spectroscopy may add to the evaluation of treatment response (Murphy *et al.*, 2004). In a recent study of low-grade oligodendroglial tumors, an objective response was denoted in 29%–52% of patients. In contrast to the relation between response to chemotherapy and loss of chromosomes 1p and 19q in high-grade oligodendroglioma, this has not been observed in all studies on LGG (Buckner *et al.*, 2003). Due to the

potential long-term adverse effects of radiation and the observation that LGG responds to chemotherapy, randomized studies comparing radiation and chemotherapy in (progressive) LGG are currently running in the USA as well as in Europe.

Neurocognitive disturbances in LGG

Neurocognitive deficits in LGG patients can be caused by the tumor, by tumor-related epilepsy (Klein *et al.*, 2003), and treatment (neurosurgery, radiotherapy, anti-epileptics, chemotherapy, or corticosteroids), as well as by psychological distress. More likely, a combination of these factors will contribute to neurocognitive dysfunction. Also tumor regrowth (either locally or diffuse), leptomeningeal metastasis, or metabolic disturbances may negatively affect neurocognitive function.

Primary tumor as a cause of neurocognitive deficits

The tumor itself is an important contributor to neurocognitive deficits, which holds true for both high-grade and low-grade tumors. Neurocognitive deficits are a prominent clinical feature in slowly growing tumors, such as LGG, or in diffusely infiltrating tumors, such as primary CNS lymphoma or gliomatosis cerebri. In rapidly growing, high-grade tumors focal neurological deficits and high intracranial pressure may overshadow more subtle cognitive deficits.

In many studies of neurocognitive function in patients with brain tumor, conclusions about the role of the tumor cannot be easily made, because data are only gathered after treatment. In a series of 139 patients with different brain tumors, neurocognitive disturbances were observed in 91% before treatment was initiated (Tucha *et al.*, 2000).

Neurocognitive testing in these studies is often directed more toward the functions of the dominant hemisphere, therefore it is not surprising that patients with tumors in the dominant hemisphere reportedly have more cognitive deficits than those with non-dominant hemisphere lesions (Hahn *et al.*, 2003; Taphoorn *et al.*, 1992).

Unlike stroke patients, who tend to have site-specific deficits, glioma patients have may have more diffuse, milder and variable deficits, which may be explained by the diffuse growth of tumor cells infiltrating normal brain tissue (Anderson *et al.*, 1990). Additionally, acute neurotransmitter changes and chronic degeneration of fiber tracts caused by damage to certain brain areas may impair neuronal responses in remote undamaged cortical regions (i.e., diaschisis).

Neurocognitive deficits may also be the first manifestation of tumor recurrence, even before structural changes are observed on imaging (Armstrong *et al.*, 2003; Meyers & Hess, 2003).

Surgery as the cause of neurocognitive deficit

Neurosurgery and peri-operative injuries may cause (transient) neurological deficits due to damage of normal surrounding tissue. Many neurosurgeons are therefore hesitant to operate on patients with brain tumors in eloquent brain areas. According to Scheibel and co-workers (1996) neurosurgery in patients with glioma leads to focal neurocognitive deficits, in contrast to more diffuse neurocognitive disturbances caused by radiation and chemotherapy. Recent studies that use intraoperative-guided imaging and functional mapping in patients with LGG in eloquent brain locations show that a high percentage of them have post-operative neurocognitive deficits (Duffau *et al.*, 2003a, 2003b). However, most of these deficits resolved within 3 months, presumably owing to the plasticity of the normal brain and recovery from the acute effects of surgery (Duffau *et al.*, 2003a, 2003b; Duffau, 2006).

In line with these data, a study on a large group of patients with LGG who had biopsy or neurosurgical tumor resection at least 1 year before indicated that neurosurgery did not contribute to neurocognitive disability (Klein *et al.*, 2002). By contrast, neurosurgery in patients with histologically proven versus suspected LGG had a negative effect on neurocog-

nitive function and health-related quality of life in a case-matched control study (Reijneveld *et al.*, 2001).

Radiation as the cause of cognitive deficit

Cranial irradiation can cause several adverse changes in normal brain tissue (Sheline *et al.*, 1980; Taphoorn & Klein, 2004). Radiation-induced white matter disease due to demyelination and/or small vessel damage may result in (severe) cognitive deterioration several months to years following cranial radiotherapy (see Chapter 7 for a more extensive discussion of radiation injury to the brain). As LGG patients have a relatively good prognosis, this long-term complication is much feared (Surma-Aho *et al.*, 2001). The risk of long-term adverse effects of radiotherapy in LGG patients has always been an important issue in the discussion of early versus delayed radiation treatment of these patients.

From a clinical and morphological point of view four types of damage caused by irradiation can be discerned: acute reaction (transient edema), early delayed reaction, late delayed reaction, and focal radiation necrosis. The type of damage and its clinical impact are time dependent. Mainly early delayed damage, occurring between 1 and 6 months after irradiation, and late delayed damage (after 6 months to several years post-irradiation) have a negative impact on neurocognitive function. The first is a reversible process of de- and remyelination, whereas the late delayed damage results in a diffuse encephalopathy, of which neurocognitive disturbances are the hallmark (Armstrong *et al.*, 2002; Béhin & Delattre, 2003; Vigliani *et al.*, 1996).

The pathophysiology of the diffuse encephalopathy following radiotherapy is not completely understood. Both vascular structures and glial cells are thought to be the target of radiation damage, as histological examination can reveal both demyelination and vascular damage. In the glial hypothesis, oligodendrocytes are the primary target of radiation damage resulting in demyelination, whereas the vascular hypothesis is based on histological proof of blood-vessel dilatation and wall thickening with hyalinization, endothelial cell loss, and a decrease in vessel density leading to white-matter necrosis. The pathogenesis is probably far more complex, and may also involve effects on neural stem cell production with resulting hippocampal dysfunction (Monje & Palmer, 2003; Monje *et al.*, 2007).

On imaging modalities late delayed encephalopathy may result in cerebral atrophy and/or diffuse white matter disease. To some extent there is a relation between the abnormalities on MRI and cognitive status (Postma *et al.*, 2002). Diffusion tensor MR imaging may be of additional value in this respect (Nagesh *et al.*, 2008).

The severity of neurocognitive deficits due to late delayed radiation encephalopathy ranges from mild or moderate neurocognitive deficits all the way to dementia. Mild to moderate neurocognitive deficits result in attention or short-term memory disturbances as the main features. Because studies on this subject vary greatly in the neuropsychological test procedures, the populations studied, and the duration of follow-up (Béhin & Delattre, 2003; Vigliani *et al.*, 1999) the clinical picture and incidence of this complication are hard to define exactly.

Following cranial irradiation, diffuse white matter changes (leukoencephalopathy on CT and MRI) may occur in as many as 40%–50% of patients (Constine *et al.*, 1988). The greater the amount of healthy brain that is exposed to irradiation, the greater the likelihood of these imaging changes and resulting neurocognitive deficits developing. Focal irradiation causes fewer imaging and neurocognitive changes compared to whole-brain irradiation (Swennen *et al.*, 2004). Therefore, caution should be used in interpreting the results of studies into the impact of cranial irradiation if the irradiated volume is not well defined: focal irradiation is current practice in the treatment of LGG, whereas in the 1980s and 1990s, some of these patients received whole-brain irradiation. These latter patients have been included in retrospective analyses, such as a study of the neurocognitive function of 160 patients treated from 1980 to 1992 (Surma-Aho *et al.*, 2001). Of these patients, 101 had received irradiation and 57 of them had died by the time of the analysis.

In contrast, 45 of the 59 non-irradiated patients were still alive, indicating that the irradiated group was highly selected. Of the 44 irradiated patients alive at the time of assessment, 28 patients had neurocognitive deficits, of whom 19 had received whole-brain irradiation (40 Gy), followed by focal irradiation up to a total dose of 64–75 Gy. Whole-brain irradiation is now obsolete in treating LGG since when it is applied in 2-Gy fractions followed by a focal boost of irradiation to a higher dose, it results in "neurocognitive disturbances." In contrast to this, Klein *et al.* (Klein *et al.*, 2002) retrospectively evaluated the impact of focal radiation on neurocognitive function in LGG patients. In this study, 195 LGG patients were compared to 100 patients with a hematological malignancy with comparable overall survival, and with 195 healthy controls. Focal radiation treatment itself was not found to be a significant factor in causing neurocognitive disturbances as long as the radiation fraction size did not exceed 2 Gy. In contrast, the presence of the tumor itself increased the risk for neurocognitive impairment compared to the hematological malignancy group. One might expect that with current focal irradiation techniques, such as three-dimensional conformal radiotherapy and intensity-modified radiotherapy, the amount of normal brain tissue irradiated will be even less compared to the patients from the Klein *et al.* (2002) study (Niël *et al.*, 2005). Studies looking at neurocognitive outcomes with these newer techniques are not yet available.

The total radiation dose given is, after volume of treatment and fraction size, the third factor that influences the amount of neurotoxicity from irradiation. In a study by Corn *et al.* (1994) the amount of white matter change (but not neurocognitive functioning) was analysed in dose escalation studies performed by the Radiation Therapy Oncology Group (RTOG). Mild white matter changes did not seem to occur more frequently with higher radiation doses than with lower doses, whereas the most severe white matter changes (necrosis) occurred significantly more frequently in the highest dose groups. A focal irradiation dose of 54 Gy resulted in less

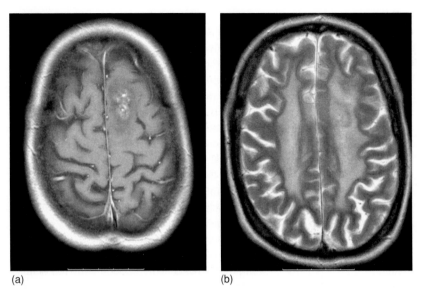

(a)   (b)

Figure 10.2. (a) A 42-year old female, who had been operated on for a left parietal low-grade oligodendroglioma 5 years before. She had focal radiation treatment (54 Gy, fraction size 1.8 Gy) when she had a regrowth of the tumor (T1-weighted image after gadolinium); (b) 2 years following radiation she experienced mental slowing, had no recurrence of tumor on imaging but had extensive white matter disease (T2-weighted image)

than 8% of moderate to severe white matter changes (Corn *et al.*, 1994).

Apart from radiation factors determining the risk of diffuse encephalopathy, such as total dose, fraction dose, volume of brain irradiated, and total duration of treatment, patient factors may also contribute to this adverse effect of treatment. These factors are age greater than 60, pre-existing white matter disease (e.g., vascular white matter disease, multiple sclerosis), vascular risk factors (smoking, diabetes, hypertension), and possibly a genetic predisposition (Peterson *et al.*, 1993; Swennen *et al.*, 2004).

In addition to the study by Klein *et al.* (2002) demonstrating that radiotherapy was not the main reason for cognitive disturbances in LGG survivors, several other studies have shown similar results. Armstrong and colleagues (2002) reported on a prospective study regarding neurocognitive function and MRI findings in 26 patients with LGG. After treatment a highly selective decline in visual

memory was demonstrated in 50% of patients. White matter abnormalities on T2-weighted MRI were observed at 6 months after treatment and beyond, but did not progress after 3 years from baseline (Armstrong *et al.*, 2002). Torres and co-workers (2003) reported subtle neurocognitive deficits in patients with LGG that were already present at the start of radiotherapy, without further decline during a 2-year follow-up (Figure 10.2). Analysis of cognitive functions in patients with LGG treated with lower dose radiation or higher dose radiation (randomly assigned to 50.4 Gy or 64.8 Gy) revealed that Mini-Mental State Examination scores in 101 patients with a median follow-up of 7.4 years after radiotherapy showed little cognitive deterioration (Brown *et al.*, 2003). Moreover, extensive psychometric testing in a subgroup of 20 patients revealed stable cognitive functioning during 3 years of follow-up (Laack *et al.*, 2005).

Despite these reassuring data regarding adverse effects of radiotherapy on cognitive functioning in

LGG patients, neurocognitive decline may still result from therapeutic irradiation, especially in the long run (Klein *et al.*, 2006). Therefore, randomized studies are underway both in the USA and Europe, comparing radiotherapy with chemotherapy in the treatment of LGG.

Medical therapy as a cause of neurocognitive disturbances

Anti-epileptic drugs

Epileptic seizures are the first symptom of an intracranial tumor in 30%–90% of patients, and this holds especially true for LGG. Among LGG patients, about 70% take one or more anti-epileptic drugs (Klein *et al.*, 2003). The older anti-epileptic drugs, such as phenytoin, carbamazepine, and valproic acid, decrease neurocognitive functioning. Impairments of attention and cognitive slowing may result in memory deficits by reducing the efficiency of encoding and retrieval (Drane & Meador, 2002; Meador, 2002). Of the newer drugs, such as lamotrigine, levetiracetam, and topiramate, data on cognitive side-effects are still scarce. Apart from anti-epileptic drugs, cognitive function may be negatively affected by the seizures themselves (Jokeit & Ebner, 1999). In a study of 156 long-term LGG survivors without signs of tumor recurrence, deficits in information-processing speed, psychomotor functioning, executive functioning, and working memory capacity were significantly related to the use of anti-epileptic drugs or the severity of epilepsy. As patients in this study who took anti-epileptic drugs had cognitive disturbances even in the absence of seizures, the use of drugs primarily seems to affect cognitive function (Klein *et al.*, 2003).

Chemotherapy

In glioma patients, combination therapy with PCV for the subset of oligodendroglial tumors proved to be a breakthrough in treatment. In LGG, both PCV chemotherapy and temozolomide have been proven to be effective treatments (Buckner *et al.*, 2003; Pace *et al.*, 2003; Quinn *et al.*, 2003; Stege *et al.*, 2005; Van den Bent *et al.*, 1998, 2003).

Cognitive side-effects of temozolomide have so far not been described, and encephalopathy with cognitive deficits caused by PCV chemotherapy has been reported only with high-dose regimens (Postma *et al.*, 1998).

The late neurotoxic effects of chemotherapy may be difficult to discern from those of radiotherapy, because many LGG patients treated with chemotherapy have already been treated with radiotherapy. In contrast to several other brain tumors, LGG is not treated with intra-arterial drug regimens, local chemotherapy or intrathecal chemotherapy. These applications may increase the likelihood of neurotoxicity, compared to systemic chemotherapy (oral or intravenous) (Wen, 2003).

Mood disorder as a cause of neurocognitive disturbances

Like any cancer patient, brain tumor patients have feelings of anxiety, depression, and future uncertainty as psychological reactions to the disease (Anderson *et al.*, 1999). As patients with extracranial tumors do not have structural brain lesions that cause cognitive deficits, neuropsychological disturbances in these patients are more likely related to mood disorders than to central nervous system lesions. LGG patients report lower levels of panic, depression, anxiety, and fear of death than do patients with high-grade tumors. These mood disturbances may lead to deficits in attention, vigilance, and motivation that subsequently affect several cognitive domains (Anderson *et al.*, 1999).

Conclusion

Compared to their high-grade counterparts, LGG may behave as rather indolent tumors with a relatively long median survival time. Due to the absence of focal neurological deficits and increased intracranial pressure in the majority of LGG patients, cognitive complaints and deficits may be very prominent. Neurotoxicity, mainly due to radiotherapy, has for a long time been thought to be the main cause of cognitive deficits in LGG patients. An important finding from several studies on LGG is that, although radiation has to some extent an adverse effect on cognitive function, other tumor and treatment factors deserve more attention. Also, cognitive function is being recognized as an independent factor in LGG patients, and may even be a first indication of tumor regrowth following treatment.

REFERENCES

Anderson SI, Taylor R, Whittle IR (1999). Mood disorders in patients after treatment for primary intracranial tumours. *Br J Neurosurg* **13**: 480–485.

Anderson SW, Damasio H, Tranel D (1990). Neuropsychological impairments associated with lesions caused by tumor or stroke. *Arch Neurol* **47**: 397–405.

Armstrong CL, Hunter JV, Ledakis GE *et al.* (2002). Late cognitive and radiographic changes related to radiotherapy: initial prospective findings. *Neurology* **59**: 40–48.

Armstrong CL, Goldstein B, Shera D *et al.* (2003). The predictive value of longitudinal neuropsychologic assessment in the early detection of brain tumor recurrence. *Cancer* **97**: 649–656.

Ashby LS, Shapiro WR (2004). Low-grade glioma: supratentorial astrocytoma, oligodendroglioma, and oligoastrocytoma in adults. *Curr Neurol Neurosci Rep* **4**: 211–217.

Béhin A, Delattre JY (2003). Neurologic sequelae of radiotherapy of the nervous system. In Schiff D, Wen PY (eds.) *Cancer Neurology in Clinical Practice* (pp. 173–192). Totowa: Humana Press.

Bondy ML, Wrensch MR (1996). Epidemiology of primary malignant brain tumours. In Yung WKA (ed.) *Cerebral Gliomas* (pp. 251–270). London: Ballière Tindall.

Brown PD, Buckner JC, O'Fallon JR *et al.* (2003). Effects of radiotherapy on cognitive function in patients with low-grade glioma measured by the Folstein mini-mental state examination. *J Clin Oncol* **21**: 2519–2524.

Brown PD, Buckner JC, O'Fallon JR *et al.* (2004). Importance of baseline mini-mental state examination as a prognostic factor for patients with low-grade glioma. *Int J Radiat Oncol Biol Phys* **59**: 117–125.

Buckner JC, Gesme D, O'Fallon JR *et al.* (2003). Phase II trial of procarbazine, lomustine, and vincristine as initial therapy for patients with low-grade oligodendroglioma and oligoastrocytoma: efficacy and associations with chromosomal abnormalities. *J Clin Oncol* **21**: 251–255.

Cairncross JG (2000). Understanding low-grade glioma: a decade of progress. *Neurology* **54**: 1402–1403.

Cairncross JG, Ueki K, Zlatescu MC *et al.* (1998). Specific chromosomal losses predict chemotherapeutic response and survival in patients with anaplastic oligodendrogliomas. *J Natl Cancer Inst* **90**: 1473–1479.

Choucair AK, Scott C, Urtasun R *et al.* (1997). Quality of life and neuropsychological evaluation for patients with malignant astrocytomas: RTOG 91–14. *Int J Radiat Oncol Biol Phys* **38**: 9–20.

Christensen HC, Schüz J, Kosteljanetz M *et al.* (2005). Cellular telephones and risk for brain tumors: a population-based, incident case-control study. *Neurology* **64**: 1189–1195.

Constine LS, Konski A, Ekholm S *et al.* (1988). Adverse effects of brain irradiation correlated with MR and CT imaging. *Int J Radiat Oncol Biol Phys* **15**(2): 319–330.

Corn BW, Yousem DM, Scott CB *et al.* (1994). White matter changes are correlated significantly with radiation dose. Obervations from a randomized dose-escalation trial for malignant glioma (Radiation Therapy Oncology Group 83-02). *Cancer* **74** (10): 2828–2835.

Drane LD, Meador KJ (2002). Cognitive and behavioural effects of antiepileptic drugs. *Epilepsy Behav* **3**: 49–53.

Dropcho EJ (2004). Low-grade gliomas in adults. *Curr Treat Options Neurol* **6**: 265–271.

Duffau H (2006). New concepts in surgery of WHO grade II glioma: functional brain mapping, connectionism and plasticity – a review. *J Neurooncol* **79**: 77–115.

Duffau H, Capelle L, Denvil D *et al.* (2003a). Functional recovery after surgical resection of low grade gliomas in eloquent brain: hypothesis of brain compensation. *J Neurol Neurosurg Psychiatry* **74**(7): 901–907.

Duffau H, Capelle L, Denvil D *et al.* (2003b). Usefulness of intraoperative electrical subcortical mapping during surgery for low-grade gliomas located within eloquent brain regions: functional results in a consecutive series of 103 patients. *J Neurosurg* **98**(4): 764–778.

Duffau H, Khalil I, Gatignol P *et al.* (2004). Surgical removal of corpus callosum infiltrated by low-grade glioma: functional outcome and oncological considerations. *J Neurosurg* **100**: 431–437.

Efird JT, Friedman GD, Sidney S *et al.* (2004). The risk for malignant primary adult-onset glioma in a large multiethnic, managed-care cohort: cigarette smoking and other lifestyle behaviors. *J Neurooncol* **68**: 57–69.

Fuller GN, Hess KR, Rhee CH *et al.* (2002). Molecular classification of human diffuse gliomas by multidimensional scaling analysis of gene expression profiles parallels morphology-based classification, correlates with survival and reveals clinically relevant novel glioma subsets. *Brain Pathol* **12**: 108–116.

Ginsberg LE, Fuller GN, Hashni M *et al.* (1998). The significance of lack of MR contrast enhancement of supratentorial brain tumors in adults: histopathological evaluation of a series. *Surg Neurol* **49**: 436–440.

Godard S, Getz G, Delorenzi M *et al.* (2003). Classification of human astrocytic gliomas on the basis of gene expression: a correlated group of genes with angiogenic activity emerges as a strong predictor of subtypes. *Cancer Res* **63**: 6613–6625.

Hahn CA, Dunn RH, Logue PE *et al.* (2003). Prospective study of neuropsychologic testing and quality-of-life assessment of adults with primary malignant brain tumors. *Int J Radiat Oncol Biol Phys* **55**: 992–999.

Hardell L, Carlberg M, Söderqvist F, Mild KH, Morgan (2007). Long-term use of cellular phones and brain tumours: increased risk associated with use for ≥ 10 years. *Occup Environ Med* **64**: 626–632.

Hemminki K, Li X (2003). Familial risks in nervous system tumors. *Cancer Epidemiol Biomarkers Prev* **12**: 1137–1142.

Herholz K, Hölzer T, Bauer B *et al.* (1998). ^{11}C-Methionine PET for differential diagnosis of low-grade gliomas. *Neurology* **50**: 1316–1322.

Hirose Y, Aldape KD, Chang S *et al.* (2003). Grade II astrocytomas are subgrouped by chromosome aberrations. *Cancer Genet Cytogenet* **142**: 1–7.

Hoang-Xuan K, Capelle L, Kujas M *et al.* (2004). Temozolomide as initial treatment for adults with low-grade oligodendrogliomas or oligoastrocytomas and correlation with chromosome 1p deletions. *J Clin Oncol* **22**: 3133–3138.

Huncharek M, Kupelnick B, Wheeler L (2003). Dietary cured meat and the risk of adult glioma: a meta-analysis of nine observational studies. *J Environ Pathol Toxicol Oncol* **22**: 129–137.

Idbaih A, Omuro A, Ducray F, Hoang-Xuan K (2007). Molecular genetic markers as predictors of response to chemotherapy in gliomas. *Curr Opin Oncol* **19**: 606–611.

Iwadate Y, Sakaida T, Hiwasa T *et al.* (2004). Molecular classification and survival prediction in human gliomas based on proteome analysis. *Cancer Res* **64**: 2496–2501.

Jackson RJ, Fuller GN, Abi-Said D *et al.* (2001). Limitations of stereotactic biopsy in the initial management of gliomas. *Neurooncology* **3**: 193–200.

Johannesen TB, Langmark F, Lote K (2003). Progress in long-term survival in adult patients with supratentorial low-grade gliomas: a population-based study of 993 patients in whom tumors were diagnosed between 1970 and 1993. *J Neurosurg* **99**: 854–862.

Jokeit H, Ebner A (1999). Long term effects of refractory temporal lobe epilepsy on cognitive abilities: a cross sectional study. *J Neurol Neurosurg Psychiatry* **67**: 44–50.

Kaloshi G, Benouaich-Amiel A, Diakite F *et al.* (2007) Temozolomide for low-grade gliomas: predictive impact of 1p/19q loss on response and outcome. *Neurology* **68**: 1831–1836.

Karim ABMF, Maat B, Hatlevoll R *et al.* (1996). A randomised trial on dose response in radiation therapy of low grade cerebral glioma: EORTC study 22844. *Int J Radiat Oncol Biol Phys* **36**: 549–556.

Karim ABMF, Afra D, Cornu P *et al.* (2002). Randomized trial on efficacy of radiotherapy for cerebral low-grade glioma in the adult. EORTC study 22845 with the MRC study BR04: an interim analysis. *Int J Radiat Oncol Biol Phys* **52**: 316–324.

Keles GE, Lamborn KR, Berger MS (2001). Low-grade hemispheric gliomas in adults: a critical review of extent of resection as a factor influencing outcome. *J Neurosurg* **95**: 735–745.

Kiebert GM, Curran D, Aaronson NK *et al.* (1998). Quality of life after radiation therapy of low-grade glioma of the adult: results of a randomised phase III trial on dose response (EORTC 22844). *Eur J Cancer* **34**: 1902–1909.

Kleihues P, Cavenee WK (eds.) (2000). *World Health Organization Classification of Tumours of the Nervous System.* Lyon: WHO/ARC Press.

Klein M Heimans JJ, Aaronson NK *et al.* (2002). Effect of radiotherapy and other treatment-related factors on mid-term to long-term cognitive sequelae in low-grade gliomas: a comparative study. *Lancet* **360**: 1361–1368.

Klein M, Engelberts NH, Van Der Ploeg HM *et al.* (2003). Epilepsy in low-grade gliomas: the impact on cognitive function and quality of life. *Ann Neurol* **54**: 514–520.

Klein M, Fagel S, Taphoorn MJB, Postma TJ, Heimans JJ (2006). Neurocognitive function in long-term low-grade glioma. Survivors: a six-year follow-up study. *Neurooncology* **8** (4): 321 (abstract).

Knopp EA, Cha S, Johnson G *et al.* (1999). Glial neoplasms: dynamic contrast-enhanced T2-weighted imaging. *Radiology* **211**: 791–798.

Komine C, Watanabe T, Katayama Y *et al.* (2003). Promotor hypermethylation of the DNA repair gene *O6*-methylguanine-DNA methyltransferase is an independent predictor of shortened progression free survival in patients with low-grade diffuse astrocytomas. *Brain Pathol* **13**: 176–184.

Kono K, Inoue Y, Nakayama K *et al.* (2001). The role of diffusion-weighted imaging in patients with brain tumors. *Am J Neuroradiol* **22**: 1081–1088.

Laack NN, Brown PD, Ivnik RJ *et al.* (2005). Cognitive function after radiotherapy for supratentorial low-grade glioma: a North Central Cancer Treatment Group prospective study. *Int J Radiat Oncol Biol Phys* **63**: 1175–1183.

Leighton C, Fisher B, Bauman G *et al.* (1997). Supratentorial low-grade glioma in adults: an analysis of prognostic factors and timing of radiation. *J Clin Oncol* **15**: 1294–1301.

Levin N, Lavon I, Zelikovitsch B *et al.* (2006). Progressive low-grade oligobendrogliomas: response to temozolomide and correlation between genetic profile and *O*-6-methyguanine DNA methyltransferase protein expression. *Cancer* **106**: 1759–1765.

Maia AC Jr., Malheiros SM, da Rocha AJ *et al.* (2005). MR cerebral blood volume maps correlated with vascular endothelial growth factor expression and tumor grade in nonenhancing gliomas. *AJNR Am J Neuroradiol* **26**: 777–783.

Mandonnet E, Delattre JY, Tnaguy ML *et al.* (2003). Continuous growth of mean tumor diameter in a subset of grade II gliomas. *Ann Neurol* **53**: 524–528.

Meador KJ (2002). Cognitive outcomes and predictive factors in epilepsy. *Neurology* **58**: 21–26.

Meyers CA, Hess KR (2003). Multifaceted end points in brain tumor clinical trials: cognitive deterioration precedes MRI progression. *Neurooncology* **5**: 89–95.

Monje ML, Palmer T (2003). Radiation injury and neurogenesis. *Curr Opin Neurol* **16**: 129–134.

Monje ML, Vogel H, Masek M, Ligon KL, Fisher PG, Palmer TD (2007). Impaired human hippocampal neurogenesis after treatment for central nervous system malignancies. *Ann Neurol* **62**: 515–520.

Murphy PS, Viviers L, Abson C *et al.* (2004). Monitoring temozolomide treatment of low-grade glioma with proton magnetic resonance spectroscopy. *Br J Cancer* **90**: 781–786.

Nagesh Y, Tsien CI, Chevenert TL *et al.* Radiation-induced changes in normal-appearing white matter in patients with cerebral tumors: a diffusion tensor imaging study. *Int J Radiat Oncol Biol Phys* **70**(4): 1002–1010.

Niël CGJH, Struikmans H, van Santvoort J (2005). Radiotherapy for primary brain tumors: clinical potential of novel treatment techniques. *Neurooncology* **7**(3): 391 (abstract).

Olson JD, Riedel E, DeAngelis LM (2000). Long-term outcome of low-grade oligodendroglioma and mixed glioma. *Neurology* **54**: 1442–1448.

Pace A, Vidiri A, Galie E *et al.* (2003). Temozolomide chemotherapy for progressive low-grade glioma: clinical benefits and radiological response. *Ann Oncol* **14**: 1722–1726.

Pahlson A, Ek L, Ahlstrom G *et al.* (2003). Pitfalls in the assessment of disability in individuals with low-grade gliomas. *J Neurooncol* **65**: 149–158.

Peterson K, Rosenblum MK, Powers JM *et al.* (1993). Effect of brain irradiation on demyelinating lesions. *Neurology* **43**: 2105–2112.

Pignatti F, van den Bent MJ, Curran D *et al.* (2002). Prognostic factors for survival in adult patients with cerebral low-grade glioma. *J Clin Oncol* **20**: 2076–2084.

Postma TJ, van Groeningen CJ, Witjes RJ *et al.* (1998). Neurotoxicity of combination chemotherapy with procarbazine, CCNU and vincristine (PCV) for recurrent glioma. *J Neurooncol* **38**: 69–75.

Postma TJ, Klein M, Verstappen CC *et al.* (2002). Radiotherapy-induced cerebral abnormalities in patients with low-grade glioma. *Neurology* **59**: 121–123.

Quinn JA, Reardon DA, Friedman AH *et al.* (2003). Phase II trial of temozolomide in patients with progressive low grade glioma. *J Clin Oncol* **21**: 646–651.

Rasheed BK, Wiltshire RN, Bigner SH *et al.* (1999). Molecular pathogenesis of malignant gliomas. *Curr Opin Oncol* **11**: 162–167.

Recht LD, Lew R, Smith TW (1992). Suspected low-grade glioma: is deferring treatment safe? *Ann Neurol* **31**: 431–436.

Rees JH (2002). Low-grade gliomas in adults. *Curr Opin Neurol* **15**: 657–661.

Reijneveld JC, Sitskoorn MM, Klein M *et al.* (2001). Cognitive status and quality of life in patients with suspected versus proven low-grade glioma. *Neurology* **56**: 618–623.

Rogers LR, Morris HH, Lupica K (1993). Effect of cranial irradiation on seizure frequency in adults with low-grade astrocytoma and medically intractable epilepsy. *Neurology* **43**: 1599–1601.

Sanai N, Berger MS (2008). Glioma extent of resection and its impact on patient outcome. *Neurosurgery* **62**(4): 753–764.

Salvati M, Artico M, Caruso R *et al.* (1991). A report on radiation-induced gliomas. *Cancer* 67: 392–397.

Scheibel RS, Meyers CA, Levin VA (1996). Cognitive dysfunction following surgery for intracerebral glioma: influence of histopathology, lesion location, and treatment. *J Neurooncol* 30(1): 61–69.

Scott JN, Brasher PM, Sevick RJ *et al.* (2002). How often are nonenhancing supratentorial gliomas malignant? A population study. *Neurology* 59: 947–949.

Shaw EG, Daumas-Duport C, Scheithauer BW *et al.* (1989). Radiation therapy in the management of low-grade supratentorial astrocytomas. *J Neurosurg* 70: 853–861.

Shaw E, Arusell R, Scheithauer B *et al.* (2002). Prospective randomized trial of low- versus high-dose radiation therapy in adults with supratentorial low-grade glioma: initial report of a NCCTG/RTOG/ECOG study. *J Clin Oncol* 20: 2267–2276.

Sheline GE, Wara WM, Smith V (1980). Therapeutic irradiation and brain injury. *Int J Radiat Oncol Biol Phys* 6: 1215–1228.

Smith JS, Perry A, Borell TJ *et al.* (2000). Alterations of chromosome arms 1p and 19q as predictors of survival in oligodendrogliomas, astrocytomas and mixed oligoastrocytoma. *J Clin Oncol* 18: 636–645.

Smith JS, Chang EF, Lamborn KR *et al.* (2008). Role of extent of resection in the long-term outcome of low-grade hemispheric gliomas. *J Clin Oncol* 26: 1338–1345.

Stege EM, Kros JM, de Bruin HG *et al.* (2005). Successful treatment of low-grade oligodendroglial tumors with a chemotherapy regimen of procarbazine, lomustine, and vincristine. *Cancer* 103: 802–809.

Surma-Aho O, Niemela M, Vilkki J *et al.* (2001). Adverse long-term effects of brain radiotherapy in adult low-grade glioma patients. *Neurology* 56: 1285–1290.

Swennen MHJ, Bromberg JEC, Witkamp TD *et al.* (2004). Delayed radiation toxicity after focal or whole brain radiotherapy for low-grade glioma. *J Neurooncol* 66: 333–339.

Takebayashi T, Varsier N, Kikuchi Y *et al.* (2008). Mobile phone use, exposure to radiofrequency electromagnetic field, and brain tumour: a case–control study. *Br J Cancer* 98: 652–659.

Taphoorn MJB, Klein M (2004). Cognitive deficits in adult brain tumour patients. *Lancet Neurol* 3: 159–168.

Taphoorn MJB, Heimans JJ, Snoek FJ *et al.* (1992). Assessment of quality of life in patients treated for low-grade glioma: a preliminary report. *J Neurol Neurosurg Psychiatry* 55: 372–376.

Torres JJ, Mundt AJ, Sweeney PJ *et al.* (2003). A longitudinal neuropsychological study of partial brain radiation in adults with brain tumors. *Neurology* 60: 1113–1118.

Tucha O, Smely C, Preier M, Lange KW (2000). Cognitive deficits before treatment among patients with brain tumors. *Neurosurgery* 47: 324–333.

Van den Bent MJ, Kros JM, Heimans JJ *et al.* (1998). Response rate and prognostic factors of recurrent oligodendroglioma treated with procarbazine, CCNU, and vincristine chemotherapy. *Neurology* 51: 1140–1145.

Van den Bent MJ, Taphoorn MJB, Brandes AA *et al.* (2003). Phase II study of first-line chemotherapy with temozolomide in recurrent oligodendroglial tumors: EORTC Brain Tumor Group Study 26971. *J Clin Oncol* 21: 2525–2528.

Van den Bent MJ, Afra D, de Witte O *et al.* (2005). Long-term efficacy of early versus delayed radiotherapy for low-grade astrocytoma and oligodendroglioma in adults: the EORTC 22845 randomised trial. *Lancet* 366: 985–990.

Vecht CJ (1993). Effect of age on treatment decisions in low-grade glioma. *J Neurol Neurosurg Psychiatry* 56: 1259–1264.

Vigliani MC, Sichez N, Poisson M, Delattre JY (1996). A prospective study of cognitive functions following conventional radiotherapy for supratentorial gliomas in young adults: 4-year results. *Int J Radiat Oncol Biol Phys* 35: 527–533.

Vigliani MC, Duyckaerts C, Hauw JJ *et al.* (1999). Dementia following treatment of brain tumors with radiotherapy administered alone or in combination with nitrosourea-based chemotherapy: a clinical and pathological study. *J Neuro Oncol* 41: 137–149.

Vuori K, Kankaanranta L, Hakkinen AM *et al.* (2004). Low-grade gliomas and focal cortical developmental malformations: differentation with proton MR spectroscopy. *Radiology* 230: 703–708.

Watanabe T, Nakamura M, Kros JM *et al.* (2002). Phenotype versus genotype correlation in oligodendroglioma and low-grade diffuse astrocytoma. *Acta Neuropathol* 103: 267–275.

Wen PY (2003). Central nervous system complications of cancer therapy. In Schiff D, Wen PY (eds.) *Cancer Neurology in Clinical Practice* (pp. 215–231. Totowa: Humana Press.

11

High-grade gliomas

Michael J. Glantz and John W. Conlee

Introduction

After more than 30 years of intensive clinical and laboratory research, high-grade gliomas (HGG) [glioblastoma multiforme (GBM), anaplastic astrocytoma (AAs), anaplastic oligodendroglioma, and anaplastic mixed glioma] retain a well-deserved reputation for poor response to therapy, rapid tumor recurrence, and short overall survival. Currently available treatments, including surgery, cranial irradiation, and chemotherapy, extend survival measurably, but are almost always non-curative, and are associated with substantial toxicity. In this context, maintaining good quality of life has assumed an increasingly prominent role in selecting treatments and in designing clinical trials (Report of the Brain Tumor Progress Review Group, 2005; Taphoorn et al., 2005), and the paradigm of compressing morbidity and "rectangularizing" the survival curve (Fries, 1980) is increasingly seen as the central goal of cancer therapy (Figure 11.1).

Traditionally, myelosuppression and its attendant problems have been the dose-limiting and most important toxicities of radiation and chemotherapy. In the late 1990s and early 2000s, however, the availability of colony stimulating factors, and dramatic improvements in transfusion medicine, antibiotic therapy, and supportive care made the bone marrow more robust. Today, a strong case can be made that the nervous system has replaced the bone marrow as the most important dose-limiting end organ for cancer therapy in general, and for therapy directed at central nervous system tumors in particular. For the large number of children (Bhat et al., 2005; Lannering et al., 1990; Packer et al., 2003), and for the still small but growing number of adult long-term survivors of malignant primary brain tumors, the nervous system rather than the hematopoietic system more frequently affects the quality of survival and the economic productivity of survivors. Thus the combination of disease-related and treatment-related nervous system insults presents a daunting challenge to patients and health care providers. The spectrum of problems includes focal neurologic deficits, cognitive impairment, affective disorders, and associated medical complications (Table 11.1). This chapter will focus on the frequency, assessment, causes, and potential therapies of cognitive impairment in adults with high-grade gliomas.

Scope of the problem

An estimated 21 810 patients will be diagnosed with primary brain tumors in the United States in 2007 (Central Brain Tumor Registry of the United States, 2005; Jemal et al., 2008). Of these, approximately 60% will be HGG (with glioblastomas comprising 50% of the total). While median survival has

Cognition and Cancer, eds. Christina A. Meyers and James R. Perry. Published by Cambridge University Press.
© Cambridge University Press 2008.

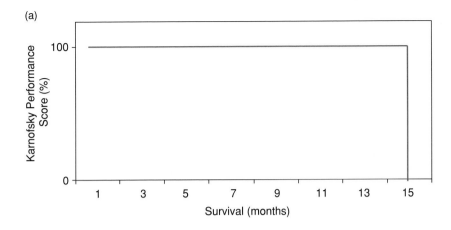

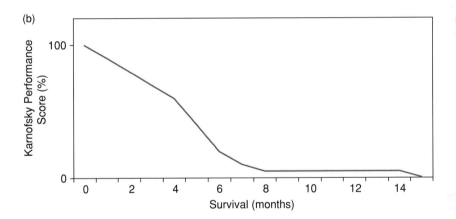

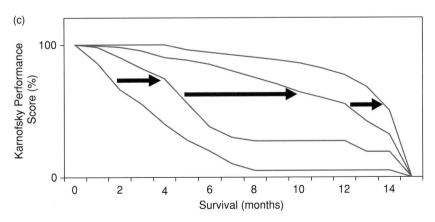

Figure 11.1. Quality of life versus survival (a) the ideal outcome, (b) the worst case, and (c) the realistic goal

Table 11.1. Spectrum of nervous system problems in patients with high-grade gliomas

Category of problem	Examples	Potential causes
Focal deficits	Hemiparesis, aphasia, hemianopsia	Tumor, surgery, radiation necrosis
Cognitive impairment	Diminished short-term memory, executive function, fine motor function, information processing	Tumor, surgery, radiation, chemotherapy
Affective disorders	Depression, anxiety	Tumor, radiation, chemotherapy, emotional response to the disease
Medical complications	Proximal myopathy, fatigue, endocrine deficiencies	Tumor, corticosteroids, chemotherapy, radiation

changed very little in the last decade (10–12 months for patients with GBM, 2–3 years for AA), a surprising variability in individual survival occurs (Carson *et al.*, 2007; Curran *et al.*, 1993). Almost two-thirds of patients with AAs survive at least 18 months, 25% of patients with AAs aged 64 or younger survive longer than 10 years, and 6% of patients with GBMs survive more than 4 years (Central Brain Tumor Registry of the United States, 2005). Similarly, the recent large, randomized EORTC/NCCI trial reported a 26.5% 2-year survival for patients with GBM (Stupp *et al.*, 2005). While increased survival is a welcome outcome of new therapeutic strategies, long-term survivors are potentially at increasing risk for developing neurocognitive deficits related to the delayed effects of therapy.

Causes of cognitive impairment in patients with high-grade gliomas

Neurocognitive dysfunction in patients with HGG is multifactorial (Table 11.2). Patients with primary brain tumors frequently report a variety of cognitive complaints, and recent studies have documented a spectrum of deficits ranging from subtle to blatant in 34% of patients when assessed by a relatively insensitive measurement tool (Folstein Mini-Mental State Examination – MMSE) (Brown *et al.*, 2006) and in 59%–100% of patients when more comprehensive cognitive assessments are performed (Klein *et al.*, 2001, 2003b; Levin *et al.*, 2002; Meyers *et al.*,

2000). Similarly, 90.5% of patients with brain metastases scored in the abnormal range on one or more tests of cognitive function prior to receiving cranial irradiation (Meyers *et al.*, 2004). Much research has focused on the role of tumor-directed therapy, particularly cranial irradiation, as a cause of cognitive deficits. As demonstrated by the almost universal presence of cognitive deficits in newly diagnosed and in post-operative patients, however, HGG themselves contribute substantially to the burden of cognitive impairment.

Neurologic and cognitive deficits related to the tumor itself may manifest as a global decline in level of alertness when the tumor is causing increased intracranial pressure or obstruction of spinal fluid pathways, or as focal deficits (for example, aphasia, verbal learning and memory difficulties, visual field defects, hemiparesis, or neglect) when the cause is local pressure effects and vascular changes related to the location of the lesion. The consequences of brain tumor surgery are also typically thought of as focal and related to the site of tumor resection (Archibald *et al.*, 1994; Imperato *et al.*, 1990; Levin *et al.*, 2002; Scheibel *et al.*, 1996). In contrast, treatment-related neurocognitive deficits (both radiation- and chemotherapy-induced) are primarily related to subcortical white matter dysfunction, and include impairment in short-term memory, executive function, sustained attention, speed of information processing, and bilateral fine motor control (Archibald *et al.*, 1994; Crossen *et al.*,

Table 11.2. Instruments available for assessing neurocognitive function in patients with high-grade gliomas

Test	Characteristic measured	Time to administer (min)
Cognitive function		
Hopkins Verbal Learning Test (Benedict *et al.*, 1998)	Verbal memory	5
Trail Making Test Part A (Lezak *et al.*, 1994)	Visual-motor speed	2
Trail Making Test Part B (Lezak *et al.*, 1994)	Executive function	5
Controlled Oral Word Association (Benton & Hamsher, 1989)	Verbal fluency	5
Digit Span Test Tota (Wechster, 1981)	Attention and concentration	10
Folstein MMSE (Folstein *et al.*, 1975)	Global cognitive function	10
Grooved Pegboard (dominant and non-dominant hands) (Lezak, 1995)	Motor dexterity and speed	2–3
Categoric Word Fluency (Benton, 1968)	Executive function	5
Overall performance		
Barthel Index (Wade & Collin, 1988)	Activities of daily living	5
Karnofsky Performance Score (Karnofsky *et al.*, 1948)	Functional Status	2
ECOG Performance Score (Oken *et al.*, 1982)	Toxicity	2
Quality of life		
Functional Assessment of Cancer Therapy (FACT) (Br) (Weitzner *et al.*, 1995)	Quality of life	5
SF-36 (Cella *et al.*, 1993; Ware & Sherbourne, 1992)	Health-related quality of life	10
Pediatric Quality of Life Inventory 4.0 (Varni *et al.*, 2007)	Health-related quality of life	<20
Edmonton Symptom Assessment Scale (Bruera *et al.*, 1991)	Multiple health-related symptoms	3
Women's Health Initiative Insomnia Rating Scale (Levine *et al.*, 2003)	Insomnia	3
EORTC Quality of Life Questionnaire Core-30 (Mauer *et al.*, 2007)	Quality of life	7
EORTC Brain Cancer Module-20 (Mauer *et al.*, 2007)	Health-related quality of life	5
Cancer Fatigue Scale (Okuyama *et al.*, 2000)	Fatigue	5
Brief Fatigue Inventory (Mendoza *et al.*, 1999)	Fatigue	3
Emotional status		
Profile of Mood States (McNair *et al.*, 1992)	Multiple subscales[a]	10
Beck Depression Inventory (Beck & Steer, 1993)	Mood (depression)	5
Hamilton Depression Rating Scale (Hamilton, 1960)	Mood (depression)	5
State-Trait Anxiety Inventory (Spielberger *et al.*, 1970)	Mood (anxiety)	5
Hamilton Anxiety Rating Scale (Hamilton, 1959)	Mood (anxiety)	5
Beck Anxiety Inventory (Beck *et al.*, 1990)	Mood (anxiety)	5

[a] Depression, anxiety, fatigue, vigor, confusion, anger, overall mood

1994; Hochberg & Slotnick, 1980; Imperato *et al.*, 1990; Salander *et al.*, 1995), as well as apathy, depression, and other alterations in personality and mood (Marin 1991, 1996). In practice, symptoms of more widespread cortical dysfunction – in particular, abulia, deficits in attention and executive function, and other characteristics of a frontal lobe dysfunction – are also common in patients with brain tumors, even when those tumors are not located in the frontal lobes (Lilja *et al.*, 1992), and even before radiation or chemotherapy has been administered. Recently, studies employing magnetoencephalography, diffusion tensor imaging, and functional MRI have started to elucidate the physiologic substrate for these clinical observations by revealing widespread loss of functional connectivity in the brains of patients with malignant gliomas, particularly when the tumor is located in the dominant hemisphere (Bartolomei *et al.*, 2006; Rozental *et al.*, 1990; Wei *et al.*, 2007; Young, 2007).

Several recent studies in patients with HGG have suggested that tumor progression contributes significantly to neurocognitive impairment, and that in the absence of tumor progression, the level of neurocognitive functioning remains relatively stable (Brown *et al.*, 2006; Steinbach *et al.*, 2006; Torres *et al.*, 2003). Similar findings have been reported in some studies of patients with brain metastases (Meyers *et al.*, 2004; Patchell *et al.*, 1998). These studies suggest that cranial irradiation, as applied with modern-day treatment-planning techniques, partial-brain treatment plans, and modest daily fraction and total dose targets, is not as neurotoxic as earlier studies suggested (Archibald *et al.*, 1994; Crossen *et al.*, 1994; DeAngelis *et al.*, 1989; Hochberg & Slotnick, 1980). Some of these studies have used insensitive measures of cognitive dysfunction. Many are retrospective; lack control groups; suffer from substantial patient drop-out, short patient follow-up, and small numbers of patients at later endpoints; include highly selected patients (for example, predominantly young patients); and have not required masked assessment. As a result, the risks of confounding (e.g., there may be shared risk factors for survival, tumor progression, and cognitive decline); selection bias (e.g., if cognitive decline is itself a risk factor for shortened survival, longer survivors are less likely to show impaired cognition); investigator bias; and lack of generalizability are considerable. Most studies have also failed to assess the contributions of patient variables (e.g., level of education; pre-existing impairment; vascular risk factors) and additional competing causes of neurocognitive dysfunction (e.g., chemotherapy, corticosteroids, anti-

convulsants). Despite these shortcomings, when taken as a group, these studies suggest that at least some of the neurocognitive deficits seen in patients with HGG are attributable to tumor progression and are not, as previously asserted, due entirely to the effects of therapy. In addition, those studies in which baseline assessments of neurocognitive status were performed prior to the start of cranial irradiation and chemotherapy have shown unequivocally that neurocognitive deficits are present, in varying degrees, in essentially all patients, even when more traditional and less sensitive measures of performance (Karnofsky Performance Score, Eastern Cooperative Oncology Group Performance Score, Barthel Index) or global cognitive function (MMSE) are normal. These findings are supported by analogous findings in patients with brain metastases and with neoplastic meningitis.

The challenge of distinguishing between tumor- and treatment-related causes of cognitive impairment in patients with HGG is further complicated by a long list of common and potentially contributory etiologies (Taphoorn & Klein, 2004) (Table 11.3). One of the most common of these is concurrent medications. As with any medical patient, anxiolytic and sedative drugs, analgesics (including non-steroidal anti-inflammatory agents), antidepressants, antihistamines, and anticholinergics are common offenders (Wen *et al.*, 2006). Anticonvulsants, particularly the first-generation agents (phenytoin, phenobarbital, and carbamazepine) are commonly implicated (Mattson, 2004), although the newer agents (in particular, topiramate) are not immune (Bosma *et al.*, 2007). Seizures themselves, sometimes subtle enough to be clinically inapparent, can produce sustained cognitive and behavioral deficits (Klein *et al.*, 2003a). Corticosteroids have also been demonstrated, both clinically and in laboratory models, to produce sustained deficits in memory and learning (Brunner *et al.*, 2006; Lupien *et al.*, 1999; Young *et al.*, 1999). A wide array of chemotherapeutic agents, including many that are frequently used in brain tumor patients, have also been associated with both acute and chronic neurocognitive deficits

Table 11.3. Differential diagnosis of behavioral in patients with cancer. *CMV*, Cytomegalovirus; *HSV*, herpes simplex virus; *JC*, John Cunningham virus; *MRI*, Magnetic resonance imaging; *SIADH*, Syndrome of inappropriate antidiuretic hormone

Etiology		Comment
Endocrinopathy		Hypothyroidism, hyperprolactinemia, cortisol, and testosterone deficiencies are all common
Infection	Meningitis	Listeria is common; ventricular reservoirs or shunts predispose
	Brain abscess	
	Sepsis	Usually in the setting of high fever, hypoxia, or hypotension
	Encephalitis	Particularly HSV, CMV, and progressive multifocal leukoencephalopathy (JC virus)
Metabolic	Hypomagnesemia	Common with cisplatin use, often 3–8 days after therapy; also after bisphosphonate administration
	Hyponatremia	Common following neurosurgery; also vincristine, carbamazepine, oxcarbazepine, SIADH, cyclophosphamide, or chemotherapy requiring co-administration of large fluid volumes
	Hypocalcemia	Following cisplatinum or bisphosphonate administration
Drug-induced	Cisplatin	Possibly related to electrolyte disturbances; may be delayed up to 2 weeks after completion of treatment
	Vincristine, Etoposide Busulfan, Methotrexate	Uncommon
	Interleukin-2, Interferon-α	Particularly during high-dose therapy
	Ifosfamide	Especially in patients with renal failure or hypoalbuminemia
	Thienamycin antibiotics (imipenem and others)	Up to 6% of all patients
Radiation-related	Radiation necrosis	MRI may be indistinguishable from recurrent tumor
Intracranial	Thrombocytopenia	Related to disease, chemotherapy, or drugs (e.g., heparin)
Hemorrhage	Coagulopathy	Disseminated intravascular coagulation
Tumor-related	New or progressive disease	Including neoplastic meningitis and brain metastases
Paraneoplastic	Encephalitis	Increasingly recognized; most common with small-cell lung cancer and ovarian teratoma
Other	Posterior reversible Leukoencephalopathy syndrome	Seen in multiple settings, including bone marrow transplant, immunosuppressive therapy with ciclosporin, tacrolimus, interferon-α, and others. Abrupt increases in blood pressure may predispose

(Cavaliere & Schiff, 2006; Hildebrand, 2006). While some of these effects are indirect (mediated through chemotherapy-associated anemia, seizures, or vasculopathy for example) many agents appear to directly produce behavioral and neurocognitive changes (Table 11.3). Increasingly, individual pharmacogenetic variations underlying these adverse cognitive effects are being identified. Examples include 5-fluorouracil (John-son et al., 1999; Raida et al., 2001; Shehata et al., 1999), methotrexate (Ulrich et al., 2001, 2003), and the selective serotonin reuptake inhibitors (SSRIs) (Murphy et al., 2003). Interactions between radiation therapy and a variety of patient risk factors (including hypercholesterolemia, diabetes, pre-existing Alzheimer's disease, hyperhomocysteinemia, and the presence of the apoE4 allele) have also been suggested. An interesting paradigm of the interaction between a chemotherapy agent and an underlying inherited condition conspiring to produce dramatic cognitive impairment can be found in patients with adult-onset fragile X syndrome who are treated with cis-platinum – a convergence of factors that may result in fulminate encephalopathy (O'Dwyer *et al.*, 2005). Other indirect effects of tumor therapy, such as infection (including chronic meningitis), radiation-related secondary and tertiary endocrinopathies, and (very rarely in patients with primary brain tumors) paraneoplastic encephalopathy, also enter the differential diagnosis. Of particular note, because of their frequency of occurrence and lack of recognition, is the contribution of fatigue, depression, and anxiety to apparent neurocognitive deficits (Cull *et al.*, 1996; Klein *et al.*, 2001; Wellisch *et al.*, 2002).

Assessment of cognitive function in patients with high-grade gliomas

Just as the differential diagnosis of cognitive impairment is complex, so too is the measurement of cognitive function in patients with HGG. Accurate assessment is complicated by the presence of competing causes of impairment (sometimes producing similar or overlapping patterns of disability); by neurologic deficits that limit the ability of patients to participate fully in testing; by the complexity of some test batteries; by limitations in time, training, and inclination on the part of health care professionals; and by deficiencies in the test instruments themselves (Brown *et al.*, 2003; Klein & Heimans, 2004; Meyers & Brown, 2006; Meyers & Wefel, 2003). Simple and widely used dementia screening tools such as the MMSE are insensitive to clinically meaningful improvements and deteriorations in cognitive function (particularly the subcortical white matter deficits most commonly produced by radiation), may be susceptible to practice effects, and are influenced significantly by the level of education and the presence of language impairment in test subjects. Nevertheless, the MMSE has been shown in some studies to presage tumor recurrence, and

to correlate with shortened survival in patients with primary and metastatic brain tumors (Brown *et al.*, 2003, 2006; Murray *et al.*, 2000; Shaw *et al.*, 2002; Taylor *et al.*, 1998). No single, simple, brief screening test currently available is capable of reliably identifying impairment; distinguishing among and apportioning responsibility between the multiple potential causes of impairment; allowing the evolution of impairment to be tracked; and predicting the ultimate course of that impairment. Relatively concise batteries of tests have, however, been composed which do fulfill these criteria, and which can be taught to and performed by health care providers without advanced training in neuropsychology (Meyers *et al.*, 2004). Neurocognitive testing (combined with a careful patient history and examination) is also reliably able to identify deficits related to alterations in mood and state such as depression, anxiety, and fatigue. Table 11.2 lists some commonly used tests of cognitive function, mood, and quality of life. These tests can be administered by anyone who has been properly trained, but can only be interpreted by an appropriate professional.

Importance of neurocognitive assessment

Neurocognitive assessment contributes in at least three essential areas to the management of patients with HGG: by providing a clinically relevant and quantifiable outcome measure for patients enrolled in clinical trials or receiving therapy outside of the investigational setting; by providing a measure of the neurotoxicity of standard or investigational therapies (Meyers *et al.*, 1997); and by refining our ability to predict patient outcomes. In diseases where therapies often differ only modestly in efficacy, neurocognitive function has the potential to become a primary endpoint in clinical trials, and is gaining acceptance from regulatory agencies for this reason (Report of the Brain Tumor Progress Review Group, 2005). In addition, in a number of recent studies, performance on neurocognitive testing in patients with low-grade (Brown *et al.*, 2003; Shaw *et al.*, 2002), and high-grade (Brown *et al.*, 2006; Meyers *et al.*, 2000; Taylor *et al.*, 1998) primary brain tumors, brain metastases (Meyers *et al.*, 2004), and neoplastic meningitis (Sherman *et al.*, 2002) has been shown to help predict both tumor recurrence and overall survival. However, caution is advised when interpreting these results as some of the studies had a large amount of missing data, used insensitive measures, lacked a control group, had only short-term follow-up assessments, or did not control for other factors that might affect cognitive function, such as the use of adjuvant medications. Similarly, a recent analysis of patients with glioblastomas participating in the EORTC phase III trial comparing cranial irradiation alone with irradiation plus daily temozolomide has raised doubts about whether cognitive functioning, social functioning, and global health status truly add predictive power to prognostic models including the more traditional variables of age, performance status, and histology (Mauer *et al.*, 2007). While additional prospective study is necessary, these findings do suggest that the results of neurocognitive function testing may help to provide a rationale for clinicians to continue or abandon therapies in the face of radiographically stable disease, and may also assist in the important role of prognostication.

Prolonging survival remains a valid long-range goal in neuro-oncology. However, when aggressive therapies are administered to patients with no or very limited curative potential, attention to alternative outcome measures becomes critical. One such alternative concept, first proposed in another context by Fries (1980), suggests that the "compression of morbidity" within a given lifespan may be equally as important as overall survival given the limitations of existing therapies. This idea of "rectangularizing" the survival curve by prolonging a high level of functioning for as much of the lifespan as possible resonates loudly with cancer patients in general, and brain tumor patients and their families in particular (Davies & Clarke, 2005; Steinbach *et al.*, 2006). Interestingly, measures of neurocognitive, social, and work-related function on the one hand and quality of life on the other have been found, in at least some studies, to correlate poorly (Steinbach *et al.*, 2006).

In part this may be related to an altered perception of functioning produced by cognitive impairments (Taphoorn *et al.*, 1992). More importantly, however, a patient's appreciation of what constitutes worthwhile "quality" evolves over the course of his or her illness, so that even in the face of mounting physical, neurological, and cognitive deficits, patients may feel that their quality of life remains good enough to justify continued tumor-directed therapy. Thus evaluation of neurocognitive function is critical in identifying treatments with less neurocognitive toxicity, and those which improve neurocognitive, economic, and social functioning, but it cannot substitute for quality of life assessments, which more directly register the patient's own appreciation of the disease process and the therapies used to fight it.

Treatment of cognitive deficits in patients with high-grade gliomas

The underlying biochemistry and neurophysiology of neurocognitive deficits in patients with HGG is still poorly understood and undoubtedly multifactorial. Radiation, chemotherapy, and the tumor itself probably conspire to produce brain injury through damage to the neurovascular endothelium and multiple cell populations (oligodendrogliocytes, neural stem cells, neurons, astrocytes, and microglia), disruption of cellular DNA, and disruption of the neuronal microenvironments, including alterations in cytokine and neurotransmitter expression (Abdallah *et al.*, 2007; Armstrong *et al.*, 1995; Belka *et al.*, 2001; O'Connor & Mayberrg, 2000; Monje *et al.*, 2002, 2007; Moulder *et al.*, 1998; Tofilon & Fike 2000). Host factors and the response of damaged tissues to injury are also involved. Nevertheless, the phenotypic similarity of some symptoms to certain neurological and psychiatric disorders in non-tumor populations, including Alzheimer's disease, has encouraged the investigative use of therapies useful in those disorders in patients with brain tumors. Thus conventional antidepressant therapy (particularly employing SSRIs and combined serotonin and norepinephrine reuptake inhibitors) has been used with success equal to that in non-brain tumor patients (Gill & Hatcher, 2000; Wen *et al.*, 2006). Improvements in energy, cognitive function, fine motor performance, depression and global measures of performance and daily functioning have all been documented in small studies using methylphenidate and modafinil. In a trial involving 30 predominantly young (mean age 40.3 years) adult patients with malignant primary brain tumors, there was a suggestion of a dose–response relationship in patients receiving 10, 20, or 30 mg of methylphenidate twice daily (Meyers *et al.*, 1998). Remarkably, improvements occurred despite radiographic evidence of tumor progression in 7 (23%) patients and treatment-related white matter injury in 8 (27%) patients. Toxicity was minimal. In particular, no worsening of seizure control was seen. A larger, randomized, placebo-controlled, double-blind crossover study in 80 pediatric long-term survivors of brain tumors (43 patients) or acute lymphoblastic leukemia also demonstrated improvements in attention, social skills, and school performance with the use of methylphenidate over the course of 3 weeks, although no difference between low (0.3 mg/kg) and moderate (0.6 mg/kg) dose therapy was identified (Mulhern *et al.*, 2004). In contrast, a short-term (7-day) randomized trial of methylphenidate in 112 patients with non-nervous-system cancer showed substantial improvement in fatigue in both the placebo and methylphenidate treatment arms, with no significant difference between treatment arms (Bruera *et al.*, 2006). Most recently, a 30-patient randomized trial of modafinil in 30 patients with a variety of high-grade and low-grade primary brain tumors showed clinically and statistically significant improvements from baseline in a comprehensive battery of neurocognitive tests and fatigue scales at doses of modafinil ranging from 200–400 mg/day for the first 3 weeks of the trial to (after a 1-week washout period) 500–600 mg/week for an additional 8-week open-label extension period. Headache (43% of patients), insomnia (27%), dizziness (23%), and dry mouth (23%) were common but generally mild in severity (Kaleita *et al.*, 2006).

A small, open-label phase II trial of donepezil (5 mg daily for 6 weeks, then 10 mg daily for 18 weeks) in 35 cognitively impaired patients with brain tumors (most low grade, all but one primary) who had survived at least 6 months from the completion of radiation therapy has recently demonstrated significant improvement in cognitive function (including measures of attention and concentration, verbal memory, and figural memory), mood, and health-related quality of life (Shaw *et al.*, 2006). Trends toward improvement were also seen in verbal fluency, fatigue, and anger, although no change in MMSE was identified. Toxicity was modest. The young age (mean 45 years), high dropout rate (11 of 35 patients), absence of a control group, and unmasked assessment represent significant problems with this study. In addition, a second study of donepezil failed to show any benefit over placebo in improving fatigue in a cohort of 142 patients with various malignancies (Bruera *et al.*, 2007). Nevertheless, the findings are encouraging enough to merit further study.

The possibility of preventing treatment-induced brain injury and the resulting neurocognitive deficits is also being actively explored. An intriguing recent series of studies in rats (Monje *et al.*, 2002) and in humans (Monje *et al.*, 2007) with medulloblastoma or acute myelogenous leukemia treated with cranial irradiation has shown that radiation inhibits hippocampal neurogenesis, diverts neural stem cell differentiation away from neuron production, and increases microglia production and inflammation – changes that can be reversed by inflammatory blockade with indomethacin (Monje *et al.*, 2003). These findings have stimulated a prophylaxis trial which is now underway.

These encouraging findings must still be treated as preliminary, but certainly underscore the urgent need for larger, well-designed, randomized trials with masked outcome assessment in a wider spectrum of patients, including pediatric and elderly individuals. Incorporation of biochemical response measures, functional imaging, and PET scanning offer the potential for more effective selection of patients and agents, and a more sophisticated understanding of the mechanisms underlying neurocognitive dysfunction in patients with brain tumors. Examination of other acetylcholinesterase inhibitors, *N*-methyl-D-aspartate (NMDA) antagonists such as memantine, dopamine agonists, and combinations of agents, as well as prophylaxis trials are all important avenues of investigation for the future. With the increasing availability of intensity-modulated radiation therapy and other highly conformal radiation techniques, the possibility of designing radiation fields that spare particularly sensitive and functionally critical structures such as the hippocampus should also be explored in the clinical trial setting.

Finally, research on effective cognitive rehabilitation strategies for brain tumor patients remains scant. The purely descriptive reports that largely populate the current literature must be replaced by studies that link neuropsychological diagnosis with specific cognitive rehabilitation interventions (Report of the Brain Tumor Progress Review Group, 2005). The cognitive deficits resulting from a brain tumor are frequently subtle and are often brought to light only by careful neuropsychological assessment (Meyers & Boake, 1993). At the same time, these psychometrically subtle deficits may produce significant functional impairments in the less structured settings of home and workplace (Mesulam, 2000). The milder and more variable cognitive impairments present in some brain tumor patients (Jagaroo *et al.*, 2000; Kayl & Meyers, 2003; Maldjian *et al.*, 2001) may make them ideal candidates for cognitive rehabilitation (Meyers & Boake, 1993; Sherer *et al.*, 1997). Cognitive rehabilitation interventions used successfully in treating patients with brain injuries and strokes may provide targeted strategies for the remediation of specific cognitive impairments in patients with brain tumors (Sohlberg & Maateer, 1989).

Summary

Neurocognitive impairment in patients with brain tumors, in particular HGG, is almost universal, and is the result of interactions between the tumor itself, direct and indirect effects of surgery, radiation, and chemotherapy, ancillary drugs such as anticonvulsants and corticosteroids, and alterations in mood and state. Recent investigations employing carefully selected neuropsychological test panels have given rise to several paradigm-altering concepts. First, neurocognitive impairment exists in most patients with HGG even prior to the start of brain tumor therapy. Second, tumor progression often contributes substantially to accumulating neurocognitive deficits during the course of therapy. Third, changes in neurocognitive performance may precede and even presage radiographic and clinical exam evidence of tumor recurrence. Finally, neurocognitive testing plays an important role in evaluating the success of conventional and investigational therapies, particularly in this setting where cures are rarely achieved, and avoidance of accumulating deficits is an important goal of treatment. Practical, validated testing batteries are currently available to clinicians and should be incorporated into both routine care and clinical trials. Several small but encouraging investigations suggest that both pharmacological and neurocognitive interventions are available which improve neurocognitive function and overall quality of life.

REFERENCES

Abdallah NM-BB, Slomianka L, Lipp H-P (2007). Reversible effect of X-irradiation on proliferation, neurogenesis, and cell death in the dentate gyrus of adult mice. *Hippocampus* **17**(12): 1230–1240.

Archibald YM, Lulnn D, Ruttan LA *et al.* (1994). Cognitive functioning in long-term survivors of high-grade glioma. *J Neurosurg* **80**: 247–253.

Armstrong C, Ruffer J, Corn B, DeVires K, Mollman J (1995). Biphasic patterns of memory deficits following moderate-dose partial-brain irradiation: neuropsychologic outcome and proposed mechanisms. *J Clin Oncol* **13**: 2263–2271.

Bartolomei F, Bosma I, Klein M *et al.* (2006). How do brain tumors alter functional connectivity? A magnetoencephalography study. *Ann Neurol* **59**: 128–138.

Beck AT, Steer RA (1993). *Beck Depression Inventory*. San Antonio, TX: Psychological Corp.

Beck AT, Brown G, Epstein N, Steer RA (1990). An inventory for measuring clinical anxiety: psychometric properties. *J Consult Clin Psychol* **56**: 893–897.

Belka C, Budach W, Kortmann RD *et al.* (2001). Radiation induced CNS toxicity – molecular and cellular mechanisms. *Br J Cancer* **85**: 1233–1239.

Benedict RHB, Schretlen D, Groninger L *et al.* (1998). Hopkins Verbal Learning Test-Revised: normative data and analysis of inter-form and test-retest reliability. *Clin Neuropsychol* **12**: 43–55.

Benton AD (1968). Differential behavioral effects in frontal lobe disease. *Neuropsychologia* **6**: 53–60.

Benton AL, Hamsher K de S (1989). *Multilingual Aphasia Examination*. Iowa City, IA: AJA Associates.

Bhat SR, Goodwin TL, Burwinkle TM *et al.* (2005). Profile of daily life in children with brain tumors: an assessment of health-related quality of life. *J Clin Oncol* **23**: 5493–5500.

Bosma I, Vos MJ, Heimans JJ *et al.* (2007). The course of neurocognitive functioning in high-grade glioma patients. *Neurooncology* **9**: 53–62.

Brown PD, Buckner JC, O'Fallon JR *et al.* (2003). Effects of radiotherapy on cognitive function in patients with low-grade glioma measured by the Folstein mini-mental state examination. *J Clin Oncol* **21**: 2519–2524.

Brown PD, Jensen AW, Felten SJ *et al.* (2006). Detrimental effects of tumor progression on cognitive function of patients with high-grade glioma. *J Clin Oncol* **24**: 5427–5433.

Bruera E, Kuehn N, Miller M, Selmser P, Macmillan K (1991). The Edmonton Symptom Assessment System (ESAS): a simple method for the assessment of palliative care patients. *J Palliative Care* **7**: 6–9.

Bruera E, Valero V, Driver L *et al.* (2006). Patient-controlled methylphenidate for cancer fatigue: a double-blind, randomized, placebo-controlled trial. *J Clin Oncol* **24**: 2073–2078.

Bruera E, Osta BE, Valero V *et al.* (2007). Donepezil for cancer fatigue: a double-blind, randomized, placebo-controlled trial. *J Clin Oncol* **25**: 3475–3481.

Brunner R, Schaefer D, Hess K, Parzer P, Resch F, Schwab S (2006). Effect of high-dose cortisol on memory functions. *Ann N Y Acad Sci* **1071**: 434–437.

Carson KA, Grossman SA, Fisher JD, Shaw EG (2007). Prognostic factors for survival in adult patients with recurrent gliomas enrolled onto the new approaches to brain tumor therapy CNS consortium phase I and II clinical trials. *J Clin Oncol* **25**: 2601–2606.

Cavaliere R, Schiff D (2006). Neurologic toxicities of cancer therapies. *Curr Neurol Neurosci Rep* **6**: 218–226.

Cella DF, Tulsky DS, Gray G *et al.* (1993). The functional assessment of cancer therapy scale: development and validation of the general measure. *J Clin Oncol* **11**: 570–577.

Central Brain Tumor Registry of the United States (2005). *Primary Brain Tumors in the United States Statistical Report 1998–2002* (pp. 8–50). Chicago, IL: Central Brain Tumor Registry of the United States.

Crossen JR, Garwood D, Glatstein E *et al.* (1994). Neurobehavioral sequelae of cranial irradiation in adults: a review of radiation-induced encephalopathy. *J Clin Oncol* **12**: 627–642.

Cull A, Hay C, Love SB *et al.* (1996). What do cancer patients mean when they complain of concentration and memory problems? *Br J Cancer* **74**: 1674–1679.

Curran WJ Jr., Scott CB, Horton J *et al.* (1993). Recursive partitioning analysis of prognostic factors in three Radiation Therapy Oncology Group malignant gliomas trials. *J Natl Cancer Inst* **85**: 704–710.

Davies E, Clarke C (2005). Views of bereaved relatives about quality of survival after radiotherapy for malignant cerebral glioma. *J Neurol Neurosurg Psychiatry* **76**: 555–561.

DeAngelis LM, Delattre J-Y, Posner JB (1989). Radiation-induced dementia in patients cured of brain metastases. *Neurology* **39**: 789–796.

Folstein MF, Folstein SE, McHugh PR (1975). "Mini-mental state": a practical method for grading the cognitive state of patients for the clinician. *J Psychiatr Res* **12**: 189–198.

Fries JF (1980). Aging, natural death, and the compression of morbidity. *N Engl J Med* **303**: 130–135.

Gill D, Hatcher S (2000). Antidepressants for depression in medical illness. *Cochrane Database Syst Rev* **4**: CD001312.

Hamilton M (1959). The assessment of anxiety state by rating. *Br J Med Psychol* **32**: 50–55.

Hamilton M (1960). A rating scale for depression. *J Neurol Neurosurg Psychiatry* **23**: 56–62.

Hildebrand J (2006). Neurological complications of cancer chemotherapy. *Curr Opin Oncol* **18**: 321–324.

Hochberg FH, Slotnick B (1980). Neuropsychologic impairment in astrocytoma survivors. *Neurology* **30**: 172–177.

Imperato JP, Palelogos NA, Vick NA (1990). Effects of treatment on long-term survivors with malignant astrocytomas. *Ann Neurol* **28**: 818–822.

Jagaroo V, Rogers MP, Black PM (2000). Allocentric visuo-spatial processing in patients with cerebral gliomas: a neurocognitive assessment. *J Neurooncol* **49**: 235–248.

Jemal A, Siegel R, Ward E *et al.* (2007). Cancer statistics, 2008. *CA Cancer J Clin* **58**: 71–96.

Johnson MR, Hageboutros A, Wand K, High L, Smith JB, Diasio RB (1999). Life-threatening toxicity in a dihydropyrimidine dehydrogenase-deficient patient after treatment with topical 5-fluorouracil. *Clin Cancer Res* **5**: 2006–2011.

Kaleita TA, Wellich DK, Graham CA *et al.* (2006). Pilot study of modafinil for treatment of neurobehavioral dysfunction and fatigue in adult patients with brain tumors. *Proc ASCO* **24**(18S): 58S, [abstract 1503].

Karnofsky DA, Abelmann WH, Craver LF (1948). The use of nitrogen mustards in the palliative treatment of carcinoma. *Cancer* **1**: 634–656.

Kayl AE, Meyers CA (2003). Does brain tumor histology influence cognitive function? *Neurooncology* **5**: 255–260.

Klein M, Heimans JJ (2004). The measurement of cognitive functioning in low-grade glioma patients after radiotherapy [Letter]. *J Clin Oncol* **22**: 966–967.

Klein M, Taphoorn MJB, Heimans JJ *et al.* (2001). Neurobehavioral status and health-related quality of life in newly diagnosed high-grade glioma patients. *J Clin Oncol* **19**: 4037–4047.

Klein M, Engelberts NHJ, van der Ploeg HM *et al.* (2003a). Epilepsy in low-grade gliomas: the impact on cognitive function and quality of life. *Ann Neurol* **54**: 514–520.

Klein M, Postma TJ, Taphoorn MJB *et al.* (2003b). The prognostic value of cognitive functioning in the survival of patients with high-grade glioma. *Neurology* **61**: 1796–1798.

Lannering B, Marky I, Lundberg A *et al.* (1990). Long-term sequelae after pediatric brain tumors: their effect on disability and quality of life. *Med Pediatr Oncol* **18**: 304–310.

Lezak MD. (1995). *Neuropsychological Assessment* (3rd edn.). New York: Academic Press.

Lezak MD, Howieson DB, Loring DW (1994). *Neuropsychological Assessment.* New York: Oxford University Press.

Levin VA, Yung WK, Bruner J *et al.* (2002). Phase II study of accelerated fractionation radiation therapy with carboplatin followed by PCV chemotherapy for the treatment of anaplastic gliomas. *Int J Radiat Oncol Biol Phys* **53**: 58–66.

Levine DW, Kripke DF, Kaplan RM *et al.* (2003). Reliability and validity of the Women's Health Initiative Insomnia Rating Scale. *Psychol Assess* **15**: 137–148.

Lilja A, Brun A, Salford LG *et al.* (1992). Neuropsychological indexes of a partial frontal syndrome in patients with nonfrontal gliomas. *Neuropsychology* **6**: 315–326.

Lupien SJ, Gillin CJ, Hauger RL (1999). Working memory is more sensitive than declarative memory to the acute effects of corticosteroids: a dose-response study in humans. *Behav Neurosci* **113**: 420–430.

Maldjian JA, Detre JA, Killgore WES *et al.* (2001). Neuropsychologic performance after resection of an activation cluster involved in cognitive memory function. *AJR Am J Roentgenol* **176**: 541–544.

Marin RS (1991). Apathy: a neuropsychiatric syndrome. *J Neuropsychiatry Clin Neurosci* **3**: 243–254.

Marin RS (1996). Apathy: concept, syndrome, neural mechanisms, and treatment. *Semin Clin Neuropsychiatry* **1**: 304–314.

Mattson RH (2004). Cognitive, affective, and behavioral side events in adults secondary to antiepileptic drug use. *Rev Neurol Dis* **1** [Suppl 1]: S10–S17.

Mauer M, Stupp R, Taphoorn MJ *et al.* (2007). The prognostic value of health-related quality-of-life data in predicting survival in glioblastoma cancer patients: results from an international randomised phase III EORTC Brain Tumour and Radiation Oncology Groups, and NCIC Clinical Trials Group study. *Br J Cancer* **97**: 302–307.

McNair DM, Lorr M, Droppleman LF (1992). *Profile of Mood States Manual.* San Diego, CA: Educational and Industrial Testing Service.

Mendoza TR, Wang XS, Cleeland CS *et al.* (1999). The rapid assessment of fatigue severity in cancer patients: use of the Brief Fatigue Inventory. *Cancer* **85**: 1186–1196.

Mesulam M (2000). Attentional networks, confusional states, and neglect syndromes. In Mesulam M (ed.) *Principles of Behavioral and Cognitive Neurology* (pp. 174–256). New York: Oxford University Press.

Meyers CA, Boake C (1993). Neurobehavioral disorders in brain tumor patients: rehabilitation strategies. *Cancer Bull* **45**: 362–364.

Meyers CA, Brown PD (2006). Role and relevance of neurocognitive assessment in clinical trials of patients with CNS tumors. *J Clin Oncol* **24**: 1305–1309.

Meyers CA, Wefel JS (2003). The use of the mini-mental state examination to assess cognitive functioning in cancer trials: no ifs, ands, buts, or sensitivity. *J Clin Oncol* **21**: 3357–3358.

Meyers CA, Kudelka AP, Conrad CA *et al.* (1997). Neurotoxicity of CI-980, a novel mitotic inhibitor. *Clin Cancer Res* **3**: 419–422.

Meyers CA, Weitzner MA, Valentine AD, Levin VA (1998). Methylphenidate therapy improves cognition, mood, and function of brain tumor patients. *J Clin Oncol* **16**: 2522–2527.

Meyers CA, Hess KR, Yung WKA, Levin VA (2000). Cognitive function as a predictor of survival in patients with recurrent malignant glioma. *J Clin Oncol* **18**: 646–650.

Meyers CA, Smith JA, Bezjak A *et al.* (2004). Neurocognitive function and progression in patients with brain metastases treated with whole-brain radiation and motexafin gadolinium: results of a randomized phase III trial. *J Clin Oncol* **22**: 157–165.

Monje ML, Mizumatsu S, Fike JR, Palmer TD (2002). Irradiation induces neural precursor-cell dysfunction. *Nat Med* **8**: 955–962.

Monje ML, Toda H, Palmer TD (2003). Inflammatory blockade restores adult hippocampal neurogenesis. *Science* **302**: 1760–1765.

Monje ML, Vogel H, Masek M, Ligon KL, Fisher PG, Palmer TD (2007). Impaired human hippocampal neurogenesis after treatment for central nervous system malignancies. *Ann Neurol* **62**(5): 515–520.

Moulder JE, Robbins ME, Cohen EP *et al.* (1998). Pharmacologic modification of radiation-induced late normal tissue injury. *Cancer Treat Res* **93**: 129–151.

Mulhern RK, Khan RB, Kaplan S *et al.* (2004). Short-term efficacy of methylphenidate: a randomized, double-blind, placebo-controlled trial among survivors of childhood cancer. *J Clin Oncol* **22**: 4795–4803.

Murphy GM, Kremer C, Rodrigues HE, Schatzberg AF (2003). Pharmacogenetics of antidepressant medication intolerance. *Am J Psychiatry* **160**: 1830–1835.

Murray KJ, Scott C, Zachariah B *et al.* (2000). Importance of the mini-mental status examination in the treatment of patients with brain metastases: a report from the Radiation Therapy Oncology Group protocol 91–04. *Int J Radiat Oncol Biol Phys* **48**: 59–64.

O'Connor NM, Mayberrg MR (2000). Effects of radiation on cerebral vasculature: a review. *Neurosurgery* **46**: 138–151.

O'Dwyer JP, Clabby C, Crown J, Barton DE, Hutchinson M (2005). Fragile X-associated tremor/ataxia syndrome presenting in a woman after chemotherapy. *Neurology* **65**: 331–332.

Oken MM, Creech RH, Tormey DC *et al.* (1982). Toxicity and response criteria of the Eastern Cooperative Oncology Group. *Am J Clin Oncol* **5**: 649–655.

Okuyama T, Akechi T, Kugaya A *et al.* (2000). Development and validation of the cancer fatigue scale: a brief, three-dimensional, self-rating scale for assessment of fatigue in cancer patients. *J Pain Symptom Manage* **19**: 5–14.

Packer RJ, Gurney JG, Punyko JA *et al.* (2003). Long-term neurologic and neurosensory sequelae in adult survivors of a childhood brain tumor: childhood cancer survivor study. *J Clin Oncol* **21**: 3255–3261.

Patchell RA, Tibbs PA, Regine WF *et al.* (1998). Postoperative radiotherapy in the treatment of single metastases to the brain: a randomized trial. *J Am Med Assoc* **280**: 1485–1489.

Raida M, Schwabe W, Hausler P *et al.* (2001). Prevalence of a common point mutation in the dihydropyrimidine dehydrogenase (DPD) gene within the 5′-splice donor site of intron 14 in patients with severe 5-fluorouracil (5-FU)-related toxicity compared with controls. *Clin Cancer Res* **7**: 2832–2839.

Report of the Brain Tumor Progress Review Group (2005). National Institute of Neurologic Disorders and Stroke. Accessed 27 March, 2008 from http://www.ninds.nih.gov/find_people/groups/brain_tumor_prg/btprgreport.htm.

Rozental JM Levine RL, Nickles RJ, Dobkin JA, Hanson JM (1990). Cerebral diaschisis in patients with malignant glioma. *J Neurooncol* **8**: 153–161.

Salander P, Karlsson T, Bergenheim T *et al.* (1995). Long-term memory deficits in patients with malignant gliomas. *J Neurooncol* **25**: 227–238.

Scheibel RS, Meyers CA, Levin VA (1996). Cognitive dysfunction following surgery for intracerebral glioma: influence of histopathology, lesion location, and treatment. *J Neurooncol* **30**: 61–69.

Shaw E, Arusell R, Scheithauer B *et al.* (2002). Prospective randomized trial of low- versus high-dose radiation therapy in adults with supratentorial low-grade glioma: initial report of a North Central Cancer Treatment Group/Radiation Therapy Oncology Group/Eastern Cooperative Oncology Group study. *J Clin Oncol* **20**: 2267–2276.

Shaw EG, Rosdhal R, D'Agostino RB Jr *et al.* (2006). Phase II study of donepezil in irradiated brain tumor patients: effect on cognitive function, mood, and quality of life. *J Clin Oncol* **24**: 1415–1420.

Shehata N, Pater A, Tang SC (1999). Prolonged severe 5-fluorouracil-associated neurotoxicity in a patient with dihydropyrimidine dehydrogenase deficiency. *Cancer Invest* **17**: 201–205.

Sherer M, Meyers CA, Bergloff P (1997). Efficacy of post-acute brain injury rehabilitation for patients with primary malignant brain tumors. *Cancer* **80**: 250–257.

Sherman AM, Jaeckle K, Meyers CA (2002). Pre-treatment cognitive performance predicts survival in patients with leptomeningeal disease. *Cancer* **95**: 1311–1316.

Sohlberg MM, Maateer CA (1989). *Introduction to Cognitive Rehabilitation.* New York: Guilford.

Spielberger C, Gorsuch R, Lushene R (1970). *State-Trait Anxiety Inventory.* Palo Alto, CA: Consulting Psychologists.

Steinbach JP, Blaicher H-P, Herrlinger U *et al.* (2006). Surviving glioblastoma for more than 5 years: the patient's perspective. *Neurology* **66**: 239–242.

Stupp R, Mason WP, van den Bent MJ *et al.* (2005). Radiotherapy plus concomitant and adjuvant temozolomide for glioblastoma. *New Engl J Med* **352**: 987–996.

Taphoorn MJ, Klein M (2004). Cognitive deficits in adult patients with brain tumours. *Lancet Neurol* **3**: 159–168.

Taphoorn MJ, Heimans JJ, Snoek FL *et al.* (1992). Assessment of quality of life in patients treated for low-grade glioma: a preliminary report. *J Neurol Neurosurg Psychiatry* **55**: 372–376.

Taphoorn MJ, Stupp R, Coens C *et al.* (2005). Health-related quality of life in patients with glioblastoma: a randomized controlled trial. *Lancet Oncol* **6**: 937–944.

Taylor BV, Buckner JC, Cascino TL *et al.* (1998). Effects of radiation and chemotherapy on cognitive function in patients with high-grade glioma. *J Clin Oncol* **16**: 2195–2201.

Tofilon PJ, Fike JR (2000). The radioresponse of the central nervous system: a dynamic process. *Radiat Res* **153**: 357–370.

Torres IJ, Mundt AJ, Sweeney PJ *et al.* (2003). A longitudinal neuropsychological study of partial brain radiation in adults with brain tumors. *Neurology* **60**: 1113–1118.

Ulrich CM, Yasui Y, Storb R *et al.* (2001). Pharmacogenetics of methotrexate: toxicity among marrow transplantation patients varies with the methylenetetrahydrofolate reductase C677T polymorphism. *Blood* **98**: 231–234.

Ulrich CM, Robien K, Sparks R (2003). Pharmacogenetics and folate metabolism – a promising direction. *Pharmacogenomics* **3**: 299–313.

Varni JW, Limbers CA, Burnwinkle TM (2007). How young can children reliably and validly self-report their health-related quality of life? An analysis of 8,591 children across age subgroups with the PedsQL 4.0 Generic Core Scales. *Health Qual Life Outcomes* **5**: 1–13.

Wade DT, Collin C (1988). The Barthel ADL Index: a standard measure of physical disability. *Int Disabil Stud* **10**: 64–67.

Ware JE, Sherbourne CD (1992). The MOS 36-item short-form health survey (SF-36): I. Conceptual framework and item selection. *Med Care* **30**: 473–483.

Wechsler D (1981). *Wechsler Adult Intelligence Scale-Revised.* San Antonio, TX: The Psychological Corporation.

Wei CW, Gui G, Mikulis DJ (2007). Tumor effects on cerebral white matter as characterized by diffusion tensor tractography. *Can J Neurol Sci* **34**: 62–68.

Weitzner MA, Meyers CA, Gelke CK *et al.* (1995). The Functional Assessment of Cancer Therapy (FACT) scale: development of a brain subscale and revalidation of the general version (FACT-G) in patients with primary brain tumors. *Cancer* **75**: 1151–1161.

Wellisch DK, Kaleita TA, Freeman D, Cloughesy T, Goldman J (2002). Predicting major depression in brain tumor patients. *Psychooncology* **11**: 230–238.

Wen PY, Schiff D, Kesari S, Drappatz J, Gigas DC, Doherty L (2006). Medical management of patients with brain tumors. *J Neurooncol* **80**: 313–332.

Young AH, Sahakian BJ, Robbns TW *et al.* (1999). The effects of chronic administration of hydrocortisone on cognitive functioning normal male volunteers. *Psychopharmacology* **145**: 260–266.

Young GS (2007). Advanced MRI of adult brain tumors. *Neurol Clin N Am* **25**: 947–973.

12

Brain metastases

Deepak Khuntia, Beela S. Mathew, Christina A. Meyers,
Sterling Johnson, and Minesh P. Mehta

Introduction

Brain metastasis is the commonest intracranial tumor in adults. In the United States, approximately 170 000 patients are diagnosed with brain metastases every year (Greenberg *et al.*, 1999; Mehta & Tremont-Lukas, 2004). The rise in incidence is attributed to a number of factors including increased life expectancy, improved control of systemic disease, and better imaging capabilities that facilitate diagnosis of smaller lesions (Wen *et al.*, 2001). While it is recognized that the overall prognosis of these patients remains poor, newer treatment methods have led to improved survival in subsets of patients. Patients with brain metastases often suffer from a variety of neurological, cognitive, and emotional difficulties. It is known that even subtle impairments of cognitive function can adversely affect the quality of life, an issue that was largely ignored earlier due to the dismal outcome. However, in the changing scenario of improved survival, recognizing the effects of the disease and its therapies on neurocognitive outcomes is important in formulating treatment modifications and strategies for rehabilitation that will enable patients to maximize their functional ability. This chapter briefly reviews the incidence and management of brain metastases as relevant to neurocognitive problems in cancer patients, discusses the etiology and pathogenesis of cognitive deficits in these patients, and suggests preventive and therapeutic strategies based on current understanding.

Overview of brain metastases

Epidemiology

Brain metastasis is a major debilitating complication affecting cancer patients. Autopsy data indicate that approximately 24% of adult cancer patients develop metastatic brain disease during the course of their cancer (Posner, 1995). The peak age group is 55–65 years, reflecting the incidence of primary cancers that occur mainly in the fifth and sixth decades of life (Lim *et al.*, 2004). Among the primary tumor types, lung cancer accounts for about 50% of all brain metastases (Ellis & Gregor, 1998; Kelly & Bunn, 1998; Postmus *et al.*, 2000). Other tumors causing brain metastases are breast cancer (15%–20%), melanoma (10%), unknown primary (10%–15%), colorectal cancer (2%–12%), kidney (1%–8%) and thyroid (1%–10%) (Cappuzo *et al.*, 2000; Lassman & DeAngelis, 2003; Wen *et al.*, 2001). In children the incidence of brain metastases is approximately 6%–10% and the most common associated solid primary tumors are sarcoma, Wilms' tumor, neuroblastoma, and germ cell tumor (Graus *et al.*, 1983; Vannucci & Baten, 1974). The majority of patients have involvement of the cerebral hemispheres (80%) while the

Table 12.1. Classification of brain metastases patients by prognosis (RPA analysis) (Gaspar *et al.*, 1997). KPS, Karnofsky Performance Scale; RPA, recursive partitioning analysis

Prognostic group	Median survival (months)
Class I (Age<65, KPS ≥70, controlled primary, no extracranial metastases)	7.1
Class II (KPS ≥70 with age ≥65 OR uncontrolled primary OR extracranial metastases)	4.2
Class III (KPS <70)	2.3

Table 12.2. Response to whole-brain radiation therapy in patients with brain metastases from various tumor types (Nieder *et al.*, 1997) (*n* = 108 patients)

Source of primary tumor	Percentage of patients showing response by CT (%)
Small-cell carcinoma	37
Breast cancer	35
Squamous cell carcinoma	25
Adenocarcinoma (non-breast)	14
Renal cell carcinoma	0
Melanoma	0

cerebellum is involved in 15% and the brainstem in <5% of patients (Sawaya & Bindal, 2001).

Clinical presentation

Brain metastases should be considered in the differential diagnosis of any cancer patient developing new neurological symptoms or signs. Common presentations include headache (24%–53%), focal weakness (16%–40%), altered mental status (24%–31%), seizures (15%), and ataxia (9%–20%) (Nussbaum *et al.*, 1996; Schellinger *et al.*, 1999).

Prognosis

The prognosis of patients with brain metastases is generally poor. The overall median survival for an untreated patient and patients receiving radiation is approximately 1 month and 4–6 months respectively (Nussbaum *et al.*, 1996; Posner, 1995; Sundstrom *et al.*, 1998; Zimm *et al.*, 1981). Retrospective recursive partitioning analysis (RPA) of prognostic factors performed on more than 1100 patients enrolled in Radiation Therapy Oncology Group (RTOG) trials identified three well-defined prognostic classes with significantly different median survivals (Gaspar *et al.*, 1997) (see Table 12.1).

Factors associated with longer survival in brain metastases patients are younger age, absence of extracranial disease, better performance status, and single lesions (Gaspar *et al.*, 1997). Improvement in cognitive function following treatment has also been reported to be a good prognostic factor (Curran *et al.*, 2002).

Response to treatment may be influenced by the tumor type being treated. Nieder and colleagues reported CT responses in 108 patients based on tumor type following whole-brain radiation therapy (WBRT) alone (Nieder *et al.*, 1997) (see Table 12.2). Complete responses were noted in 24% of all patients after WBRT with partial responses in 35%. Small cell lung cancers had the best response rate with 37% being responders, while renal cell and malignant melanoma were the worst with 0%.

Despite higher response rates with small cell lung cancer that has metastasized to the brain, patients do similarly poorly, with median survival ranging 6.5–8.5 months after treatment (Quan *et al.*, 2004). For patients undergoing surgery, however, histology has not been found to be an important factor (Agboola *et al.*, 1998).

Treatment

The aims of treatment of brain metastases are to maintain quality of life and functional status while maximizing duration of survival (Renschler *et al.*,

2003). Traditionally the mainstay of treatment has consisted of fractionated external WBRT. Phase III trials have reported that WBRT results in a median survival of 4–6 months and improves neurologic function in about half of patients (Borgelt *et al.*, 1980; Gaspar *et al.*, 1997). Common fractionation schemes include 30 Gy in 10 fractions, 37.5 Gy in 15 fractions, and 40 Gy in 20 fractions. Randomized trials by Kondzoilka *et al.* (1999) and Patchell *et al.* (1990) indicate that actuarial local control at 1 year after WBRT alone ranges from 0% to 14%. These data suggest that long-term control of gross brain metastases after WBRT alone is unlikely. Owing to the poor survival outcomes with WBRT alone, newer surgical, radiation, and chemotherapeutic approaches have been tried with promising results in subsets of patients.

Patchell *et al.* (1990) demonstrated superior local control (20% vs. 52%, $p < 0.02$) and median survival (40 vs. 15 weeks, $p < 0.01$) as well as prolonged time to brain metastases recurrence (59 vs. 21 weeks, $p < 0.005$) with the addition of surgery for patients with solitary brain metastases. Likewise another study of 63 patients also reported improvement in overall survival and functional independence for combined treatment with surgery and radiation compared to radiation alone (Noordjik *et al.*, 1994). Patchell and colleagues (1998) have also compared surgery alone versus surgery and WBRT. This study noted significant differences in favor of combined treatment for patients with tumor recurrence (18% vs. 70%, $p < 0.001$), median time to recurrence (220 weeks vs. 26 weeks, $p < 0.001$) and fewer deaths due to neurological causes (14% vs. 44%, $p = 0.003$). Currently surgical resection followed by WBRT is recommended for patients with a single brain metastasis who have none or minimal systemic disease and a Karnofsky Performance Score (KPS) higher than 70.

Radiosurgery, a technique that delivers accurately targeted highly conformal radiation to a defined lesion, has been evaluated as a non-invasive alternative to surgery in solitary brain metastases and more recently in multiple lesions too. High doses, generally in a single treatment, are prescribed

and several retrospective and prospective trials have proven that radiosurgery along with WBRT improves local control and survival for patients with unresectable solitary or multiple brain metastases if they have favorable characteristics (Alexander & Loeffler, 1999; Aoyama *et al.*, 2006; Breneman *et al.*, 1997; Chougule *et al.*, 2000; Kondzoilka *et al.*, 1999; Mehta & Tremont-Lukas, 2004; Seung *et al.*, 1998; Young, 1998). Sanghavi *et al.* (2001) analyzed radiosurgical data from 10 institutions and stratified 502 patients into three RPA classes as defined by the RTOG. Patients treated with radiosurgery boost in addition to WBRT showed improved median survival ($p < 0.05$) in all three classes compared to patients who received WBRT alone. Three prospective randomized trials comparing stereotactic radiosurgery plus WBRT to WBRT have been conducted (Andrews *et al.*, 2004; Chougule *et al.*, 2000; Kondzoilka *et al.*, 1999). Two studies with 27 and 104 patients respectively demonstrated improved local control rates favoring the radiosurgery arm but showed no significant difference in median survival (Chougule *et al.*, 2000; Kondzoilka *et al.*, 1999). However, results from a phase III multi-institutional trial (RTOG 9508) of 333 patients reported statistically significant improvement in median survival with the addition of radiosurgery to WBRT for patients with solitary brain metastases (6.5 vs. 4.9 months, $p = 0.039$), higher local control at 1 year (82% vs. 71%, $p = 0.01$) and an increase in the likelihood of stable or improved KPS and decreased steroid use at 6 months (43% vs. 27%, $p = 0.03$) for all patients. No differences were seen when assessing mental status, largely because only the Mini-Mental Status Examination was used for evaluation. On multivariate analysis RPA class I patients ($p < 0.0001$) and those with favorable histology ($p = 0.0121$) did significantly better (Andrews *et al.*, 2004). Thus radiosurgery boost is recommended as a standard treatment for patients with a single unresectable brain metastasis or for RPA class I patients. A phase III trial comparing radiosurgery alone to radiosurgery and WBRT has recently been completed in Japan (Aoyama *et al.*, 2006). In this trial, Aoyama and colleagues have demonstrated that the addition of

WBRT to radiosurgery decreased local recurrence from 46.8% in the WBRT + stereotactic radiosurgery (SRS) group compared to 76.4% for the SRS-alone group ($p < 0.001$). Furthermore, salvage treatments were less likely in patients receiving the whole-brain radiation. Despite the improvement in local control, no difference in overall survival was realized. Another study comparing SRS with or without WBRT is currently accruing patients through the American College of Surgeons Oncology Group (ACOSOG-Z0300).

It is generally believed that most chemotherapeutic agents are not useful in brain tumors due to their inability to penetrate the blood–brain barrier (BBB). Recent understanding that metastatic tumor growth causes the upregulation of angiogenic factors and neovascularization with a disrupted BBB in the new vessels has led to a renewed interest in using chemotherapy for brain metastases. Temozolomide, a novel alkylating agent with 100% bioavailability after oral administration and high cerebrospinal fluid (CSF) penetrability, has been tested with promising results (Abrey *et al.*, 2001; Antonadou *et al.*, 2002a, 2002b; Christodoulou *et al.*, 2001; Verger *et al.*, 2003).

Radiosensitizers are agents that enhance the effects of radiation. Two agents – motexafin gadolinium (MGd), a redox modulator that induces apoptosis, and RSR13, an allosteric modifier of hemoglobin that augments oxygenation of hypoxic tissues – have been tested in brain metastases patients (Bradley & Mehta, 2004; Mehta *et al.*, 2002, 2003, 2006). Although neither agent could demonstrate an overall survival advantage over WBRT alone, cohorts of patients who may benefit have been identified, and prospective trials evaluating the efficacy of radiosensitizers in these subsets are underway.

Neurocognitive impairment in brain metastases

The majority of brain metastases patients suffer from some degree of neuropsychological impairment. Our knowledge about the nature, severity, and course of cognitive dysfunction is limited owing to a lack of formal and systematic evaluation of neuropsychometric morbidity in a population of patients expected to have short longevity. Newer treatment approaches have clearly demonstrated improved survival in subpopulations of brain metastases patients with favorable prognostic factors. In this context neurocognitive and quality of life issues are a growing concern for survivors. Further, neurocognitive function has been demonstrated to be a predictor of survival for patients with brain metastases and primary brain tumor patients, and is considered to be a sensitive, viable and important endpoint that measures clinical benefit on patient functioning (Meyers & Hess, 2003).

Incidence

Although comprehensive data on the magnitude of cognitive dysfunction in patients with brain metastases are limited, it has been demonstrated that the majority have significant neurocognitive defects compromising their quality of life. Neurocognitive impairment affecting functional independence may even be more common than physical disability (Meyers & Boake, 1993). Deficits range from subtle problems with concentration, memory, affect, and personality to severe dementia. One of the early reports of cognitive decline in patients with brain metastases documented dementia in 11% patients who survived 1 year after WBRT (DeAngelis *et al.*, 1989). This was considered to be a function of the large fraction sizes employed for WBRT at that time; in fact none of the patients treated with conventional schedules and doses developed serious long-term dementia. Prospective studies conducted in small cell lung carcinoma (SCLC) patients receiving prophylactic cranial irradiation (PCI) demonstrated cognitive dysfunction prior to radiotherapy. Komaki *et al.* (1995) reported impaired cognitive tests in 97% patients at baseline. Two large randomized trials of PCI that incorporated neuropsychometric testing into the protocols found that 40%–60% patients showed significant abnormalities at the time of randomization (Arriagada *et al.*, 1995; Gregor *et al.*, 1997). Cognitive deficits were unrelated to age, gender or previous therapy (Gregor *et al.*, 1997). That being said, recent data from Li *et al.* (2006) have shown that with treatment and subsequent reduction in tumor burden in the brain, neurocognitive function can be improved with time.

Recognizing the importance of neurobehavioral outcome measures in brain tumor trials, the RTOG conducted a phase II feasibility study (BR0018) of systematic neurocognitive assessments in 55 brain metastases patients with excellent compliance rates prior to (95%), upon completion of (84%), and 1 month after (70%) WBRT (Regine *et al.*, 2004). Another single institution study in 30 patients reported 100% compliance, proving the feasibility of conducting such assessments in a routine clinical context (Herman *et al.*, 2003). Subsequently, prospective cognitive testing was incorporated into a large randomized pharmaceutical trial of 401 brain metastases patients in which Meyers *et al.* (2004) demonstrated baseline cognitive impairment in 90.5% of patients, with multiple abnormalities in most patients. This study establishes that neurocognitive dysfunction is a significant problem for brain metastases patients.

Etiology and pathogenesis

The etiology of neurocognitive impairment in brain metastases patients is diverse. Etiologies include direct damage due to the cancer, indirect effects of cancer (paraneoplastic), and effects of cancer treatments on the brain. In addition, these patients often have co-existing neurological and psychiatric disorders that affect their cognition and mood.

Neurocognitive deficits due to cancer

Cognitive problems in brain tumor patients preceding cancer treatments such as surgery, radiation or chemotherapy are typically related to the damage inflicted by the tumor itself. The evidence

of cognitive deficits in a significant number of patients prior to treatment and correlation of cognitive decline with tumor progression in patients who have received WBRT both clearly indicate that the cancer itself is an important cause of cognitive dysfunction in brain metastases patients. In some instances the cognitive deficits pre-date the development of metastatic disease to the brain, possibly suggesting the presence of unidentified paraneoplastic processes (Arriagada *et al.*, 1995; Komaki *et al.*, 1995; Regine *et al.*, 2001). The type and degree of deficits depend on the location of the lesion, but they also correlate with the total volume of brain metastatic disease (as opposed to the number of brain metastases alone) (Turkheimer *et al.*, 1990). Patients with left hemispheric tumors generally have language dysfunction, verbal, learning, memory and right-sided motor dexterity impairment. Right hemispheric tumors cause impairment of visual-perception skills and left-sided motor dexterity. Changes in mentation are common with tumors of the frontal lobe (Scheibel *et al.*, 1996). Cerebellar cancers are also implicated in cognitive malfunction (Gottwald *et al.*, 2004; Karatekin *et al.*, 2000).

Tumor-related events such as edema and hemorrhage cause disruption of sensitive afferent and efferent connections between the frontal region and other parts of the brain (Herman *et al.*, 2003). This accounts for the impairment in executive frontal lobe functions manifested as apathy, lack of motivation and spontaneity, impaired attention and memory, which are noted even in the absence of a frontal tumor (Lilja *et al.*, 1992).

Apart from the direct insult exerted by the tumor, neuropsychiatric difficulties could also be a result of other processes such as paraneoplastic effects particularly in patients with lung cancer (Komaki *et al.*, 1995). Central nervous system (CNS) paraneoplastic disorders are grouped into a clinico-pathological entity of paraneoplastic encephalomyelitis (PEM) characterized by multifocal autoimmune injury to the brain, spinal cord, dorsal root ganglia, and autonomic ganglia. Patients with brain lesions often present with memory loss, affective disorders, and cognitive deterioration (Dropcho, 2005).

Cognitive sequelae of cancer therapy

Brain damage consequent to cancer therapy is a well-recognized cause of cognitive decline in cancer patients. Contributory factors include specific antineoplastic treatments such as radiation, chemotherapy, hormonal therapy, immunotherapy, and surgery as well as supportive medications such as corticosteroids and anticonvulsants.

Radiotherapy

Most patients with brain metastases receive whole-brain radiotherapy in current practice. The deleterious effects of radiation on the CNS are well documented. The response to irradiation of the brain has been classically divided into three categories based on the timing of the onset of symptoms (Sheline et al., 1980). Acute effects occur during the first few weeks of treatment and are characterized by drowsiness, headache, nausea, vomiting, and worsening focal deficits. These symptoms are believed to be due to cerebral edema and are reversed by treatment with corticosteroids. Subacute encephalopathy (early delayed reaction) occurring at 1–6 months after completion of radiation is thought to be secondary to diffuse demyelination (Boldrey & Sheline, 1967; Van der Kogel, 1986). Typical symptoms include headache, somnolence, fatigability, and deterioration of pre-existing deficits that resolve within several months. Late delayed effects appear more than 6 months after radiation and are irreversible and progressive (Kramer, 1968). This is thought to be a result of white matter damage due to vascular injury, demyelination, and necrosis. Symptoms range from mild lassitude to significant memory loss, and severe dementia (Schultheiss et al., 1995). The pathophysiology of radiation-induced neurocognitive impairment thus involves dynamic, complex processes including inter- and intracellu-

lar interactions between vasculature and parenchymal cells particularly oligodendrocytes, which are important for myelination. Oligodendrocyte death occurs due to either a direct p53-dependent radiation apoptosis, or exposure to radiation-induced tumor necrosis factor α (TNF-α) (Cammer, 2000; Chow et al., 2000). Post-radiation injury to the vasculature involves damage to the endothelium leading to platelet aggregation and thrombus formation initially, followed by abnormal endothelial proliferation and intraluminal collagen deposition (Burger et al., 1979; Crossen et al., 1994). Hippocampal-dependent functions of learning, memory, and spatial information processing seem to be preferentially affected by radiation (Monje & Palmer, 2003). Animal studies have shown that doses as low as 2 Gy produce apoptosis in the proliferating cells in the hippocampus leading to decreased repopulative capacity (Peissner et al., 1999). The reader is directed to Chapter 7 for a more detailed review of the biological bases of radiation injury to the brain.

Studies of neurocognitive functioning in patients surviving 1 year after radiation yield conflicting results. DeAngelis and colleagues reported dementia in 11% patients who received WBRT using daily fractions of 3–6 Gy (DeAngelis et al., 1989). No patients receiving <3 Gy per fraction experienced this. Likewise no significant cognitive decline was reported for treatments with 40 Gy in 20 fractions (Penitzka et al., 2002), 30 Gy in 10 fractions or 54.4 Gy in an accelerated hyperfractionated regimen (Regine et al., 2001). Data from prospective trials of PCI in SCLC patients showed no significant cognitive deterioration following radiotherapy with fraction sizes of less than 3 Gy (Arriagada et al., 1995; Gregor et al., 1997; Komaki et al., 1995; Van Oosterhout et al., 1995). Fraction size, advanced age (>60 years), higher total dose, volume of brain irradiated, chemotherapy, and co-morbid vascular risk factors such as diabetes mellitus influence the incidence of radiation-induced injury to the brain and may account for the differences in reported incidences of cognitive deficits (Crossen et al., 1994; Lee et al., 2002).

Systemic anti-cancer therapy

The majority of brain metastases patients receive systemic anticancer therapies for control of primary or extracranial metastatic disease, either before or after the diagnosis of brain metastases. Many agents administered are known to have effects on brain function.

Chemotherapy-related cognitive impairment has been reported in 17%–75% patients (Ahles *et al.*, 2002; Brezden *et al.*, 2000; Schagen *et al.*, 1999; Wieneke & Dienst, 1995): rather than dementia, subtle neurocognitive variations are more common. A prospective trial evaluating neuropsychological function in breast cancer patients undergoing chemotherapy reported cognitive decline between baseline and short-term (6 months post chemotherapy) assessments in 61% of patients (Wefel *et al.*, 2004b). The most commonly affected domains included attention, learning, and processing speed, consistent with disruption of frontal network systems (Wefel *et al.*, 2004b). Etiologic mechanisms underlying chemotherapy-induced cognitive dysfunction may differ according to the agents used. Drugs such as methotrexate and 5-fluorouracil are particularly neurotoxic. Cisplatin, etoposide and vincristine may cause white matter injury (Komaki *et al.*, 1995). Potential reasons for brain damage include direct injury to the gray and white matter, microvascular injury, and secondary insults due to immune-mediated inflammatory responses (Wefel *et al.*, 2004a).

Alterations of an individual's hormonal milieu are associated with neurocognitive impairments (Wefel *et al.*, 2004a). Hormonal manipulation for control of systemic cancer is common in cancers of the breast and prostate. Estrogen receptors have been detected in areas of the brain important for cognitive functioning including the hypothalamus, anterior pituitary, amygdala, and hippocampus (McEwen & Alves, 1999). Assessments of neurocognitive function in women receiving anti-estrogens have demonstrated impairment in memory, executive function, and motor coordination (Rich & Maki, 1999; Varney *et al.*, 1998).

Positron emission tomography (PET) imaging has demonstrated greater prefrontal hypometabolism in women treated with chemotherapy and tamoxifen compared to chemotherapy alone (Silverman *et al.*, 2003). The hippocampus contains testosterone receptors as well as estradiol receptors. Hormonal challenges through luteinizing-hormone-releasing (LHRH) agonists thus have the potential to affect hippocampal function. However, there are inconsistent findings regarding neurocognitive dysfunction in the patients treated with LHRH agonists (Green *et al.*, 2002; Salminen *et al.*, 2003).

Other systemic antineoplastic agents that have the potential to produce neurotoxic effects include cytokines such as interferons and interleukins. Cytokines are reported to have direct and indirect effects on CNS function through alteration of, for example, neurotransmitters and neuroendocrine function (Kelley *et al.*, 2003). More than 50% of patients receiving cytokine therapy are reported to have neurocognitive impairment (Meyers & Abbruzzese, 1992). Functional neuroimaging studies have demonstrated frontal region abnormalities consistent with the neurocognitive deficits in such patients (Juengling *et al.*, 2000; Meyers *et al.*, 1994). The interested reader is directed to Chapter 8 for a more detailed review of chemotherapy-related cognitive impairment.

Surgery

Surgery has the potential to induce cognitive dysfunction secondary to brain injury and is most likely related to the tumor's location. There are conflicting reports as to the contribution of surgery to cognitive decline in brain tumor patients. While there are reports of cognitive decline after neurosurgery in children (Fontanella *et al.*, 2003; Grill *et al.*, 2004; Peace *et al.*, 1997), other investigators could not demonstrate any impairment of cognitive function following surgery compared to the pre-operative status (Friedman *et al.*, 2003; Hutter *et al.*, 1997; Tucha *et al.*, 2003). There are no data regarding the effect of surgery on cognitive function in brain metastases patients.

Adjuvant medications

Apart from the neurotoxic effects of specific anti-cancer therapy, other medications such as steroids, anticonvulsants, and pain medications used as adjuncts in brain metastases patients may cause neurocognitive and behavioral symptoms. Glucocorticoids are associated with a 5%–50% incidence of psychiatric syndromes including euphoria, mania, insomnia, restlessness, and increased motor activity and memory dysfunction (Kershner & Wang-Cheng, 1989; Wefel et al., 2004a; Wolkowitz et al., 1990). Anticonvulsants are associated with a sixfold increased risk of deficits in perception, psychomotor speed, attention and executive functioning (Taphoorn, 2003). Klein et al. (2003) demonstrated that both seizure frequency and the use of anticonvulsants have an adverse impact on neurocognitive function. Pain medications may cause sedation and associated difficulties in neurocognitive function.

Management of neurocognitive deficits

Knowledge of management strategies for therapy-induced neurocognitive deficits is limited. Since standard therapy has traditionally resulted in poor survival, few patients live long enough to develop late side-effects of therapy. Though no standard exists for the management of neurocognitive deficits, medical management, oxygen therapy, and astrocyte cell transplantation have been investigated.

Methylphenidate

Methylphenidate, a dopamine agonist used in patients with narcolepsy and attention deficit disorder, has been studied in patients with primary brain tumors experiencing neurocognitive dysfunction. The drug acts as a stimulant, which is useful in addressing fatigue, concentration, and depression in patients with side-effects from brain irradiation (Weitzner et al., 1995). The main toxicities of this agent include insomnia, cardiac symptoms, and anxiety or nervousness. It inhibits the metabolism of certain drugs such as warfarin and tricyclic antidepressants, and therefore plasma levels of these agents must be monitored. The drug also holds a relative contraindication in patients receiving monamine oxidase inhibitors.

In a series by Meyers et al. (1998), 30 patients with primary brain tumors with evidence of neurocognitive deficits were administered methylphenidate at doses between 10 mg and 30 mg twice daily (bid). In this study, subjective improvement was seen in all patients receiving 30 mg bid. This included improvement in energy, concentration, mood, and ambulation. Toxicity from the drug in this trial was quite minimal. The presumed mechanism for this improvement in neurocognitive function relates to the dopaminergic innervation of the mesolimbic system, which mediates subcortical function, and methylphenidate could help with improvement in motivation and drive by stimulating this system. Therefore, methylphenidate could be considered in the management of neurocognitive deficits in brain metastasis patients. Certainly, larger trials will be necessary to evaluate the use of methylphenidate in the adjuvant setting.

Donepezil

Donepezil, a cholinesterase inhibitor, has shown efficacy in Alzheimer's disease (Feldman et al., 2005). This drug inhibits acetylcholinesterase, allowing for increased availability of the neurotransmitter acetylcholine. It is relatively safe, with headaches, fatigue, dizziness, and gastrointestinal upset being the most common toxicities. Because of its metabolism through the liver, caution must be used when prescribed with drugs that block liver enzymes responsible for its metabolism (e.g., ketoconazole, quinidine). Also, the activity of this drug can be decreased when combined with agents such as carbamazepine, phenytoin, and rifampin, which increase its metabolism in the body.

As a result of its efficacy in Alzheimer's disease, efforts have been made to test the drug in cancer patients. Recently, a prospective randomized double-blind placebo control study was attempted to evaluate the efficacy of this drug in patients with SCLC (Jatoi *et al.*, 2005). However, because of poor accrual (only 9 of 104 patients) the study was closed prematurely.

Currently, the National Cancer Institute (NCI) is sponsoring a phase II trial looking at donepezil and EGb761 as agents that may improve neurocognitive function in patients who have undergone radiation for either primary brain tumors or brain metastases. EGb761 is an extract from *Ginkgo biloba* that has been found to have efficacy in the management of dementia and improvement in general cognition (Hoerr, 2003; LeBars, 2003; Mix & Crews, 2002). A more detailed discussion is presented in Chapter 22.

Hyperbaric oxygen

Radiation can decrease perfusion of tissues because of narrowing of the vasculature. As a result, tissues may be deficient of oxygen and other nutrients that are necessary to help with the tissue's recovery process (Kohshi *et al.*, 2003; Roman, 2000). Oxygenation increases tissue oxygen levels and results in increased fibroblast proliferation, which promotes angiogenesis allowing for neovascularization (Knighton *et al.*, 1983; Marx *et al.*, 1985). Generally, patients are given 100% oxygen at above-sea-level pressures in an enclosed chamber. These sessions are referred to as dives (as they simulate below-sea-level pressure). Each dive takes about 2 h and often 20–30 treatments are necessary. Because of the expense and labor necessary to do this, it is only offered in select institutions in the United States.

Data showing efficacy in improving radiation-related toxicities following soft-tissue and bone injury after head and neck radiotherapy are relatively well established, but few data are available showing the efficacy of hyperbaric oxygen for neurotoxicity following cranial irradiation. In a phase I-II trial conducted in the Netherlands, seven patients experiencing post-radiation neurocognitive deficits were treated with 30 sessions of hyperbaric oxygen.

All patients underwent a comprehensive battery of baseline neuropsychological testing and were then randomized to either immediate hyperbaric treatment with post-therapy neurocognitive testing versus delayed treatment (by 3 months) (Hulshof *et al.*, 2002). Six of the seven patients ultimately realized a benefit from the therapy, however there was no statistically significant benefit to earlier versus later intervention. As response to this therapy may take months, this therapy should only be considered in patients who have reasonable performance status and no active extracranial disease.

Transplantation of purified oligodendrocytes

In addition to vascular changes induced by radiation, there may also be direct damage to neural tissue. Classical teachings suggest that neural cells are incapable of repair. However, more recent data suggest that the introduction of transplanted oligodendrocytes may allow for remyelination of damaged neural cells (Groves *et al.*, 1993). Groves and colleagues described a process by which they were able to expand purified populations of oligodendrocyte type-2 astrocytes (O-2A) *in vitro*. These cells were injected into demyelinated lesions of rat spinal cords. They observed remyelination of the damaged cords. Others have described similar experiences in animal models where transplanted oligodendrocytes can either promote remyelination or even prevent white matter damage (Bambakidis & Miller, 2004; Blakemore *et al.*, 2003; Magy *et al.*, 2003). However, few data currently exist with transplantation in humans.

NMDA receptor

The NMDA (*N*-methyl-D-aspartate) receptor assists in a variety of functions in the mammalian CNS. Of particular interest is the long-term potentiation of synapses within the hippocampus (Kauer *et al.*, 1988). This process plays a critical role in memory and learning (Izquierdo *et al.*, 1992; Levin *et al.*, 2003; Riedel & Reymann, 1996). Memantine is a drug approved by the FDA for use in the management

Table 12.3. Randomized trials of whole-brain radiation therapy alone for brain metastases (adapted from Shaw *et al.*, 2003)

Study	Year	No. of patients	Randomization Gy/fractions	Median survival time (months)
Harwood & Simson, 1977	1977	101	30/10 vs. 10/1	4.0–4.3
Kurtz *et al.*, 1981	1981	255	30/10 vs. 50/20	3.9–4.2
Borgelt *et al.*, 1980	1980	138	10/1 vs. 30/10 vs. 40/20	4.2–4.8
Borgelt *et al.*, 1981	1981	64	12/2 vs. 20/5	2.8–3.0
Chatani *et al.*, 1986	1986	70	30/10 vs. 50/20	3.0–4.0
Haie-Meder *et al.*, 1993	1993	216	18/3 vs. 36/6 or 43/13	4.2–5.3
Chatani *et al.*, 1994	1994	72	30/10 vs. 50/20 or 20/5	2.4–4.3
Murray *et al.*, 1997	1997	445	54.4/34 vs. 30/10	4.5

of moderate to severe Alzheimer's disease (Danysz *et al.*, 2000). The drug acts as an NMDA-receptor antagonist, which may assist in the excitation of the NMDA receptor, resulting in improvement of memory and learning. Currently, the use of this drug in the management of neurocognitive deficits following treatment of brain metastases remains investigational.

A more detailed discussion with regards to pharmacologic interventions is presented in Chapter 22.

Prevention of neurocognitive deficits

Radiation dose and fractionation

A variety of WBRT treatment schedules, from hypofractionation to hyperfractionation, from low dose (10 Gy) to high dose (54 Gy), and from small fields to large fields have been evaluated. Table 12.3 shows the variation in radiation treatment schedules studied by the RTOG. The finding of these studies suggests that differences in dose, timing, and fractionation have not significantly altered the median survival time following WBRT treatment of brain metastases. As described earlier, patients with fraction sizes greater than 3 Gy are at higher risk of developing neurotoxicity from whole-brain therapy (DeAngelis *et al.*, 1989); therefore, hypofractionated regimens should be avoided. No significant cognitive decline was reported for treatments with 40 Gy in 20 fractions, 30 Gy in 10 fractions, or 54.4 Gy in

an accelerated hyperfractionated regimen (Penitzka *et al.*, 2002; Regine *et al.*, 2001).

Radiosurgery alone

The use of radiosurgery alone is controversial, but may be reasonable in the appropriately selected patient. For patients with solitary lesions, in whom there is a high degree of certainty that there are no other intracranial metastases, radiosurgery alone may be adequate treatment. Also, patients with significant small vessel disease with few metastases may also be candidates for radiosurgery alone to reduce the neurocognitive toxicities of WBRT. Pirzkall and colleagues, in a retrospective study of 236 patients, found no survival difference between patients with radiosurgery plus WBRT versus radiosurgery alone (Pirzkall *et al.*, 1998). However, there was a trend for improved survival in those patients without extracranial disease who received both WBRT and radiosurgery, suggesting that such an approach should involve careful selection of patients.

Recently, a report from the Japanese Radiation Oncology Study Group randomized patients with brain metastases to either radiosurgery alone or radiosurgery plus whole-brain radiation (Aoyama *et al.*, 2006). As mentioned earlier, patients receiving radiosurgery alone were at a higher risk of developing recurrence not only in the untreated brain,

Table 12.4. Up-front WBRT decreases risk of brain and local relapse. NS, Not significant; RS, radiosurgery, WBRT, whole-brain radiation therapy

Treatment	RS	RS + WBRT	P value	Risk ratio
n	67	65	–	–
Median survival (months)	7.6	7.9	NS	–
Local control (%)	70	86	0.0001	1.22
Brain failure (%)	52	18	0.0001	1.7

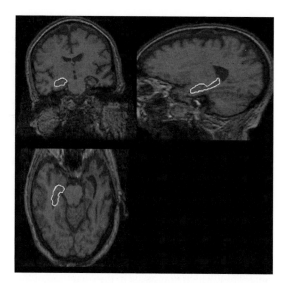

Figure 12.1. Identification of the hippocampus. Area in white denotes the mapped out hippocampus on MRI

but also at the site of radiosurgery. There was no difference in overall survival, neurological function, or cause of death (see Table 12.4). Therefore, it is not unreasonable to consider radiosurgery alone in the carefully selected patient with a solitary brain metastasis, as long as they are followed closely.

Erythropoietin

Recently, erythropoietin (EPO) has been described as a possible radiation protectant in the brain (Senzer, 2002). Reactive oxygen and nitrogen intermediates resulting from radiation treatment play a role in the development of neurotoxicity. In a mouse model, EPO has been found to improve performance and prevent cognitive impairment. Erythropoietin is an ideal drug for neurotoxicity prevention, as it crosses the BBB and also because receptors for EPO are present on astrocytes, neurons, and endothelial cells in the brain. Recently, however, the use of EPO in patients with metastatic breast cancer receiving first-line chemotherapy was found to decrease survival (Leyland-Jones *et al.*, 2005). Therefore, routine use of this drug in patients is not recommended, as further investigations are necessary to validate its efficacy.

Conformal avoidance of the hippocampus

As mentioned earlier, the hippocampus plays a vital role in memory and learning. Very low doses of

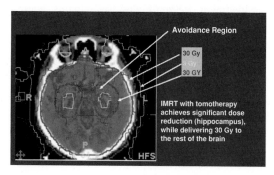

Figure 12.2. Hippocampus avoidance with intensity modulated radiotherapy (provided by Drs. Hazim Jaradat and Wolfgang Tome, University of Wisconsin). See color version in color plate section

radiation (2 Gy or less) can damage the hippocampus (Peissner *et al.*, 1999). Current investigations are looking at means of using image-guided technology to avoid the hippocampus in the delivery of WBRT. Because the hippocampus can be difficult to identify (see Figure 12.1), autocontouring algorithms are being developed to make this type of delivery practical on a large scale. With the use of intensity-modulated radiotherapy, it may be possible to treat the entire brain to standard doses of whole-brain radiation, while keeping the radiation dose to the hippocampus very low (see Figure 12.2). Clinical trials implementing this new technology are currently under development.

Further details on neuroprotection can be found in Chapter 22.

Conclusion

Cognitive dysfunction is an important component of many malignancies, and occurs in the vast majority of patients with brain metastases. This results in major quality of life disruption, and recent data suggest that the level of neurocognitive dysfunction may be predictive of overall outcome. Decline in neurocognition is commonly encountered in these patients and the etiology of this is multifactorial, including the disease process itself, treatment effects, the consequences of supportive treatment measures, and underlying physiological processes such as anemia, etc. The incidence and severity of neurocognitive deficits are generally underestimated, as few studies have prospectively rigorously evaluated cognitive function. With the development of "user-friendly" test batteries, it is now relatively easy to measure and follow deficits and changes in neurocognitive function. As management for brain metastasis continues to evolve, whole-brain radiotherapy remains a mainstay of treatment. Though efficacy is realized with WBRT, survival is short, and toxicities are real. As multimodal approaches including WBRT, radiosurgery, systemic, and local chemotherapy evolve and outcomes improve, long-term toxicities will become even more of an issue. Knowledge of mechanisms of this toxicity is expanding. This understanding, along with advances in radiation technology, will likely improve our outcomes with this difficult disease. In particular, newer pharmacologic interventions, based on seminal research in Alzheimer's disease, a better appreciation of the exquisite radiosensitivity of the hypothalamus and the development of "hippocampus-avoidance" radiotherapy techniques, the recognition of regenerative stem cells as a possible source of ameliorating this condition, the possibility of oligodendrocytic/astrocytic cell transplantation, and other approaches promise possible future interventional avenues.

REFERENCES

Abrey LE, Olson JD, Raizer JJ *et al.* (2001). A phase II trial of temozolomide for patients with recurrent or progressive brain metastases. *J Neurooncol* 53: 259–265.

Agboola O, Benoit B, Cross P *et al.* (1998). Prognostic factors derived from recursive partitioning analysis (RPA) of Radiation Therapy Oncology Group (RTOG) brain metastases trials applied to surgically resected and irradiated brain metastatic cases. *Int J Radiat Oncol Biol Phys* 42: 155–159.

Ahles TA, Saykin AJ, Furstenberg CT *et al.* (2002). Neuropsychologic impact of standard dose systemic chemotherapy in long-term survivors of breast cancer and lymphoma. *J Clin Oncol* 20: 485–493.

Alexander E, Loeffler JS (1999). The case for radiosurgery. *Clin Neurosurg* 45: 32–40.

Andrews DW, Scott CB, Sperduto PW *et al.* (2004). Whole brain radiation therapy with or without stereotactic radiosurgery boost for patients with one to three brain metastases: phase III results of the RTOG 9508 randomized trial. *Lancet* 363(9422): 1665–1672.

Antonadou D, Coliarakis N, Paraskevaidis M *et al.* (2002a). Whole brain radiotherapy alone or in combination with temozolomide for brain metastases. A phase III study [abstract]. *Int J Radiat Oncol Biol Phys* 54: 93–94.

Antonadou D, Paraskevaidis M, Sarris G *et al.* (2002b). Phase II randomized trial of temozolomide and concurrent radiotherapy in patients with brain metastases. *J Clin Oncol* 20: 3644–3650.

Aoyama H, Shirato H, Tago M *et al.* (2006). Stereotactic radiosurgery plus whole-brain radiation therapy vs stereotactic radiosurgery alone for treatment of brain metastases: a randomized controlled trial. *J Am Med Assoc* 295(25): 2483–2491.

Arriagada R, LeChevalier T, Borie F *et al.* (1995). Prophylactic cranial irradiation for patients with small cell lung cancer in complete remission. *J Natl Cancer Inst* 87: 183–190.

Bambakidis NC, Miller RH (2004). Transplantation of oligo-dendrocyte precursors and sonic hedgehog results in improved function and white matter sparing in the spinal cords of adult rats after contusion. *Spine J* 4(1):16–26.

Blakemore WF, Gilson JM, Crang AJ (2003). The presence of astrocytes in areas of demyelination influences remyelination following transplantation of oligodendrocyte progenitors. *Exp Neurol* 184(2): 955–963.

Boldrey E, Sheline G (1967). Delayed transitory clinical manifestation after radiation treatment of intracranial tumors. *Acta Radiol* 5: 5–10.

Borgelt B, Gelber R, Kramer S *et al.* (1980). The palliation of brain metastases: final results of the first two studies by the Radiation Therapy Oncology Group. *Int J Radiat Oncol Biol Phys* 6: 1–9.

Borgelt B, Gelber R, Larson M *et al.* (1981). Ultra-rapid high dose irradiation schedules for the palliation of brain metastases: final results of the first two studies by the Radiation Therapy Oncology Group. *Int J Radiat Oncol Biol Phys* 7: 1633–1638.

Bradley KA, Mehta MP (2004). Management of brain metastases. *Semin Oncol* 31: 693–701.

Breneman JC, Warnick RE, Albright REJ *et al.* (1997). Stereotactic radiosurgery for the treatment of brain metastases. Results of a single institution series. *Cancer* 79: 551–557.

Brezden CB, Phillips KA, Abdolell M (2000). Cognitive function in breast cancer patients receiving adjuvant chemotherapy. *J Clin Oncol* 18: 2695–2701.

Burger PC, Mahaley MS Jr., Dudka L *et al.* (1979). The morphologic effects of radiation administered therapeutically for intracranial gliomas: a postmortem study of 25 cases. *Cancer* 44: 1256–1279.

Cammer W (2000). Effects of TNFalpha on immature and mature oligodendrocytes and their progenitors invitro. *Brain Res* 864(2): 213–219.

Cappuzo F, Mazzoni F, Maestri A *et al.* (2000). Medical treatment of brain metastases from solid tumors. *Forum (Genova)* 10: 137–148.

Chatani M, Teshima T, Hata K *et al.* (1986). Prognostic factors in patients with brain metastases from lung carcinoma. *Strahlenther Onkol* 162: 157–161.

Chatani M, Matayoshi Y, Masaki N *et al.* (1994). Radiation therapy for brain metastases from lung carcinoma. Prospective randomized trial according to the level of lactate dehydrogenase. *Strahlenther Onkol* 170: 155–161.

Chougule PB, Burton-Williams M, Saris S *et al.* (2000). Randomized treatment of brain metastases with gamma knife radiosurgery, whole brain radiotherapy or both [abstract]. *Int J Radiat Oncol Biol Phys* 48: 114

Chow BM, Li YQ, Wong CS. (2000). Radiation-induced apoptosis in the adult central nervous system is p53-dependent. *Cell Death Differ* 7(8): 712–720.

Christodoulou C, Bafaloukos D, Kosmidis P *et al.* (2001). Phase II study of temozolomide in heavily pretreated cancer patients with brain metastases. *Ann Oncol* 12: 249–254.

Crossen JR, Garwood D, Glatstein E *et al.* (1994). Neurobehavioral sequelae of cranial irradiation in adults: a review of radiation induced encephalopathy. *J Clin Oncol* 12: 627–642.

Curran W, Mehta MP, Terhaard C *et al.* (2002). Predictors of Survival for Patients with Brain Metastases: Results of a Randomized Phase III Trial [abstract 155]. *Int J Radiat Oncol Biol Phys* 54: 93.

Danysz W, Parsons CG, Mobius JH *et al.* (2000). Neuroprotective and symptomatological action of memantine relevant for Alzheimer's disease: a unified glutamatergic hypothesis on the mechanism of action. *Neurotoxicity Res* 2: 85–97.

DeAngelis LM, Delattre JY, Posner JB (1989). Radiation induced dementia in patients cured of brain metastases. *Neurology* 39: 789–796.

Dropcho EJ (2005). Paraneoplastic disorders of the nervous system. In Black PM, Loeffler JS (eds.) *Cancer of the Nervous System*, (pp. 691–714). Philadelphia, PA: Lippincott Williams & Wilkins.

Ellis R, Gregor A (1998). The treatment of brain metastases from lung cancer. *Lung Cancer* 20: 81–84.

Feldman H, Gauthier S, Hecker J *et al.* (2005). Efficacy and safety of donepezil in patients with more severe Alzheimer's disease: a subgroup analysis from a randomized placebo-controlled trial. *Int J Geriatr Psychiatry* 20(6): 559–569.

Fontanella M, Perozzo P, Ursone R *et al.* (2003). Neuropsychological assessment after microsurgical clipping or endovascular treatment for anterior communicating artery aneurysm. *Acta Neurochir* 145: 867–872.

Freidman MA, Meyers CA, Sawaya R (2003). Neuropsychological effects of third ventricular tumor surgery. *Neurosurgery* 52: 791–798.

Gaspar L, Scott C, Rotman M *et al.* (1997). Recursive partitioning analysis (RPA) of prognostic factors in three Radiation Therapy Oncology Group (RTOG) brain metastases trials. *Int J Radiat Oncol Biol Phys* 37(4): 745–751.

Gottwald B, Wilde B, Mihajlovic Z *et al.* (2004). Evidence for distinct cognitive deficits after focal cerebellar lesions. *J Neurol Neurosurg Psychiatry* **75**: 1524–1531.

Graus F, Walker RW, Allen JC (1983). Brain metastases in children. *J Pediatr* **103**(4): 558–561.

Green HJ, Pakenham KI, Headley BC *et al.* (2002). Altered cognitive function in men treated for prostate cancer with luteinising hormone-releasing hormone analogues and cyproterone acetate: a randomized controlled trial. *Br J Urol* **90**: 427–432.

Greenberg H, Chandler WF, Sandler HM (1999). Brain metastases. In: Greenberg H, Chandler WF, Sandler HM (eds.) *Brain Tumors*, (pp. 299–317, Vol. 54). New York: Oxford University Press.

Gregor A, Cull A, Stephens RJ *et al.* (1997). Prophylactic cranial irradiation is indicated following complete response to induction therapy in small cell lung cancer: results of a multicenter randomized trial. United Kingdom Coordinating Committee for Cancer Research (UKCCCR) and the European Organisation for Research and Treatment of Cancer (EORTC). *Eur J Cancer* **33**: 1752–1758.

Grill J, Viguier D, Kieffer V *et al.* (2004). Critical risk factors for intellectual impairment in children with posterior fossa tumors: the role of cerebellar damage. *J Neurosurg* **101**: 152–158.

Groves AK, Barnett SC, Franklin RJ *et al.* (1993). Repair of demyelinated lesions by transplantation of purified O-2A progenitor cells. *Nature* **362**(6419): 453–455.

Haie-Meder C, Pellae-Cosset B, Laplanche A *et al.* (1993). Results of a randomized clinical trial comparing two radiation schedules in the palliative treatment of brain metastases. *Radiother Oncol* **26**: 111–116.

Harwood AR, Simson WJ (1977). Radiation therapy of cerebral metastases: a randomized prospective clinical trial. *Int J Radiat Oncol Biol Phys* **2**: 1091–1094.

Herman MA, Tremont-Lukats I, Meyers CA *et al.* (2003). Neurocognitive and functional assessment of patients with brain metastases. *Am J Clin Oncol* **26**(3): 273–279.

Hoerr R (2003). Behavioral and psychological symptoms of dementia (BPSD): effects of EGb 761. *Pharmacopsychiatry* **36** [Suppl. 1]: S56–S61.

Hulshof MC, Stark NM, van der Kleij A *et al.* (2002). Hyperbaric oxygen therapy for cognitive disorders after irradiation of the brain. *Strahlenther Onkol* **178**(4): 192–198.

Hutter BO, Spetzger U, Bertalanffy H *et al.* (1997). Cognition and quality of life in patients after transcallosal microsurgery for midline tumors. *J Neurosurg Sci* **41**: 123–129.

Izquierdo I, da Cunha C, Rosat R *et al.* (1992). Neurotransmitter receptors involved in post-training memory processing by the amygdala, medial septum, and hippocampus of the rat. *Behav Neural Biol* **58**(1): 16–26.

Jatoi A, Kahanic SP, Frytag S *et al.* (2005). Donepezil and vitamin E for preventing cognitive dysfunction in small cell lung cancer patients: preliminary results and suggestions for future study designs. *Support Care Cancer* **13**(1): 66–69.

Juengling FD, Ebert D, Gut O *et al.* (2000). Prefrontal cortical hypometabolism during low-dose interferon alpha treatment. *Psychopharmacology (Berl)* **152**: 383–389.

Karatekin C, Lazareff JA, Asarnow RF (2000). Relevance of cerebellar hemispheres for executive functions. *Pediatr Neurol* **22**: 106–112.

Kauer JA, Manlenka RC, Nicoll RA (1988). NMDA application potentiates synaptic transmission in the hippocampus. *Nature* **334**(6179): 250–252.

Kelly K, Bunn PAJ (1998). Is it time to reevaluate our approach to the treatment of brain metastases in patients with non-small cell lung cancer? *Lung Cancer* **20**: 85–91.

Kelley KW, Bluthé RM, Dantzer R *et al.* (2003). Cytokine-induced sickness behavior. *Brain Behav Immun* **17**: S112–S118.

Kershner P, Wang-Cheng R (1989). Psychiatric side-effects of steroid therapy. *Psychosomatics* **30**: 135–139.

Klein M, Engelberts NHJ, van der Ploeg HM *et al.* (2003). Epilepsy in low grade gliomas: the impact on cognitive function and quality of life. *Ann Neurol* **54**: 514–520.

Knighton DR, Hunt TK, Schenestuhl H *et al.* (1983). Oxygen tension regulates the expression of angiogenesis factor by macrophages. *Science* **221**: 1283–1289.

Kohshi K, Imada H, Nomoto S *et al.* (2003). Successful treatment of radiation-induced brain necrosis by hyperbaric oxygen therapy. *J Neurol Sci* **209**(1–2): 115–117.

Komaki R, Meyers CA, Shin DM *et al.* (1995). Evaluation of cognitive function in patients with limited small cell lung cancer prior to and shortly following prophylactic cranial irradiation. *Int J Radiat Oncol Biol Phys* **33**(1): 179–182.

Kondzoilka D, Patel A, Lunsford LD *et al.* (1999). Stereotactic radiosurgery plus whole brain radiotherapy versus radiotherapy alone for patients with multiple brain metastases. *Int J Radiat Oncol Biol Phys* **45**(2): 427–434.

Kramer S (1968). The hazards of therapeutic irradiation of the central nervous system. *Clin Neurosurg* **15**: 301–318.

Kurtz JM, Gelber R, Brady LW *et al.* (1981). The palliation of brain metastases in a favorable patient population:

a randomized clinical trial by the Radiation Therapy Oncology Group. *Int J Radiat Oncol Biol Phys* 7: 891–895.

Lassman AB, DeAngelis LM (2003). Brain metastases. *Neurol Clin* 21(I): I,vii.

LeBars PL (2003). Response patterns of EGb 761 in Alzheimer's disease: influence of neuropsychological profiles. *Pharmacopsychiatry* Jun; 36 [Suppl 1]: S44–S49.

Lee AW, Kwong DLW, Leung SF *et al.* (2002). Factors affecting risk of symptomatic temporal lobe necrosis: significance of fractional dose and treatment time. *Int J Radiat Oncol Biol Phys* 53: 75–85.

Levin ED, Sledge D, Baruah A *et al.* (2003). Ventral hippocampal NMDA blockade and nicotinic effects on memory function. *Brain Res Bull* 61(5): 489–495.

Leyland-Jones B, Semiglazov V, Pawlicki M *et al.* (2005). Maintaining normal hemoglobin levels with epoetin alfa in mainly nonanemic patients with metastatic breast cancer receiving first-line chemotherapy: a survival study. *J Clin Oncol* 23: 5960–5972.

Li J, Bentzen SM, Renschler M, Mehta MP (2006). Improvement in neurocognitive function (NCF) correlates with tumor regression after whole brain radiation therapy (WBRT) for brain metastases (BM) [abstract]. *Proc Am Soc Clin Oncol* 24 [Suppl. 18S]: 1504.

Lilja A, Smith GJ, Salford LG (1992). Microprocesses in perception and personality. *J Nerv Ment Dis* 180: 82–88.

Lim LC, Rosenthal MA, Maartens N *et al.* (2004). Management of brain metastases. *Intern Med J* 34: 270–278.

Magy L, Mertens C, Avellana-Adalid V *et al.* (2003). Inducible expression of FGF2 by a rat oligodendrocyte precursor cell line promotes CNS myelination in vitro. *Exp Neurol* 184(2): 912–922.

Marx RE, Johnson RP, Kline SN (1985). Prevention of osteoradionecrosis: a randomized prospective clinical trial of hyperbaric oxygen versus penicillin. *J Am Dent Assoc* 111; 49–54.

McEwen BS, Alves SE (1999). Estrogen actions in the central nervous system. *Endocr Rev* 20: 279–307.

Mehta MP, Tremont-Lukas I (2004). Radiosurgery for single and multiple metastases. In Sawaya R (ed.) *Intracranial Metastases: Current Management Strategies*, (pp. 139–164). Malden MA: Blackwell.

Mehta MP, Shapiro WR, Glantz M *et al.* (2002). Lead-in phase to randomized trial of Motexafin Gadolinium and whole brain radiation for patients with brain metastases. Centralized assessment of magnetic resonance imaging, neurocognitive and neurologic end points. *J Clin Oncol* 20: 3445–3453.

Mehta MP, Rodrigus P, Terhaard CHJ et al: (2003). Survival and neurologic outcomes in a randomized trial of Motexafin Gadolinium and whole brain radiation therapy in brain metastases. *J Clin Oncol* 21: 2529–2536.

Mehta MP, Gervais R, Chabot P *et al.* (2006). Motexafin gadolinium (MGd) combined with prompt whole brain radiation therapy (RT) prolongs time to neurologic progression in non-small cell lung cancer (NSCLC) patients with brain metastases: Results of a phase III trial [abstract]. *Proc Am Soc Clin Oncol* 24 [Suppl. 18S]: 7014.

Meyers CA, Abbruzzese JL (1992). Cognitive functioning in cancer patients: effect of previous treatment. *Neurology* 42: 434–436.

Meyers CA, Boake C (1993). Neurobehavioral disorders experienced by brain tumor patients: rehabilitation strategies. *Cancer Bull* 45: 362–364.

Meyers CA, Hess KR (2003). Multifaceted endpoints in brain tumor clinical trials: cognitive deterioration precedes MRI progression. *Neurooncology* 5: 89–95.

Meyers CA, Valentine AD, Wong FCL *et al.* (1994). Reversible neurotoxicity of interleukin-2 and tumor necrosis factor: correlation of SPECT with neuropsychological testing. *J Neuropsychiatry Clin Neurosci* 6: 285–288.

Meyers CA, Weitzner MA, Valentine *et al.* (1998). Methylphenidate therapy improves cognition, mood, and function of brain tumor patients. *J Clin Oncol* 16(7): 2522–2527.

Meyers CA, Smith JA, Bezjak A *et al.* (2004). Neurocognitive function and progression in patients with brain metastases treated with whole brain radiation and Motexafin Gadolinium: results of a randomized phase III trial. *J Clin Oncol* 22(1): 157–165.

Mix JA, Crews WD (2002). A double-blind, placebo-controlled, randomized trial of *Ginkgo biloba* extract EGb 761 in a sample of cognitively intact older adults: neuropsychological findings. *Hum Psychopharmacol* 17(6): 267–277.

Monje ML, Palmer T (2003). Radiation injury and neurogenesis. *Curr Opin Neurol* 16: 129–134.

Murray KJ, Scott C, Greenberg HM *et al.* (1997). A randomized phase III study of accelerated hyperfractionation versus standard in patients with unresected brain metastases: a report of the Radiation Therapy Oncology Group (RTOG) 9104. *Int J Radiat Oncol Biol Phys* 39: 571–574.

Nieder C, Berberich W, Schnabel K (1997). Tumor-related prognostic factors for remission of brain metastases after radiotherapy. *Int J Radiat Oncol Biol Phys* 39: 25–30.

Noordjik EM, Vecht CJ, Haaxma-Reiche H *et al.* (1994). The choice of treatment of single brain metastases should be based on extracranial tumor activity and age. *Int J Radiat Oncol Biol Phys* **29**: 711–717.

Nussbaum ES, Djalilian HR, Cho K *et al.* (1996). Brain metastases: histology, multiplicity, surgery and survival. *Cancer* **78**(8): 1781–1788.

Patchell RA, Tibbs PA, Walsh JW *et al.* (1990). A randomized trial of surgery in the treatment of single metastases to the brain. *N Eng J Med* **322**(8): 494–500.

Patchell RA, Tibbs PA, Regine WF *et al.* (1998). Postoperative radiotherapy in the treatment of single metastases to the brain: a randomized trial. *J Am Med Assoc* **280**: 1485–1489.

Peace KA, Orme SM, Thompson AR (1997). Cognitive dysfunction in patients treated for pituitary tumors. *J Clin Exp Neuropsychol* **19**: 1–6.

Peissner W, Kocher M, Treuer H (1999). Ionizing radiation-induced apoptosis of proliferating stem cells in the dentate gyrus of the adult rat hippocampus. *Brain Res Mol Brain Res* **71**(1): 61–68.

Penitzka S, Steinvorth S, Sehlleier S *et al.* (2002). Assessment of cognitive function after preventive and therapeutic whole brain irradiation using neuropsychological testing. *Strahlenther Onkol* **178**: 252–258.

Pirzkall A, Debus J, Lohr F *et al.* (1998). Radiosurgery alone or in combination with whole-brain radiotherapy for brain metastases. *J Clin Oncol* **16**: 3563–3569.

Posner JB (1995). *Neurologic Complications of Cancer.* Philadelphia, PA: FA Davis.

Postmus PE, Haaxma-Reiche H, Smit EF *et al.* (2000). Treatment of brain metastases of small-cell lung cancer: comparing teniposide and teniposide with whole-brain radiotherapy. A phase III study of the European Organization for the Research and Treatment of Cancer Lung Cancer Cooperative Group. *J Clin Oncol* **18**: 3400–3408.

Quan AL, Videtic GM, Suh JH (2004). Brain metastases in small cell lung cancer. *Oncology* **18**: 961–72.

Regine WF, Scott C, Murray K *et al.* (2001). Neurocognitive outcome in brain metastases patients treated with accelerated-fractionation vs accelerated hyperfractionated radiotherapy: an analysis of RTOG study 91–04. *Int J Radiat Oncol Biol Phys* **51**: 711–717.

Regine WF, Schmitt FA, Scott CB *et al.* (2004). Feasibility of neurocognitive outcome evaluations in patients with brain metastases in a multi-institutional cooperative group setting: results of Radiation Therapy Oncology Group trial BR-0018. *Int J Radiat Oncol Biol Phys* **58**(5): 1346–1352.

Renschler M, Mehta MP, Donald DM *et al.* (2003). Treatment intent for brain metastases: surveys of medical and radiation oncologists indicate that maintaining neurologic and neurocognitive function is more important than prolonging survival. *Proc Am Soc Clin Oncol* **22**: 552 (no. 2222).

Rich JB, Maki P (1999). Estrogen, testosterone and the brain: a review of neuropsychological, aging and neuroimaging studies. *J Int Neuropsychol Soc* **6**: iii.

Riedel G, Reymann KG (1996). Metabotropic glutamate receptors in hippocampal long-term potentiation and learning and memory. *Acta Physiol Scand* **157**(1): 1–19.

Roman G (2000). Perspectives in the treatment of vascular dementia. *Drugs Today (Barc)* **36**(9): 641–653.

Salminen E, Porten R, Korpela J *et al.* (2003). Androgen deprivation and cognition in prostate cancer. *Br J Cancer* **89**: 971–976.

Sanghavi SN, Miranpuri SS, Chappell R *et al.* (2001). Radiosurgery for patients with brain metastases: a multi-institutional analysis stratified by the RTOG recursive partitioning analysis method. *Int J Radiat Oncol Biol Phys* **51**: 426–434.

Sawaya R, Bindal R (2001). Metastatic brain tumors. In Laws E, Kaye AH (eds.) *Brain Tumors: an Encyclopedic Approach* (pp. 923–946). Edinburgh: Churchill Livingstone.

Schagen SB, vanDam FS, Muller MJ *et al.* (1999). Cognitive deficits after postoperative chemotherapy for breast cancer. *Cancer* **85**: 640–650.

Scheibel RS, Meyers CA, Levin VA (1996). Cognitive dysfunction following surgery for intracerebral glioma: influence of histopathology, lesion location and treatment. *J Neurooncol* **30**: 61–69.

Schellinger PD, Meinck HM, Thron A (1999). Diagnostic accuracy of MRI compared to CCT in patients with brain metastases. *J Neurooncol* **44**(3): 275–281.

Schultheiss TE, Kun LE, Ang KK *et al.* (1995). Radiation response of the central nervous system. *Int J Radiat Oncol Biol Phys* **31**: 1093–1112.

Senzer N (2002). Rationale for a phase III study of erythropoietin as a neurocognitive protectant in patients with lung cancer receiving prophylactic cranial irradiation. *Semin Oncol* **6** [Suppl. 19]: 47–52.

Seung SK, Sneed PK, McDermott MW *et al.* (1998). Gamma Knife radiosurgery for malignant melanoma brain metastases. *Cancer J Sci Am* **4**: 103–109.

Shaw E, Scott C, Suh J *et al.* (2003). RSR13 plus cranial radiation therapy in patients with brain metastases: comparison with the Radiation Therapy Oncology

Group recursive partitioning analysis brain metastases database. *J Clin Oncol* 21: 2364–2371.

Sheline GE, Wara WM, Smith V (1980). Therapeutic irradiation and brain injury. *Int J Radiat Oncol Biol Phys* 6: 1215–1228.

Silverman DH, Castellon SA, Abraham L *et al.* (2003). Abnormal regional brain metabolism in breast cancer survivors after adjuvant chemotherapy is associated with cognitive changes. *Proc Am Soc Clin Oncol* 22: 12.

Sundstrom JT, Minn H, Lertola KK *et al.* (1998). Prognosis of patients treated for intracranial metastases with whole-brain irradiation. *Ann Med* 30: 296–299.

Taphoorn MJB (2003). Neurocognitive sequelae in the treatment of low grade gliomas. *Semin Oncol* 30 [6 Suppl. 19] 45–48.

Tucha O, Smely C, Preier M (2003). Preoperative and post-operative cognitive functioning in patients with frontal meningioma. *J Neurosurg* 98: 21–31.

Turkheimer E, Yeo RA, Jones CL *et al.* (1990). Quantitative assessment of covariation between neuropsychological function and location of naturally occurring lesions in human. *J Clin Exp Neuropsychol* 12: 549–565.

Van Der Kogel AJ (1986). Radiation-induced damage in the central nervous system: an interpretation of target cell responses. *Br J Cancer* 7: 207–217.

Van Oosterhout AG, Boon PJ, Houx PJ *et al.* (1995). Follow up of cognitive functioning in patients with small cell lung cancer. *Int J Radiat Oncol Biol Phys* 31: 911–914.

Vannucci RC, Baten M (1974). Cerebral metastatic disease in childhood. *Neurology* 24(10): 981–985.

Varney NR, Syrop C, Kubu CS *et al.* (1998). Neuropsychologic dysfunction in women following leuprolide acetate induction of hypoestrogenism. *J Assist Reprod Genet* 10: 53–57.

Verger E, Gil M, Yaya R *et al.* (2003). Concomitant temozolomide (TMZ) and whole brain radiotherapy (WBRT) in patients with brain metastases (BM): randomized multi-centric phase II study [abstract]. *Proc Am Soc Clin Oncol* 22: 101.

Wefel JS, Kayl AE, Meyers CA (2004a). Neuropsychological dysfunction associated with cancer and cancer therapies: a conceptual review of an emerging target. *Br J Cancer* 90: 1691–1696.

Wefel JS, Lenzi R, Theriault RL *et al.* (2004b). The cognitive sequelae of standard-dose adjuvant chemotherapy in women with breast carcinoma: results of a prospective randomized longitudinal trial. *Cancer* 100(11): 2292–2299.

Weitzner MA, Meyers CA, Valentine AD (1995). Methylphenidate in the treatment of neurobehavioral slowing associated with cancer and cancer treatment. *J Neuropsychiatry Clin Neurosci* 7: 347–350.

Wen PY, Black PM, Loeffler JS (2001). Metastatic brain cancer. In Devita VT Jr., Hellman S, Rosenberg SA (eds.) *Cancer: Principles and Practice of Oncology* (6th edn.) (pp. 2655–2670). Philadelphia PA: Lippincott Williams & Wilkins.

Wieneke MH, Dienst ER (1995). Neuropsychological assessment of cognitive functioning following chemotherapy for breast cancer. *Psychooncology* 4: 61–66.

Wolkowitz OM, Reus VI, Weingartner H *et al.* (1990). Cognitive aspects of corticosteroids. *Am J Psychiatry* 147: 1297–1303.

Young RF (1998). Radiosurgery for the treatment of brain metastases. *Semin Surg Oncol* 14: 70–78.

Zimm S, Wampler GL, Stablein D *et al.* (1981). Intracerebral metastases in solid tumor patients: natural history and results of treatment. *Cancer* 48: 384–394.

13

Primary central nervous system lymphoma

Denise D. Correa

Introduction

Primary central nervous system lymphoma (PCNSL) is a relatively rare non-Hodgkin's lymphoma that arises within the CNS. Until recently, it accounted for only 1% of all primary brain tumors, but its incidence increased threefold in immunocompetent populations from 1988 to the time of writing (Eby *et al.*, 1988). With a median age at diagnosis of 60 years (Peterson & DeAngelis, 1997), PCNSL is a disease of middle and late adult life, and it is slightly more common in males (O'Neill & Illig, 1989). It is an infiltrative tumor most often located in the periventricular region and subcortical gray matter (Grant & Isaacson, 1992) (Figure 13.1). Leptomeningeal involvement is present in approximately one-third of patients at diagnosis (Peterson & DeAngelis, 1997), and the eye is another site of multifocal CNS involvement in about 25% of patients (Peterson *et al.*, 1993). On neuroimaging studies, PCNSL is identified as contrast-enhancing in 90% of cases, and multifocal lesions occur in approximately 40% of patients (DeAngelis, 1995).

Diagnosis and treatment

Patients may present with focal neurological signs, such as weakness, gait disturbance, language dysfunction, or seizures. Generalized symptoms of increased intracranial pressure, headache, or progressive cognitive decline may also occur at presentation. The diagnosis of PCNSL involves stereotactic brain biopsy or demonstration of malignant lymphocytes in the cerebrospinal fluid (CSF) or vitreous in cases of ocular involvement. Surgical resection is often not beneficial, and the deep-seated nature of most lesions increases the risk of possible surgical complications (DeAngelis *et al.*, 1990). Glucocorticoids produce only temporary clinical and radiographic response.

Conventional treatment of PCNSL has consisted of whole-brain radiation therapy (WBRT) due to the multifocal growth and spread of the disease. A dose of 40–50 Gy is used in most centers, yielding a median survival of 12–24 months (DeAngelis *et al.*, 1992; Nelson, 1999). Most patients have a complete or major partial response to this treatment, but the tumor typically relapses within the first year post-WBRT (DeAngelis *et al.*, 1990). Unlike primary glial tumors, PCNSL often relapses at a location distant from the original site of disease and may show widespread infiltration. In recent years, chemotherapy in conjunction with radiotherapy has been more frequently used to treat this disease. The use of agents that cross the blood–brain barrier (BBB) has been found to be necessary in order to gain access to disease residing behind an intact BBB. Regimens that include high-dose methotrexate (HD-MTX), high-dose cytarabine (HD-ARA-C),

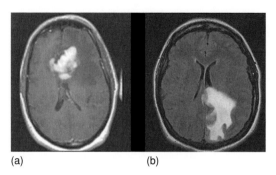

(a)   (b)

Figure 13.1. (a, b) T1-weighted axial MRIs revealing gadolinium-enhancing lesions in two patients with primary central nervous system lymphoma (PCNSL)

as well as intrathecal MTX and WBRT have shown favorable results, with a median survival of 3–4 years and a 30% 5-year survival (Abrey *et al.*, 1998; Boiardi *et al.*, 1993; DeAngelis *et al.*, 1992). Most prospective trials have used chemotherapy followed by WBRT, as there is some evidence that HD-MTX administered subsequent to WBRT increases the risk of late neurotoxicity (Blay *et al.*, 1998). Although combined modality regimens prolong survival, there is an increased risk for long-term neurotoxicity that increases with advanced age and in patients with prolonged disease-free survival (Abrey *et al.*, 1998; Pels & Schlegel, 2006).

Chemotherapy based on HD-MTX without WBRT is efficacious in the treatment of PCNSL and reduces the risk of delayed neurotoxicity (Freilich *et al.*, 1996; Kraemer *et al.*, 2002); it has been used more frequently in elderly PCNSL patients (Abrey *et al.*, 2000; Hoang-Xuan *et al.*, 2003). In prospective trials, HD-MTX alone produced a 52%–100% response rate and a 2-year survival rate of about 60% (Cher *et al.*, 1996; Guha-Thakurta *et al.*, 1999; Herrlinger *et al.*, 2002); HD-MTX-based polychemotherapy regimens resulted in a 65%–100% response rate and a 2-year survival rate of 65%–78% (Sandor *et al.*, 1998; Schlegel *et al.*, 2001). Considering that MTX does not readily cross an intact BBB, Neuwelt and colleagues (1991) have used intra-arterial MTX administration after transiently opening the BBB. A complete response to this treatment

was reported in 74% of patients and median survival was 40 months (Dahlborg *et al.*, 1996; Doolittle *et al.*, 2000; McAllister *et al.*, 2000). However, the long-term efficacy of HD-MTX-based regimens with or without BBB disruption remains to be confirmed (Ferreri *et al.*, 2002; Herrlinger *et al.*, 2005), as many patients relapse and require additional treatment with radiotherapy or chemotherapy (Abrey *et al.*, 2000; Pels *et al.*, 2003; Sandor *et al.*, 1998).

Treatment-related delayed neurotoxicity

Radiotherapy often produces irreversible and progressive damage to the CNS through vascular injury causing ischemia of surrounding tissue, and demyelination of white matter and necrosis (Sheline *et al.*, 1980). These are delayed effects of radiation that become apparent a few months to many years after treatment (Sheline, 1980). Pathological changes include multifocal areas of coagulative necrosis in the deep white matter with loss of myelin, axonal swelling, fragmentation, and gliosis. Suggested mechanisms include depletion of glial progenitor cells and perpetuation of oxidative stress induced by radiation (Tofilon & Fike, 2000). Radiation may diminish the reproductive capacity of the O-2A progenitors of oligodendrocytes, disrupting the normal turnover of myelin (Van Der Maazen *et al.*, 1993). This progressive demyelination may take months to produce symptoms, contributing to the latency in onset of neurotoxicity and its progressive nature. The prevalence of radiation-induced brain injury appears to increase with volume of radiated tissue, dose of radiation, dose per fraction, concomitant administration of chemotherapy, and age (Constine *et al.*, 1988). See Chapter 7 for a detailed discussion of radiation injury to the brain.

The interactions between radiation and HD-MTX are the most clearly demonstrated (Keime-Guibert *et al.*, 1998), as WBRT may have a synergistic effect when combined with HD-MTX (Crossen *et al.*, 1992). Other chemotherapy agents that when combined with radiation may produce CNS damage are nitrosoureas, cytosine arabinoside, and

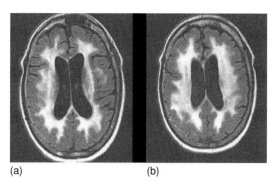

(a)   (b)

Figure 13.2. (a, b) T1-weighted axial MRI showing diffuse white matter abnormalities in a 61-year-old PCNSL patient 5 years post-WBRT and HD-MTX-based chemotherapy (HD-MTX, High-dose methotrexate; WBRT, whole-brain radiation therapy)

vincristine (DeAngelis & Shapiro, 1991). In PCNSL patients treated with combined modality therapy, magnetic resonance imaging (MRI) studies most commonly show diffuse white matter abnormalities (Figure 13.2), but cerebral atrophy, communicating hydrocephalus, and radionecrotic lesions can also be seen. Several chemotherapeutic agents, particularly HD-MTX and HD-ARA-C, have been shown to produce periventricular white matter abnormalities, but often less extensive than seen after combined modality treatment. The pathophysiological mechanisms of chemotherapeutic agents are not well understood, but several have been hypothesized including demyelination, secondary inflammatory response, and microvascular injury. In a recent series of five autopsied PCNSL patients treated with WBRT and chemotherapy (i.e., HD-MTX, HD-ARA-C, doxorubicin, or etoposide) who died of leukoencephalopathy (Lai *et al.*, 2004), there was myelin and axonal loss, pallor, rarefaction, spongiosis, and gliosis of the cerebral hemispheric white matter. In addition, all patients had fibrotic thickening of small blood vessels in the deep white matter, and four patients had atherosclerosis of the large cerebral blood vessels in the circle of Willis.

Delayed neurotoxicity has been recognized as a significant problem as effective treatment for PCNSL has increased survival rates (Abrey *et al.*,

1998; Peterson & DeAngelis, 1997; Poortmans *et al.*, 2003). The specific contribution of the disease itself and of various treatment modalities to the development of neurotoxicity remains to be elucidated, as the neurotoxic potential of combined treatments is difficult to determine when each modality can produce CNS damage individually (DeAngelis & Shapiro, 1991). Neurological sequelae of treatment usually develop more than 1 year after therapy, and can only be established in the absence of tumor (DeAngelis *et al.*, 1989). Therefore, its incidence is proportional to the percentage of patients with disease-free survival (DeAngelis *et al.*, 1992), and is related to both long-term survival and advanced age (DeAngelis & Hormigo, 2004). When a combination of WBRT and chemotherapy is used, the incidence of delayed neurotoxicity ranges from 8% to 50% of patients in different PCNSL clinical trials (Abrey *et al.*, 1998; Glass *et al.*, 1994; O'Brien *et al.*, 2000; Sarazin *et al.*, 1995). It has been recognized as a significant problem in long-term survivors over 60 years of age (Abrey *et al.*, 1998; Batchelor & Loeffler, 2006; Besell *et al.*, 2001; Blay *et al.*, 1998; Ferreri *et al.*, 2002; Peterson & DeAngelis, 1997; Poortmans *et al.*, 2003), and reported to range between 50% and 80% in older patients treated with WBRT and HD-MTX-based chemotherapy, and between 5% and 8% in patients treated with MTX-based chemotherapy alone (Abrey *et al.*, 2000; Hoang-Xuan *et al.*, 2003). The variability in the reported incidence of neurotoxicity across studies may be in part related to differences in both the type and severity of symptoms documented.

Cognitive functions in PCNSL

The development of cognitive dysfunction in PCNSL patients is most likely related to multiple factors including the effects of the tumor itself given its infiltrative pattern, age (i.e., median age at diagnosis is 60 years), and the delayed effects of treatment with WBRT and HD-MTX-based chemotherapy either combined or alone (O'Neill, 2004). It is currently considered the most frequent complication among long-term survivors (Behin & Delattre, 2003), and may interfere with the patient's ability to function at pre-morbid levels professionally and socially, despite adequate disease control (Correa *et al.*, 2004; Harder *et al.*, 2004). Consistent with the current status of the research on patients with other brain tumor histologies, there is also a paucity of information regarding cognitive functioning in PCNSL patients. The majority of studies reported performance status, patients' complaints, clinical observations, and mental status examinations (Corry *et al.*, 1998; Herrlinger *et al.*, 1998), but systematic cognitive evaluations have rarely been included. These methods have low sensitivity to detect cognitive dysfunction in patients with brain tumors (Meyers & Wefel, 2003; Weitzner & Meyers, 1997). Therefore, only severe neurotoxicity resulting in significant disability was documented in most clinical trials, suggesting that the true incidence of cognitive dysfunction in PCNSL is most probably higher than reported (Blay *et al.*, 1998; Keime-Guibert *et al.*, 1998; Laack & Brown, 2004). The few studies that described cognitive outcome in PCNSL involved a relatively small number of patients at follow-up, mostly as a result of increased drop-out rates due to disease relapse or death.

Prospective studies

Neuwelt and his colleagues have investigated neuropsychological abilities in PCNSL patients who were treated with osmotic BBB disruption with or without radiotherapy, and performed pre-treatment and long-term follow-up on several patients (Crossen *et al.*, 1992; Dahlborg *et al.*, 1996, 1998; Neuwelt *et al.*, 1991; Roman-Goldstein *et al.*, 1995). Initial studies (Dahlborg *et al.*, 1996; Neuwelt *et al.*, 1991) showed that PCNSL patients who obtained a complete response to treatment with HD-MTX-based chemotherapy with BBB disruption ($n = 15$) had no significant overall cognitive decline over a period of several years (median survival = 41 months) regardless of age. In contrast, patients whose disease has recurred after initial radiotherapy and who subsequently received chemotherapy with

BBB disruption ($n = 7$ with complete response) displayed cognitive deterioration despite limited survival (i.e., 16 months). The investigators used an extensive battery of neuropsychological tests and included pre- and post-treatment evaluations, but only a small number of patients were available for long-term follow-up in these studies. In addition, the findings were discussed regarding the presence or absence of cognitive decline (i.e., overall summary index of change from baseline), and little information about specific cognitive domains that may have been differentially affected by treatment was reported. In a more recent study, McAllister and colleagues (2000) reported the results of pre- and post-therapy cognitive evaluations on 23 PCNSL patients who had a complete response at least 1 year after treatment with HD-MTX chemotherapy with BBB disruption. The mean time interval between the two evaluations was 16.5 months (SD = 10.9 months). All patients showed improvement in overall cognitive functions (summary z-scores) at follow-up. However, an evaluation of individual test scores revealed no significant changes from baseline in verbal learning, cognitive flexibility, and motor skills; in seven patients there was a mild decline in motor performance (at least 1 SD below the mean) at follow-up.

Fliessbach and colleagues (2003) performed longitudinal neuropsychological evaluations on a group of PCNSL patients treated with a poly-chemotherapy regimen that included HD-MTX. Although 20 patients were available for pre-treatment evaluations, only 10 patients (median age = 60 years, range = 27–67) achieved durable remissions without relapse more than 1 year after completion of treatment (median follow-up = 36 months). The authors assessed verbal learning and recall, non-verbal recognition memory, word fluency, visuoconstruction, and attention. There was evidence of cognitive improvement (i.e., primarily in attention and verbal memory) in 4 of the 5 patients who had impaired performance at baseline, and no change at follow-up was noted in the 3 patients who had intact cognition prior to therapy; 2 patients could not be assessed at base-line. In the 4 patients who relapsed within 1 year after treatment, significant cognitive impairment was noted in 3 patients after additional treatment (i.e., 2 had chemotherapy, 1 had WBRT). A subsequent study including 5 additional patients treated with the same regimen (Pels et al., 2003) reported no significant cognitive decline at long-term follow-up.

In a more recent study, Fliessbach and colleagues (2005) reported the results of prospective cognitive evaluations in 23 PCNSL patients (median age = 54 years, range = 28–68) who achieved a complete remission after treatment with HD-MTX-based polychemotherapy. At baseline, 16 patients had moderate to severe cognitive impairments (i.e., reduced verbal fluency, attention/executive, and memory abilities), 3 had mild impairment, and 4 had intact cognitive abilities. At long-term follow-up (median follow-up = 44 months, range = 17–96), 6 patients had moderate to severe cognitive impairment, 5 had mild cognitive difficulties, and 12 had intact cognitive functions; only 4 patients reported diminished quality of life. The authors concluded that cognitive functions either improved or remained stable at follow-up, suggesting that HD-MTX-based chemotherapy is not associated with long-term neurotoxicity. However, not all patients received the same tests, and timed measures of psychomotor speed, cognitive flexibility, and working memory were given only to a subset of patients. It is possible that the limited assessment of executive abilities in these two studies underestimated the degree of cognitive dysfunction in their patient cohort.

Schlegel and colleagues (2001) assessed cognitive outcome in 20 PCNSL patients (median age = 64 years, range = 27–71) treated with HD-MTX and HD-ARA-C. The neuropsychological test battery included measures of attention, verbal and non-verbal memory, verbal fluency, and visuoconstruction; a global index score of cognitive function was generated by transforming raw scores into standard values according to normative data and averaging them (mean = 100). Ten patients were eval-uated at baseline, 4 months, 12 months, and 15–41 months after completion of treatment (8 patients had a complete response); these patients showed stable or improved summary cognitive test scores at the last follow-up (median = 95, range = 89–107; 100 $\pm$ 10 as reference value). Nine patients also had preserved cognitive functions during follow-up, but no specific intervals or summary scores were reported. One patient required additional chemotherapy due to disease relapse and developed severe cognitive impairment 21 months after therapy. No information was available regarding the patients' performance on each cognitive test domain.

In a prospective study of patients with PCNSL treated with high-dose chemotherapy and stem cell transplantation without WBRT (Abrey et al., 2003), 14 patients (mean age = 53.6 years, SD = 6.8) received prospective neuropsychological evaluations. Patients performed in the impaired range (z-scores 2 SD below normative sample means) prior to treatment on several cognitive domains including executive function, memory, and psychomotor speed. Improvements across all cognitive domains were documented after induction chemotherapy with HD-MTX and HD-ARA-C for the 7 patients who had no progressive disease and were available for initial follow-up (Correa et al., 2003); this was consistent with neuroimaging evidence of reduction in lesion size in response to treatment. Three patients who had a complete response to treatment remained cognitively stable up to 18 months post-transplant (i.e., scores within 1 SD below the normative mean). The small number of patients seen for long-term cognitive follow-up in this study precludes any conclusions regarding the possible neurotoxicity of this treatment regimen.

Retrospective studies

Pels and colleagues (2000) described a series of 27 PCNSL patients (age range = 27–74 years) treated with various regimens including WBRT, high-dose chemotherapy (i.e., HD-MTX, HD-ARA-C), or combined modality therapy. Patients' survival time ranged from 2 to 95 months. The cognitive evaluations were conducted subsequent to treatment, but the follow-up intervals were not reported. There was evidence of cognitive deficits in 8 of the 13 patients who received WBRT alone or in combination with high-dose chemotherapy; however, 4 of these patients had either disease progression or only a partial response to therapy, suggesting that both the tumor and treatment may have contributed to the cognitive impairment. Of the 14 patients treated with high-dose chemotherapy alone, 10 had cognitive deficits; 8 of these patients had a complete response to treatment. The authors included no information regarding specific cognitive tests used or the cognitive domains affected by tumor and/or treatment.

Herrlinger and colleagues (2005) studied neuropsychological functions and quality of life in 6 PCNSL patients (age range = 56 to 63 years) who survived for at least 48 months and had no active disease (follow-up range = 55–69 months); all patients were treated with HD-MTX and one patient also had WBRT. There was evidence of mild to moderate cognitive impairment in all patients, particularly in attention and memory functions. Cognitive dysfunction was more pronounced in the two patients with marked leukoencephalopathy (one had combined modality therapy). Three patients reported moderate restriction in quality of life, particularly in cognitive and social functioning; the patient treated with WBRT described significantly decreased quality of life.

Harder and colleagues (2004) studied cognitive abilities in 19 PCNSL patients (median age = 44 years, range = 24–63) treated with HD-MTX-based chemotherapy followed by WBRT; patients were evaluated at least 6 months after treatment completion and had no recurrent disease (mean = 23 months, SD = 14). It was reported that 63% of patients showed mild to moderate cognitive impairments (i.e., four to six test indices 2 SD below the normative mean). In comparison to matched controls with hematological malignancies treated with systemic chemotherapy or non-CNS radiotherapy, PCNSL patients obtained lower scores on cognitive domains involving verbal and non-verbal memory,

attention, executive function, and motor speed. Ten patients were on disability, four worked at a lower level, and two worked less than before diagnosis.

Correa and colleagues (2004) investigated cognitive functioning in 28 survivors of PCNSL who were treated with WBRT and HD-MTX-based chemotherapy, or high-dose chemotherapy alone, and had no disease recurrence. In the study, 18 patients received WBRT ± HD-MTX-based chemotherapy (median age = 53 years, range = 36–73; mean post-treatment interval = 61 months, SD = 40), and 10 patients had HD-MTX-based chemotherapy alone (median age = 71 years, range = 59–82; mean post-treatment interval = 18 months, SD = 16). Patients who received combined modality treatment showed mild to moderate cognitive impairments (i.e., scores at least 1.5 SD below the normative sample) on tests of complex attention and executive functions, memory, psychomotor speed, and naming. In comparison to patients treated with chemotherapy alone, their performance was more impaired on tests of memory, and attention and executive functions, regardless of time since completion of treatment. Patients treated with HD-MTX-based chemotherapy alone had moderate impairment in psychomotor speed, but performed within 1 SD below the normative sample on other cognitive domains. The memory performance of patients treated with WBRT ± chemotherapy did not differ according to time since treatment completion (≤60 months, n = 9; ≥60 months, n = 9), but was significantly (p < 0.05) more impaired than the performance of patients treated with chemotherapy alone (≤60 months), who were also older. Evaluation of quality of life showed that half of the patients were either not employed or were working at a lower capacity as a consequence of their disease and treatment. The findings suggested that combined modality therapy was associated with more severe cognitive impairment than chemotherapy alone, regardless of time since treatment completion. The assessment of the specific contributions of the disease and treatment, and time of onset and course of neurotoxicity is relatively limited in this study given its retrospective nature.

Overall, the findings suggest that combined modality treatment for PCNSL with WBRT and HD-MTX-based chemotherapy results in more severe cognitive impairment than chemotherapy alone, particularly in the areas of attention, executive function, memory, and psychomotor speed. Studies involving patients treated with MTX-based chemotherapy with or without BBB disruption reported variable findings ranging from no significant cognitive decline or improvement from baseline to cognitive impairment in some patients. However, these trials included a relatively small number of patients who completed long-term follow-up, some studies evaluated patients with recurrent disease, and in some studies patients treated with combined modality therapy had a history of relapse or partial response to therapy suggesting a possible selection bias. In addition, not all studies assessed or described the specific cognitive domains that may have been differentially affected by treatment, such as executive functions and motor speed.

Cognitive outcome and treatment-related white matter abnormalities

The association between diffuse treatment-related white matter abnormalities and the presence or severity of neuropsychological dysfunction in brain tumor patients is unclear. It may vary in severity, ranging from no abnormal clinical findings to progressive global cognitive decline (Dropcho, 1991). A moderate association between treatment-related white matter changes and cognitive impairment was found in some but not all studies involving PCNSL patients (Correa *et al.*, 2004; Fliessbach *et al.*, 2003, 2005; Harder *et al.*, 2004; Pels *et al.*, 2000).

Fliessbach and colleagues (2003) documented the development of white matter changes in four of ten patients who received a polychemotherapy regimen; in three patients there were confluent subcortical white matter changes; cognitive functions were within the normal range. In a subsequent study (Fliessbach *et al.*, 2005), the authors observed bilateral confluent white mat-

ter abnormalities in eight patients after HD-MTX-based polychemotherapy, but these were not correlated with cognitive performance. Roman-Goldstein and colleagues (1995) documented white matter abnormalities in only one of nine PCNSL patients following treatment with chemotherapy with BBB disruption; there was no evidence of cognitive impairment in any of the patients. Schlegel and colleagues (2001) reported that 6 of 20 PCNSL patients treated with HD-MTX and ARA-C developed confluent white matter lesions 1–6 months after initiation of treatment; only 1 of these patients had cognitive impairment. Neuwelt and colleagues (2005) documented that peri-tumor-enhancing abnormalities were associated with cognitive dysfunction at diagnosis in 15 PCNSL patients, but not after a complete response to MTX-based chemotherapy with BBB disruption. Long-term follow-up ($n = 9$) showed that some patients developed post-treatment diffuse or focal bilateral periventricular abnormalities, but these were not associated with cognitive performance (overall summary score), which remained stable or improved more than 2 years after diagnosis.

Pels and colleagues (2000) reported that 5 of 13 PCNSL patients treated with WBRT alone or in combination with high-dose chemotherapy developed confluent white matter lesions and marked cognitive deficits following treatment. Three patients treated with chemotherapy alone developed white matter disease but it was not associated with cognitive dysfunction; 10 of the 14 patients treated with this regimen had cognitive dysfunction without evidence of significant white matter disease. In a subsequent study (Pels *et al.*, 2003), 20 of 57 patients developed white matter abnormalities during treatment with HD-MTX-based chemotherapy, and these remained stable at follow-up; only 2 of these patients had severe cognitive dysfunction. Harder and colleagues (2004) reported white matter abnormalities and cortical atrophy in 14 PCNSL patients (78% of the patient sample) following treatment with HD-MTX-based chemotherapy and WBRT; cortical atrophy, but not white matter disease, was significantly correlated with cognitive impairment, age, and Karnofsky Performance Score. Correa and colleagues (2004) found that more extensive white matter abnormalities on MRI were significantly correlated with greater impairment in executive function, memory, and language abilities in 28 PCNSL patients; white matter changes were more extensive in the 18 patients treated with WBRT and HD-MTX-based chemotherapy than in the 10 patients who received HD-MTX-based chemotherapy alone.

The variable findings in the literature may be attributed in part to methodological factors (Desmond, 2002), as different scales and MRI sequences were used to measure white matter abnormalities across studies. In addition, several studies reported cognitive function as a summary score, and no correlations between white matter abnormalities and specific cognitive functions (e.g., executive function, processing speed) were reported. Nevertheless, the results suggest that in comparison to chemotherapy-alone regimens, WBRT alone or in combination with HD-MTX-based chemotherapy produces more extensive white matter abnormalities, which are associated with cognitive impairment. These observations are consistent with evidence that more extensive white matter disease may be necessary to produce measurable cognitive deficits, and that only specific cognitive domains, such as executive functions and processing speed, are disrupted by diffuse white matter disease (Tullberg *et al.*, 2004).

Conclusion

Treatment-related neurotoxicity has been recognized as a significant problem as therapy regimens for PCNSL have prolonged survival. However, the incidence of cognitive dysfunction in this population may have been underestimated as only a small number of clinical trials have included formal neuropsychological assessment as an outcome measure. The studies reviewed suggest that treatment involving a combination of WBRT and HD-MTX-based chemotherapy is associated with cognitive impairment and diffuse white matter abnormalities. Cognitive dysfunction after treatment with high-dose chemotherapy alone was reported in some but not all studies; it is also unclear if this regimen results in a compromise of long-term disease control. Future collaborative, prospective longitudinal studies are required to determine the incidence of cognitive dysfunction associated with various treatment modalities in patients with PCNSL. At present, there is no effective therapy for treatment-related cognitive dysfunction, but recent studies have reported some benefit from psychopharmacological interventions (Chapter 22) and cognitive rehabilitation (Chapter 20).

REFERENCES

Abrey LE, DeAngelis LM, Yahalom J (1998). Long-term survival in primary CNS lymphoma. *J Clin Oncol* **16**: 859–863.

Abrey LE, Yahalom J, DeAngelis LM (2000). Treatment of primary CNS lymphoma: the next step. *J Clin Oncol* **18**: 3144–3150.

Abrey L, Moskowitz CH, Mason WP *et al.* (2003). Intensive methotrexate and cytarabine followed by high-dose chemotherapy with autologous stem-cell rescue in patients with newly diagnosed primary CNS lymphoma: an intent-to-treat analysis. *J Clin Oncol* **21**: 4151–4156.

Batchelor T, Loeffler JS (2006). Primary CNS lymphoma. *J Clin Oncol* **24**: 1281–1288.

Behin A, Delattre J-Y (2003). Neurologic sequelae of radiotherapy on the nervous system. In Schiff D, Wen PY (eds.) *Cancer Neurology in Clinical Practice* (pp. 173–191). Totowa, NJ: Humana Press Inc.

Besell EM, Graus F, Lopez-Guillermo A *et al.* (2001). CHOD/BVAM regimen plus radiotherapy in patients with primary CNS non-Hodgkin's lymphoma. *Int J Radiat Oncol Biol Phys* **50**: 457–464.

Blay J-Y, Conroy T, Chevreau C *et al.* (1998). High-dose methotrexate for the treatment of primary cerebral lymphomas: analysis of survival and late neurologic toxicity in a retrospective series. *J Clin Oncol* **16**: 864–871.

Boiardi A, Silvani A, Valentini S *et al.* (1993). Chemotherapy as a first treatment for primary non-Hodgkin's lymphoma of the central nervous system: preliminary data. *J Neurol* **241**: 96–100.

Cher L, Glass J, Harsh GR *et al.* (1996). Therapy of primary CNS lymphoma with methotrexate-based chemotherapy and deferred chemotherapy: preliminary results. *Neurology* **46**: 1757–1759.

Constine LS, Konski A, Ekholm S *et al.* (1988). Adverse effects of brain irradiation correlated with MR and CT imaging. *Int J Radiat Oncol Biol Phys* **15**: 319–330.

Correa DD, Anderson ND, Glass A *et al.* (2003). Cognitive functions in primary central nervous system lymphoma patients treated with chemotherapy and stem cell transplantation: preliminary findings. *Clin Adv Hematol Oncol* **1**: 490.

Correa DD, DeAngelis LM, Shi W *et al.* (2004). Cognitive functions in survivors of primary central nervous system lymphoma. *Neurology* **62**: 548–555.

Corry J, Smith JG, Wirth A *et al.* (1998). Primary central nervous system lymphoma: age and performance status are more important than treatment modality. *Int J Radiat Oncol* **41**: 615–620.

Crossen JR, Goldman DL, Dahlborg SA *et al.* (1992). Neuropsychological asssessment outcomes of nonacquired immunodeficiency syndrome patients with primary central nervous system lymphoma before and after blood-brain barrier disruption chemotherapy. *Neurosurgery* **30**: 23–29.

Dahlborg SA, Henner WD, Crossen JR *et al.* (1996). Non-AIDS primary CNS lymphoma: first example of a durable response in a primary brain tumor using enhanced chemotherapy delivery without cognitive loss and without radiotherapy. *Cancer J Sci Am* **2**: 166–174.

Dahlborg SA, Petrillo A, Crossen JR *et al.* (1998). The potential for complete and durable response in nonglial primary brain tumors in children and young adults with enhanced chemotherapy delivery. *Cancer J Sci Am* **4**(2): 110–124.

DeAngelis LM (1995). Current management of primary central nervous system lymphoma. *Oncology* **9**: 63–71.

DeAngelis LM, Hormigo A (2004). Treatment of primary central nervous system lymphoma. *Semin Oncol* **31**: 684–692.

DeAngelis LM, Shapiro WR (1991). Drug/radiation interactions and central nervous system injury. In Gutin PH, Leibel SA, Sheline GE (eds.) *Radiation Injury to the Nervous System* (pp. 361–382). New York: Raven Press.

DeAngelis LM, Delattre J-Y, Posner JB (1989). Radiation-induced dementia in patients cured of brain metastases. *Neurology* **39**: 789–796.

DeAngelis LM, Yahalom J, Heinemann MH, Cirrincione C, Thaler HT, Krol G (1990). Primary CNS lymphoma: combined treatment with chemotherapy and radiotherapy. *Neurology* **40**(1): 80–86.

DeAngelis LM, Yahalom J, Thaler HT *et al.* (1992). Combined modality therapy for primary CNS lymphoma. *J Clin Oncol* **10**: 635–643.

Desmond DW (2002). Cognition and white matter lesions. *Cerebrovasc Dis* **13**: 53–57.

Doolittle ND, Miner ME, Siegal T *et al.* (2000). Safety and efficacy of a multicenter study using intraarterial chemotherapy in conjunction with osmotic opening of the blood-brain barrier for the treatment of patients with malignant brain tumors. *Cancer* **88**: 637–647.

Dropcho EJ (1991). Central nervous system injury by therapeutic irradiation. *Neurol Clin* **9**: 69–88.

Eby NL, Grufferman S, Flannelly CM *et al.* (1988). Increasing incidence of primary brain lymphoma in the U.S. *Cancer* **62**: 2461–2465.

Ferreri AJM, Reni M, Pasini F *et al.* (2002). A multicenter study of treatment of primary CNS lymphoma. *Neurology* **58**: 1513–1520.

Fliessbach K, Urbach H, Helmstaedter C *et al.* (2003). Cognitive performance and magnetic resonance imaging findings after high-dose systemic and intraventricular chemotherapy for primary central nervous system lymphoma. *Arch Neurol* **60**: 563–568.

Fliessbach K, Helmstaedter C, Urbach H *et al.* (2005). Neuropsychological outcome after chemotherapy for primary CNS lymphoma: a prospective study. *Neurology* **64**: 1184–1188.

Freilich RJ, Delattre J-Y, Monjour A, DeAngelis LM (1996). Chemotherapy without radiation therapy as initial treatment for primary CNS lymphoma in older patients. *Neurology* **46**: 435–439.

Glass J, Gruber ML, Cher L, Hochberg F (1994). Preirradiation methotrexate chemotherapy of primary central nervous system lymphoma: long-term outcome. *J Neurosurg* **81**: 88–195.

Grant JW, Isaacson PG (1992). Primary central nervous system lymphoma. *Brain Pathol* **2**: 97–109.

Guha-Thakurta N, Damek D, Pollack C *et al.* (1999). Intravenous methotrexate as initial treatment for primary central nervous system lymphoma: response to therapy and quality of life of patients. *J Neurooncol* **43**: 259–268.

Harder H, Holtel H, Bromberg JEC *et al.* (2004). Cognitive status and quality of life after treatment for primary CNS lymphoma. *Neurology* **62**: 544–547.

Herrlinger U, Schabet M, Clemens M *et al.* (1998). Clinical presentation and therapeutic outcome in 26 patients with primary CNS lymphoma. *Acta Neurol Scand* **97**: 257–264.

Herrlinger U, Schabet M, Brugger W *et al.* (2002). German Cancer Society Neuro-Oncology Working Group NOA-03 multicenter trial of single-agent high-dose methotrexate for primary central nervous system lymphoma. *Ann Neurol* **51**: 247–252.

Herrlinger U, Kuker W, Uhl M *et al.* (2005). NOA-03 trial of high-dose methotrexate in primary central nervous system lymphoma: final report. *Ann Neurol* **57**: 843–847.

Hoang-Xuan K, Taillandier L, Chinot O *et al.* (2003). Chemotherapy alone as initial treatment for CNS lymphoma in patients older than 60 years: a multicenter phase II study (26952) of the European Organization for Research and Treatment of Cancer Brain Control Group. *J Clin Oncol* **21**: 2726–2731.

Keime-Guibert F, Napolitano M, Delattre JY (1998). Neurological complications of radiotherapy and chemotherapy. *J Neurol* **245**: 695–708.

Kraemer DF, Fortin D, Neuwelt EA (2002). Chemotherapeutic dose intensification for treatment of malignant brain tumors: recent developments and future directions. *Curr Neurol Neurosci Rep* **2**: 216–224.

Laack NN, Brown PD (2004). Cognitive sequelae of brain radiation in adults. *Semin Oncol* **31**: 702–713.

Lai R, Abrey LE, Rosenblum MK, DeAngelis LD (2004). Treatment-induced leukoencephalopathy in primary CNS lymphoma. *Neurology* **62**: 451–456.

McAllister LD, Doolittle ND, Guastadisegni PE *et al.* (2000). Cognitive outcomes and long-term follow-up results after enhanced chemotherapy delivery for primary central nervous system lymphoma. *Neurosurgery,* **46**: 51–61.

Meyers CA, Wefel JS (2003). The use of the mini-mental state examination to assess cognitive functioning in cancer trials: no ifs, ands, buts, or sensitivity. *J Clin Oncol* **21**: 3557–3558.

Nelson DF (1999). Radiotherapy in the treatment of primary central nervous system lymphoma (PCNSL). *J Neurooncol* **43**: 241–247.

Neuwelt EA, Goldamn DA, Dahlborg SA *et al.* (1991). Primary CNS lymphoma treated with osmotic blood-brain barrier disruption: prolonged survival and preservation of cognitive function. *J Clin Oncol* **9**: 1580–1590.

Neuwelt EA, Guastadisegni PE, Varallyay P *et al.* (2005). Imaging changes and cognitive outcome in primary CNS lymphoma after enhanced chemotherapy delivery. *Am J Neuroradiol* **26**: 258–265.

O'Brien P, Roos D, Pratt G *et al.* (2000). Phase II multicenter study of a brief single agent methotrexate followed by irradiation in primary CNS lymphoma. *J Clin Oncol* **18**: 519–526.

O'Neill BP (2004). Neurocognitive outcomes in primary CNS lymphoma (PCNSL). *Neurology* **62**: 532–533.

O'Neill BP, Illig JJ (1989). Primary central nervous system lymphoma. *Mayo Clinic Proc* **64**: 1005–1020.

Pels H, Schlegel U (2006). Primary central nervous system lymphoma. *Curr Treat Options Neurol* **8**: 346–357.

Pels H, Deckert-Schulter M, Glasmacher A *et al.* (2000). Primary central nervous system lymphoma: a clinicopathological study of 28 cases. *Hematol Oncol* **18**: 21–32.

Pels H, Schmidt-Wolf IGH, Glasmacher A *et al.* (2003). Primary central nervous system lymphoma: results of a pilot study and phase II study of systemic and intraventricular chemotherapy with deferred radiotherapy. *J Clin Oncol* **21**: 4489–4495.

Peterson K, DeAngelis LM (1997). Primary cerebral lymphoma. In Vecht CJ (ed.) *Handbook of Clinical Neurology* (Vol. 24, pp. 257–268). Part II: Neuro-Oncology. Amsterdam: Elsevier Science.

Peterson K, Gordon KB, Heinemann M-H *et al.* (1993). The clinical spectrum of ocular lymphoma. *Cancer* **72**: 843–849.

Poortmans PMP, Kluin-Nelemans HC, Haaxma-Reiche H *et al.* (2003). High-dose methotrexate-based chemotherapy followed by consolidating radiotherapy in non-AIDS-related primary central nervous system lymphoma: European Organization for Research and Treatment of Cancer Lymphoma Group phase II Trial 20962. *J Clin Oncol* **21**: 4483–4488.

Roman-Goldstein SM, Mitchell P, Crossen JR *et al.* (1995). MR and cognitive testing of patients undergoing osmotic blood-brain barrier disruption with intraarterial chemotherapy. *Am J Neuroradiol* **16**: 543–553.

Sandor V, Stark-Vancs V, Pearson D *et al.* (1998). Phase II trial of chemotherapy alone for primary CNS and intraocular lymphoma. *J Clin Oncol* **16**: 3000–3006.

Sarazin M, Ameri A, Monjour A *et al.* (1995). Primary central nervous system lymphoma: treatment with chemotherapy and radiotherapy. *Eur J Cancer* **31A**: 2003–2007.

Schlegel U, Pels H, Glasmacher A *et al.* (2001). Combined systemic and intraventricular chemotherapy in primary CNS lymphoma: a pilot study. *J Neurol Neurosurg Psychiatry* **71**: 118–122.

Sheline G (1980). Irradiation injury of the human brain: a review of clinical experience. In Gilbert HA, Kagan AR (eds.) *Radiation Damage to the Nervous System* (pp. 39–68). New York: Raven Press.

Sheline G, Wara WM, Smith V (1980). Therapeutic irradiation and brain injury. *Int J Radiat Oncol Biol Physics* **6**:
1215–1228.

Tofilon PJ, Fike JR (2000). The radioresponse of the central
nervous system: a dynamic process. *Radiat Res* **153**: 357–
370.

Tullberg M, Fletcher E, DeCarli C *et al.* (2004). White matter lesions impair frontal lobe function regardless of their
location. *Neurology* **63**: 246–253.

Van Der Maazen RW, Kleiboer BJ, Verhagen I *et al.* (1993).
Repair capacity of adult rat glial progenitor cells determined by an in vitro clonogenic assay after in vitro or
in vivo fractionated irradiation. *Int J Radiat Biol* **63**: 661–
666.

Weitzner MA, Meyers CA (1997). Cognitive functioning and quality of life in malignant glioma patients:
a review of the literature. *Psychooncology* **6**: 169–
177.

14

Childhood brain tumors

H. Stacy Nicholson, Louise Penkman Fennell, and Robert W. Butler

In long-term survivors of childhood and adolescent central nervous system (CNS) tumors, neuropsychological and psychosocial late effects of therapy occur in a milieu of numerous medical late complications (Anderson *et al.*, 2001). With improvements in treatment and survival rates for these patients since the 1980s, most children and adolescents with CNS tumors currently diagnosed will become long-term survivors (Pollack, 1994). This is particularly true for children with medulloblastoma or low-grade astrocytoma. Therefore, concerns about late complications of therapy are increasingly important to survivors and their families. In addition to the late consequences of radiation therapy and chemotherapy, which are similar for all survivors of childhood cancer, the singular susceptibility of the brain and spinal cord to injury causes several late consequences unique to long-term survivors of CNS tumors.

Late complications may be due to the tumor, surgery, radiation therapy, chemotherapy, or the psychological trauma of dealing with a malignancy, and the late effects following CNS tumors include medical, psychological, neuropsychological, and psychosocial problems. Some late effects may be life threatening. In fact, long-term survivors of CNS tumors have an excess risk of mortality relative to survivors of other cancers (Mostow *et al.*, 1991; Nicholson *et al.*, 1994). In a large cohort study of childhood cancer survivors (Oeffinger *et al.*, 2006),

CNS tumor survivors were among the most likely to have chronic health conditions and multiple other chronic conditions; in addition, they often have functional impairments (Ness *et al.*, 2005). Long-term medical surveillance of survivors is critically important so that late effects of therapy may be detected while still possibly amenable to intervention (Oeffinger *et al.*, 2004).

Medical late effects

Although 5-year disease-free survival is the outcome measure most often used in clinical trials, it may not correlate with a normal life expectancy. In one large cohort study of adult survivors of childhood cancer (Nicholson *et al.*, 1994), survivors of CNS tumors were much more likely to die during adulthood than were survivors of all other childhood and adolescent malignancies, except for those with Hodgkin's disease. In this study CNS tumor survivors had a 9.2-fold excess risk of death from causes other than their primary cancer diagnosis during their thirties. Non-tumor causes of death included trauma, pneumonia and other respiratory diseases, cerebrovascular disease, and aspiration of emesis. In a more recently treated cohort, CNS tumor survivors had an almost 16-fold increase in mortality, and survivors were still experiencing an excess risk of mortality

25 years after diagnosis (Mertens *et al.*, 2001). These mortality data underscore the serious nature of late complications in this population.

Secondary malignancies

Secondary malignancies are increasingly problematic for cancer survivors (Goldstein *et al.*, 1997; Peterson *et al.*, 2005; Stavrou *et al.*, 2001; Travis *et al.*, 2006). In CNS tumor survivors, the most frequent secondary malignancy is another brain tumor (Neglia *et al.*, 2006). These are typically associated with radiotherapy, and the most common radiation-induced tumors are high-grade gliomas and meningiomas. In addition, radiation may also invoke thyroid cancer (Ronckers *et al.*, 2006). Also, as chemotherapy has been increasingly used, secondary leukemia has occurred (Packer *et al.*, 1994).

Estimates of the risk of a subsequent cancer after CNS tumors are best based on epidemiologic studies. In a population-based study of 1262 histologically confirmed cases of medulloblastoma in the United States and Sweden (Goldstein *et al.*, 1997), 20 secondary malignancies occurred. This corresponded to a 5.4-fold excess of secondary neoplasms (95% confidence interval, CI: 3.3–8.4) relative to the number expected based on population data, and the median latency between the medulloblastoma and the secondary malignancy was 73 months (range 8 months to 36 years). These second malignancies included cancers of the salivary glands, uterine cervix, CNS, thyroid gland, and acute lymphoblastic leukemia (ALL); 46% of secondary malignancies occurred in or near the radiation field. In another study, secondary carcinomas were less problematic for survivors of CNS tumors when compared to other childhood cancer survivors (Bassal *et al.*, 2006). The cumulative risk of secondary malignancies will likely increase with time as survivor cohorts age. Latency periods of more than six decades for radiation-induced CNS tumors have been reported (Kleinschmidt-DeMasters & Lillehei, 1995).

Similarly, follow-up beyond the usual 5-year disease-free survival outcome for clinical trials will be important because severe late effects, such as secondary cancers, may impact future treatment decisions. In a study with excellent treatment outcomes for 63 children with medulloblastoma treated with chemotherapy [lomustine (CCNU), cisplatin, and vincristine] and craniospinal radiotherapy, three patients developed secondary malignancies [two CNS tumors and one acute myelogenous leukemia (AML)] (Packer *et al.*, 1994). The risk of a secondary malignancy may also be due to factors other than the anticancer therapy, such as an underlying genetic predisposition to malignancy (Goldstein *et al.*, 1994). For such patients, the risk of a secondary cancer will likely be greater than it is for other children with the same primary cancer. Although most children with brain tumors do not have a known genetic predisposition to cancer, there are rare genetic syndromes associated with pediatric brain tumors (Goldstein *et al.*, 1994; Hamilton *et al.*, 1995). These include Gorlin syndrome, in which children tend to be diagnosed with medulloblastoma at a particularly young age. These children are particularly susceptible to basal cell carcinomas in the radiation fields. Turcot syndrome includes brain tumors and multiple colonic polyps (Hamilton *et al.*, 1995). A family history can be particularly helpful in ascertaining which patients are at increased risk of secondary malignancies. The family history should be updated at each annual follow-up visit for long-term survivors.

Cardiac complications

Although anthracycline-induced cardiomyopathy is of concern for most childhood cancer survivors (Lipshultz *et al.*, 1991), these agents are not routinely used to treat brain tumors. Therefore, this serious toxicity usually does not occur in survivors of CNS tumors. However, other chemotherapeutic agents, such as cyclophosphamide, have also been associated with cardiac dysfunction. Radiation is also known to damage the heart and lead to premature atherosclerosis. This is particularly true for long-term survivors of Hodgkin's disease treated with high doses of radiation (Donaldson & Kaplan, 1982). Children with brain tumors who received spinal irradiation have had some cardiac abnormalities documented, presumably due to the exit beam. In one study that included 26 patients who had received spinal radiotherapy, cardiac evaluations included electrocardiography, 24-h ambulatory electrocardiography, echocardiography, and exercise testing. Of the 16 patients who were exercise-tested, 75% achieved a maximal cardiac index below the fifth percentile. In addition, 31% had pathologic Q waves, and there was an excess of elevated posterior wall stress (Jakacki *et al.*, 1993). Although the long-term significance of these findings is not yet known, this study points out that cardiac function needs to be followed in survivors who received spinal radiotherapy. In the Childhood Cancer Survival Study (CCSS) cohort, 18% of survivors reported a cardiovascular complication, including stroke (relative risk, RR = 42.8), blood clots (RR = 5.7) and angina (RR = 2) (Gurney *et al.*, 2003a). These findings have been confirmed by others (Bowers *et al.*, 2002). Whether CNS tumor survivors have an increased risk of obesity is debated (Gurney *et al.*, 2003b; Heikens *et al.*, 2000), but those who are overweight would be at increased risk of cardiovascular disease.

Pulmonary complications

Few data exist regarding late pulmonary complications in long-term survivors of pediatric CNS tumors. However, many patients, including those with astrocytoma and medulloblastoma, are exposed to the nitrosoureas, which are known to be associated with pulmonary fibrosis. The risk apparently does not decline with time, and fatal pulmonary fibrosis has been described as long as 17 years after exposure (O'Driscoll *et al.*, 1990). In addition to the nitrosoureas, other chemotherapeutic agents are known to have pulmonary fibrosis as a potential complication, including cyclophosphamide. The risk from agents other than the nitrosoureas is not likely to be high.

Pulmonary fibrosis may also be associated with spinal radiotherapy. In a study of 28 survivors of childhood brain tumors, half had significant pulmonary fibrosis. Although the sample sizes are small, 1 of 7 patients (14%) who received CCNU without spinal radiotherapy, compared with 13 of 21 of those (62%) who received spinal radiotherapy (with or without lomustine), developed pulmonary fibrosis (Jakacki *et al.*, 1995). This included 4 of 8 who did not receive CCNU. In this study, pulmonary fibrosis was most associated with a history of spinal irradiation and not with CCNU exposure. Thus, survivors who received spinal radiotherapy for their CNS tumor have a risk of late pulmonary complications. In a large study not limited to CNS tumor survivors (Mertens *et al.*, 2002), those who had received chest radiotherapy had a 3.5% 20-year cumulative incidence of pulmonary fibrosis. More precise estimates of risk in CNS tumor survivors are needed.

Endocrine complications

Hormonal deficiencies are among the most common late effects of therapy in long-term survivors of childhood brain tumors (Oberfield *et al.*, 1996; Sklar, 1995, 1997; Sklar & Constine, 1995), with 43% of survivors reporting at least one endocrine abnormality in the CCSS cohort (Gurney *et al.*, 2003a). Endocrine late effects can result from the tumor itself, surgery, or radiotherapy. Tumors of the pituitary or hypothalamic region often present with pituitary dysfunction. Furthermore, the surgical treatment of tumors in this region also poses a risk of pituitary damage. In these patients, either the tumor itself or surgery may result in panhypopituitarism. However, by far the most common cause of late endocrinologic sequelae is radiotherapy (Sklar & Constine, 1995). Focal radiotherapy that includes the pituitary gland, whole-brain radiotherapy, and/or craniospinal radiotherapy all involve the pituitary and carry a risk of hormonal deficiencies. The deficiencies, which are dose-dependent, most commonly include growth hormone deficiency. In addition, low-dose cranial irradiation (18 Gy) may be associated with the premature onset of puberty, and higher doses of irradiation (more than 40 Gy) may lead to deficiencies of gonadotropins and thyroid-hormone-releasing hormone, as well as hyperprolactinemia (Oberfield *et al.*, 1996). Furthermore, the risk of developing hormonal complications of irradiation does not appear to decrease with time. Thus, careful follow-up of growth, pubertal development, and thyroid function is critical because hormonal deficiencies are universally treatable.

Thyroid function should be followed for life in all children who received irradiation to the thyroid gland, regardless of whether or not the brain was irradiated, and regardless of the radiotherapy dose to the pituitary gland (Sklar & Constine, 1995). As with other hormonal deficiencies, the risk of hypothyroidism does not appear to decrease over time (Hancock *et al.*, 1991). In addition, radiation therapy may be associated with both benign and malignant thyroid nodules. Thus, as part of the annual checkup, these patients should have careful thyroid palpation.

In general, hormonal deficiencies can be treated with replacement therapy (Hancock *et al.*, 1991; Oberfield *et al.*, 1996; Sklar, 1995, 1997; Sklar & Constine, 1995; Vassilopoulou *et al.*, 1995). In fact, children with growth hormone deficiency due to radiotherapy respond to replacement therapy as well as do children with idiopathic growth hormone deficiency (Vassilopoulou *et al.*, 1995), although those survivors who have received spinal radiotherapy will not respond as well as those who have not (Brownstein *et al.*, 2004). The use of growth hormone appears not to be associated with an increased risk of relapse, although there may be a slight increase in risk of secondary malignancies (Ergun-Longmire *et al.*, 2006). Consultation with an endocrinologist is important if endocrine deficits are known or suspected.

Disorders of hearing and sight

Depending on tumor location, either hearing or sight can be affected. In addition, chemotherapy with cisplatin can also cause sensorineural hearing loss in virtually all patients (Skinner *et al.*, 1990). This hearing loss is irreversible and is likely to be exacerbated by radiation therapy to the inner ear.

However, severe cisplatin ototoxicity in the speech frequencies can often be prevented with careful monitoring and dose adjustment during therapy. In the CCSS, a retrospective cohort study comparing survivors to a control group of siblings without a history of cancer, childhood brain tumor survivors had an elevated risk of hearing impairment (RR = 17.3), legal blindness in at least one eye (RR = 14.8), cataracts (RR = 11.9), and double vision (RR = 8.8) (Packer *et al.*, 2003).

As part of routine follow-up, all children who received cisplatin should have their hearing tested because hearing loss can occur or worsen even when audition was previously documented to be sufficient; furthermore, many survivors can benefit from amplification. Also, as hearing impairment may affect school performance, the results of the hearing evaluation should be shared with the neuropsychologist so that neurocognitive results can be effectively integrated with educational recommendations.

Renal complications

Some chemotherapeutic agents used in the treatment of CNS tumors are nephrotoxic, such as cisplatin and ifosfamide (Daugaard & Abildgaard, 1991). Cisplatin can both decrease the glomerular filtration rate (GFR) and cause electrolyte abnormalities. Also, wasting of magnesium and potassium are common in children who have received cisplatin, and some of these survivors may require long-term supplementation. Similarly, patients who receive ifosfamide may develop renal Fanconi syndrome, including renal tubular acidosis, phosphaturia, and glucosuria. The development of electrolyte abnormalities long after chemotherapy has ended is not expected, and whether the GFR decreases with time is not well understood.

Gastrointestinal and hepatic complications

There is generally little risk of late gastrointestinal sequelae in long-term survivors of brain tumors. As noted above, rarely patients may have their brain tumor as the initial manifestation of Turcot syndrome (Hamilton *et al.*, 1995); therefore, any patient with obstructive symptoms or bloody stool should be considered to be at risk for colonic polyps. As with other cancer survivors who received blood products, there is a small risk of blood-borne infections, including hepatitis. Patients transfused prior to 1992, when routine screening for hepatitis C was implemented, should be screened for hepatitis C (Luban, 1998).

Neurological complications

Children with brain tumors have malignancies and therapy that both directly affect the brain, and neurological sequelae are common. These include seizures, paralysis, radiation necrosis, and migraine-like symptoms (Martins *et al.*, 1977; Shuper *et al.*, 1995). Some of the neurological complications may be severe and life-threatening (Mostow *et al.*, 1991; Nicholson *et al.*, 1994).

Although the tumor and surgery can also cause neurological damage, most late neurological complications can be traced to radiation therapy (Kramer & Lee, 1974). Whether injuries result from direct radiation damage to neurons and/or glial cells, or to the vasculature, or to a combination of both is not well understood. Radiation necrosis can be a particular problem for the survivor of CNS tumors requiring steroids or surgery (Martins *et al.*, 1977). These lesions often mimic a tumor, and whether a new mass in the radiation bed represents recurrent tumor or radiation necrosis can be difficult to ascertain by CT or MRI. This complication usually occurs between 9 months and 2 years after radiation, and symptoms vary, depending on the location in the brain. Radiation necrosis can cause headache, behavioral changes, seizures, lethargy, hemiparesis, ataxia, and/or increased intracranial pressure.

In addition, vascular changes may occur following radiation and in the most severe cases may lead to a stroke (Reinhold *et al.*, 1990). Moyamoya disease, in which the small blood vessels have the abnormal appearance of a "puff of smoke," can also occur in this setting. In the CCSS cohort, the risk of stroke in survivors was 39 times greater than that in sibling controls (Bowers *et al.*, 2006), with a rate of nearly 268 events per 100 000 person-years. The risk increased with increasing doses of radiotherapy.

Neurological complications in survivors are quite common. In the CCSS cohort, 49% of survivors reported co-ordination problems, 26% had motor problems, and 25% had seizures (Packer *et al.*, 2003). Finally, in a large retrospective cohort study, survivors of brain tumors were at increased risk of being hospitalized for psychiatric problems (Ross *et al.*, 2003).

Neuropsychological late effects

The neuropsychological and psychosocial sequelae of childhood brain tumors and their treatment remain one of the most significant challenges to managing late effects. Disease-free survival in this population is increasing (Ries *et al.*, 2005). Unfortunately, the incidence of childhood brain tumors also appears to be increasing. Treatment for childhood leukemias has evolved to a point where craniospinal irradiation is largely avoided as a CNS prophylactic treatment. This has, correspondingly, resulted in fewer neuropsychological late effects in this population (Mulhern & Butler, 2004). However, treatment for the more common childhood brain tumors involves relatively high doses of whole and focal brain irradiation. Correspondingly, neuropsychological and psychosocial late effects continue to be prominent, and the nature of the deficits is reasonably well understood at this time. Current research efforts are increasingly being directed towards the development and testing of interventions designed to lessen cognitive and social impairment (Penkman, 2004).

Neurocognitive late effects

Earlier studies were summarized in a review paper authored by Nicholson and Butler (2001). It is important to keep in mind that cranial irradiation is not the only CNS insult associated with brain tumors as identified above. In terms of irradiation (RT), a pattern of deficits that includes attentional dysfunction (particularly under conditions of vigilance), non-dominant hemisphere deficits (such as visual-motor integration difficulties), declines in performance intelligence, and spatial awareness impairments frequently result in the presentation of a non-verbal learning disability (Butler *et al.*, 1994; Packer *et al.*, 1989; Radcliffe *et al.*, 1992; Ris & Noll, 1994). Other related insults such as resection and chemotherapy are poorly understood.

The majority of childhood brain tumors, as noted previously, are posterior fossa in nature. Nevertheless, supratentorial tumors that are located in the cortex do occur. Correspondingly, cognitive impairment and declines are associated with tumor location. Thus, memory impairment, language deficits, and motor dysfunction can also be present.

More current literature has further advanced our understanding of tumor- and treatment-related neurocognitive late effects in the pediatric malignancy population. There is considerable research evidencing the significant cognitive declines and subsequent academic failures experienced by children who are treated with RT (Mulhern *et al.*, 2001; Ris *et al.*, 2001). In fact, radiation injury to the brain is regarded as one of the most serious complications of this treatment, and is considered the major limitation in delivering high-dose radiation (Strother *et al.*, 2002). Radiation-induced brain injury includes edema formation, damage to glial cells that inhibits the development of myelin, and vascular damage leading to white matter necrosis. Magnetic resonance imaging studies have shown less white matter in children treated with RT as compared to children treated with surgery alone (Mulhern *et al.*, 1999) or healthy controls (Reddick *et al.*, 2005). Radiation-induced injury is believed to be a progressive process, as opposed to a static injury, as evidenced by the observation that most children do not manifest measurable deficits until 1–3 years after RT has been completed, and because their measured deficit appears to increase over time (Hoppe-Hirsch *et al.*, 1995; Mulhern & Butler, 2004, 2005).

Age is a significant risk factor for neuropsychological dysfunction following treatment with RT. Mulhern and colleagues (Mulhern *et al.*, 2001) examined the role of age and white matter loss in young children treated for medulloblastoma. Children receiving RT for treatment of medulloblastoma prior to 4 years of age were at the greatest risk for neuronal and glial cell damage. In another study by this group (Reddick *et al.*, 2005), age at time of RT and the eventual non-development of normal appearing white matter (NAWM) were shown to be significantly related. They suggest that the process of myelination is halted at an earlier stage for young children, and likely results in more severe intellectual impairment.

As the research base examining the neurocognitive outcomes of treatment for brain tumors accumulates, an evolution in focus of study has occurred. Initially, researchers primarily investigated global intellectual functioning (IQ scores) as the sum measure of neuropsychological outcome (Ellenberg *et al.*, 1987; Jannoun & Bloom, 1990; Mulhern *et al.*, 1992). This was followed by a more detailed and comprehensive approach with tests assessing many areas of specific cognitive function (see Ris & Noll, 1994, for a comprehensive review of the earlier literature). As knowledge amasses, studies are now beginning to implement theory-driven approaches examining processes that would be expected to be compromised, given the underlying neuropathology of radiation-induced injury.

It is now well accepted that global IQ is significantly impacted by RT in children with brain tumors. The estimates vary, but 22-point (Walter *et al.*, 1999) and 17.4-point drops in full-scale IQ have been reported in the literature (Ris *et al.*, 2001). Ris and colleagues (2001) estimated the rate of change per year to be a reduction of 4 IQ points within verbal, performance, and full-scale IQ domains in a group of 43 children with average-risk tumors of the posterior fossa treated with reduced-dose RT and adjuvant chemotherapy. More recently, Reimers and colleagues (Reimers *et al.*, 2003) reported a mean full-scale IQ score nearly 1 SD below the population mean of 100 in a large group of pediatric brain tumor survivors. This decrement in IQ scores has been shown to be due to a decline in rate of learning rather than a loss of previously acquired skills (Palmer *et al.*, 2001). The decline in IQ has also been demonstrated to correlate with degree of white matter loss (Mulhern *et al.*, 2001; Reddick *et al.*, 2003).

Studies using neuropsychological test batteries have identified deficits in a number of areas beyond global IQ. Impairment has been identified in visuomotor and visual perceptual skills, attention, memory, language, and executive functions (Anderson *et al.*, 2001; Bordeaux *et al.*, 1988; Butler *et al.*, 1994; Copeland *et al.*, 1999; Ris *et al.*, 2001; Riva *et al.*, 1989). These children also seem to struggle with math at school more than they do with the acquisition and maintenance of reading abilities (Buono *et al.*, 1998; Butler *et al.*, 1994; Fletcher & Copeland, 1988; Jankovic *et al.*, 1994). As described above, some have likened the deficits observed in this group of children to a non-verbal learning disability (NVLD) because they evidence a high rate of difficulties with visual-spatial problem solving and arithmetic (Anderson *et al.*, 2000; Buono *et al.*, 1998). This implicates greater dysfunction of the non-dominant hemisphere.

It is now evident that brain tumor survivors treated with RT evidence deficits in core neuropsychological processes such as attention, processing speed, and working memory skills that result in the secondarily observed deficits in knowledge acquisition and ultimately academic performance. Attention, memory, and processing speed have been implicated as areas of deficit that emerge several years following RT for treatment of a brain tumor (Mulhern *et al.*, 1998). Processes such as attention and speed of processing are thought to rely on distributed neural networks that are dependent on white matter tracts for efficient processing. Therefore, it follows that deficits in these areas would be observed. Reeves and colleagues (Reeves *et al.*, 2006) reported impaired sustained attention in the context of no impairment in verbal memory in a group of survivors of medulloblastoma. Mulhern and colleagues (Mulhern *et al.*, 2004) assessed

sustained attention abilities of survivors of malignant brain tumors treated with RT using the Conners' Continuous Performance Test. Their group demonstrated poor performance and reduced white matter volume in the prefrontal cortex and cingulate gyrus, areas typically activated during attention tasks. A model has been proposed whereby intellectual and academic deficits could be explained by core deficits in attention and memory. It was reported that the primary consequence of reduced NAWM in a group of pediatric patients treated for brain tumors with RT was decreased attentional abilities, and that this deficit led to reduced IQ and academic achievement (Reddick *et al.*, 2003). Others have examined attention, working memory, and processing speed in a group of children treated for malignant brain tumors with RT and chemotherapy, a group of children treated with surgery alone, and a group of children treated for a non-CNS cancer as a control group (Mabbott *et al.*, 2005). Although there were trends for the RT group to evidence lower scores in all areas, only processing speed resulted in a statistically significant difference, with the children receiving RT evidencing the poorest performance. Hierarchical regression analysis revealed that processing speed accounted for unique variance in intellectual functioning.

Very recent published research from Dr. Mulhern's group and others is further elucidating the relationship between memory, attention, and new learning following treatment for medulloblastoma, the most common brain tumor in children. It is becoming increasingly apparent that damage to normal white matter following irradiation, and possibly chemotherapy treatments are primarily responsible for neurocognitive deficits in children. These individuals clearly suffer deficits in sustained attention, reaction time, and processing speed (Reeves *et al.*, 2006). The neuropsychological pattern of attentional difficulties with reduced processing speed and slowed reaction time is undoubtedly due to white matter damage (Filley, 2001). Sustained attention and processing speed, in addition to reaction time difficulties, are clearly present in the majority of children who receive treatment for the most common pediatric brain tumors. These neurocognitive deficits are being recognized as having a clear impact on intellectual and adaptive functioning (Beebe *et al.*, 2005; Palmer *et al.*, 2003).

Taken together, this growing literature suggests that intellectual functioning is impacted in children treated for malignant brain tumors with RT. Mounting evidence is implicating impairment in several core cognitive processes as underlying the decline in functioning. This appears to be primarily related to disruption in the normal development of white matter by RT. We do not, however, have evidence regarding the relative impact of resection and chemotherapy independent of RT at this time. Next, we will summarize some of the significant psychosocial deficits that are suffered by pediatric brain tumor survivors.

Psychosocial late effects

Preliminary evidence provided clues that pediatric brain tumor survivors were at extremely high risk for difficulties in psychosocial adjustment (Mostow *et al.*, 1991; Mulhern *et al.*, 1989). A very frequently cited study (Hoppe-Hirsch *et al.*, 1990) indicated that nearly one-half of pediatric brain tumor survivors, specifically those who had been treated for medulloblastoma, displayed significant deficits in social competence, adjustment, and also continued to have behavioral and adaptive deficits as they transitioned into adulthood. Unfortunately, few studies have attempted to replicate these findings, and many childhood brain tumor survivors are lost to follow-up as they become adults. Little is known about vocational status, which is particularly relevant given that many of these individuals are not able to enter college/university. The first and third authors of this chapter have begun a research project that is specifically designed to assess vocational readiness in adolescents and young adult survivors of brain tumors, due to this gap in our knowledge.

The importance of familial integrity is becoming increasingly relevant for survivors of brain tumors. Eiser (2004) has emphasized the need to view the

child/adolescent patient from a systems perspective. The system extends inside and outside of the household. As Eiser comments, "not only are parents unprepared and disappointed, but also confronted by lack of sympathy. Teachers who understandably know little about the disease and treatment may be at a loss as to why the child makes so little progress. They also have to deal with many other children with learning or behavioral difficulties and may pay more attention to those showing disruptive tendencies rather than worry about the child treated for cancer." In support of Dr. Eiser's impressions, there is an excellent study that identified predictors of child behavior problems and adaptive functioning in the pediatric brain tumor population (Carlson-Green *et al.*, 1995). This study demonstrated that not only illness-related issues, but also family variables were predictive of eventual intellectual functioning. More specifically, family stress, the ability of the mother to cope with the stress, the number of parents in the home, and socio-economic status were all related to psychosocial adjustment in the child/adolescent survivor.

A recent review of behavioral, social, and psychological adjustment in childhood brain tumor survivors has identified a total of 31 published manuscripts that addressed social, emotional, and behavioral functioning in children who had been diagnosed and treated for a CNS tumor (Fuemmeler *et al.*, 2002). A rather wide discrepancy between significant adjustment difficulties was noted across the various studies. More specifically, the authors reported a range of 25%–93% significant distress among participants. While the authors described difficulties in summary interpretations, there did appear to be an increased risk for internalizing problems as opposed to externalizing problems in brain tumor survivors. Internalizing psychopathology is typically characterized by disorders in the depression and anxiety groupings. Externalizing problems refer to behavior control and conduct disturbances. Overall, it was concluded that children treated for a brain tumor are at increased risk for socialization difficulties, and problems with peer relationships. This appears to be present both on parent- and teacher-rated measures. The overall impression is that these competence deficits are associated with degree of CNS impairment. It was further concluded that survivors continue to exhibit deficits in adjustment following the transition to adulthood. Employment, marriage, parenthood, and post-secondary academic placements all are areas in which the survivors lag behind their peers. Diagnosis and treatment prior to the age of 3–5 years increases the risk for eventual significant late effects.

The review further identified a number of directions for future research. More specifically, they recommend three areas that are in need of increased attention: first, assessment of more specific neurological deficits as they relate to psychosocial issues; second, greater attention to the environmental demands that children treated for a CNS malignancy experience; and, third, increased attention to parental and family adjustment. In support of this latter point, there is an emerging literature within childhood traumatic brain injury that is clearly implicating family adjustment as an important moderator of improvement and recovery from injury in the child/adolescent (Yeates *et al.*, 2004). These findings are likely to be extremely relevant to all childhood brain injury populations, including the CNS cancer patients.

Interventions

We would like to emphasize the need for treatment and rehabilitation efforts with this population. As identified in this chapter, these survivors are at an extremely high risk for neurocognitive and psychosocial difficulties. Researchers must begin to devote more attention to treatment in addition to assessment. Butler and Mulhern (2005) have summarized intervention efforts directed towards childhood cancer survivors, and most participants in the reviewed studies were brain tumor survivors. Therapeutic efforts have generally been directed towards traditional cognitive remediation methods, psychoactive medications (mainly the stimulant drugs), or a holistic approach as described by Butler

and Copeland (2002). There is an increasing interest in hybrid approaches that will, for example, combine stimulant medication with holistic cognitive rehabilitation. Given that family issues are becoming increasingly apparent, direct treatment towards the parents and siblings is also gaining interest.

Progress in the area of brain injury rehabilitation, both with children/adolescents and adults, is traditionally slow and laborious. Nevertheless, this is an exciting field, and the authors are very pleased to be describing increased efforts towards treatment of late effect disabilities, as opposed to continued description of severity of impairment, and patterns of impairment. In sum, while treatment progress regarding neurocognitive and psychosocial late effects remains in its infancy, a greater number of researchers are directing their attention towards rehabilitation. This is a much needed trend because it will further serve a growing group of courageous survivors, parents, and siblings.

Summary

Survivors of childhood and adolescent CNS tumors have an increased risk of multiple medical consequences and neuropsychological problems compared to other cancer survivors. These issues have serious consequences for survivors' quality of life and contributions to society. Although many problems have multifactorial causes, radiotherapy underlies many of the most severe late effects, including the cognitive issues that these survivors face. Future treatment strategies that decrease the use of radiotherapy would benefit this survivor population. In addition, lifelong annual medical follow-up for all, and periodic neuropsychological evaluation and rehabilitative treatment for those experiencing educational or vocational difficulties are important. To facilitate such follow-up, the Children's Oncology Group has developed evidence-based screening guidelines that advise clinicians on screening tests to include in the medical evaluation, based on therapy received (Landier *et al.*, 2004); these guidelines can be downloaded from www.survivorshipguidelines.org.

REFERENCES

Anderson DM, Rennie KM, Ziegler RS *et al.* (2001). Medical and neurocognitive late effects among survivors of childhood central nervous system tumors. *Cancer* **92(10)**: 2709–2719.

Anderson VA, Godber T, Smibert E *et al.* (2000). Cognitive and academic outcome following cranial irradiation and chemotherapy in children: a longitudinal study. *Br J Cancer* **82(2)**: 255–262.

Bassal M, Mertens AC, Taylor L *et al.* (2006). Risk of selected subsequent carcinomas in survivors of childhood cancer: a report from the Childhood Cancer Survivor Study. *J Clin Oncol* **24(3)**: 476–483.

Beebe DW, Ris MD, Armstrong FD *et al.* (2005). Cognitive and adaptive outcome in low-grade pediatric cerebellar astrocytomas: evidence of diminished cognitive and adaptive functioning in National Collaborative Research Studies (CCG 9891/POG 9130). *J Clin Oncol* **23(22)**: 5198–5204.

Bordeaux JD, Dowell RE Jr., Copeland DR *et al.* (1988). A prospective study of neuropsychological sequelae in children with brain tumors. *J Child Neurol* **3(1)**: 63–68.

Bowers DC, Mulne AF, Reisch JS *et al.* (2002). Nonperioperative strokes in children with central nervous system tumors. *Cancer* **94**: 1094–1101.

Bowers DC, Liu Y, Leisenring W *et al.* (2006). Late-occurring stroke among long-term survivors of childhood leukemia and brain tumors: a report from the Childhood Cancer Survivor Study. *J Clin Oncol* **24(33)**: 5277–5282.

Brownstein CM, Mertens AC, Mitby PA *et al.* (2004). Factors that affect final height and change in height standard deviation scores in survivors of childhood cancer treated with growth hormone: a report from the childhood cancer survivor study. *J Clin Endocrinol Metab* **89(9)**: 4422–4427.

Buono L, Morris M, Morris R *et al.* (1998). Evidence for the syndrome of nonverbal learning disabilities in children with brain tumors. *Child Neuropsychol* **4(2)**: 144–157.

Butler RW, Copeland DR (2002). Attentional processes and their remediation in children treated for cancer: a literature review and the development of a therapeutic approach. *J Int Neuropsychol Soc* **8(1)**: 115–124.

Butler RW, Mulhern RK (2005). Neurocognitive interventions for children and adolescents surviving cancer. *J Pediatr Psychol* **30(1)**: 65–78.

Butler RW, Hill JM, Steinherz PG *et al.* (1994). Neuropsychologic effects of cranial irradiation, intrathecal methotrexate, and systemic methotrexate in childhood cancer. *J Clin Oncol* **12(12)**: 2621–2629.

Carlson-Green B, Morris RD, Krawiecki N (1995). Family and illness predictors of outcome in pediatric brain tumors. *J Pediatr Psychol* **20(6)**: 769–784.

Copeland DR, deMoor C, Moore BD 3rd *et al.* (1999). Neurocognitive development of children after a cerebellar tumor in infancy: a longitudinal study. *J Clin Oncol* **17(11)**: 3476–3486.

Daugaard G, Abildgaard U (1991). *Renal Morbidity of Chemotherapy*. Oxford: Butterworth-Heinemann.

Donaldson SS, Kaplan HS (1982). Complications of treatment of Hodgkin's disease in children. *Cancer Treat Rep* **66(4)**: 977–989.

Eiser C (2004). Neurocognitive sequelae of childhood cancers and their treatment: a comment on Mulhern and Butler. *Pediatr Rehabil* **7(1)**: 15–16.

Ellenberg L, McComb JG, Siegel SE *et al.* (1987). Factors affecting intellectual outcome in pediatric brain tumor patients. *Neurosurgery* **21(5)**: 638–644.

Ergun-Longmire B, Mertens AC, Mitby P *et al.* (2006). Growth hormone treatment and risk of second neoplasms in the childhood cancer survivor. *J Clin Endocrinol Metab* **91(9)**: 3494–3498.

Filley CM (2001). *The Behavioral Neurology of White Matter*. New York: Oxford University Press.

Fletcher JM, Copeland DR (1988). Neurobehavioral effects of central nervous system prophylactic treatment of cancer in children. *J Clin Exp Neuropsychol* **10(4)**: 495–537.

Fuemmeler BF, Elkin TD, Mullins LL (2002). Survivors of childhood brain tumors: behavioral, emotional, and social adjustment. *Clin Psychol Rev* **22(4)**: 547–585.

Goldstein AM, Pastakia B, DiGiovanna JJ *et al.* (1994). Clinical findings in two African-American families with the nevoid basal cell carcinoma syndrome (NBCC). *Am J Med Genet* **50(3)**: 272–281.

Goldstein AM, Yuen J, Tucker MA (1997). Second cancers after medulloblastoma: population-based results from the United States and Sweden. *Cancer Causes Control* **8(6)**: 865–871.

Gurney J, Kadan-Lottick N, Packer R *et al.* (2003a). Endocrine and cardiovascular late effects among adult survivors of childhood brain tumors: Childhood Cancer Survivor Study. *Cancer* **97**: 663–673.

Gurney JG, Ness KK, Stovall M *et al.* (2003b). Final height and body mass index among adult survivors of childhood brain cancer: childhood cancer survivor study. *J Clin Endocrinol Metab* **88(10)**: 4731–4739.

Hamilton SR, Liu B, Parsons RE *et al.* (1995). The molecular basis of Turcot's syndrome. *N Engl J Med* **332**(13): 839–847.

Hancock SL, Cox RS, McDougall IR (1991). Thyroid diseases after treatment of Hodgkin's disease. *N Engl J Med* **325**(9): 599–605.

Heikens J, Ubbink M, van der Pal H *et al.* (2000). Long term survivors of childhood brain cancer have an increased risk for cardiovascular disease. *Cancer* **88**: 2116–2121.

Hoppe-Hirsch E, Renier D, Lellouch-Tubiana A *et al.* (1990). Medulloblastoma in childhood: progressive intellectual deterioration. *Childs Nerv Syst* **6**(2): 60–65.

Hoppe-Hirsch E, Brunet L, Laroussinie F *et al.* (1995). Intellectual outcome in children with malignant tumors of the posterior fossa: influence of the field of irradiation and quality of surgery. *Childs Nerv Syst* **11**(6): 340–345; discussion 345–346.

Jakacki RI, Goldwein JW, Larsen RL *et al.* (1993). Cardiac dysfunction following spinal irradiation during childhood. *J Clin Oncol* **11**(6): 1033–1038.

Jakacki RI, Schramm CM, Donahue BR *et al.* (1995). Restrictive lung disease following treatment for malignant brain tumors: a potential late effect of craniospinal irradiation. *J Clin Oncol* **13**(6): 1478–1485.

Jankovic M, Brouwers P, Valsecchi MG *et al.* (1994). Association of 1800 cGy cranial irradiation with intellectual function in children with acute lymphoblastic leukaemia. ISPACC. International Study Group on Psychosocial Aspects of Childhood Cancer. *Lancet* **344**(8917): 224–227.

Jannoun L, Bloom HJ (1990). Long-term psychological effects in children treated for intracranial tumors. *Int J Radiat Oncol Biol Phys* **18**(4): 747–753.

Kleinschmidt-DeMasters BK, Lillehei KO (1995). Radiation-induced meningioma with a 63-year latency period. Case report. *J Neurosurg* **82**(3): 487–488.

Kramer S, Lee KF (1974). Complications of radiation therapy: the central nervous system. *Semin Roentgenol* **9**(1): 75–83.

Landier W, Bhatia S, Eshelman DA *et al.* (2004). Development of risk-based guidelines for pediatric cancer survivors: the Children's Oncology Group Long-Term Follow-Up Guidelines from the Children's Oncology Group Late Effects Committe and Nursing Discipline. *J Clin Oncol* **22**(24): 4979–4990.

Lipshultz SE, Colan SD, Gelber RD *et al.* (1991). Late cardiac effects of doxorubicin therapy for acute lymphoblastic leukemia in childhood. *N Engl J Med* **324**(12): 808–815.

Luban NL (1998). An update on transfusion-transmitted viruses. *Curr Opin Pediatr* **10**(1): 53–59.

Mabbott D, Penkman L, Witol A *et al.* (2005). Attention, working memory and processing speed in children with posterior fossa tumours. Poster presented at the 2005 International Neuropsychological Society Meeting, Dublin, Ireland, 6–9 July, 2005.

Martins AN, Johnston JS, Henry JM *et al.* (1977). Delayed radiation necrosis of the brain. *J Neurosurg* **47**(3): 336–345.

Mertens AC, Yasui Y, Neglia JP *et al.* (2001). Late mortality experience in five-year survivors of childhood and adolescent cancer: the Childhood Cancer Survivor Study. *J Clin Oncol* **19**(13): 3163–3172.

Mertens AC, Yasui Y, Liu Y *et al.* (2002). Pulmonary complications in survivors of childhood and adolescent cancer. A report from the Childhood Cancer Survivor Study. *Cancer* **95**(11): 2431–2441.

Mostow EN, Byrne J, Connelly RR *et al.* (1991). Quality of life in long-term survivors of CNS tumors of childhood and adolescence. *J Clin Oncol* **9**(4): 592–599.

Mulhern RK, Butler RW (2004). Neurocognitive sequelae of childhood cancers and their treatment. *Pediatr Rehabil* **7**(1): 1–14; discussion 15–16.

Mulhern R, Butler RW (2005). Neuropsychological late effects. In Brown RT (ed.) *Pediatric Hematology/ Oncology: A Biopsychosocial Approach.* New York: Oxford University Press.

Mulhern RK, Wasserman AL, Friedman AG *et al.* (1989). Social competence and behavioral adjustment of children who are long-term survivors of cancer. *Pediatrics* **83**(1): 18–25.

Mulhern RK, Hancock J, Fairclough D *et al.* (1992). Neuropsychological status of children treated for brain tumors: a critical review and integrative analysis. *Med Pediatr Oncol* **20**(3): 181–191.

Mulhern RK, Kepner JL, Thomas PR *et al.* (1998). Neuropsychologic functioning of survivors of childhood medulloblastoma randomized to receive conventional or reduced-dose craniospinal irradiation: a Pediatric Oncology Group study. *J Clin Oncol* **16**(5): 1723–1728.

Mulhern RK, Reddick WE, Palmer SL (1999). Neurocognitive deficits in medulloblastoma survivors and white matter loss. *Ann Neurol* **46**(6): 834–841.

Mulhern R, Palmer S, Reddick W *et al.* (2001). Risks of young age for selected neurocognitive deficits in medulloblastoma are associated with white matter loss. *J Clin Oncol* **19**(2): 472–479.

Mulhern RK, White HA, Glass JO *et al.* (2004). Attentional functioning and white matter integrity among survivors of malignant brain tumors of childhood. *J Int Neuropsychol Soc* **10(2)**: 180–189.

Neglia JP, Robison LL, Stovall M *et al.* (2006). New primary neoplasms of the central nervous system in survivors of childhood cancer: a report from the Childhood Cancer Survivor Study. *J Natl Cancer Inst* **98(21)**: 1528–1537.

Ness KK, Mertens AC, Hudson MM *et al.* (2005). Limitations on physical performance and daily activities among long-term survivors of childhood cancer. *Ann Intern Med* **143(9)**: 639–647.

Nicholson HS, Butler R (2001). Late effects of therapy in long-term survivors. In Keating R, Goodrich J, Packer R (eds.) *Tumors of the Pediatric Central Nervous System.* New York: Thieme.

Nicholson HS, Fears TR, Byrne J (1994). Death during adulthood in survivors of childhood and adolescent cancer. *Cancer* **73(12)**: 3094–3102.

Oberfield SE, Soranno D, Nirenberg A *et al.* (1996). Age at onset of puberty following high-dose central nervous system radiation therapy. *Arch Pediatr Adolesc Med* **150(6)**: 589–592.

O'Driscoll BR, Hasleton PS, Taylor PM *et al.* (1990). Active lung fibrosis up to 17 years after chemotherapy with carmustine (BCNU) in childhood. *N Engl J Med* **323(6)**: 378–382.

Oeffinger KC, Mertens AC, Hudson MM *et al.* (2004). Health care of young adult survivors of childhood cancer: a report from the Childhood Cancer Survivor Study. *Ann Fam Med* **2(1)**: 61–70.

Oeffinger KC, Mertens AC, Sklar CA *et al.* (2006). Chronic health conditions in adult survivors of childhood cancer. *N Engl J Med* **355(15)**: 1572–1582.

Packer RJ, Sutton LN, Atkins TE *et al.* (1989). A prospective study of cognitive function in children receiving whole-brain radiotherapy and chemotherapy: 2-year results. *J Neurosurg* **70(5)**: 707–713.

Packer RJ, Sutton LN, Elterman R *et al.* (1994). Outcome for children with medulloblastoma treated with radiation and cisplatin, CCNU, and vincristine chemotherapy. *J Neurosurg* **81(5)**: 690–698.

Packer R, Gurney J, Punyko J *et al.* (2003). Long-term neurologic and neurosensory sequelae in adult survivors of a childhood brain tumor: Childhood Cancer Survivor Study. *J Clin Oncol* **21**: 3255–3261.

Palmer SL, Goloubeva O, Reddick WE *et al.* (2001). Patterns of intellectual development among survivors of pediatric medulloblastoma: a longitudinal analysis. *J Clin Oncol* **19(8)**: 2302–2308.

Palmer SL, Gajjar A, Reddick WE *et al.* (2003). Predicting intellectual outcome among children treated with 35–40 Gy craniospinal irradiation for medulloblastoma. *Neuropsychology* **17(4)**: 548–555.

Penkman L (2004). Remediation of attention deficits in children: a focus on childhood cancer, traumatic brain injury and attention deficit disorder. *Pediatr Rehabil* **7(2)**: 111–123.

Peterson K, Shao C, McCarter R *et al.* (2005). An analysis of SEER data of increasing risk of secondary malignant neoplasms among long-term survivors of childhood brain tumors. *Pediatric Blood Cancer* **47**: 83–88.

Pollack IF (1994). Brain tumors in children. *N Engl J Med* **331(22)**: 1500–1507.

Radcliffe J, Packer RJ, Atkins TE *et al.* (1992). Three- and four-year cognitive outcome in children with noncortical brain tumors treated with whole-brain radiotherapy. *Ann Neurol* **32(4)**: 551–554.

Reddick WE, White HA, Glass JO *et al.* (2003). Developmental model relating white matter volume to neurocognitive deficits in pediatric brain tumor survivors. *Cancer* **97(10)**: 2512–2519.

Reddick WE, Glass JO, Palmer SL *et al.* (2005). Atypical white matter volume development in children following craniospinal irradiation. *Neurooncology* **7(1)**: 12–19.

Reeves CB, Palmer SL, Reddick WE *et al.* (2006). Attention and memory functioning among pediatric patients with medulloblastoma. *J Pediatr Psychol* **31**: 272–280.

Reimers TS, Ehrenfels S, Mortensen EL *et al.* (2003). Cognitive deficits in long-term survivors of childhood brain tumors: identification of predictive factors. *Med Pediatr Oncol* **40(1)**: 26–34.

Reinhold HS, Calvo W, Hopewell JW *et al.* (1990). Development of blood vessel-related radiation damage in the fimbria of the central nervous system. *Int J Radiat Oncol Biol Phys* **18(1)**: 37–42.

Ries LAG, Eisner M, Kosary C *et al.* (2005). *SEER Cancer Statistics Review, 1975–2002.* Bethesda, MD: National Cancer Institute. http://seer.cancer.gov/CSR/1975_2002/, based on November 2004 SEER data submission, posted to the SEER website, 2005.

Ris MD, Noll RB (1994). Long-term neurobehavioral outcome in pediatric brain-tumor patients: review and methodological critique. *J Clin Exp Neuropsychol* **16(1)**: 21–42.

Ris MD, Packer R, Goldwein J *et al.* (2001). Intellectual outcome after reduced-dose radiation therapy plus adjuvant chemotherapy for medulloblastoma: a Children's Cancer Group study. *J Clin Oncol* **19**(15): 3470–3476.

Riva D, Pantaleoni C, Milani N *et al.* (1989). Impairment of neuropsychological functions in children with medulloblastomas and astrocytomas in the posterior fossa. *Childs Nerv Syst* **5**(2): 107–110.

Ronckers CM, Sigurdson AJ, Stovall M *et al.* (2006). Thyroid cancer in childhood cancer survivors: a detailed evaluation of radiation dose response and its modifiers. *Radiat Res* **166**(4): 618–628.

Ross L, Johansen C, Dalton S *et al.* (2003). Psychiatric hospitalizations among survivors of cancer in childhood or adolescence. *New Engl J Med* **349**: 650–657.

Shuper A, Packer RJ, Vezina LG *et al.* (1995). "Complicated migraine-like episodes" in children following cranial irradiation and chemotherapy. *Neurology* **45**(10): 1837–1840.

Skinner R, Pearson AD, Amineddine HA *et al.* (1990). Ototoxicity of cisplatinum in children and adolescents. *Br J Cancer* **61**(6): 927–931.

Sklar CA (1995). Growth following therapy for childhood cancer. *Cancer Invest* **13**(5): 511–516.

Sklar CA (1997). Growth and neuroendocrine dysfunction following therapy for childhood cancer. *Pediatr Clin North Am* **44**(2): 489–503.

Sklar CA, Constine LS (1995). Chronic neuroendocrinological sequelae of radiation therapy. *Int J Radiat Oncol Biol Phys* **31**(5): 1113–1121.

Stavrou T, Bromley C, Nicholson HS *et al.* (2001). Prognostic factors and secondary malignancies in childhood medulloblastoma. *J Pediatr Hematol Oncol* **23**: 431–436.

Strother D, Pollack I, Fisher PG *et al.* (2002). Tumors of the central nervous system. In Poplack PA (ed.) *Principles and Practice of Pediatric Oncology* (4th edn.). Philadelphia, PA: Lippincott Williams & Wilkins.

Travis LB, Rabkin CS, Brown LM *et al.* (2006). Cancer survivorship – genetic susceptibility and second primary cancers: research strategies and recommendations. *J Natl Cancer Inst* **98**(1): 15–25.

Vassilopoulou S, Klein MJ, Moore BD *et al.* (1995). Efficacy of growth hormone replacement therapy in children with organic growth hormone deficiency after cranial irradiation. *Horm Res* **43**(5): 188–193.

Walter AW, Mulhern RK, Gajjar A *et al.* (1999). Survival and neurodevelopmental outcome of young children with medulloblastoma at St Jude Children's Research Hospital. *J Clin Oncol* **17**(12): 3720–3728.

Yeates KO, Swift E, Taylor HG *et al.* (2004). Short- and long-term social outcomes following pediatric traumatic brain injury. *J Int Neuropsychol Soc* **10**(3): 412–426.

15

Neurofibromatosis

Bartlett D. Moore, III and John M. Slopis

Introduction

History

Neurofibromatosis (NF) is a common neurocutaneous disorder that has an incidence of approximately 1 in 4000 (Mulvihill *et al.*, 1990). Although NF has been postulated to have as many as eight different forms (Riccardi & Eichner, 1986), this classification system has not been widely adopted. Neurofibromatosis is a group of genetic disorders including NF type I (NF-I), NF type II (NF-II), and multiple schwannomatosis, each with distinctly different genetic mutations and pathologic bases. The NF-I gene is nearly ubiquitous in human tissues and so impacts virtually all organ systems. NF-I is particularly interesting to neurocognitive scientists because of its characteristic phenotypical abnormalities in development of form and function in brain. NF-II and multiple schwannomatosis are essentially disorders of cranial nerves, peripheral nerves, and meningeal tissues with no associated cognitive abnormalities and so these disorders will be excluded from this discussion.

The original term neurofibromatosis was derived at the turn of the last century but the disorder is also called von Recklinghausen's disease because the condition was described in the late 1800s clinically and scientifically by Friedrich Daniel von Recklinghausen (Cawthon *et al.*, 1990; Crump, 1981;

Viskochil *et al.*, 1990). The molecular genetic basis of distinguishing clinical features of NF-I was localized to chromosome 17 in 1990 by two teams of investigators (Viskochil *et al.*, 1990; Wallace *et al.*, 1990).

John Merrick, the so-called Elephant Man, was perhaps the most famous individual to be diagnosed with NF-I although recent reports suggest that a more likely diagnosis for Mr Merrick is Proteus syndrome, an unrelated condition that resembles NF-I externally but which arises from a genetic mutation on a different chromosome (Ablon, 1995).

Phenotype and genotype

NF-I is a disorder that has been shrouded in confusion over the years because the symptoms and clinical outcome of the disorder vary greatly from patient to patient. Approximately 50% of all cases result from a spontaneous mutation in the NF gene region and so only half of all known cases are familial. The phenotype of NF-I is highly variable between unrelated individuals and even within affected families (von Deimling *et al.*, 1995), despite the fact that the gene produces near-complete penetrance. Ethnic, racial, and gender grouping shows no predominance in NF-I. When the gene was localized to chromosome 17 (Viskochil *et al.*, 1990; Wallace *et al.*, 1990) a new era of refined definition of the phenotypic profile of NF-I ensued, allowing

Cognition and Cancer, eds. Christina A. Meyers and James R. Perry. Published by Cambridge University Press.

segregation of NF-II and multiple schwannomatosis patients from study groups. This distinction particularly sharpened clinical definition of the cognitive abnormalities brought about by the NF-I gene, as childhood developmental specialists and neuroscientists recognized the learning disabilities and behavioral abnormalities common to patients with NF-I. This cognitive profile is characterized by a high incidence of learning disabilities (LD), behavioral problems such as attention deficit hyperactivity disorder (ADHD), and neurocognitive deficits in visual spatial abilities. The cognitive phenotype is considered to be an important predictor of the diagnosis by some investigators and will be discussed in detail later.

The phenotypic variability of NF-I results in many individuals who live normal lives and experience relatively little impact from the disorder, often unaware that they even carry the NF-I gene mutation. The presence of these mildly affected individuals calls into question the accuracy of the incidence and prevalence estimates of NF-I. The presence of cognitive disability in this segment of the population is unknown but may represent the etiology of a significant proportion of LD in the "general population." Chronic, progressive, and debilitating morbidity with severe disfigurement as well as multiple types of cancers affect a minority of patients with NF-I. However in the case of severely affected individuals these complications generally progress in prevalence and severity with advancing age resulting in reduced life span of the group (Riccardi, 1981). The psychological stress of illness in this segment of the population is an important clinical issue, but will not be a topic of this review.

Initial symptoms of NF evolve with age and early diagnosis is often problematic, especially in cases of spontaneous mutation. In families where NF-I is already present, each child born will have a 50% chance of having the mutation. NF-I can present with congenital anomalies that are obvious at birth or with clinical features conspicuous within the first few years of life. Although biochemical and genetic testing techniques have been developed, clinical assessment is the most reliable approach to the

Table 15.1. Diagnostic criteria of NF, type I

---

1. Six or more café-au-lait spots greater than 5 mm in diameter in pre-pubertal children or greater than 15 mm in diameter in post-pubertal individuals
2. Two or more neurofibromas of any form or one plexiform neurofibroma
3. Freckling in the axillary or inguinal regions
4. Optic glioma
5. Two or more Lisch nodules (iris hamartomas)
6. A distinctive osseous lesion such as sphenoid dysplasia or thinning of long bone cortex with or without pseudoarthrosis
7. A first-degree relative with NF-I by the above criteria
8. The presence of two or more criteria constitutes a definitive diagnosis in an individual. If an individual has a first-degree relative with NF-I, then only one additional criterion is required for the diagnosis

---

diagnosis of NF-I. The diagnostic criteria for NF-I (see Table 15.1) are based on a consensus statement developed by the National Institutes of Health in 1988 (1988) and reaffirmed in 1997 (Gutmann *et al.*, 1997) as representing the most frequent clinical features of NF-I. The diagnosis of NF-I is established when two or more features from this list are identified in the patient. Therefore, if one family member carries the diagnosis, only a single criterion is needed for the diagnosis in additional family members.

The most promising development in genetic testing for NF-I is DNA sequencing of the NF-I coding region on chromosome 17. This technology has revealed great variability in DNA sequences in the NF-I gene region as might be expected in a disorder with great clinical variability. Several hundred distinct mutations, deletions, and rearrangements have been found in DNA samples from individuals who meet clinical diagnostic criteria. These findings demonstrate the complexity of the disorder on a molecular level and define the need for extensive future research in genotype/phenotype correlation. To date, no specific patterns of mutation in the NF-I gene are predictive of phenotype, severity, or long-term outcome for any affected individual. In time

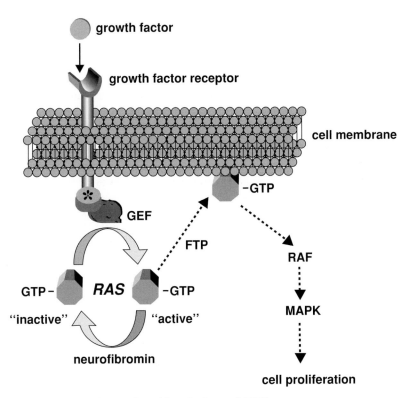

Figure 15.1. Ras pathway. Adapted from Packer *et al.* (2002)

this growing body of information will provide useful prognostic information to predict relative risks and outcomes, including neurocognitive morbidity, for individuals who carry the NF-I gene.

The NF-I gene

Localization of the NF-I gene led to the isolation of the gene product named "neurofibromin." The role of the protein neurofibromin was discovered through study of chronic monocytic myelogenous leukemia, a disorder seen in disproportionately high frequency in patients with NF-I. This protein product is now recognized to have a central role in signal transduction in the Ras system, which regulates cellular growth in Schwann cells as well as numerous other cell types (Figure 15.1).

The Ras "oncogene" is linked to extracellular receptors that bind various "first messenger" hormones including human growth hormone and nerve growth factors. The Ras system serves as the "second messenger" in the signal pathway by induced phosphorylation, changing configuration and binding to the inner cell membrane through cytoskeletal bonds. These bonds are promoted by the process of farnesylation via the intracellular enzyme system farnesyltransferase. Neurofibromin is a constituent component of the reversible phosphorylation enzyme guanosine 5′-triphosphatase (GTP-ase), accelerating the process to proceed forward toward cell activation and/or growth. Mutations in the gene coding region produce mutated or "truncated" copies of the protein neurofibromin leading to defective Ras signaling and the uncontrolled schwann cell growth seen in neurofibromas.

The enzyme system farnesyltransferase has been the subject of intense investigation as a potential target to interrupt dysregulated growth and cellular activation in NF-I. Pharmacologic agents known as farnesyltransferase inhibitors are currently under clinical trial to inhibit the growth of the benign Schwann cell tumors called neurofibromas in NF-I and these agents may ultimately play a role in the treatment of neurofibromas that undergo malignant transformation.

Systemic impact

Focal growth dysregulation in benign tumors

Neurofibromas are complex benign tumors containing multiple tissue elements including neural tissue, connective tissue, and vascular components. Researchers have long recognized the abnormal patterns of growth in these various tissues suggesting that the influence of the NF gene is widespread. Neurofibromin has now been identified in multiple tissues that are derived from virtually all embryonic tissue lines including mesoderm, ectoderm, neuroectoderm, and neural crest. Mature tissues known or presumed likely to be affected by NF-I mutations are listed in Table 15.2. The gene product has been isolated from fetal ectoderm tissues as early as at 6 weeks of gestation. This early presentation suggests that the NF gene is a critical factor in embryonic development and therefore is a clue to the widespread systemic nature of the disorder. Developmental and functional anomalies of the brain in NF-I are best understood within this larger view of the impact of the gene on embryogenesis.

Brain malformation in animal models of NF-I and humans

Development of the human central nervous system involves interactions with virtually all embryonic primitive tissues. The NF-I gene appears to influence central nervous system development during embryogenesis and mutations in this gene produce malformations of brain in animal models and in humans.

Developing gray matter and white matter elements in the brain interact in the process of neu-

Table 15.2. Embryonic tissues giving rise to mature tissues as features of NF-I

Neural crest
Lisch nodules – pigmented iris hamartoma
Café-au-lait – disordered cutaneous migration of
    melanocytes
Axillary freckles – disordered cutaneous migration of
    melanocytes at limb buds
Cardiac conduction bundle – murine models of failed
    cardiac septal fusion
Neuroectoderm
Eye – optic nerve glioma and congenital "glaucoma"
Brain – astrocyte/oligodendroglial defects producing brain
    tumor and unidentified bright object
Spinal cord – astrocyte – spinal cord tumors
Spinal root – Schwann cell defects producing radicular
    neurofibroma
Peripheral nerve – Schwann cell defects producing
    peripheral neurofibroma
Ectoderm
Dermis – neural elements producing cutaneous
    neurofibroma
Epidermis
Mesoderm
Long bone – limb bud defects, hypertrophy,
    pseudoarthrosis
Spinal bone – vertebral body anomalies, meningiocoels
Muscle – neurofibroma
Adipocyte – neurofibroma
Vascular elements – neurofibroma

ronal migration in normal brain development. The NF-I gene appears to function in roles of both signal transduction and environment sensing (Uhlmann & Gutmann, 2001) as well as programmed apoptosis. This concept supports the idea that disorders in developing cellular apoptotic signals result in excess neuronal and astrocytic populations in the mature brain in NF-I. Malformations of cortical development and white matter are the end result of abnormal apoptotic signaling. The interactions between gray and white matter precursors appear to be disarrayed, perhaps as a consequence of defective cell-to-cell signaling, resulting in abnormalities of oligodendrogliocyte myelin production and maturation in NF-I with the consequence that areas of hyperintense signal are commonly seen on brain magnetic resonance imaging (MRI). Finally, nests of persistent astrocyte precursors that were not eliminated by apoptosis remain as potential foci of brain tumor development over time. Numerous clinical features of NF-I are explained by these concepts.

One of the most easily recognized malformations in NF-I is aqueductal stenosis, which is seen in approximately 15% of patients. The mechanism of this malformation remains unclear although low-grade glioma or hamartoma may appear within the brainstem as age progresses. This common disorder is easily identified by neuroimaging, is frequently asymptomatic, and appears to have no distinct impact upon cognition. The association between malformation and latent brain tumor development suggests two independent but interrelated processes that occur in brain development. Benign macrocephaly, another common clinical feature of NF-I, also implies that the NF-I gene has an impact on the brain during embryogenesis. Volumetric MRI studies indicate significant increases in gray matter volumes in patients with NF-I (Moore *et al.*, 2000). Morphologic studies of brain in NF-I also demonstrate abnormal development of the corpus callosum (Kayl *et al.*, 2000).

Frontal brain structural malformation (including forebrain fusion and holoprosencephaly) has been modeled in mice using multiple specific gene knock-out animals developed and studied in conjunction with an additional NF-I knock-out. The NF-I gene appears to have a significant influence on neuronal migration and frontal cortex formation (Zhu *et al.*, 2001) in these models. These models predict the presence of the cortical malformations that are reported in NF-I and human clinical descriptions. Gross malformations of cortex have been reported in humans with NF-I (Balestri *et al.*, 2003). Three mentally retarded patients were evaluated with MRI scans of the brain that defined right hemispheric transmantle cortical dysplasia, periventricular band cortical dysplasia with overlying pachygyria, and polymicrogyria in these individuals. These major brain malformations seem a certain cause of mental retardation and seizure in these three individuals but they are not common features of NF-I. More significant is the fact that these various malformations are presumed to result from different pathological mechanisms, supporting the role of neurofibromin in early brain development.

In contrast, minor malformations in cortical development occur with much greater frequency. Minor malformation of frontal cortex development has been studied in NF-I as a feature associated with reading disability (Billingsley *et al.*, 2003b). MRI-based anatomic studies of patients with dyslexia in the general population reveal specific patterns of cortical gyral formation in humans within the inferior frontal gyrus (Leonard *et al.*, 2001). MRI-based analysis of reading-disabled patients with NF-I shows a similar occurrence of these pathological patterns within the inferior frontal gyrus with an approximately 40% rate of occurrence of these minor malformations (Billingsley *et al.*, 2002).

Common clinical experience in the management of NF-I also supports the concept that aberrant cell signaling with disordered cell-to-cell neurotransmission occurs. Approximately 40%–60% of children with NF-I demonstrate behavioral features of ADHD. This frequency is five- to sixfold greater than in the general population. Dopamine reuptake inhibitor stimulant therapy is commonly used effectively in this population for the management of ADHD. Whether this high incidence of ADHD is a consequence of neuropharmacologic disorder or frontal/callosal dysmorphism (Kayl *et al.*, 2000), or both, remains uncertain at this time.

Brain tumors in NF-I

Development of optic nerve glioma may occur in association with plexiform neurofibroma and focal dysplasia of the tissues of the orbit and periorbital regions. These complex tumors represent the focal or mosaic impact of the NF-I gene localized to the developing cranium. The formation of these tumors is an example of anomalous cell-to-cell interaction in NF-I during embryogenesis of the eye. During brain formation, the eye buds develop from the anterior telencephalon. The eye buds migrate forward and induce the surrounding primitive

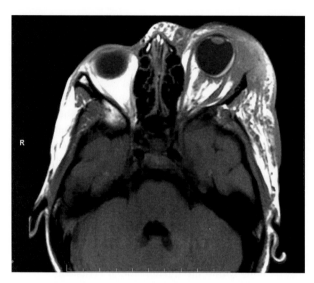

Figure 15.2. Axial MRI image of a 7-year-old boy with NF-I showing a large orbital plexiform neurofibroma

embryonic tissues to form the mature eye. This process occurs in a cascade of events in which mesodermal elements ultimately give rise to the bone of the orbit, vasculature, and extra-ocular muscles; neural crest elements give rise to the iris ciliary body; neuroectodermal elements give rise to the optic nerve and oculomotor nerves; and ectodermal elements give rise to the eyelid. Disruption of one or more of the elements of this cascade results in dysplastic formation of the eye, forming either isolated optic nerve glioma or more extensive disfiguring orbital plexiform neurofibroma (Figure 15.2).

Astrocytic brain tumors of all types occur in patients with NF-I with a similar or slightly higher incidence than in the general population. The exception is optic pathway glioma, which develops in approximately 15% of individuals with NF-I. Optic pathway glioma is primarily a tumor of childhood, usually identified before the age of 6 years with a peak incidence occurring around 2 years of age. Optic pathway glioma may arise within the orbital segment of the optic nerve, within the optic chiasm, or within the brain parenchyma in the optic pathways, usually limited to the anterior visual pathways and not extending to the occipi-

tal lobes. The majority of these tumors are non-progressive and asymptomatic (Listernick et al., 1997). Tumors limited to the orbit often represent overgrowth of the optic nerve sheath without a progressive astrocytic component. Tumors of the chiasm and optic pathways are typically juvenile pilocytic astrocytomas. The highly stereotyped profile of these tumors appears directly related to the presence of the NF-I gene and its impact on central nervous system development in utero.

Optic nerve tumors are also fairly stereotyped in associated symptomatology in patients with NF-I. Tumors of the optic chiasm frequently involve the adjacent hypothalamus causing precocious puberty by unknown endocrine mechanisms. It is interesting to note that tumors of the optic chiasm are usually not related directly to the short stature that is seen in approximately 15% of the NF-I population. A significant body of evidence suggests that short stature is a systemic disorder of growth hormone and growth factor receptors in NF-I.

The majority of optic nerve tumors in NF-I are low grade, non-progressive, and do not require intervention. Treatment of symptomatic or progressive optic glioma in NF-I is similar to treatment of optic glioma in the general population with the exception of the use of cranial radiation (RT). Surgical intervention is rare but may be required if the tumor is exerting a mass effect within the orbit or within the suprasellar region. The most common effective treatment is combination chemotherapy using vincristine and carboplatin, in some cases followed by tamoxifen. Cranial radiation is now considered to be contraindicated in NF-I. Several groups have shown that secondary tumor formation occurs with a higher frequency in the presence of the NF gene (Kortmann et al., 2003). These secondary tumors are usually higher-grade infiltrative astrocytes or malignant nerve sheath tumors, both often fatal (Sharif et al., 2006). In addition to secondary tumors, children with NF-I also appear to develop central nervous system vascular malformations at a higher than expected rate after RT leading to cerebral infarction (Kortmann et al., 2003). As recently as the early 1990s RT was routinely utilized in the treatment of optic glioma and found to produce a high incidence of hypothalamic dysfunction. No comprehensive studies of the effects of RT specific to NF-I are available but clinicians generally suspect that the known impact of RT on the developing brain may compound the cognitive deficits known to occur in NF-I. Optic pathway glioma has no known independent correlation with cognitive deficit in NF-I (De Winter *et al.*, 1999).

Systemic impact on function

The impact of the NF-I gene clearly extends far beyond the promotion of the growth of benign nerve sheath fibromas. The goal of current clinical trials of farnesyltransferase inhibitors is to interrupt intercellular transmission of the growth message and so to inhibit the growth of benign neurofibromas. Of perhaps greater interest, however, is the recent demonstration that these agents have a positive impact upon learning deficits in NF-I knock-out mice (Costa *et al.*, 2002). Knock-out mice that are haplo-insufficient for the NF-I gene demonstrate visual-spatial memory deficits that model human NF-I learning disabilities in a limited way. These mice were studied in a Morris water maze system and found to have significant visual-spatial learning impairments. The mice were then treated with a farnesyltransferase inhibitor, which led to significant reductions in learning time and improvement in overall learning efficiency (Costa *et al.*, 2002).

The role of the NF-I gene has also been studied in NF haplo-insufficient *Drosophila*. The *Drosophila* NF-I protein is highly conserved showing 60% identity with human neurofibromin (Guo *et al.*, 2000). The fruit fly depends heavily upon olfaction for survival, so models of learning must distinguish between behavioral patterns that include or exclude olfaction. These models include olfactory-guided avoidance, olfactory-guided learning, and electric shock avoidance. Studies indicate that *Drosophila* NF-I protein acts as both a Ras GTP-ase-activating protein (GAP) and as a regulator of the AMP pathway that involves the *rutabaga-* (*rut-*) encoded adenylyl cyclase. G-protein-activated adenylyl cyclase activity in the fruitfly appears to occur in NF-I-dependent and NF-I independent mechanisms. The mechanism of NF-I-dependent activation of the Rut adenylyl cyclase pathway is essential for *Drosophila* learning and memory (Guo *et al.*, 2000).

The implications of these animal studies are far-reaching with respect to learning disabilities in humans with NF-I. The functionally disordered GTP-ase of the Ras signaling system has the potential to be present as a common defective second messenger in numerous signaling systems throughout the body, including the brain. These animal studies suggest that abnormal cell signaling in the brain leads to defects in neurotransmission and subsequent learning disabilities that respond to pharmacological intervention.

Neurocognitive status of children with NF-I

From a neuropsychological standpoint, NF-I is an exceptionally interesting medical disorder. NF-I is associated with much higher incidences of learning disability (LD), neuropsychological deficits, behavioral problems, and brain tumors in comparison with the general population. In addition, those with NF-I have a wide range of neuroanatomical abnormalities. Neuropsychological studies of children and adolescents with NF-I have revealed a wide range of cognitive sequelae associated with the disorder. Visual-spatial deficits and learning disabilities are two of the most commonly reported problems, but speech disarticulation, language deficits, and motor inco-ordination are also typical features (Brewer *et al.*, 1997; Eldridge *et al.*, 1989; Eliason, 1986; Hofman *et al.*, 1994; Moore & Denckla, 1999; Moore *et al.*, 1994; North *et al.*, 1997).

Intellectual functioning

It was once widely believed that NF-I was associated with a high incidence of mental retardation. This idea has been widely discounted by numerous studies that have instead found a slight downward shift of the distribution of IQ (Figure 15.3) and

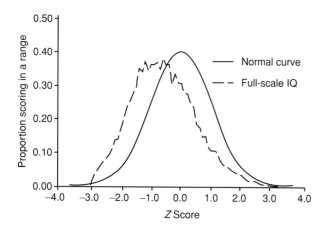

Figure 15.3. Full-scale IQ distribution in 84 children with NF-I compared to the normal curve

only a slightly elevated incidence of mental retardation over population estimates (Eldridge *et al.*, 1989; Moore *et al.*, 1994; North *et al.*, 1997). Some early studies reported a discrepancy between verbal and performance intellectual abilities favoring verbal abilities (Eliason, 1986, 1988; Wadsby *et al.*, 1989). This led to the belief that the LD in NF-I are similar to the classic non-verbal learning disability (NVLD) syndrome (Rourke, 1989). The NF-I Cognitive Disorders Task Force review of studies for which both verbal and performance IQ data were reported found no significant trend for verbal or performance intellectual advantage or disadvantage (North *et al.*, 1997). The Task Force reviewed 10 studies with a total of 416 patients with NF-I. Of the 6 studies that reported data on the incidence of mental retardation ($n = 350$), the average rate (defined as IQ < 70) was 7.1% with a range of 4.8%–11.2%. This is higher than the estimated rate in the general population of 2%–3%, but not as high as once thought. The average full-scale IQ was 92.9 in the 9 studies with objective standardized measures of IQ with a range of 88.6–94.8. Whereas the ranges of IQ reported in these studies are somewhat similar, it is important to note that children with NF-I cover the entire range of intellectual abilities that is seen in the general population: some show severe intellec-

tual deficiency while others are highly gifted intellectually.

Learning and academic achievement profile

Difficulties with academic performance are often reported to be the most significant morbidity associated with childhood NF-I (Coude *et al.*, 2004). The NF Consensus Task Force reported variable rates of LD with an average rate of 44.3% and a range of from 30% to 61% in the 6 studies reporting this information (North *et al.*, 1997). However, not all studies used the same criteria for defining what constitutes a LD. The *Diagnostic and Statistical Manual of Mental Disorders* (DSM-IV; American Psychiatric Association, 2000) does not list "learning disability" per se but describes specific disorders in reading, mathematics, and written expression. The criterion for a disorder in one of these areas is that academic achievement, as measured by standardized tests, must be substantially below expectations for the child's chronological age, intelligence, and age-appropriate education. This is the standard discrepancy model of LD and, while controversial and in need of change, it is what most school districts now use. However, in many studies of NF-I, formal criteria for LD have not been applied when arriving at incidence levels. Many children are underachievers, are in special classes, or have had to repeat a grade. Others may have behavioral issues such ADHD that interfere with academic success. Thus many children with NF-I are given the LD label even when they may not meet objective diagnostic criteria.

Visual-spatial deficits are a common characteristic of children with NF-I (discussed below) (Eldridge *et al.*, 1989; Eliason, 1986), therefore, some have speculated that they suffer from NVLD. Learning disabilities in this population, however, are not exclusively non-verbal, as more recent studies have shown that verbal deficits are also common. Mazzocco and colleagues (1995) examined reading disability in NF-I and found a higher incidence in children with NF-I (53%) compared to their non-affected siblings (26%). Children with NF-I, in comparison to their siblings without NF-I, had weaknesses in vocabulary and phonetic abilities, reading and mathematics, in addition to their visual-spatial deficits (Mazzocco *et al.*, 1995). Cutting *et al.* (2000) compared the cognitive profiles of children with NF-I to those of an LD clinic population. While both groups performed worse than non-disabled controls on measures of sight reading and reading comprehension, the NF-I group had more global language impairments compared to the LD clinic group. Cutting also found that children with NF-I scored significantly lower than an LD control group on visual-spatial measures, indicating that children with NF-I have visual-spatial deficits that are not representative of the broader reading-disabled population (Cutting *et al.*, 2000).

Others have also suggested that the academic profile does not seem to fit the typical types of LD or dyslexia. For example, Descheemaeker *et al.* (2005) reported that half of a relatively small sample (*n* = 17) of children with NF-I had LD a figure in keeping with other reports. Of those with documented LD (*n* = 8) one-half had spelling deficits but only one had a pure arithmetic deficit (Descheemaeker *et al.*, 2005). Brewer and colleagues (1997) used cluster analysis to document the neurocognitive profile in a large cohort (*N* = 105) of children with NF-I. She found that, among 72 children with academic difficulties, 3 groups emerged. One group had a normal neurocognitive profile (39%), another had general academic deficits (47%), and the third had primarily visual-spatial/motor deficits (14%). The low incidence of visual-spatial deficits was surprising given the often-reported high incidence of deficits in this area. However, this study did not include the Judgment of Line Orientation (JLO) test (Lindgren & Benton, 1980), which is often reported as the most impaired test of visual perceptual skills in this population (Schrimsher *et al.*, 2003).

When taken together, reports of cognitive deficits in children and adolescents with NF-I show that this disorder is characterized by a complex range of both verbal and visual-spatial deficits, and does not lead to a strictly non-verbal LD syndrome, insofar as this syndrome has been described in other populations (Rourke, 1989).

Visual-spatial abilities and their impact on academic achievement

Dyslexic readers in the general population have deficits in the rapid processing of visual stimuli (Eden *et al.*, 1996a, 1996c; Temple *et al.*, 2000). Deficiencies in the rapid identification of letters may also contribute to reading problems in children and adolescents with NF-I. Visual-spatial processing problems, including the rapid identification of objects (Cutting *et al.*, 2000) and the accurate identification of similar lines and angles (Eldridge *et al.*, 1989; Moore *et al.*, 1996), have been identified children and adolescents with NF-I, as well as in poor readers without NF-I (Eden *et al.*, 1996a). Functional neuroimaging studies of the visual-spatial processing of letters and other stimuli in healthy individuals have shown significant activity in bilateral inferior parietal and posterior-superior parietal cortex, as well as in lateral frontal and extrastriate cortex (Alivisatos & Petrides, 1997; Booth *et al.*, 2000; Greenlee *et al.*, 2000).

Children with NF-I have visual-spatial deficits that are not representative of the broader LD population (Cutting *et al.*, 2000), but may be related to deficits in reading. Adults with NF-I have also been found to have visual-spatial deficits. Using discriminant function analyses, the JLO test accurately classified adults with NF-I from controls (Pavol *et al.*, 2006). Nevertheless, the role of visual-spatial deficits in the learning deficits of children with NF-I is far from clear (Brewer *et al.*, 1997). We have found that the deficit in visual-spatial abilities is somewhat specific rather than general. For example, the JLO test is impaired in approximately 70% of children with NF-I and it bears a strong relation with academic performance in general (Figure 15.4).

Although performance by most children with NF-I on the JLO test is impaired (Lindgren & Benton, 1980), not all areas of visual-spatial processing are affected in children with NF-I. For example, the ability to discriminate among two-dimensional drawings of similar geometric figures is not impaired relative to normal control subjects (Figure 15.5).

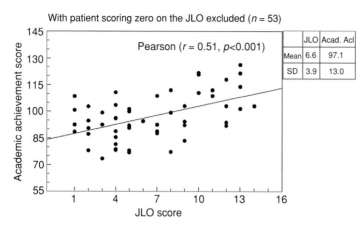

Figure 15.4. Correlation between standard score on the Judgment of Line Orientation (JLO) test and general academic achievement

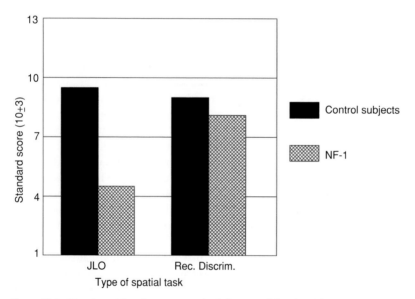

Figure 15.5. Visual spatial performance on the Judgment of the Line Orientation (JLO) versus the Recognition-Discrimination test tasks

Schrimsher and colleagues (2003) reported that the multivariate combination of visual-spatial/motor tasks was highly discriminative of the NF-I diagnosis in that it correctly identified 90% of individuals with clinically identified NF-I. Four visual processing tests (JLO, Orientation, Block Design, Recognition-Discrimination Test, Beery Visual-Motor Integra-

tion Test) were a significant predictor of NF-I diagnostic status ($p = 0.000\,000\,4$). Two of these tests are purely visual spatial and two are visual perceptual/motor. The JLO (a purely visual-spatial task) by itself, but not the other tests, was still highly predictive of NF diagnostic status. Although the diagnosis of NF-I is usually made on the basis of the clinical features presented in Table 15.1, additional information may be provided by performance on tests of visual-spatial abilities, especially when the diagnosis based on clinical characteristics is marginal (e.g., 5, but not 6 café-au-lait spots). Schools and entities testing large numbers of school-aged children should be aware that a profile consisting of visual-spatial deficits, ADHD, and learning deficits in the context of intact intellectual abilities is often associated with NF-I. For medical personnel caring for children with diagnosed NF-I, a comprehensive neurocognitive evaluation should become part of their standard of care. Since visual-spatial functioning influences reading and academic abilities in general, tests of visual-spatial abilities should be included. A brief screening examination is even warranted for suspected NF-I should school or medical personnel have suspicions of the diagnosis.

Brain structure/function correlates

NF-I presents with a unique combination of white matter abnormalities, low-grade, or sometimes malignant, brain tumors, and abnormalities in brain morphology. These morphological differences can be seen in both gross and regional brain development and have been widely investigated for their role in the neuropsychological and learning deficits seen in NF-I. The relationship between brain MR hyperintensities, brain tumors, and macrocephaly with neuropsychological functioning in NF-I is an area of intense research interest.

Brain tumors

Approximately 15% of children and adolescents with NF-I will be diagnosed with a brain tumor, usually an optic glioma. Only 20% of optic gliomas are symptomatic however. Although optic gliomas in NF-I are usually benign and are often left untreated, one might surmise that an optic glioma is still a pathological condition of the central nervous system, and therefore might be associated with other less conspicuous brain abnormalities that could play a role in learning and cognitive difficulties. However, the severity of cognitive and learning deficits in children with NF-I is not exacerbated by the presence of a brain tumor unless cranial radiation therapy is given (De Winter *et al.*, 1999; Moore *et al.*, 1994).

MR hyperintensities

Areas of hyperintense signal on T2-weighted and, more conspicuously, on fluid-attenuated inversion recovery (FLAIR) MRI sequences are observed in the brains of most children and adolescents with NF-I. These "MR hyperintensities," as we will refer to them, are benign, do not appear to occupy space, and may occur in multiple regions in the same individual. Their most common locations are the basal ganglia, cerebellum, brainstem, and diencephalon. Uncertainty continues with regard to the makeup and clinical significance of MR hyperintensities in children with NF-I. One report of three children with NF-I seen at autopsy documented that MR hyperintensities consisted of spongiotic tissue with fluid-filled vacuoles, which accounts for their appearance on MRI (DiPaolo *et al.*, 1995). Using magnetization transfer ratio measurement techniques, MR hyperintensities were characterized as areas of hypomyelination or structurally abnormal myelin (Margariti *et al.*, 2007). Because of their uncertain nature, these areas of MR hyperintensity have been informally referred to as "unidentified bright objects" (UBOs). However, because they are bright only on MRI and because they are not space-occupying objects, we prefer the label MR hyperintensities. It has been estimated that between 50% and 70% of children and adolescents with NF-I have MR hyperintensities, leading some to predict that they are markers for more extensive, albeit unobservable, white matter abnormalities (Moore *et al.*, 1996; North *et al.*, 1994). Several studies have reported that MR hyperintensities disappear or diminish in size with advancing age (Aoki *et al.*, 1989; Itoh *et al.*, 1994; Sevick *et al.*, 1992), strengthening the case that they are an anomaly of the normal developmental process of myelination.

Correlative neuropsychological studies of MR hyperintensities have generally been disappointing however, because few consistent relations with cognitive functioning have been observed. Early studies failed to find a significant association between learning disabilities and MR hyperintensities in the brain (Duffner *et al.*, 1989; Dunn & Roos, 1989; Ferner *et al.*, 1993). More recent studies have reported significant associations between the presence (North *et al.*, 1994), number (Denckla *et al.*, 1996; Hofman *et al.*, 1994), and location (Moore *et al.*, 1996) of MR hyperintensities and neurocognitive functioning. These conflicting results suggest that MR hyperintensities are not *consistent* predictors of cognitive deficits or learning disabilities across samples of the NF-I population, but may represent a neurocognitive burden if found in sufficient numbers and in certain locations. MR hyperintensities in the thalamus are associated with lower scores on tests of visual-spatial and memory ability (Moore *et al.*, 1996) and with lower IQ (Goh *et al.*, 2004). When located in the globus pallidus, MR hyperintensities are associated with relatively low attention scores (Goh *et al.*, 2004).

Macrocephaly

Macrocephaly occurs in 30%–50% of patients with NF-I (Bale *et al.*, 1991) and is associated with increased clinical and physical severity (Zvulunov *et al.*, 1998) but not increased neuropsychological impairment (Ferner *et al.*, 1996). The relationship between macrocephaly and learning disabilities in NF-I has been a focus of several recent studies using quantitative volumetric imaging techniques. Said and colleagues (1996) reported greater overall brain volume, specifically cortical white matter, using quantitative imaging techniques. Using the magnetization transfer ratio, Margariti and colleagues concluded that macrocephaly results from increased volumes of gray matter *and* white matter in children with NF-I (Margariti *et al.*, 2007). Our group, however, found significantly larger overall brain volumes, due to gray but not white matter differences. In addition, a higher gray-to-white

matter ratio and significantly larger corpus callosa were reported in this group of 52 children with NF-I (Kayl *et al.*, 2000; Moore *et al.*, 2000). Greater volume of gray matter and size of the corpus callosum was positively correlated with the degree of discrepancy between IQ and academic achievement in children with NF-I but not controls (Moore *et al.*, 2000). The differences between these studies may be related to the selection of brain structures included in the volumetric calculations (Moore *et al.*, 2000).

Congenital malformation

In proficient readers there is a left-greater-than-right superior temporal lobe asymmetry. Measurement of specific regions of the superior temporal lobe, the planum temporale (PT) and planum parietale (PP), has been reported in 24 children and adolescents with NF-I and an equal number of controls (Billingsley *et al.*, 2002). Intelligence-based discrepancy scores of reading and math achievement, which are commonly used to define learning disabilities, were significantly related to PT asymmetry in the NF-I group. Specifically, boys with NF-I had an absence of the normal asymmetry seen in proficient readers. In addition, the left PT in boys with NF-I was smaller than in girls with NF-I and in non-NF-I controls (Billingsley *et al.*, 2002).

Functional imaging studies

Structural neuroanatomy is an important approach to studying disorders such as NF-I because of the high incidence of morphological abnormalities (discussed above). However, this approach may have limitations for determining the etiology of the cognitive effects also commonly observed in individuals with NF-I. Structural abnormalities may only be an indirect indication of function. A more complete understanding of learning disabilities in NF-I requires methods that can associate underlying neuronal activity with cognitive operations in a time-linked fashion. Hemodynamic imaging methods, such as functional MRI (fMRI), provide a way to analyze regional brain function that is temporally linked to cognitive processing. Functional MRI detects blood oxygen level dependent (BOLD) responses in the brain during cognitive activity. These BOLD responses are temporally linked to changes in underlying neuronal activity resulting from cognitive activity. Functional MRI has been used to study reading and visual-spatial processing associated with learning disabilities, including dyslexia, in healthy individuals as well as in a variety of patient populations with neurological disorders (Billingsley *et al.*, 2001; Eden *et al.*, 1996b; Paulesu *et al.*, 1996; Shaywitz *et al.*, 1998; Temple *et al.*, 2001).

Developmental reading impairments involve problems in learning to relate visual input to phonological representations. Phonological discrimination, which requires an individual to identify distinct sounds that make up words and letters, has been shown to be a core component of learning to read (Fletcher *et al.*, 1994; Stanovich, 1988). Functional MRI studies in other populations have implicated inferior frontal, dorsolateral prefrontal, and temporal cortices in phonological processing skills (Pugh *et al.*, 1996; Shaywitz *et al.*, 1998; Temple *et al.*, 2001). Previous fMRI investigations of phonological processing in poor readers who do not have NF-I have shown differential neural responses to phonological stimuli (Temple *et al.*, 2000, 2001). Children with dyslexia were found to have reduced neural activity in left temporal-parietal cortex during a phonological decision task that required them to determine whether two letters rhymed. Activity in left inferior frontal cortex, a region that has been identified as critical to phonological processing in neurologically normal individuals (Pugh *et al.*, 1996), was similar in dyslexic children compared with controls (Temple *et al.*, 2001).

Phonological processing is one of the most basic skills involved in learning to read and the inferior frontal cortex is integral to this skill. Using an fMRI paradigm that involved phonological processing, Billingsley and colleagues (2003a) found that children with NF-I activate inferior frontal relative to posterior cortex to a greater extent than controls, especially in the right hemisphere. These results agree with previous morphological studies indicating inferior frontal cortex malformations in adults with developmental language disorders (Clark & Plante, 1998).

As discussed above, visual-spatial impairments are a hallmark of NF-I. Just as in phonological processing, children with NF-I appear to have different activation patterns from controls during visual-spatial processing. Relative to lateral and inferior frontal cortex, children with NF-I activate posterior cortex (occipital, parietal, and middle temporal) to a greater extent than controls (Billingsley *et al.*, 2004). Patterns of activation were associated not only with their accuracy during the activation task during fMRI, but also with their standardized reading scores in a normal testing environment.

Summary

Neurofibromatosis is more common than other high profile disorders such as muscular dystrophy, Tay-Sachs disease, cystic fibrosis, and Huntington's disease *combined* (Korf & Rubenstein, 2005) and yet it remains virtually unknown to the public. The underlying molecular pathogenesis of NF was discovered almost a century after its first clinical descriptions. Advances in the understanding of the NF gene mutation have led to insights into specific tumor suppressor gene function as well as insights into the impact of growth dysregulation upon embryonic development, including structural and functional brain development.

The vast size and complexity of the NF gene results in a broad spectrum of distinct human NF mutations and so the disorder is expressed with variable manifestations of physical and behavioral phenotypes. Individuals with mild symptoms are often unaware that they even carry the disordered gene. This is a particular problem in childhood as the morbidity of NF-I increases with age and early detection of developing problems is important.

The neurocognitive phenotype of NF-I consists of average or slightly below average intellectual abilities, difficulties in school achievement, visual-spatial processing deficits, ADHD, and frequently low self-esteem. Some children with NF have none of these neurocognitive features, a fact that demonstrates the variability of the phenotype. The neurocognitive phenotype ranges from severe mental deficiency to superior intellect, and yet any individual with NF may exhibit a LD. The NF population includes children who struggle in special education hoping to graduate from high school and children who attain top academic achievement despite competition from their non-NF peers. Whether learning disability is a cause of social dysfunction and failure in personal achievement remains to be studied, but one could argue that learning disability is the greatest morbidity of NF.

The reasons for the high incidence of LD in the NF population remain largely unknown. MRI-based morphologic studies of the brains of children with NF-I have revealed both gross and fine structural abnormalities of brain development similar to abnormalities seen in idiopathic dyslexia and ADHD. Much of this evidence suggests both structural and functional disorders of frontal cortex.

Undoubtedly mutation of the NF-I gene plays a role in these specific disorders of neural development in children with NF-I and thereby indirectly influences their learning and neurocognitive profile. Genetically engineered murine and insect models bearing NF-I mutations provide excellent surrogates that mimic the human conditions of learning deficits. NF-I haplo-insufficient mice model deficits in spatial learning (Costa *et al.*, 2002; Silva *et al.*, 1997), while the NF-I haplo-insufficient *Drosophila* models deficits in olfactory learning and independent mechanisms of memory. These models provide behavioral platforms for pharmacological trials with a direct molecular genetic window into correlative studies of signal transduction in the brain. In this way the ubiquitous nature of the NF gene provides a rare opportunity to study neural signal transduction in models that correlate a specific genotype with stereotyped behavioral and developmental patterns.

ACKNOWLEDGMENTS

The authors wish to acknowledge the support of Cheniere Energy, Inc., Houston, Texas, Kirk Gentle, and Chris Shaw for helping to make this work possible.

REFERENCES

Ablon J (1995). "The Elephant Man" as "self" and "other": the psycho-social costs of a misdiagnosis. *Soc Sci Med* **40**: 1481–1489.

Alivisatos B, Petrides M (1997). Functional activation of the human brain during mental rotation. *Neuropsychologia* **35**: 111–118.

American Psychiatric Association (2000). *Diagnostic and Statistical Manual of Mental Disorders* (4th edn.) (Test Revision). DSM-IV-TR. Arlington, VA: American Psychiatric Association.

Aoki S, Barkovich AJ, Nishimura K *et al.* (1989). Neurofibromatosis types 1 and 2: cranial MR findings. *Radiology* **172**: 527–534.

Bale SJ, Amos CI, Parry DM *et al.* (1991). Relationship between head circumference and height in normal adults and in the nevoid basal cell carcinoma syndrome and neurofibromatosis type I. *Am J Med Genet* **40**: 206–210.

Balestri P, Vivarelli R, Grosso S *et al.* (2003). Malformations of cortical development in neurofibromatosis type 1. *Neurology* **61**: 1799–1801.

Billingsley RL, McAndrews MP, Crawley AP *et al.* (2001). Functional MRI of phonological and semantic processing in temporal lobe epilepsy. *Brain* **124**: 1218–1227.

Billingsley RL, Schrimsher GW, Jackson EF *et al.* (2002). Significance of planum temporale and planum parietale morphologic features in neurofibromatosis, type I. *Arch Neurol* **59**: 616–622.

Billingsley RL, Jackson EF, Slopis JM *et al.* (2003a). Functional magnetic resonance imaging of phonologic processing in neurofibromatosis 1. *J Child Neurol* **18**: 731–740.

Billingsley RL, Slopis JM, Swank PR *et al.* (2003b). Cortical morphology associated with language function in neurofibromatosis, type I. *Brain Lang* **85**: 125–139.

Billingsley RL, Jackson EF, Slopis JM *et al.* (2004). Functional MRI of visual-spatial processing in neurofibromatosis, type I. *Neuropsychologia* **42**: 395–404.

Booth JR, MacWhinney B, Thulborn KR *et al.* (2000). Developmental and lesion effects in brain activation during sentence comprehension and mental rotation. *Dev Neuropsychol* **18**: 139–169.

Brewer VR, Moore BD, Hiscock M (1997). Learning disability subtypes in children with neurofibromatosis. *J Learn Disabil* **30**: 521–533.

Cawthon RM, Weiss R, Xu GF *et al.* (1990). A major segment of the neurofibromatosis type 1 gene: cDNA sequence, genomic structure, and point mutations [published erratum appears in *Cell* 1990 Aug 10:62(3):following 608]. *Cell* **62**: 193–201.

Clark MM, Plante E (1998). Morphology of the inferior frontal gyrus in developmentally language-disordered adults. *Brain Lang* **61**: 288–303.

Costa RM, Federov NB, Kogan JH *et al.* (2002). Mechanism for the learning deficits in a mouse model of neurofibromatosis type 1. *Nature* **415**: 526–530.

Coude FX, Mignot C, Lyonne S *et al.* (2004). Academic impairment is the most frequent complication of neurofibromatosis type-1 (NF1) in children. *Behav Genet* **34**: 635.

Crump T (1981). Translation of case reports in *Ueber die multiplen Fibrome der Haut und ihre Beziehung zu den multiplen Neuromen* [On Multiple Fibromas of the Skin and their Relationship to Multiple Neuromas] by F. V. Recklinghausen. In Riccardi VM, Mulvihill J (eds.) *Neurofibromatosis (von Recklinghausen Disease): Genetics, Cell Biology, and Biochemistry* (Vol. **23**, pp. 259–275). New York: Raven Press.

Cutting LE, Koth CW, Denckla MB (2000). How children with neurofibromatosis type 1 differ from "typical" learning disabled clinic attenders: nonverbal learning disabilities revisited. *Dev Neuropsychol* **17**: 29–47.

De Winter AE, Moore BD, Slopis JM *et al.* (1999). Brain tumors in children with neurofibromatosis: additional neuropsychological morbidity? *Neurooncology* **1**: 275–281.

Denckla MB, Hofman K, Mazzocco MM *et al.* (1996). Relationship between T2-weighted hyperintensities (unidentified bright objects) and lower IQs in children with neurofibromatosis-1. *Am J Med Genet* **67**: 98–102.

Descheemaeker MJ, Ghesquiere P, Symons H *et al.* (2005). Behavioural, academic and neuropsychological profile of normally gifted neurofibromatosis type 1 children. *J Intellect Disabil Res* **49**: 33–46.

DiPaolo DP, Zimmerman RA, Rorke LB *et al.* (1995). Neurofibromatosis type 1: pathologic substrate of high-signal-intensity foci in the brain. *Radiology* **195**: 721–724.

Duffner P, Cohen M, Seidel F *et al.* (1989). The significance of MRI abnormalities in children with neurofibromatosis. *Neurology* **39**: 373–378.

Dunn DW, Roos KL (1989). Magnetic resonance imaging evaluation of learning difficulties and incoordination in neurofibromatosis. *Neurofibromatosis* **2**: 1–5.

Eden GF, Stein JF, Wood HM *et al.* (1996a). Differences in visuospatial judgement in reading-disabled and normal children. *Percept Motor Skills* **82**: 155–177.

Eden GF, VanMeter JW, Rumsey JM *et al.* (1996b). Abnormal processing of visual motion in dyslexia revealed by functional brain imaging [see comments]. *Nature* **382**: 66–69.

Eden GF, VanMeter JW, Rumsey JM *et al.* (1996c). The visual deficit theory of developmental dyslexia. *Neuroimage* **4**: S108–S117.

Eldridge R, Denckla MB, Bien E *et al.* (1989). Neurofibromatosis type 1 (Recklinghausen's disease). Neurologic and cognitive assessment with sibling controls. *Am J Dis Child* **143**: 833–837.

Eliason MJ (1986). Neurofibromatosis: implications for behavior and learning. *Neurofibromatosis* **7**: 175–179.

Eliason MJ (1988). Neuropsychological patterns: neurofibromatosis compared to developmental learning disorders. *Neurofibromatosis* **1**: 17–25.

Ferner RE, Chaudhuri R, Bingham J *et al.* (1993). MRI in neurofibromatosis 1: the nature and evolution of increased intensity T2 weighted lesions and their relationship to intellectual impairment. *J Neurol Neurosurg Psychiatry* **56**: 492–495.

Ferner RE, Hughes RA, Weinman J (1996). Intellectual impairment in neurofibromatosis 1. *J Neurol Sci* **138**: 125–133.

Fletcher JM, Shaywitz SE, Shankweiler DP *et al.* (1994). Cognitive profiles of reading disability: comparisons of discrepancy and low achievement definitions. *J Educ Psychol* **86**: 6–23.

Goh WHS, Khong PL, Leung CSY *et al.* (2004). T2-weighted hyperintensities (unidentified bright objects) in children with neurofibromatosis 1: Their impact on cognitive function. *J Child Neurol* **19**: 853–858.

Greenlee MW, Magnussen S, Reinvang I (2000). Brain regions involved in spatial frequency discrimination: evidence from fMRI. *Exp Brain Res* **132**: 399–403.

Guo HF, Tong JY, Hannan F *et al.* (2000). A neurofibromatosis-1-regulated pathway is required for learning in Drosophila. *Nature* **403**: 895–898.

Gutmann DH, Aylsworth A, Carey JC *et al.* (1997). The diagnostic evaluation and multidisciplinary management of neurofibromatosis 1 and neurofibromatosis 2. *J Am Med Assoc* **278**: 51–57.

Hofman KJ, Harris EL, Bryan RN *et al.* (1994). Neurofibromatosis type 1: the cognitive phenotype. *J Pediatr* **124**: S1–S8.

Itoh T, Magnaldi S, White RM *et al.* (1994). Neurofibromatosis type 1: the evolution of deep gray and white matter MR abnormalities. *AJNR Am J Neuroradiol* **15**: 1513–1519.

Kayl AE, Moore B, Slopis JM *et al.* (2000). Quantitative morphology of the corpus callosum in children with neurofibromatosis and attention deficit hyperactivity disorder. *J Child Neurol* **15**: 90–96.

Korf BR, Rubenstein AE (2005). *Neurofibromatosis: A Handbook for Patients, Families, and Health Care Professionals* (2nd edn.). New York: Thieme Medical Publications.

Kortmann RD, Timmermann B, Taylor RE *et al.* (2003). Current and future strategies in radiotherapy of childhood low-grade glioma of the brain. Part II: Treatment-related late toxicity. *Strahlenther Onkol* **179**: 585.

Leonard CM, Eckert MA, Lombardino LJ *et al.* (2001). Anatomical risk factors for phonological dyslexia. *Cerebral Cortex* **11**: 148–157.

Lindgren SD, Benton AL (1980). Developmental patterns of visuospatial judgment. *J Pediatr Psychol* **5**: 217–225.

Listernick R, Louis DN, Packer RJ *et al.* (1997). Optic pathway gliomas in children with neurofibromatosis 1: consensus statement from the NF1 Optic Pathway Glioma Task Force. *Ann Neurol* **41**: 143–149.

Margariti PN, Blekas K, Katzioti FG *et al.* (2007). Magnetization transfer ratio and volumetric analysis of the brain in macrocephalic patients with neurofibromatosis type 1. *Eur Radiol* **17**: 433–438.

Mazzocco MM, Turner JE, Denckla MB *et al.* (1995). Language and reading deficits associated with neurofibromatosis type 1: evidence for a not-so-nonverbal learning disability. *Dev Neuropsychol* **11**: 503–522.

Moore BD, Denckla MB (1999). Neurofibromatosis. In Yeates K, Ris M, Taylor H (eds.) *Pediatric Neuropsychology: Research, Theory, and Practice.* New York: Guilford Publications, Inc.

Moore BD, Ater JL, Needle MN *et al.* (1994). Neuropsychological profile of children with neurofibromatosis, brain tumor, or both. *J Child Neurol* **9**: 368–377.

Moore BD, Slopis JM, Schomer D *et al.* (1996). Neuropsychological significance of areas of high signal intensity on brain MRIs of children with neurofibromatosis. *Neurology* **46**: 1660–1668.

Moore BD, Slopis JM, Jackson EF *et al.* (2000). Brain volume in children with neurofibromatosis, type 1: relation to neuropsychological status. *Neurology* **54**: 914–920.

Mulvihill JJ, Parry DM, Sherman JL *et al.* (1990). Neurofibromatosis-1 (Recklinghausen Disease) and neurofibromatosis-2 (bilateral acoustic neurofibromatosis) – an update. *Ann Int Med* **113**: 39–52.

National Insitutes of Health (1988). Consensus development conference: neurofibromatosis conference statement. *Arch Neurol* **45**: 575–578.

North K, Joy, P, Yuille D *et al.* (1994). Specific learning disability in children with neurofibromatosis type 1: significance of MRI abnormalities [see comments]. *Neurology* **44**: 878–883.

North KN, Riccardi V, Samango-Sprouse C *et al.* (1997). Cognitive function and academic performance in neurofibromatosis. 1: consensus statement from the NF1 Cognitive Disorders Task Force. *Neurology* **48**: 1121–1127.

Packer RJ, Gutmann DH, Rubenstein A *et al.* (2002). Plexiform neurofibromas in NF1: toward biologic-based therapy. *Neurology* **58**(10): 1461.

Paulesu E, Frith U, Snowling M *et al.* (1996). Is developmental dyslexia a disconnection syndrome? Evidence from PET scanning. *Brain* **119** (Pt 1): 143–157.

Pavol M, Hiscock M, Massman P *et al.* (2006). Neuropsychological function in adults with von Recklinghausen's neurofibromatosis. *Dev Neuropsychol* **29**: 509–526.

Pugh KR, Shaywitz BA, Shaywitz SE *et al.* (1996). Cerebral organization of component processes in reading. *Brain* **119**: 1221–1238.

Riccardi VM (1981). Von Recklinghausen neurofibromatosis. *N Engl J Med* **305**: 1617–1627.

Riccardi V, Eichner J (1986). Neurofibromatosis: *Phenotype, Natural History, and Pathogenesis.* Baltimore, MD: Johns Hopkins University.

Rourke BP (1989). *Nonverbal Learning Disabilities.* New York: Guilford Press.

Said SM, Yeh TL, Greenwood RS *et al.* (1996). MRI morphometric analysis and neuropsychological function in patients with neurofibromatosis. *Neuroreport* **7**: 1941–1944.

Schrimsher GW, Billingsley RL, Slopis JM *et al.* (2003). Visual-spatial performance deficits in children with neurofibromatosis type-1. *Am J Med Genetics Part A* **120A**: 326–330.

Sevick RJ, Barkovich AJ, Edwards MS *et al.* (1992). Evolution of white matter lesions in neurofibromatosis type 1: MR findings. *AJR Am J Roentgenol* **159**: 171–175.

Sharif S, Ferner R, Birch JM *et al.* (2006). Second primary tumors in neurofibromatosis I patients treated for optic glioma: substantial risks after radiotherapy. *J Clin Oncol* **24**: 2570–2575.

Shaywitz SE, Shaywitz BA, Pugh KR *et al.* (1998). Functional disruption in the organization of the brain for reading in dyslexia. *Proc Natl Acad Sci USA* **95**: 2636–2641.

Silva AJ, Frankland PW, Marowit Z *et al.* (1997). A mouse model for the learning and memory deficits associated with neurofibromatosis type I. *Nat Genet* **15**: 281–284.

Stanovich KE (1988). Explaining the differences between the dyslexic and the garden-variety poor reader: the phonological-core variable-difference model. *J Learn Disabil* **21**: 590–604.

Temple E, Poldrack RA, Protopapas A *et al.* (2000). Disruption of the neural response to rapid acoustic stimuli in dyslexia: evidence from functional MRI. *Proc Natl Acad Sci USA*, **97**: 13907–13912.

Temple E, Poldrack RA, Salidis J *et al.* (2001). Disrupted neural responses to phonological and orthographic processing in dyslexic children: an fMRI study. *Neuroreport* **12**: 299–307.

Uhlmann EJ, Gutmann DH (2001). Tumor suppressor gene regulation of cell growth – recent insights into neurofibromatosis 1 and 2 gene function. *Cell Biochem Biophys* **34**: 61–78.

Viskochil D, Buchberg AM, Xu G *et al.* (1990). Deletions and a translocation interrupt a cloned gene at the neurofibromatosis type 1 locus. *Cell* **62**: 187–192.

von Deimling A, Krone W, Menon AG (1995). Neurofibromatosis type 1: pathology, clinical features and molecular genetics. *Brain Pathol* **5**: 153–162.

Wadsby M, Lindehammar H, Eeg-Olofsson O (1989). Neurofibromatosis in childhood: neuropsychological aspects. *Neurofibromatosis* **2**: 251–260.

Wallace MR, Marchuk DA, Andersen LB *et al.* (1990). Type 1 neurofibromatosis gene: identification of a large transcript disrupted in three NF1 patients [published erratum appears in *Science* 1990 Dec 21; **250**(4988): 1749]. *Science* **249**: 181–186.

Zhu Y, Romero MI, Ghosh P *et al.* (2001). Ablation of NF1 function in neurons induces abnormal development of cerebral cortex and reactive gliosis in the brain. *Genes Dev* **15**: 859–876.

Zvulunov A, Weitz R, Metzker A (1998). Neurofibromatosis type 1 in childhood: evaluation of clinical and epidemiologic features as predictive factors for severity. *Clin Pediatr (Phila)* **37**: 295–299.

16

Hematological malignancies

Melissa Friedman and Mercedes Fernandez

Introduction

Development of effective treatments for cancer has significantly improved survival rates for hematological cancer patients. For example, in 1964 the 5-year survival rate for acute lymphoblastic leukemia (ALL) was 3%; in 1995–2001, it was 86% (Leukemia and Lymphoma Society, 2005; Ries *et al.*, 2005). However, survival is often associated with negative effects on cognitive functioning which interfere with patients' current and future functional status.

In patients with hematological malignancies, risk factors for cognitive disorders are present during all stages of the disease and treatment process. Risk factors include cancer treatments, anemia and fatigue, immune response activity, central nervous system (CNS) involvement of the primary malignancy (especially in the case of ALL), disease and treatment complications affecting the CNS such as infection, hemorrhage, degeneration and leukoencephalopathy, and cognitive and psychiatric disorders that occur in the general population independent of having cancer.

Information on the long-term neuropsychological effects of cancer therapies is an important component of not only the informed consent process, but also the treatment planning process. In the risk-benefit analysis for selecting treatment, survival rates alone may be insufficient because some treatments are associated with significant depletion of cognitive and functional abilities.

Neurological complications independent of cognitive deficits

Neurological complications, independent of cognitive complaints, are common in hematological cancer patients. Neurological complications have been reported in 11%–65% of hematopoietic stem cell transplantation (HSCT) patients (Faraci *et al.*, 2002; Gallardo *et al.*, 1996; Graus *et al.*, 1996; Harder *et al.*, 2002; Sostak *et al.*, 2003) and may be the main cause of death in 8.5%–26% of recipients (Faraci *et al.*, 2002; Gallardo *et al.*, 1996; Snider *et al.*, 1994; Sostak *et al.*, 2003). White matter abnormalities or focal lesions have been observed on MRI in up to 50% of cases (Harder *et al.*, 2002; Sostak *et al.*, 2003).

Neurological complications may include neoplasms, infections, encephalopathy, seizures, and strokes. Neoplasms of hematopoietic or lymphoid origin may compress brain structures, the extradural region, peripheral nerves, or may directly invade the meninges (i.e., leptomeningeal infiltration). Acute lymphoblastic leukemia is associated with a particular propensity for leptomeningeal involvement; routine prophylactic CNS treatment is frequently instituted in cases of ALL. In addition to neoplasms, viral or fungal infections (e.g.,

Cognition and Cancer, eds. Christina A. Meyers and James R. Perry. Published by Cambridge University Press.
© Cambridge University Press 2008.

aspergillus) may occur as a result of treatment-induced immunosuppression and may lead to encephalitis, meningitis or peripheral neuropathies (Recht & Mrugala, 2003). Metabolic encephalopathy has been reported in 3%–37% of HSCT patients. Progressive, treatment-induced leukoencephalopathy has been reported in 1%–2% of patients (Antonini et al., 1998; Antunes et al., 2000; Graus et al., 1996). Seizures occur in approximately 10% of HSCT patients, and cerebrovascular infarctions or hemorrhages in 6% (Gallardo et al., 1996).

Identified risk factors for neurological complications in HSCT patients include older age, prior treatment with intrathecal methotrexate (MTX), long-term use of ciclosporin, use of total body irradiation (TBI) in the conditioning regimen, corticosteroid medication (Faraci et al., 2002; Sostak et al., 2003), and allogeneic transplantation. Among allogeneic recipients, those with a donor who has a matching human leukocyte antigen (HLA) display the lowest risk for complications (De Brabander et al., 2000). Neurological complications have been associated with acute and severe graft verses host disease (GVHD) (Faraci et al., 2002; Sostak et al., 2003), as well as chronic GVHD which has been linked to hypertension and small vessel disease (Padovan et al., 1998).

Methotrexate, used as a systemic or intrathecal cancer treatment for hematological malignancy, is associated with symptoms ranging from fatigue and dizziness to encephalopathy, with encephalopathic symptoms including hemiparesis, ataxia, and seizures. Methotrexate neurotoxicity can become chronic, lasting months to years, and may include leukoencephalopathy, which can lead to coma and death (Vezmer et al., 2003).

Ciclosporin, administered as an immunosuppressive agent to minimize GVHD, has been associated with a range of neurological complications and symptoms. These include cerebellar symptoms, confusion (Atkinson et al., 1984), tremor, EEG and MRI abnormalities (Shah, 1999), posterior leukoencephalopathy evidenced by severe oculogyric crisis (Antunes et al., 1999), and seizures leading to death (Velu et al., 1985). Discontinuing ciclosporin treatment may allow for reversal of neurological symptoms (Atkinson et al., 1984; Shah, 1999). Yet, discontinuing or lowering ciclosporin dose, or implementing new medications to manage neurological side-effects, may place patients at increased risk for other life-threatening complications (Uckan et al., 2005).

Cognitive deficits

Studies have provided valuable information that quantifies the impact of hematological cancer and treatment on patients' cognitive functioning, and can lead to improvement in interventions and outcomes. Nevertheless, methodological challenges of studies in this population warrant caution in their interpretation. Most studies do not use random assignment of patients to treatment groups, and treatments are often inextricably confounded with disease variables, such as severity, co-morbidity or underlying disease process. Small sample sizes may lead to underestimation of group differences due to low statistical power, or overestimation of group differences when multiple statistical tests or comparisons are conducted. Cross-sectional studies that compare outcome between groups after treatment do not allow the identification of pre-treatment group differences, and do not allow for the identification of intra-individual factors that may account for post-treatment findings. In longitudinal studies, subject attrition carries the confound that patients evaluated at follow-up represent a different group than those who do not complete the study. Finally, many patients receive multiple treatments or experience multiple disease complications, which makes it difficult to attribute any identified cognitive impairments to a single cause.

Cognitive effects of treatment

Most patients with hematological malignancies are exposed at various phases in their illness to neurotoxic cancer therapies, including chemotherapy, radiation, HSCT, and biological therapies, all of which have been associated with adverse effects on cognition (Harder *et al.*, 2005; for reviews, see Anderson-Hanley *et al.*, 2003; Armstrong, 2001; Lee *et al.*, 2004; Meyers & Valentine, 1995; Mulhern & Butler, 2004). In addition, the reader is referred to Chapters 7–9 in this volume discussing treatment effects.

Chemotherapy

In cancer patients, systemic chemotherapy has been associated with cognitive dysfunction not only in the scientific medical literature but also in the popular media, which has referred to such dysfunction as *chemobrain* and *chemofog*. Systemic chemotherapy agents are generally introduced through oral or intravenous routes. In addition, patients with ALL may receive intrathecal chemotherapy or cranial radiotherapy (RT) in addition to systemic chemotherapy, to prevent CNS metastatic disease.

In adults, chemotherapy is associated with cognitive effects on psychomotor function and memory which are subtle but interfere with everyday functioning, and may still be present 10 years after chemotherapy is completed (Ahles & Saykin, 2001; Ahles *et al.*, 2002). In a cross-sectional comparison of neuropsychological performance in breast cancer and lymphoma patients receiving systemic chemotherapy versus local radiation therapy, systemic chemotherapy was associated with lower performance in a subset of patients, particularly on measures of psychomotor functioning and verbal memory. Despite the group differences, however, both treatment groups performed within normal limits overall, suggesting that the effects of chemotherapy on cognition were subtle. Group differences were not accounted for by depression, anxiety or fatigue (Ahles *et al.*, 2002), but may have been related to disease factors necessitating systemic chemotherapy as opposed to localized treatment.

Another study (Harder *et al.*, 2005) evaluated neuropsychological functioning of 183 hematological cancer patients, 101 of whom were scheduled to undergo HSCT, and nearly all ($n = 173$) of whom had received at least one course of chemother-

apy. A subset of these patients displayed cognitive impairments on tests assessing psychomotor functions, and the ability to copy and to later recall a complex figure. However, in contrast to previous findings (Ahles *et al.*, 2002), these investigators did not identify significant differences between patients with a history of systemic chemotherapy as compared to those with local radiation only. Neither did they observe differences between patients who had received only one course of systemic chemotherapy as compared to those who had received multiple courses. The investigators concluded that chemotherapy was probably not the only contributor to the observed cognitive deficits in this hematological cancer population.

In children, cognitive deficits observed at a given time point should be viewed in the context of neuropsychological development. Although some studies do not document chemotherapy-related changes on neuropsychological tests (Rodgers *et al.*, 2003) or MRI measures of hippocampal volume (Hill *et al.*, 2004), other studies associate chemotherapy with modest cognitive deficits (Espy *et al.*, 2001; Kaemingk *et al.*, 2004; Kingma *et al.*, 2002). In children with ALL, receiving MTX (intrathecal and/or high-dose IV administration) without RT is associated with slowed processing speed, but little or no effect on accuracy or on attentional and information-processing tasks (Buizer *et al.*, 2005; Mennes *et al.*, 2005). Kaemingk *et al.* (2004) documented math weaknesses in survivors of ALL who had completed treatment with systemic chemotherapy and intrathecal prophylaxis including cytosine arabinoside, hydrocortisone and MTX, to prevent CNS metastases. Survivors performed below normal limits on one math test, and lower than their matched controls but within normal limits on four other math tests. Of note, illness-related school absences may contribute to or even account for the modest deficits in these patients.

The modest findings identified in research studies may underestimate the true effect of chemotherapy on patients' lives. The quiet and controlled neuropsychological testing environment does not mimic the distractions and multiple cognitive demands often present in everyday situations. Additionally, the neuropsychological tests used may not be sensitive enough to detect cognitive impairments affecting patients' functioning. In children, cognitive deficits may manifest themselves at a time point in academic development beyond the testing. Finally, it may be that only a subset of patients in these studies is vulnerable to chemotherapy-induced deficits. Research on lymphoma and breast cancer patients suggests that the ε4 allele of the apolipoprotein E (APOE) gene, which predisposes people to Alzheimer's disease (Richard & Amouyel, 2001), may also predispose some patients to chemotherapy-induced cognitive deficits (Ahles et al., 2003).

Radiation therapy

Cranial radiotherapy (CRT), like intrathecal MTX, is used as prophylaxis in the treatment of ALL to prevent CNS metastases. Most studies evaluating the neuropsychological effects of RT in hematological patients are conducted on children with ALL. Some research suggests that treatment in young children (i.e., before 36 months of age) is associated with greater cognitive deficits than treatment in older children (i.e., after 36 months of age) (Waber et al., 2001).

Until the 1980s, 24 Gy was the standard RT dose for children with ALL. Due to the recognition of cognitive deficits associated with this, lower doses (e.g., 12–18 Gy) are now used (Oeffinger & Hudson, 2004). At these lower doses of RT, cognitive deficits have been detected. One study assessed the intellectual, academic, attention and memory performance in children at least 5 years after their diagnosis of ALL (Spiegler et al., 2006), all of whom were treated with a uniform chemotherapy protocol and intrathecal therapy. Those whose CNS prophylaxis consisted additionally of RT performed more poorly on most cognitive measures compared with those receiving high- or very-high-dose intravenous MTX; the authors concluded that avoidance of RT in the treatment strategy is associated with good long-term neurocognitive outcomes (Spiegler

et al., 2006). Nevertheless, the effect of RT is difficult to quantify because it is often administered in combination with intrathecal MTX (Waber et al., 1995), and there may be a synergistic effect of treatments. In fact, RT may not induce negative cognitive effects (Mulhern et al., 1992), and any negative impact of RT in ALL treatment should be evaluated relative to the improved protection that it provides against CNS relapse (Langer et al., 2002). Also, consistent with an emerging literature on genetic vulnerability to treatment-induced neurotoxicity (e.g., Ahles et al., 2003), particular genotypes may predispose ALL patients to RT-induced cognitive deficits (Krajinovic et al., 2005).

Hematopoietic stem cell transplantation

Hematopoetic stem cell transplantation (HSCT) refers to the two-part process of administering a conditioning regimen of intensive high-dose chemotherapy or radiation, followed by infusing the patient with stem cells obtained from a donor's marrow or peripheral blood, for the purposes of hematopoietic rescue. HSCT is based on the rationale that eradication of cancer cells is more likely if the chemotherapy and radiation doses are not limited by their lethal effects on the patient's blood production system. In HSCT, patients are administered treatment regimens (conditioning regimens) in intensive doses, which leave patients severely vulnerable to infection, anemia, and hemorrhage (due to lack of platelets). After administration of such otherwise lethal treatment doses, patients are infused with a donor's blood stem cells as a method of restoring normal blood cell production.

Timing of HSCT during the course of a patient's disease varies according to medical and practical considerations, including the disease, prognosis, medical status, history of complications, availability of a compatible donor, and age. Although occasionally patients receive HSCT prior to any other cancer treatment, patients frequently receive HSCT during first remission, first relapse, second remission, and so on. Therefore, many patients who undergo HSCT have been exposed to potentially neurotoxic treatments before their transplant.

In adults, cross-sectional and prospective studies indicate that many HSCT patients display pre-transplant cognitive deficits in the areas of memory, complex attention, and psychomotor speed (Andrykowski *et al.*, 1992; Friedman, 2001; Harder *et al.*, 2005, 2006; Peper *et al.*, 2000), which worsen during the hospital stay (Ahles *et al.*, 1996; Meyers *et al.*, 1994) but are not significantly different from baseline at or beyond a 1-year post-HSCT follow-up (Friedman, 2001; Harder *et al.*, 2006). Despite post-HSCT improvements, cognitive abilities may not return to normal levels; memory impairments have been documented 8 months after transplantation (Meyers *et al.*, 1994), and executive and information processing deficits up to 8 years afterwards (Harder *et al.*, 2002). Patients also experience effects on quality of life indices, including sleep and energy deficits noted 18 months after transplantation (Andrykowski *et al.*, 1997), and inability to work (Stalfelt & Zettervall, 1997).

In children, prospective studies indicate cognitive deficits associated with HSCT. Kramer *et al.* (1997) found that IQ and behavioral adaptation declined from pre-transplant to a 1-year follow-up evaluation with no additional decline detected after 3 years. Phipps *et al.* (2000) did not identify decline in IQ or achievement measures between the pre-transplant baseline and the 1- and 3-year follow-up evaluations, but found that achievement scores were generally one-half to two-thirds of a standard deviation below the normative mean, and this was not attributable to prior therapy. Data suggest that younger children (under 36 months of age) at the time of transplantation display greater vulnerability to cognitive impairment than older children (6 years or older) (Kramer *et al.*, 1997; Phipps *et al.*, 2000). Younger children may be more vulnerable to the effects of psychosocial variables, such as isolation and hospitalization, on neuropsychological functioning and behavioral adaptation. Additionally, brain development may be more susceptible to treatment side-effects at earlier stages of development than at later stages.

Biological treatments

Biological response modifiers such as interferon alpha (IFN-α), commonly used to treat chronic myelogenous leukemia, and interleukin-2 (IL-2) have been associated with a higher risk for cognitive impairment than other forms of treatment (Meyers & Abbruzzese, 1992). Patients treated with IFN-α display poorer cognitive speed and mood than those treated with chemotherapy (Pavol *et al.*, 1995). Neurotoxic effects are seen at low doses of IFN-α, and cognitive and mood functioning are correlated with length of time on treatment (Meyers, 1999).

Treatment with IFN-α has been associated with memory and executive dysfunction and slowed processing speed that cannot be accounted for by the frequently co-occurring cytokine-induced depression. These deficits are severe enough to interfere with occupational and daily functioning, and may be exacerbated by a high cumulative IFN-α dose or concurrent chemotherapy. The memory deficits are associated with executive and information-processing dysfunction, rather than hippocampal damage (Scheibel *et al.*, 2004). This pattern is consistent with frontal-subcortical pathology as seen in Parkinson's disease, and, in fact, some patients on IFN-α treatment have been reported to display extrapyramidal signs including rigidity, tremor, and masked facies (Meyers *et al.*, 1991).

Patients receiving IFN-α experience neurovegetative symptoms such as appetite change and fatigue around the 2nd week of treatment, with mood and cognitive disturbance appearing around the 8th to 12th weeks of treatment (Capuron *et al.*, 2002). Neuropsychological impairments have been observed from 3 weeks to 2 years after discontinuation of the treatment, and the deficits may not always be reversible (Meyers *et al.*, 1991).

Anemia and iron deficiency

Anemia is a concern for hematological cancer patients due to the effects of both the cancer itself and the treatment on the blood production system. Anemia is associated with increased fatigue and cognitive decline particularly in functions related to attention and memory. Jacobsen *et al.* (2004) examined the relationship between hemoglobin levels, fatigue, and cognitive functioning in adult cancer patients undergoing repeated chemotherapy administrations. In patients whose hemoglobin declined to below normal levels, the amount of hemoglobin decline was related to the level of fatigue and to deficits in attention, executive functioning, and visual memory. In elderly cancer patients, chemotherapy-related anemia may adversely affect not only cognitive but also functional status, and successful anemia treatment with recombinant human erythropoeitin (rHuEPO) supplementation over the course of chemotherapy may help to preserve functional independence (Mancuso *et al.*, 2006).

In non-cancer patients, reports of mental status changes associated with anemia date back to the 1830s (Stivelman, 2000). Thalassemia, an inherited form of anemia associated with faulty synthesis of hemoglobin, has been associated with transient ischemic attacks, silent infarctions, and in rare cases stroke (Armstrong, 2005). In end-stage renal disease, anemia has been associated with changes not only in cognitive functioning (Martin-Lester, 1997; Temple *et al.*, 1995) but also in measures of event related brain potentials (ERPs) (Brown *et al.*, 1991; Marsh *et al.*, 1991; Nissenson, 1992), which are direct electrophysiological measures of brain functioning. Furthermore, successful treatment of anemia with rHuEPO in renal patients is associated with improved neuropsychological performance on measures of attention and working memory (Marsh *et al.*, 1991) and with increased amplitudes and decreased latencies of the P300 component of the ERP (Singh *et al.*, 2006). In healthy adults, artificially induced anemia has been associated with increased latency of the P300 (Weiskopf *et al.*, 2005); it has also been linked to slowed performance on the Digit-Symbol Substitution Test, which may be reversed by transfusing individuals with either fresh or stored autologous erythrocytes (Weiskopf *et al.*, 2006).

In children, cognitive deficits may improve once the anemia resolves (Bruner *et al.*, 1996;

Metallinos-Katsaras *et al.*, 2004), although deficits are not always reversible. For instance, Walter (1994) described two studies, one conducted in Chile and the other in Costa Rica, demonstrating the negative cognitive effects of anemia in infants. Fewer anemic children than controls successfully completed tasks assessing language comprehension and balance. Follow-up studies at 5 years of age revealed that those who were anemic as infants scored lower on neuropsychological tests than controls, suggesting that anemia during critical periods of neural development may have enduring negative effects.

Immune response

The normal immune response to illness consists of inflammatory cytokine activity, which may underlie neuropsychological changes in cancer patients (Lee *et al.*, 2004). Cytokines are chemicals secreted in the body which act as messengers between immune cells. Proinflammatory cytokines, including tumor necrosis factor alpha (TNF-α), IL-1 β, and IL-6, are proteins that augment the body's immune response by helping to speed the elimination of pathogens and the resolution of the inflammatory challenge. They communicate with white blood cells, causing them to become activated and to respond to infection and inflammation. They have also been linked to stress reactions, hormone and neurotransmitter activity, and "sickness behaviors" such as increased sleep, decreased appetite and decreased sexual drive (Watkins, 2000). Proinflammatory cytokines and their receptors have been detected in various areas of the brain, including the hippocampus and hypothalamus. They may enter the brain from outside of the CNS, or may be synthesized and released from within the CNS. Hematopoietic cytokines, such as IL-3, IL-5 and colony-stimulating factors, are involved in altering the hematopoietic response, and may play a role in hematological malignancies (see Kronfol & Remick, 2000 for a review).

The immune response alone, independent of cancer treatment, may have an impact on cognition. In a group of patients with acute myelogenous leukemia or myelodysplastic syndrome, cognitive impairment and fatigue were observed before the initiation of treatment, and poorer cognitive performance was associated with higher levels of circulating cytokines (Meyers *et al.*, 2005). Increased levels of proinflammatory cytokines and poorer performance status rating have been observed in untreated Hodgkin's disease patients (Seymour *et al.*, 1997).

In healthy humans, experimental activation of the immune response produces memory disturbance, anxiety and depression, even in the absence of subjective symptoms of sickness, and these neuropsychological changes are correlated with cytokine secretion levels (Reichenberg *et al.*, 2001). In neonates, cytokine secretion levels have been associated with impaired cerebral metabolism during the neonatal period and with abnormal neurodevelopment at 30 months of age (Bartha *et al.*, 2004).

Treatment for cognitive and emotional dysfunction

Due to the multiple contributing etiological factors in cancer-related symptomatology, an individualized, multidisciplinary treatment approach addressing cognitive, emotional, and physical symptoms is recommended.

Psychosocial interventions often play an important role in remediation of cognitive deficits or overall functioning. Stress management techniques, breathing exercises, and aerobic exercise may be useful for improving fatigue and quality of life (Kim & Kim, 2005; Wilson *et al.*, 2006). Patient and caregiver education about cancer- and treatment-related cognitive symptoms are also recommended. Children with cognitive and behavioral problems following cancer treatment should be identified for special education services whenever possible, especially since the rate of utilization of special education services is not always consistent with the need in this population (Buizer *et al.*, 2006). In childhood cancer survivors, exercises for remediating atten-

tion and information processing may help improve these abilities (Butler & Copeland, 2002).

Regarding psychiatric medications, paroxetine has been found effective at reducing symptoms of depression, anxiety, cognitive dysfunction, and pain in melanoma patients receiving IFN-α therapy, in a double-blind, placebo-controlled randomized trial (Capuron *et al.*, 2002). Methylphenidate has been found effective at reducing social and attentional deficits in children with ALL and brain tumors (Mulhern *et al.*, 2004). Treatment issues are addressed in greater detail in Chapter 18.

Summary

Cognitive deficits have been documented in hematological cancer patients. Such deficits may be attributable to cancer treatment, underlying disease factors such as anemia, or immune response mechanisms. Additionally, co-occurring psychiatric or neurological conditions independent of the cancer may contribute to cognitive deficits. The studies reviewed suggest that cognitive deficits attributable to the cancer or its treatment are often subtle as detected on neuropsychological testing, but severe enough to interfere with everyday or occupational functioning. However, not all patients experience neuropsychological deficits, and any deficits should be evaluated in the context of the increased opportunity for survival and sometimes cure that many treatments offer. Additionally, many interventions exist to minimize the impact of neuropsychological disturbances on the daily lives of patients.

REFERENCES

Ahles TA, Saykin A (2001). Cognitive effects of standard-dose chemotherapy in patients with cancer. *Cancer Invest* **19(8)**: 812–820.

Ahles TA, Tope DM, Furstenberg C, Hann D, Mills L (1996). Psychologic and neuropsychologic impact of autologous bone marrow transplantation. *J Clin Oncol* **14**: 1457–1462.

Ahles TA, Saykin AJ, Furstenberg CT *et al.* (2002). Neuropsychologic impact of standard dose systemic chemotherapy in long term survivors of breast cancer and lymphoma. *J Clin Oncol* **20**: 485–493.

Ahles TA, Saykin AJ, Noll WW *et al.* (2003). The relationship of APOE genotype to neuropsychological performance in long-term cancer survivors treated with standard dose chemotherapy. *Psychooncology* **12**: 612–619.

Anderson-Hanley C, Sherman ML, Riggs R, Agocha VB, Compas BE (2003). Neuropsychological effects of treatments for adults with cancer: a meta-analysis and review of the literature. *J Int Neuropsychol Soc* **9**: 967–982.

Andrykowski MA, Schmitt FA, Gregg ME, Brady MJ, Lamb DG, Henslee-Downey PJ (1992). Neuropsychologic impairment in adult bone marrow transplant candidates. *Cancer* **70**: 2288–2297.

Andrykowski MA, Carpenter JS, Greiner CB *et al.* (1997). Energy level and sleep quality following bone marrow transplantation. *Bone Marrow Transplant* **20**: 669–679.

Antonini G, Ceschin V, Morino S *et al.* (1998). Early neurologic complications following allogeneic bone marrow transplant for leukemia: a prospective study. *Neurology* **50**: 1441–1445.

Antunes NL, Small TN, George D, Farid B, Lis E (1999). Posterior leukoencephalopathy syndrome may not be reversible. *Pediatr Neurol* **20**: 241–243.

Antunes NL, Boulad FL, Prasad V, Rosenblum M, Lis E, Souweidane M (2000). Rolandic encephalopathy and epilepsia partialis continua following bone marrow transplant. *Bone Marrow Transplant* **26**: 917–919.

Armstrong FD (2001). Acute and long term neurodevelopmental outcomes in children following bone marrow transplantation. *Front Biosci* **6**: 6–12.

Armstrong FD (2005). Thalassemia and learning: neurocognitive functioning in children. *Ann N Y Acad Sci* **1054**: 283–289.

Atkinson K, Biggs J, Darveniza P, Boland J, Concannon A, Dodds A (1984). Cyclosporine associated central nervous system toxicity after allogeneic bone marrow transplantation. *Transplantation* **38**: 34–37.

Bartha AI, Foster-Barber A, Miller SP *et al.* (2004). Neonatal encephalopathy: association of cytokines with MR spectroscopy and outcome. *Pediatr Res* **56**(6): 960–966.

Brown WS, Marsh JT, Wolcott D *et al.* (1991). Cognitive function, mood and P3 latency: effects of the amelioration of anemia in dialysis patients. *Neuropsychologia* **29**: 35–45.

Bruner AB, Joffe A, Duggan AK, Casella JF, Brandt J (1996). Randomised study of cognitive effects of iron supplementation in non-anaemic iron-deficient adolescent girls. *Lancet* **348**: 992–996.

Buizer AI, de Sonneville LMJ, Van Den Heuvel-Eibrink MM, Veerman AJP (2005). Chemotherapy and attentional dysfunction in survivors of childhood acute lymphoblastic leukemia: effect of treatment intensity. *Pediatr Blood Cancer* **45**: 281–290.

Buizer AI, de Sonneville LMJ, Van Den Heuvel-Eibrink MM, Veerman AJP (2006). Behavioral and educational limitations after chemotherapy for childhood acute lymphoblastic leukemia or Wilms tumor. *Cancer* **106**: 2067–2075.

Butler RW, Copeland DR (2002). Attentional processes and their remediation in children treated for cancer: a literature review and the development of a therapeutic approach. *J Int Neuropsychol Soc* **8**: 115–124.

Capuron L, Gumnick JF, Musselman DL, Lawson DH *et al.* (2002). Neurobehavioral effects of interferon alpha in cancer patients: phenomenology and paroxetine responsiveness of symptom dimensions. *Neuropsychopharmacology* **26**: 643–652.

De Brabander C. Cornelissen J, Smitt, P, Vecht CJ, van den Bent MJ (2000). Increased incidence of neurological complications in patients receiving an allogenic bone marrow transplantation from alternative donors. *J Neurol Neurosurg Psychiatry* **68**: 36–40.

Espy KA, Moore IM, Kaufmann PM, Kramer JH, Matthay K, Hutter JJ (2001). Chemotherapeutic CNS prophylaxis and neuropsychologic change in children with acute lymphoblastic leukemia: a prospective study. *J Pediatr Psychol* **26**: 1–9.

Faraci M, Lanino E, Dini G *et al.* (2002). Severe neurologic complications after hematopoietic stem cell transplantation in children. *Neurology* **59**: 1895–1904.

Friedman MA (2001). Neuropsychological functioning in hematopoietic stem cell transplantation. Dissertation Abstracts. Houston, TX: University of Houston.

Gallardo D, Ferra C, Berlanga JJ *et al.* (1996). Neurologic complications after allogeneic bone marrow transplantation. *Bone Marrow Transplant* **18**: 1135–1139.

Graus F, Saiz A, Sierra J *et al.* (1996). Neurologic complications of autologous and allogeneic bone marrow transplantation in patients with leukemia. *Neurology* **46**: 1004–1009.

Harder H, Cornelissen JJ, Van Gool AR *et al.* (2002). Cognitive functioning and quality of life in long-term adult survivors of bone marrow transplantation. *Cancer* **95**: 183–192.

Harder H, van Gool AR, Cornelissen JJ *et al.* (2005). Assessment of pre-treatment cognitive performance in adult bone marrow or haematopoietic stem cell transplantation patients: a comparative study. *Eur J Cancer* **41**: 1007–1016.

Harder H, Duivenvoorden HJ, van Good AR *et al.* (2006). Neurocognitive functions and quality of life in haematological patients receiving haematopoietic stem cell grafts: a one-year follow-up pilot study. *J Clin Exp Neuropsychol* **28**: 283–293.

Hill DE, Ciesielski KT, Hart BL, Jung RE (2004). MRI morphometric and neuropsychological correlates of long-term memory in survivors of childhood leukemia. *Pediatr Blood Cancer* **42**: 611–617.

Jacobsen PB, Garland LL, Booth-Jones M *et al.* (2004). Relationship of hemoglobin levels to fatigue and cognitive functioning among cancer patients receiving chemotherapy. *J Pain Symptom Manage* **28**: 7–18.

Kaemingk KL, Carey ME, Moore IM, Herzer M, Hutter JJ (2004). Math weaknesses in survivors of acute lymphoblastic leukemia compared to healthy children. *Child Neuropsychol* **10**: 14–23.

Kim S-D, Kim H-S (2005). Effects of a relaxation breathing exercise on fatigue in haemopoietic stem cell transplantation patieints. *J Clin Nurs* **14**: 51–55.

Kingma A, Van Dommelen RI, Mooyaart EL, Wilmink JT, Deelman BG, Kamps WA (2002). No major cognitive impairment in young children with acute lymphoblastic leukemia using chemotherapy only: a prospective longitudinal study. *J Pediatr Hematol-Oncol* **24**: 106–114.

Krajinovic M, Robaey P, Chiasson S *et al.* (2005). Polymorphisms of genes controlling homocysteine levels and IQ score following the treatment for childhood ALL. *Pharmacogenomics* **6**: 293–302.

Kramer JH, Crittenden MR, DeSantes K, Cowan MJ (1997). Cognitive and adaptive behavior one and three years following bone marrow transplantation. *Bone Marrow Transplant* **19**: 607–613.

Kronfol Z, Remick DG (2000). Cytokines and the brain: implications for clinical psychiatry. *Am J Psychiatry* **157**: 683–694.

Langer T, Martus P, Ottensmeier H, Hertzberg H, Beck JD, Meier W (2002). CNS late-effects after ALL therapy in childhood. Part III: Neuropsychological performance in long-term survivors of childhood ALL: impairments of concentration, attention, and memory. *Med Pediatr Oncol* **38**: 320–328.

Lee BN, Dantzer R, Langley KE *et al.* (2004). A cytokine-based neuroimmunologic mechanism of cancer-related symptoms. *Neuroimmunomodulation* **11**: 279–292.

Leukemia and Lymphoma Society (2005). Facts 2005. Available online at www.leukemia-lymphoma.org, accessed 4 April 2008.

Mancuso A, Migliorino M, De Santis S, Saponiero A, De Marinis F (2006). Correlation between anemia and functional/cognitive capacity in elderly lung cancer patients treated with chemotherapy. *Ann Oncol* **17**(1): 146–150.

Marsh JT, Brown WS, Wolcott D *et al.* (1991). rHuEPO treatment improves brain and cognitive function of anemic dialysis patients. *Kidney Int* **39**: 155–163.

Martin-Lester M (1997). Cognitive function in dialysis patients. *ANNA J* **24**: 359–365.

Mennes M, Stiers P, Vandenbussche E *et al.* (2005). Attention and information processing in survivors of childhood acute lymphoblastic leukemia treated with chemotherapy only. *Pediatr Blood Cancer* **44**: 478–486.

Metallinos-Katsaras E, Valassi-Adamn E, Dewey KG, Lonnerdal B, Stamoulakatou A, Pollitt E (2004). Effect of iron supplementation on cognition in Greek preschoolers. *Eur J Clin Nutri* **58**: 1532–1542.

Meyers CA (1999). Mood and cognitive disorders in cancer patients receiving cytokine therapy. In Dantzer R (ed.) *Cytokines, Stress and Depression.* New York: Kluwer Academic/Plenum Publishers.

Meyers CA, Abbruzzese JL (1992). Cognitive functioning in cancer patients: effect of previous treatment. *Neurology* **42**: 434–436.

Meyers CA, Valentine AD (1995). Neurological and psychiatric adverse effects of immunological therapy. *CNS Drugs* **3**: 56–68.

Meyers CA, Scheibel RS, Forman AD (1991). Persistent neurotoxicity of systematically administered interferon alpha. *Neurology* **41**: 672–676.

Meyers CA, Weitzner M, Byrne K, Valentine A, Champlin RE, Przepiorka D (1994). Evaluation of the neurobehavioral functioning of patients before, during, and after bone marrow transplantation. *J Clin Oncol* **12**: 820–826.

Meyers CA, Albitar M, Estey E (2005). Cognitive impairment, fatigue, and cytokine levels in patients with acute myelogenous leukemia or myelodysplastic syndrome. *Cancer* **104**: 788–793.

Mulhern RK, Butler RW (2004). Neurocognitive sequelae of childhood cancers and their treatment. *Pediatr Rehabit* **7**: 1–14.

Mulhern RK, Ochs J, Fairclough D (1992) Deterioration of intellect among children surviving leukemia: IQ test changes modify estimates of treatment toxicity. *J Consult Clin Psychol* **60**: 477–480.

Mulhern RK, Khan RB, Kaplan S *et al.* (2004). Short term efficacy of methylphenidate: a randomized double-blind, placebo-controlled trial among survivors of childhood cancer. *J Clin Oncol* **22**: 4795–4803.

Nissenson AR (1992). Epoetin and cognitive function. *Am J Kidney Dis* **20**: 21–24.

Oeffinger KC, Hudson MM (2004). Long term complications following childhood and adolescent cancer: foundations for providing risk-based health care for survivors. *CA Cancer J Clin* **54**: 208–236.

Padovan CS, Yousry TA, Schleuning M, Holler E, Kolb H-J, Straube A (1998). Neurological and neuroradiological findings in long-term survivors of allogeneic bone marrow transplantation. *Ann Neurol* **43**: 627–633.

Pavol MA, Meyers CA, Rexer JL, Valentine AD, Mattis PJ, Talpaz M (1995). Pattern of neurobehavioral deficits associated with interferon alfa therapy for leukemia. *Neurology* **45**: 947–950.

Peper M, Steinvorth S, Schraube P *et al.* (2000). Neurobehavioral toxicity of total body irradiation: a follow-up in long-term survivors. *Int J Radiat Oncol Biol Phys* **46**(2): 303–311.

Phipps S, Dunavant M, Srivastava DK, Bowman L, Mulhern RK (2000). Cognitive and academic functioning in survivors of pediatric bone marrow transplantation. *J Clin Oncol* **18** (5): 1004–1011.

Recht L, Mrugala M (2003). Neurologic complications of hematologic neoplasms. *Neurol Clin* **21**: 87–105.

Reichenberg A, Yirmiya R, Schuld A *et al.* (2001). Cytokine-associated emotional and cognitive disturbances in humans. *Arch Gen Psychiatry* **58**: 445–452.

Richard F, Amouyel P (2001). Genetic susceptibility factors for Alzheimer's disease. *Eur J Pharmacol* **412**: 1–12.

Ries LAG, Eisner MP, Kosary CL *et al.* (2005). *SEER Cancer Statistics Review, 1975–2002*. Bethesda, MD: National Cancer Institute. http://seer.cancer.gov/csr/1975_2002/, based on November 2004 SEER data submission, posted to the SEER website, 2005.

Rodgers J, Marckus R, Kearns P, Windebuck K (2003). Attentional ability among survivors of leukaemia treated without cranial irradiation. *Arch Dis Child* **88**: 147–150.

Scheibel RS, Valentine AD, O'Brien S, Meyers CA (2004). Cognitive dysfunction and depression during treatment with interferon-alpha and chemotherapy. *J Neuropsychiatry Clin Neurosci* **16**: 185–191.

Seymour JF, Talpaz M, Hagemeister FB, Cabanillas F, Kurzrock R (1997). Clinical correlates of elevated serum levels of interleukin-6 in patients with untreated Hodgkin's disease. *Am J Med* **102**: 21–28.

Shah AK (1999). Cyclosporine A neurotoxicity among bone marrow transplant recipients. *Clin Neuropharmacol* **22**: 67–73.

Singh NP, Sahni V, Wadhwa A *et al.* (2006). Effect of improvement in anemia on electroneurophysiological markers (P300) of cognitive dysfunction in chronic kidney disease. *Hemodial Int* **10**(3): 267–273. Erratum in *Hemodial Int* 2006; **10**(4): 408.

Snider S, Bashir R, Bierman P (1994). Neurologic complications after high-dose chemotherapy and autologous bone marrow transplantation for Hodgkin's disease. *Neurology* **44**: 681–684.

Sostak P, Padovan CS, Yousry TA, Ledderose G, Kolb HJ, Straube A (2003). Prospective evaluation of neurological complications after allogeneic bone marrow transplantation. *Neurology* **60**: 842–848.

Spiegler BJ, Kennedy K, Maze R *et al.* (2006). Comparison of long-term neurocognitive outcomes in young children with acute lymphoblastic leukemia treated with cranial radiation or high-dose or very high-dose intravenous methotrexate. *J Clin Oncol* **24**: 3858–3864.

Stalfelt AM, Zettervall O (1997). Quality of life in young patients with chronic myelocytic leukaemia during intensive treatment including interferon. *Leukemia Res* **21**(8): 775–783.

Stivelman JC (2000). Benefits of anaemia treatment on cognitive function. *Nephrol Dial Transplant* **15**(3): 29–35.

Temple RM, Deary IJ, Winney RJ (1995). Recombinant erythropoietin improves cognitive function in patients maintained on chronic ambulatory peritoneal dialysis. *Nephrol Dial Transplant* **10**: 1733–1738.

Uckan D, Cetin M, Yigitkanli I *et al.* (2005). Life-threatening neurological complications after bone marrow transplantation in children. *Bone Marrow Transplant* **35**: 71–76.

Velu T, Debusscher L, Stryckmans PA (1985). Cyclosporin-associated fatal convulsions. *Lancet* Jan 26; **1**(8422): 219.

Vezmer S, Becker A, Bode, U, Jaehde U (2003). Biochemical and clinical aspects of methotrexate neurotoxicity. *Chemotherapy* **49**: 92–104.

Waber DP, Tarbell NJ, Fairclough D *et al.* (1995). Cognitive sequelae of treatment in childhood acute lymphoblastic leukemia: cranial radiation requires an accomplice. *J Clin Oncol* **13**: 2490–2496.

Waber DP, Shapiro BL, Carpentieri SC *et al.* (2001). Excellent therapeutic efficacy and minimal late neurotoxicity in children treated with 18 grays of cranial radiation therapy for high-risk acute lymphoblastic leukemia. *Cancer* **92**: 15–22.

Walter T (1994). Effect of iron-deficiency anaemia on cognitive skills in infancy and childhood. *Baillieres Clin Haematol* **7**: 815–827.

Watkins LR (2000). The pain of being sick: implications of immune-to-brain communication for understanding pain. *Annu Rev Psychol* **51**: 29–57.

Weiskopf RB, Toy P, Hopf HW *et al.* (2005). Acute isovolemic anemia impairs central processing as determined by P300 latency. *Clin Neurophysiol* **116**: 1028–1032.

Weiskopf RB, Feiner J, Hopf H *et al.* (2006). Fresh blood and aged stored blood are equally efficacious in immediately reversing anemia-induced brain oxygenation deficits in humans. *Anesthesiology* **104**: 911–920.

Wilson RW, Taliaferro LA, Jacobsen PB (2006). Pilot study of a self-administered stress management and exercise intervention during chemotherapy for cancer. *Support Care Cancer* **14**: 928–935.

17

Paraneoplastic disorders

Edward Dropcho

Introduction

Neurological paraneoplastic disorders refer to non-metastatic disorders that are not attributable to the toxicity of cancer therapy, cerebrovascular disease, coagulopathy, infection, or toxic and metabolic causes. Paraneoplastic disorders can affect any part(s) of the central (CNS) or peripheral (PNS) nervous systems (Table 17.1). Patients can be roughly grouped into those with pure or relatively pure clinical involvement of one part of the nervous system, such as cerebellar degeneration or sensory neuronopathy, and those with signs and symptoms of a diffuse and multifocal "paraneoplastic encephalomyelitis" (Dropcho, 2002; Graus *et al.*, 2004). Several syndromes should always raise the possibility of a paraneoplastic etiology, including Lambert–Eaton myasthenic syndrome, subacute cerebellar degeneration, severe sensory neuronopathy, limbic encephalopathy, and opsoclonus-myoclonus. None of the clinical syndromes, however, have an absolute association with neoplasia, and each can occur in patients without tumors.

For any paraneoplastic neurological disorder, there is a clear over-representation of one or a few particular neoplasms. Overall, small cell lung carcinoma is the tumor most often associated with paraneoplastic phenomena in adults, although the actual incidence of paraneoplastic disorders among patients with this tumor is probably no more than 1%–3%. Other tumors over-represented among adults with paraneoplastic syndromes include breast carcinoma, ovarian carcinoma, Hodgkin's lymphoma, thymoma, and testicular germ cell tumors. Except for opsoclonus-myoclonus associated with neuroblastoma, paraneoplastic disorders in children are rare.

Paraneoplastic disorders are far less common than nervous system metastases and are relatively rare compared to other non-metastatic neurological complications of systemic cancer, but they are clinically important for several reasons. First, in most patients with paraneoplastic disorders, the neurological symptoms are the presenting feature of an otherwise undiagnosed tumor. Physicians must therefore be able to identify the disorder as paraneoplastic and to initiate the appropriate search for the tumor. Second, paraneoplastic disorders often cause severe and permanent neurological morbidity. Third, prompt recognition of a paraneoplastic disorder maximizes the likelihood of successful tumor treatment and a favorable neurological outcome.

Most neurological paraneoplastic disorders are believed to be autoimmune diseases. The central theory of autoimmunity postulates that tumor cells express "onconeural" antigen(s) that are identical or antigenically related to molecules normally expressed by neurons, and that in rare instances an autoimmune response initially arising

Table 17.1. Neurologic paraneoplastic disorders

Central nervous system	Peripheral nervous system
Multifocal encephalomyelitis	Sensory neuronopathy
Cerebellar degeneration	Nerve vasculitis
Limbic encephalitis	Sensorimotor polyneuropathy
Opsoclonus-myoclonus	Motor neuropathy
Extrapyramidal syndrome	Neuromyotonia
Brainstem encephalitis	Autonomic insufficiency
Myelopathy	Lambert–Eaton syndrome
Motorneuron disease	Inflammatory myopathy
Stiff person syndrome	Necrotizing myopathy
Optic neuritis	
Retinal degeneration	

against the tumor "spills over" to attack neurons expressing the same or related antigen(s) (Dropcho, 2002; Roberts & Darnell, 2004). If true, this theory should be supported by several lines of evidence: (1) the neuropathology should be consistent with an immune or inflammatory process; (2) affected patients should have specific antibody or cellular immune autoreactivity; (3) tumor cells in affected patients should express the onconeural antigen(s); (4) there should be a demonstrable antitumor immune response; (5) immunosuppressive treatment should produce a beneficial clinical effect; (6) the clinical and neuropathological features should be reproducible in an experimental model.

Many patients with neurological paraneoplastic disorders have one or more of a steadily growing list of circulating antineuronal antibodies (Dropcho, 2002). The neuronal molecular targets of several of these autoantibodies have been cloned and characterized. Protein antigens reacting with antineuronal antibodies are known to be expressed by tumors from affected patients, supporting the general theory of an autoimmune response arising against shared onconeural antigens. Some paraneoplastic antibodies have selective neuronal reactivity and are found only in patients with a particular clinical syndrome, such as anti-recoverin antibodies in patients with retinal degeneration, and anti-Yo antibodies in patients with cerebellar degeneration. Most paraneoplastic autoantibodies show

more widespread or pan-neuronal reactivity and are associated with a variety of clinical neurological syndromes, or with multifocal encephalomyelitis. The most prevalent such antibodies are anti-Hu and anti-CV2 (Pittock *et al.*, 2004).

There are good but not perfect correlations among particular paraneoplastic syndromes, antineuronal antibody specificities, and associated tumor types. Antineuronal antibodies are useful diagnostic tools because, when present, they greatly increase the index of suspicion for a paraneoplastic condition, and the type of antibody can help guide the search for the underlying tumor. Antineuronal antibody assays do, however, have important practical clinical limitations. First, a given clinical syndrome (e.g., limbic encephalitis) may be associated with one of several autoantibodies; conversely, a given autoantibody (e.g., anti-Hu) may be associated with a variety of clinical presentations. Second, for several of the syndromes, a few patients have high-titer antineuronal autoantibodies and yet never develop a demonstrable tumor. The presence of antibodies does not absolutely indicate an underlying neoplasm. Third, several of the autoantibodies are present at low titers in tumor patients without any accompanying clinical neurological manifestations. Fourth, patients with a suspected paraneoplastic syndrome may not have demonstrable antineuronal antibodies, or may have "atypical" or incompletely characterized antibodies not detected in commercially available assays. A negative antibody assay, therefore, does not rule out the possibility of a paraneoplastic disorder and the presence of an underlying neoplasm.

For a few neurological paraneoplastic syndromes the antineuronal autoantibodies are directly involved in causing clinical disease (Dropcho, 2002). Prime examples are Lambert–Eaton myasthenic syndrome caused by antibodies against P/Q-type voltage-gated calcium channels at the pre-synaptic neuromuscular junction, and neuromyotonia caused by antibodies against voltage-gated potassium channels at pre-synaptic nerve terminals. Antibodies may also directly mediate neuronal dysfunction or injury for some CNS syndromes.

Examples include anti-recoverin antibodies in carcinoma-associated retinal degeneration, antibodies against P/Q-type voltage-gated calcium channels or glutamate receptors in some patients with paraneoplastic cerebellar degeneration, and anti-voltage-gated potassium channel antibodies in a subset of patients with paraneoplastic or non-paraneoplastic limbic encephalitis (see below).

For most paraneoplastic syndromes associated with antineuronal antibodies, the antibodies are probably an epiphenomenon or they play a minor indirect role in causing neuronal injury. Recent studies of two of the most common CNS paraneoplastic syndromes, i.e., encephalomyelitis/sensory neuronopathy associated with small cell lung cancer and cerebellar degeneration associated with breast or ovarian carcinoma, implicate cell-mediated immune effectors in causing neuronal injury. For these disorders it is postulated that onconeural antigens released by apoptotic tumor cells are presented to T lymphocytes in draining peripheral lymph nodes, initiating a Th1 helper response that eventually gains access to the CNS and attacks neurons expressing the antigens (Roberts & Darnell, 2004). There are many unanswered questions regarding exactly how this happens. Presently there is no fully successful animal model for any cell-mediated paraneoplastic syndrome affecting the CNS.

The clinical neurological outcome of patients with paraneoplastic syndromes varies considerably among different disorders and among patients with a given disorder. With very few exceptions neurological paraneoplastic syndromes do not remit spontaneously. For several syndromes the neurological outcome is linked to the associated tumor type and antineuronal antibody type. Successful treatment of the underlying tumor can bring about significant neurological improvement, at least for some syndromes and for some but not all patients. Unfortunately, many patients are left with severe and permanent neurological disability despite response or apparent cure of the associated tumor.

If paraneoplastic disorders are autoimmune diseases they should theoretically respond to immunosuppressive or immunomodulatory treatment (Dropcho, 2005). Several factors make it difficult to interpret the published literature regarding immunotherapy for paraneoplastic disorders:

1. These syndromes are relatively rare – for some of the syndromes there is only a handful of well-characterized published cases
2. Most reports are anecdotal and nearly all single-institution or multi-institution series are retrospective
3. There is a reporting bias, in that studies on patients who respond to treatment are more likely to be published than those on patients who do not respond
4. For some syndromes there are pharmacological treatments that improve neurological symptoms independent of tumor treatment or immunotherapy. Examples include Lambert–Eaton syndrome treated with pyridostigmine or 3,4-diaminopyridine, or stiff person syndrome treated with diazepam and baclofen
5. Patients with paraneoplastic encephalomyelitis, cerebellar degeneration, and other syndromes often stabilize spontaneously (although at a level of severe neurological disability), so that it is difficult to interpret reports of "neurological stabilization" with immunotherapy
6. Patients often receive concomitant tumor treatment and immunotherapy, making it difficult to discern the impact of each therapy on the neurological outcome. For many syndromes immunotherapy is more likely to be effective when the tumor is also treated successfully.

Factors that interact in influencing the response to immunotherapy include the neuroanatomical site (central versus peripheral), the cellular location of the onconeural target antigen(s) (neuronal cell surface versus intracellular), and the proven or presumed mechanism(s) of neuronal injury (antibody-mediated versus cell-mediated). In general, syndromes affecting the PNS are more likely to improve with tumor treatment and/or immunosuppressive treatment than are CNS syndromes. Lambert–Eaton myasthenic syndrome and other syndromes caused by autoantibodies reacting with ion channels or cell surface receptors are likely to respond to immunotherapy, probably because the antibodies do not usually cause axonal degeneration or neuronal cell death.

Unfortunately, the two most prevalent paraneoplastic CNS syndromes in adults, i.e., encephalomyelitis/sensory neuronopathy associated with small cell lung cancer and cerebellar degeneration associated with breast or ovarian carcinoma, have a poor prognosis. Fewer than 10% of these patients show significant neurological improvement despite aggressive tumor treatment and a variety of immunosuppressive therapies (Dropcho, 2002, 2005). Patients with other CNS syndromes including opsoclonus-myoclonus, limbic encephalitis, or stiff person syndrome have a somewhat higher likelihood of neurological improvement, suggesting that the immune-mediated neuronal dysfunction or injury is less severe or of a sort more likely to be reversible.

Even for the "unfavorable" syndromes such as encephalomyelitis and cerebellar degeneration, there are a few patients who do show a meaningful neurological response to immunotherapy. For these few responders, the only factors that sometimes correlate with neurological improvement are successful tumor treatment, and the duration and severity of neurological deficits prior to diagnosis and initiation of therapy. For patients who have already stabilized at a plateau of severe neurological disability for more than several weeks, subsequent improvement with any intervention is not impossible but extremely unlikely. The decision whether to use immunosuppressive therapies must therefore be based on the particular syndrome and on the individual patient's circumstances.

There are several potential explanations for the disappointingly poor response to immunotherapy in many patients. The continuing presence of even a small tumor burden seems to provide an "antigenic drive" for further neuronal injury. It is also likely that current immunotherapies do not adequately gain access to the CNS, and do not effectively abrogate an ongoing autoimmune response that is "sequestered" in the CNS. Unfortunately, for many if not most central syndromes it is likely that patients have already suffered neuronal death or irreversible injury by the time the diagnosis of a paraneoplastic disorder is made.

There is theoretical concern that if paraneoplastic disorders arise from an immune response directed against the tumor, attempts to treat the neurological disorder with immunosuppression may adversely affect the evolution of the tumor. At this time, there is no definite evidence that patients given immunosuppressive treatment have a worse tumor outcome than those who are not (Keime-Guibert *et al.*, 1999; Rojas *et al.*, 2000).

Two paraneoplastic disorders cause significant cognitive dysfunction in cancer patients and will be discussed in detail. These are paraneoplastic limbic encephalitis associated with a variety of neoplasms in adults, and the syndrome of paraneoplastic opsoclonus-myoclonus occurring in children with neuroblastoma.

Paraneoplastic limbic encephalitis

Limbic encephalitis as a clinicopathological entity was first described by Brierley in 1960 (Brierley *et al.*, 1960), and its frequent association with neoplasia was documented over the next several years (Corsellis *et al.*, 1968; Henson *et al.*, 1965). Paraneoplastic limbic encephalitis (PLE) may occur either as part of a multifocal encephalomyelitis, or less commonly as an isolated clinicopathological syndrome.

Approximately 50%–60% of reported patients with PLE have small cell lung carcinoma (Alamowitch *et al.*, 1997; Gultekin *et al.*, 2000; Lawn *et al.*, 2003). Other associated neoplasms include testicular germ cell tumors (Dalmau *et al.*, 2004; Rosenfeld *et al.*, 2001), thymoma (Ances *et al.*, 2005; Antoine *et al.*, 1995; Fujii *et al.*, 2001; Rickman *et al.*, 2000), Hodgkin's lymphoma (Deodhare *et al.*, 1996; Duyckaerts *et al.*, 1985), non-Hodgkin's lymphoma (Mihara *et al.*, 2005; Thuerl *et al.*, 2003), non-small cell lung cancer (Bakheit *et al.*, 1990; Benke *et al.*, 2004), breast carcinoma (Fakhoury *et al.*, 1999; Lawn *et al.*, 2003; Sutton *et al.*, 2000), ovarian teratoma (Aydiner *et al.*, 1998; Nokura *et al.*, 1997; Taylor *et al.*, 1999; Vitaliani *et al.*, 2005), endometrial carcinoma (Petit *et al.*, 1997), colon carcinoma (Tsukamoto *et al.*, 1993), renal carcinoma (Bell *et al.*, 1998; Kararizou *et al.*, 2005), and prostate carcinoma (Modrego *et al.*, 2002; Stern & Hulette, 1999). Because of the tumor associations, PLE occurs most commonly in middle-aged or older adults, although it may occur in adolescents or young adults when associated with Hodgkin's lymphoma, thymoma, ovarian teratoma, or testicular tumors (Lee *et al.*, 2003; Okamura *et al.*, 1997; Rosenbaum *et al.*, 1998).

Pathology

Patients with subacute neurological symptoms referable to the temporal lobes or limbic system may have a brain biopsy to rule out herpes encephalitis or other infection, and are subsequently diagnosed with PLE. Biopsy specimens in these patients show a variable degree of non-specific changes including neuronal loss, astrogliosis, or perivascular and leptomeningeal mononuclear cell infiltrates (Dalmau *et al.*, 2004; Deodhare *et al.*, 1996; Gultekin *et al.*, 2000; Ingenito *et al.*, 1990; Rosenbaum *et al.*, 1998).

The most consistent and severe neuropathological abnormalities in autopsied cases of PLE are extensive neuronal loss, gliosis, and microglial nodules in the hippocampus and amygdala (Brierley *et al.*, 1960; Corsellis *et al.*, 1968; Dalmau *et al.*, 2004; Gultekin *et al.*, 2000). Similar but less severe changes are often present in the parahippocampal gyrus, cingulate gyrus, insular cortex, orbital frontal cortex, basal ganglia, and diencephalon. Perivascular lymphocytic cuffing and leptomeningeal mononuclear cell infiltrates are patchy and variable. In some patients with clinically "pure" PLE the pathological changes at autopsy are entirely confined to the limbic system (Bakheit *et al.*, 1990; Duyckaerts *et al.*, 1985; Farrugia *et al.*, 2005; Fujii *et al.*, 2001). Most patients with PLE and small cell lung cancer, and many patients with other associated tumors, have multifocal encephalomyelitis, with patchy neuronal loss or inflammatory infiltrates in any or all areas of the nervous system, including the cerebral hemispheres, basal ganglia, diencephalon, brainstem, cerebellum, gray matter of the spinal cord, dorsal root ganglia, and autonomic ganglia (Brierley *et al.*, 1960; Ingenito *et al.*, 1990; Kinirons *et al.*, 2003). The pathological changes may be more widespread than would have been predicted based on patients' signs and symptoms.

Clinical features

In the majority of patients with PLE the neurological symptoms are the presenting feature of the associated neoplasm, often preceding discovery of the tumor by several months or longer. Exceptional patients have been reported to develop limbic encephalitis after apparent cures of a previously diagnosed tumor (Kodama *et al.*, 1991; Lacomis *et al.*, 1990); in these patients the association between limbic encephalitis and the previous tumor may be fortuitous.

Paraneoplastic limbic encephalitis generally has a subacute onset evolving over days to weeks. Patients typically present either with an amnestic syndrome or with psychiatric symptoms; most patients eventually develop features of both (Alamowitch *et al.*, 1997; Gultekin *et al.*, 2000; Lawn *et al.*, 2003). The memory loss includes short-term anterograde amnesia and a variable period of retrograde amnesia. Denial of the deficit and confabulation are common. The psychiatric disorder usually includes some combination of depression, anxiety, emotional lability, and personality change. Hallucinations and paranoid delusions may occur. Generalized or partial complex seizures occur in most patients, may be the initial neurological feature, and can be medically intractable.

Less common manifestations of limbic or diencephalic dysfunction include abnormal sleep-wake cycles, disturbed temperature regulation, labile blood pressure, inappropriate secretion of antidiuretic hormone, and elements of the Kluver–Bucy syndrome, such as hyperphagia and hypersexuality (Aydiner *et al.*, 1998; Dalmau *et al.*, 2004; Overeem *et al.*, 2004; Rosenbaum *et al.*, 1998).

In addition to the limbic encephalopathy, most patients with small cell lung carcinoma and many patients with other tumors develop manifestations of a more generalized, multifocal paraneoplastic encephalomyelitis. These include varied combinations of signs and symptoms referable to the extralimbic cerebral cortex, basal ganglia, brainstem, cerebellum, dorsal root ganglia, spinal cord, and autonomic system (Alamowitch *et al.*, 1997; Gultekin *et al.*, 2000; Hirayama *et al.*, 2003; Kinirons *et al.*, 2003; Lawn *et al.*, 2003; Rickman *et al.*, 2000). Patients with small cell lung carcinoma may develop PLE concurrent with peripheral neuropathy or Lambert–Eaton myasthenic syndrome. Other extralimbic clinical features have particular associations with certain tumors and antineuronal antibodies (see below).

Diagnostic studies

Brain magnetic resonance imaging is abnormal in at least two-thirds of patients with PLE, showing areas of abnormal T2-weighted and/or fluid-attenuated inversion recovery (FLAIR) signal in the mesial temporal lobe and amygdala bilaterally, and less commonly in the hypothalamus and basal frontal cortex (Alamowitch *et al.*, 1997; Gultekin *et al.*, 2000; Kodama *et al.*, 1991; Lawn *et al.*, 2003). The lesions enhance with gadolinium in a minority of cases. Some patients additionally have extratemporal cortical or subcortical lesions (Ances *et al.*, 2005; Hirayama *et al.*, 2003; Lawn *et al.*, 2003; Rickman *et al.*, 2000; Rosenbaum *et al.*, 1998). There is a single report of bilateral T2-weighted hyperintensity in the posterior thalamus ("pulvinar sign") in a patient with non-Hodgkin's lymphoma (Mihara *et al.*, 2005). Patients with anti-Ma2 antibodies (see below) may have MR lesions in the thalamus, hypothalamus, and/or brainstem in addition to the mesial temporal lobes (Bennett *et al.*, 1999; Dalmau *et al.*, 2004). In some patients the MR lesions subsequently resolve with or without concomitant clinical improvement, sometimes eventuating in temporal lobe atrophy (Benke *et al.*, 2004; Dirr *et al.*, 1990; Kodama *et al.*, 1991; Rosenbaum *et al.*, 1998).

At some time during the course of illness, the cerebrospinal fluid (CSF) in about two-thirds of patients with PLE shows a mild lymphocytic pleocytosis and/or slightly elevated protein (Alamowitch *et al.*, 1997; Dalmau *et al.*, 2004; Gultekin *et al.*, 2000; Lawn *et al.*, 2003). Some patients additionally have oligoclonal bands and/or an elevated CSF IgG index. Normal CSF does not rule out PLE.

Approximately 75% of patients with PLE have an abnormal electroencephalogram (EEG) during the course of their illness (Gultekin *et al.*, 2000; Lawn *et al.*, 2003). The most common EEG abnormality is slowing, either diffuse or localized to the frontal or temporal regions. There may be superimposed paroxysmal sharp waves and spikes with or without clinical seizures.

Fluorodeoxyglucose positron emission tomography (PET scanning) may demonstrate unilateral or bilateral hippocampal hypermetabolism in patients with PLE (Ances *et al.*, 2005; Fakhoury *et al.*, 1999; Na *et al.*, 2001; Provenzale *et al.*, 1998; Scheid *et al.*, 2004b). The hypermetabolic areas do not necessarily correspond to lesions seen on MR scans. The findings on PET scanning do not distinguish PLE from other causes of limbic encephalitis.

Autoimmunity

Most but not all patients with PLE have one or more circulating antineuronal autoantibodies (Table 17.2). Several antineuronal antibodies associated with PLE have pan-neuronal reactivity and are present in patients with a variety of clinical neurological syndromes. The most common of these are polyclonal IgG anti-Hu antibodies found in patients with various clinical manifestations of multifocal encephalomyelitis, reflecting involvement of the cerebral hemispheres, limbic system, cerebellum, brainstem, spinal cord, dorsal root ganglia, and autonomic ganglia (Graus *et al.*, 2001; Gultekin *et al.*, 2000; Sillevis Smitt *et al.*, 2002; Vernino *et al.*, 2002). More than 90% of patients with anti-Hu antibodies and paraneoplastic encephalomyelitis have small cell lung carcinoma, with reports of other tumors including non-small cell lung cancer,

Table 17.2. Antineuronal antibodies in paraneoplastic limbic encephalitis

Autoantibody	Associated tumor(s)	Antibody reactivity
anti-Hu (ANNA-1) (Alamowitch *et al.*, 1997; Graus *et al.*, 2001; Gultekin *et al.*, 2000; Sillevis Smitt *et al.*, 2002)	Small cell lung carcinoma, others	Pan-neuronal nuclear > cytoplasmic staining; 35- to 40-kDa RNA-binding proteins
Anti-CV2 (CRMP-5) (Kinirons *et al.*, 2003; Lawn *et al.*, 2003; Rickman *et al.*, 2000; Yu *et al.*, 2001)	Small cell lung carcinoma, thymoma, others	Cytoplasm of neurons; 66-kDa CV2 protein, 62-kDa CRMP-5 protein
Anti-Ma2 (anti-Ta) (Dalmau *et al.*, 2004; Rosenfeld *et al.*, 2001; Voltz *et al.*, 1999)	Germ cell tumors, breast carcinoma, non-small cell lung carcinoma	Pan-neuronal nuclei and nucleoli; 40- to 42-kDa Ma1 and Ma2 proteins
Anti-VGKC (Buckley *et al.*, 2001; Pozo-Rosich *et al.*, 2003; Vernino & Lennon, 2004)	Thymoma, small cell lung carcinoma	Voltage-gated potassium channels
Novel neuropil antibodies (Ances *et al.*, 2005; Vitaliani *et al.*, 2005)	Ovarian teratoma, others	Hippocampal dendrites and synapses
Anti-amphiphysin (Antoine *et al.*, 1999; Dorresteijn *et al.*, 2002; Pittock *et al.*, 2005)	Breast, small cell lung carcinoma	Neuropil; 125-kDa synaptic vesicle-associated protein
ANNA-3 (Chan *et al.*, 2001)	Small cell lung carcinoma	Nuclei of Purkinje cells and dentate neurons; 170-kDa protein
Anti-VGCC (Lawn *et al.*, 2003)	Small cell lung carcinoma, others	P/Q-type and N-type calcium channels
PCA-2 (Vernino & Lennon, 2000)	Small cell lung carcinoma	Neuronal cytoplasm; 280-kDa protein
Anti-Zic (Bataller *et al.*, 2004)	Small cell lung carcinoma	35- to 55-kDa zinc finger proteins
"Atypical" (Antoine *et al.*, 1995; Fujii *et al.*, 2001; Scheid *et al.*, 2004a, b; Tsukamoto *et al.*, 1993)	Thymoma, small cell lung carcinoma, others	Varied
Antibody-negative	Various	

neuroblastoma, carcinoma of the breast or prostate, or thymoma.

Limbic encephalitis is an early and prominent feature in 10%–20% of patients with paraneoplastic encephalomyelitis and anti-Hu antibodies; most of these patients develop other multifocal signs and symptoms during the course of their illness (Dalmau *et al.*, 1992; Graus *et al.*, 2001; Gultekin *et al.*, 2000; Sillevis Smitt *et al.*, 2002). Among patients with PLE and small cell lung carcinoma, approximately one-half have anti-Hu antibodies, a few patients have other antibodies, and the remainder have no identifiable antibodies (Alamowitch

et al., 1997; Gultekin *et al.*, 2000). Anti-Hu-positive patients usually show additional signs and symptoms of multifocal paraneoplastic encephalomyelitis, whereas patients with small cell lung cancer but without anti-Hu antibodies are more likely to have "pure" limbic system involvement.

Anti-Hu antibodies are a valuable clinical marker for PLE or paraneoplastic encephalomyelitis, but it is currently thought that cellular immune effectors and not the anti-Hu antibodies are the mediators of neuronal injury. Evidence to support cell-mediated autoimmune neuronal injury includes the presence of CD8+ T lymphocytes clustered around neurons in the brain and dorsal root ganglia (Bernal *et al.*, 2002), and the presence of oligoclonal T lymphocytes in the blood and dorsal root ganglia (Plonquet *et al.*, 2002). T lymphocytes from patients' peripheral blood recognize and respond to peptides derived from the HuD onconeural antigen (Plonquet *et al.*, 2003; Rousseau *et al.*, 2005).

Several other antineuronal antibodies associated with PLE or with other CNS syndromes have a pan-neuronal or widespread reactivity. These include anti-CV2 (CRMP-5) antibodies, anti-amphiphysin antibodies, PCA-2 antibodies, anti-voltage-gated calcium channel antibodies, and ANNA-3 antibodies (Table 17.2). Any of these antibodies can be present in patients with PLE, but none of them has a particular association with PLE versus other neurological syndromes. Small cell lung cancer is by far the tumor most commonly associated with these antibodies. It is not unusual for patients with small cell lung carcinoma and PLE (or other CNS syndromes) to have more than one type of antineuronal antibody (Pittock *et al.*, 2004). At this time it is not known whether any of these antibodies is directly involved in causing neuronal injury.

A few antineuronal antibodies have a specific linkage to PLE and are not commonly associated with other neurological syndromes. Anti-Ma2 (anti-Ta) antibodies mainly occur in young men with testicular germ cell tumors (Dalmau *et al.*, 2004; Rosenfeld *et al.*, 2001; Voltz *et al.*, 1999). There are a few reported cases of anti-Ma2 (anti-Ta) antibodies in women with breast carcinoma or non-small cell lung carcinoma (Sahashi *et al.*, 2003; Sutton *et al.*, 1993). Some patients with anti-Ma2 antibodies have a clinically "pure" limbic encephalitis, while the majority present with a combined syndrome reflecting involvement of the limbic system, diencephalon (e.g., sleep disorder or autonomic dysfunction), and brainstem (especially ocular motor disturbance) (Bennett *et al.*, 1999; Dalmau *et al.*, 2004; Overeem *et al.*, 2004; Waragi *et al.*, 2006). Patients whose antibodies react with the Ma1 protein in addition to the Ma2 protein tend to have more severe cerebellar and brainstem dysfunction (Dalmau *et al.*, 2004).

The mechanisms of autoimmune neuronal injury in anti-Ma2-associated PLE are not known. Interstitial and perivascular infiltration of T lymphocytes in affected brain areas suggests cellular immune effectors (Dalmau *et al.*, 2004). In one attempted animal model, adoptive transfer of rat T lymphocytes specific for the Ma1 onconeural protein caused meningeal and perivascular inflammatory infiltrates in recipient rats, but the recipient animals did not develop neuronal loss or clinical disease (Pelkofer *et al.*, 2004).

Some patients with limbic encephalitis have circulating antibodies against voltage-gated potassium channels (VGKC). To date, most of the small number of reported patients with limbic encephalitis and anti-VGKC antibodies do not have an identifiable neoplasm (Thieben *et al.*, 2004; Vincent *et al.*, 2004). In some patients the limbic encephalitis occurs as a paraneoplastic syndrome, usually in association with thymoma (Buckley *et al.*, 2001; Vernino & Lennon, 2004) or small cell lung carcinoma (Pozo-Rosich *et al.*, 2003). Voltage-gated potassium channels comprise hetero-oligomers of different subunits. Subtypes of VGKCs are widely distributed throughout the brain and PNS. Anti-VGKC antibodies are also found in patients with paraneoplastic or non-paraneoplastic neuromyotonia (Hart *et al.*, 2002), and in patients with the syndrome of "Morvan's fibrillary chorea" featuring neuromyotonia, hyperhidrosis and other dysautonomia, insomnia, hallucinations, and limbic encephalopathy (Lee *et al.*, 1998; Liguori *et al.*, 2001). Unlike many other paraneoplastic antineuronal antibodies that are believed to be markers of autoimmunity but do not directly mediate neuronal injury, anti-VGKC antibodies may directly cause neuronal dysfunction. In an experimental model of neuromyotonia, patients' anti-VGKC antibodies were shown to cross-link the receptors and reduce potassium channel currents (Tomimitsu *et al.*, 2004). Less is known about the effects of anti-VGKC antibodies on CNS neuronal function. Presumably, differences in the fine specificity of reactivity of anti-VGKC antibodies account for the heterogeneous clinical presentation among patients with limbic encephalitis, neuromyotonia, and Morvan's syndrome (Kleopa *et al.*, 2006).

The newest autoantibodies associated with PLE are "novel neuropil antibodies," which stain the dendritic network and synaptic-enriched regions in the neuropil of the hippocampus (Ances *et al.*, 2005; Vitaliani *et al.*, 2005). Associated neoplasms include ovarian teratoma and thymic tumors. Some patients present with a "typical" limbic encephalopathy, while others have a more severe clinical course with acute psychosis, seizures, lethargy, and central hypoventilation requiring extended ventilatory support. The latter patients usually have evidence for multifocal extralimbic involvement based on MR imaging, PET scans, or autopsy.

Several reported patients with PLE have "atypical" or incompletely characterized antineuronal antibodies. Most reports are of single patients, with one of a variety of tumors including thymoma, small cell lung cancer, and breast carcinoma (Fujii *et al.*, 2001; Scheid *et al.*, 2004a). It is important to keep in mind that some patients with PLE, regardless of tumor association, do not have identifiable autoantibodies.

Differential diagnosis

Differential diagnosis in patients with suspected PLE partly depends on whether there is a known cancer diagnosis and on the tumor histology. Among patients with a prior cancer diagnosis who develop cognitive dysfunction, the level of suspicion for a paraneoplastic disorder is much higher for patients with small cell lung carcinoma, thymoma, Hodgkin's lymphoma, and testicular germ cell tumors than for patients with other tumors. Tumor metastases and neurotoxicity of cancer treatments are far more common than paraneoplastic disorders and should always be considered, as should metabolic derangements and CNS infection. Methotrexate, procarbazine, ifosfamide, and other chemotherapeutic drugs can cause a diffuse or multifocal encephalopathy (Dropcho, 2004). Diffuse cerebral injury may occur following cranial radiation therapy for primary or metastatic brain

tumors (Behin & Delattre, 2004). This condition generally presents with global cognitive dysfunction and gait apraxia, rather than the selective memory loss seen in prototypic cases of limbic encephalitis, but there is some overlap. Limbic encephalitis associated with human Herpes virus type 6 has occurred in patients following allogeneic stem cell transplantation (Ogata *et al.*, 2006; Wainwright *et al.*, 2001). Varicella zoster virus may also cause a selective limbic encephalitis in immunocompromised patients (Tattevin *et al.*, 2001).

For patients without a previous cancer diagnosis who present with limbic encephalitis, the level of suspicion for a paraneoplastic etiology depends on the patient's age, gender, risk factors (especially cigarette smoking), and the presence of antineuronal antibodies. The most common alternative diagnoses are Herpes simplex encephalitis, a primary psychiatric disorder, or non-paraneoplastic limbic encephalitis. Patients with PLE who have early and prominent affective symptoms or hallucinations are often initially diagnosed as having a primary psychiatric condition, especially when accompanying "hard" neurological findings are absent, missed, or misinterpreted.

There is increasing recognition of patients whose clinical presentations are indistinguishable from those of PLE, but in whom no tumor is ever discovered, even at autopsy (Bien *et al.*, 2000; Kohler *et al.*, 1988; Mori *et al.*, 2002). Some patients with non-paraneoplastic limbic encephalitis have anti-VGKC antibodies (Ances *et al.*, 2005; Buckley *et al.*, 2001; Fauser *et al.*, 2005; Pozo-Rosich *et al.*, 2003; Thieben *et al.*, 2004; Vincent *et al.*, 2004). Patients with anti-VGKC antibodies often improve with plasma exchange, intravenous immunoglobulin, or corticosteroids. There are reports of a few patients with limbic encephalitis and anti-Hu, anti-Ma2, or other antineuronal antibodies in whom no tumor was ever discovered (Ances *et al.*, 2005; Dalmau *et al.*, 2004; Gultekin *et al.*, 2000). No clinical features or laboratory studies (including CSF, EEG, MR imaging, or PET) reliably distinguish paraneoplastic from non-paraneoplastic limbic encephalitis.

Patient management

Any middle-aged patient with a history of cigarette smoking who develops limbic encephalitis should be suspected of harboring a small cell lung carcinoma. Chest CT or MR scanning is clearly more sensitive than a "plain" chest X-ray in detecting a small neoplasm. If present, anti-Hu, anti-CV2, or other serum antineuronal antibodies (Table 17.2) are a highly specific marker for small cell lung carcinoma (rarely another tumor). Total body PET scanning may detect lung or other neoplasms in patients who are suspected of having paraneoplastic syndromes and yet have unrevealing or equivocal chest CT or MR scans (Linke *et al.*, 2004; Younes-Mhenni *et al.*, 2004). If a patient's initial evaluation for an occult tumor is unrevealing, which is not at all uncommon, the workup should be repeated at regular intervals.

In young adults or non-smokers presenting with limbic encephalitis, the most common neoplasms to consider are thymoma, Hodgkin's lymphoma, testicular germ cell tumor, and ovarian teratoma. These patients should have a thorough physical examination and CT or MR scanning of the chest and abdomen. Anti-VGKC antibodies should raise suspicion for an associated thymoma, although many if not most patients with limbic encephalitis and anti-VGKC antibodies do not have an underlying tumor. Young men should also have testicular ultrasound, which can show a small tumor even after negative clinical examinations (Wingerchuk *et al.*, 1998). Elevated serum alpha-fetoprotein or human chorionic gonadotropin in young men may indicate a non-seminomatous germ cell tumor. Serum anti-Ma2 antibodies are a marker for testicular germ cell tumors, although a negative assay does not rule out a tumor (Dalmau *et al.*, 2004). There are reports of young men with brainstem or limbic encephalitis, anti-Ma2 antibodies, and negative or equivocal testicular ultrasound, in whom orchiectomy revealed a microscopic intratubular germ cell tumor (Dalmau *et al.*, 2004). Young women should additionally have a pelvic examination and imaging to look for an ovarian teratoma.

The course of PLE is variable and rather unpredictable. A few patients with clinically "pure" PLE show spontaneous remission of the neurological condition prior to any treatment (Sillevis Smitt *et al.*, 2002). Paraneoplastic limbic encephalitis is rather unusual among CNS paraneoplastic disorders in that a significant proportion of patients have major neurological improvement after successful treatment of the associated tumor. Approximately one-half of patients with PLE and small cell lung cancer improve after tumor treatment (Alamowitch *et al.*, 1997; Bak *et al.*, 2001; Dalmau *et al.*, 1992; Dorresteijn *et al.*, 2002; Gultekin *et al.*, 2000; Kaniecki & Morris, 1993). Patients with small cell lung cancer but without antineuronal antibodies are more likely to improve than those with anti-Hu antibodies. Among patients with anti-Hu antibodies in whom limbic encephalitis is a component of multifocal encephalomyelitis, the "limbic" features may improve after tumor treatment, whereas the other neurological features rarely do so.

Among patients with PLE, testicular germ cell tumors, and anti-Ma2 antibodies who receive tumor treatment and/or immunosuppressive therapy, approximately 25% have neurological improvement and about another 25% have neurological stabilization (Dalmau *et al.*, 2004; Landolfi & Nadkarni, 2003). Successful tumor treatment is correlated with a better neurological outcome. Some patients have improved memory and cognition but continue to have chronic intractable seizures.

Approximately one-half of reported patients with PLE and thymoma, including those with anti-VGKC or anti-CV2 antibodies, have significant neurological improvement following successful tumor treatment, with or without immunotherapy (Ances *et al.*, 2005; Antoine *et al.*, 1995; Buckley *et al.*, 2001; Gultekin *et al.*, 2000). There are also reports of partial or complete reversal of PLE after treatment of the underlying Hodgkin's lymphoma (Deodhare *et al.*, 1996), ovarian teratoma (Ances *et al.*, 2005; Nokura *et al.*, 1997; Vitaliani *et al.*, 2005), renal carcinoma (Bell *et al.*, 1998), or ovarian carcinoma (Bloch *et al.*, 2004).

As outlined above, the responsiveness of PLE to immunosuppressive therapy is difficult to judge precisely from the literature. Many reported patients received tumor treatment concurrently with immunosuppressive therapy including oral or intravenous pulse corticosteroids, cyclophosphamide, intravenous immunoglobulin, or plasmapheresis (Alamowitch *et al.*, 1997; Gultekin *et al.*, 2000; Vitaliani *et al.*, 2005). There are reports of definite responses to immunotherapy. These include patients with thymoma (and anti-VGKC or anti-CV2 antibodies) (Buckley *et al.*, 2001; Rickman *et al.*, 2000), testicular tumors (anti-Ma2 antibodies) (Dalmau *et al.*, 2004; Scheid *et al.*, 2003), small cell lung cancer (anti-VGKC antibodies) (Pozo-Rosich *et al.*, 2003), patients with ovarian teratoma (Lee *et al.*, 2003; Taylor *et al.*, 1999), and patients with novel neuropil antibodies (Ances *et al.*, 2005), who improved following some combination of corticosteroids, intravenous immunoglobulin, or plasmapheresis.

Roughly one-half of patients with PLE fail to improve with tumor treatment, with or without immunosuppressive therapy, regardless of tumor association (Dalmau *et al.*, 2004; Gultekin *et al.*, 2000). These patients are usually left with moderate or severe neurological disability. Less commonly, patients may become progressively demented with eventual obtundation and fatal coma.

Paraneoplastic opsoclonus-myoclonus

Clinical features

The syndrome of "myoclonic encephalopathy of infancy" or opsoclonus-myoclonus was first clearly described by Kinsbourne in 1962 (Kinsbourne, 1962). The association between opsoclonus-myoclonus and neuroblastoma in children was identified in two publications in 1968 (Dyken & Kolar, 1968; Solomon & Chutorian, 1968). Since that time approximately one-half of the reported cases of opsoclonus-myoclonus syndrome in children occurred in association with neuroblastoma. This

is probably an overestimate of the true frequency of paraneoplastic opsoclonus (POM) due to reporting bias; POM occurs in approximately 2%–3% of children with neuroblastoma (Gambini *et al.*, 2003; Rudnick *et al.*, 2001). The median age at onset of POM is 18–24 months. In nearly all cases it is the neurological syndrome that leads to discovery of an otherwise occult neuroblastoma. Paraneoplastic opsoclonus can rarely occur months to years after successful neuroblastoma treatment, without evidence of tumor recurrence.

Paraneoplastic opsoclonus-myoclonus typically has an abrupt onset. The cardinal feature, opsoclonus, is continuous multidirectional rapid eye movements (saccadic oscillations) without an intersaccadic interval. In addition to opsoclonus, children have some combination of myoclonus, ataxia, and altered sensorium (Gambini *et al.*, 2003; Rudnick *et al.*, 2001; Telander *et al.*, 1989). Myoclonic jerks are arrhythmic, multifocal, spontaneous and/or stimulus triggered, and vary in severity from mild to incapacitating. Ataxia may involve limbs, trunk, and gait, and again may be mild to severe. Nearly all children are irritable in the acute phase. Other signs and symptoms can include nausea and vomiting, dysarthria, facial diplegia, hearing loss, and upper motor neuron findings. A high percentage of children have residual long-term motor, neurocognitive, and behavioral problems (see below).

The majority of children with POM have mild elevation of CSF protein, lymphocytic pleocytosis, oligoclonal IgG bands, and an elevated IgG index. Brain MR scans are usually normal; there are individual case reports of cerebellar vermal lesions in the acute phase (Telander *et al.*, 1989) or of eventual diffuse cerebellar atrophy (Hayward *et al.*, 2001). The main differential diagnosis of POM is opsoclonus-myoclonus occurring during an acute viral infection (e.g., enterovirus or Coxsackie virus) (Kuban *et al.*, 1983; Tabarki *et al.*, 1998) or as a syndrome following infection with agents including Epstein–Barr virus (Sheth *et al.*, 1995) or *Streptococcus* (Candler *et al.*, 2006). There are no clinical, neuroimaging, or CSF findings that reliably differentiate

POM from "post-infectious" or idiopathic opsoclonus-myoclonus syndrome in children or adults (Boltshauser *et al.*, 1979; Pohl *et al.*, 1996).

Pathology

The pathological substrate of childhood POM remains unclear, as there are no distinctive or uniformly present lesions. Some of the very few published autopsied cases show partial loss of cerebellar Purkinje cells (Moe & Nellhaus, 1970; Ziter *et al.*, 1979). Among adult patients with paraneoplastic opsoclonus associated with small cell lung cancer, breast carcinoma or other tumors, autopsies have shown mild to severe dropout of Purkinje cells, and/or patchy neuronal loss and perivascular mononuclear cell infiltrates in the inferior olivary nuclei and other areas of the brainstem (Anderson *et al.*, 1988; Wong *et al.*, 2001). In a significant proportion of autopsied children and adults with POM there are no identifiable histopathological abnormalities in either the cerebellum or brainstem (Hersh *et al.*, 1994; Ridley *et al.*, 1987). Disturbance of the tonic inhibitory control of saccadic burst neurons by the "omnipause" neurons in the pontine reticular formation has been postulated as the key pathophysiological event in producing opsoclonus, but the pons may not show any histological changes (Ridley *et al.*, 1987). An alternative model postulates that opsoclonus is the result of cerebellar Purkinje cell injury, which disinhibits the fastigial oculomotor region (Wong *et al.*, 2001).

One of the many unanswered questions in paraneoplastic childhood POM is why affected children develop cognitive and behavioral problems if the autoimmune response is seemingly directed against the brainstem and cerebellum. One possible explanation is that POM is actually a diffuse or multifocal encephalitis that also involves supratentorial structures. Another possibility is that cerebellar injury is the source of the neurocognitive deficits in children with POM; this derives from recent studies of neurocognitive sequelae in children with cerebellar

neoplasms (Konczak *et al.*, 2005; Ravizza *et al.*, 2006; Ronning *et al.*, 2005).

Autoimmunity

The pathological and biological features of neuroblastomas in children with POM are generally favorable. The tumors of a disproportionately high percentage of children with POM are classified as ganglioneuroblastoma and are in a favorable histological group. Patients with POM are less likely to have advanced-stage neuroblastoma at diagnosis compared to neuroblastoma patients in general (Rudnick *et al.*, 2001; Russo *et al.*, 1997). Perivascular and interstitial infiltrates of B lymphocytes and T lymphocytes are more frequent and more intense in POM patients than in neuroblastoma patients without POM (Cooper *et al.*, 2001; Gambini *et al.*, 2003; Mitchell & Snodgrass, 1990; Telander *et al.*, 1989). Amplification of the *N-myc* oncogene is relatively rare (Gambini *et al.*, 2003). The occurrence of POM in a child with neuroblastoma generally carries a good prognosis for survival independent of patient's age, tumor site, or tumor stage (Rudnick *et al.*, 2001; Russo *et al.*, 1997), although a good oncological outcome is not universal (Hiyama *et al.*, 1994). These observations indirectly support the theory that POM occurs when an anti-neuroblastoma immune response causes tumor regression or differentiation, but simultaneously attacks cross-reacting neuronal antigens. It has been postulated that some cases of "idiopathic" or "post-infectious" opsoclonus-myoclonus represent instances of an occult neuroblastoma that is obliterated by a cross-reacting antitumor/antineuronal immune response.

Some patients with POM have serum autoantibodies that react with shared neuronal-neuroblastoma antigens. A small percentage of patients have anti-Hu antibodies (Fisher *et al.*, 1994; Hayward *et al.*, 2001; Korfei *et al.*, 2005). Other patients have one of a number of antibodies with heterogeneous reactivities on immunocytochemical staining and immunoblots (Antunes *et al.*, 2000; Blaes *et al.*, 2005; Connolly *et al.*, 1997; Korfei *et al.*, 2005). The identity of the onconeural antigens remains to be shown. There is no universally observed antibody or antigen in published studies. Some of the antibodies are also present in children with non-paraneoplastic opsoclonus-myoclonus, and in children with neuroblastoma but no neurological symptoms. In one study IgG antibodies from POM patients exerted an antiproliferative and cytotoxic effect on neuroblastoma cells *in vitro* (Korfei *et al.*, 2005). Other evidence supporting an autoimmune etiology for POM includes an abnormally increased number of B lymphocytes and T lymphocyte subsets in the CSF (Pranzatelli *et al.*, 2004b), and elevated CSF neopterin, which is a marker for cellular immune activation (Pranzatelli *et al.*, 2004a). These CSF abnormalities do not distinguish between patients with paraneoplastic or non-paraneoplastic opsoclonus-myoclonus.

To date there is no successful animal model for POM, and the actual immunopathogenetic mechanism(s) of neuronal injury or dysfunction are unclear.

Patient management

All children who present with opsoclonus should have a workup for neuroblastoma including chest radiograph, abdominal CT scan, and a 24-h urine collection for vanillylmandelic acid, homovanillic acid, and metanephrine (Telander *et al.*, 1989). Nuclear medicine imaging with the norepinephrine analog metaiodobenzylguanidine (MIBG) may demonstrate a tumor in the absence of a radiographic lesion (Parisi *et al.*, 1993; Shapiro *et al.*, 1994). If initially unrevealing, the workup should be repeated at regular intervals. In at least 75% of children with POM the neuroblastoma is diagnosed within 6 months after onset of neurological symptoms (Rudnick *et al.*, 2001; Russo *et al.*, 1997).

The majority of children with POM have a localized neuroblastoma and undergo tumor resection. Some of these children show post-operative neurological improvement without any other treatment (Hayward *et al.*, 2001). Whether given before or after surgical resection, adrenocorticotropin (ACTH)

produces rapid and dramatic neurological improvement in at least two-thirds of children (Hammer *et al.*, 1995). Oral or intravenous (IV) corticosteroids are also used but are probably less effective than ACTH (Hammer *et al.*, 1995; Rostasy *et al.*, 2005). Patients may also show improvement with IV Ig, either given alone or in combination with ACTH/corticosteroids (Fisher *et al.*, 1994; Petruzzi & Alarcon, 1995; Rudnick *et al.*, 2001; Veneselli *et al.*, 1998). Plasmapheresis (Yiu *et al.*, 2001) or rituximab (Pranzatelli *et al.*, 2005d; Tersak *et al.*, 2005) may be effective in patients refractory to other therapies. In one study, the addition of intravenous cyclophosphamide to ACTH/IV Ig did not improve the short-term or long-term neurological outcome for patients over that associated with ACTH/IV Ig alone (Pranzatelli *et al.*, 2005c). In one small series chronic mycophenolate allowed reduced corticosteroid doses and produced a reduction in activated T lymphocytes and T cell cytokines in the CSF (Pranzatelli *et al.*, 2005b).

At least one-half of children with POM have a protracted or fluctuating course. Exacerbations of neurological symptoms may occur when ACTH or corticosteroids are tapered or discontinued, or during febrile illnesses (Hammer *et al.*, 1995; Mitchell & Snodgrass, 1990; Mitchell *et al.*, 2005; Telander *et al.*, 1989). Unfortunately, at least two-thirds of children are left with some combination of residual motor deficits, speech delay, learning disability, impulsive or aggressive behavior, and sleep disturbance (Hayward *et al.*, 2001; Mitchell *et al.*, 2002; Papero *et al.*, 1995; Pranzatelli *et al.*, 2005a). An initially good neurological response to tumor treatment and/or immunotherapy does not necessarily predict a better long-term neurological outcome (Hammer *et al.*, 1995; Hayward *et al.*, 2001; Rudnick *et al.*, 2001; Russo *et al.*, 1997). In one retrospective study the minority of patients with POM who received chemotherapy had a more favorable long-term neurological outcome (Russo *et al.*, 1997), but this was not seen in other series. A long-term longitundinal neurodevelopmental study showed that patients who had a monophasic course had a better long-term outcome than those with exacer-bations or relapses (Mitchell *et al.*, 2005).

REFERENCES

Alamowitch S, Graus F, Uchuya M *et al.* (1997). Limbic encephalitis and small cell lung cancer: clinical and immunological features. *Brain* **120**: 923–928.

Ances BM, Vitaliani R, Taylor RA *et al.* (2005). Treatment-responsive limbic encephalitis identified by neuropil antibodies: MRI and PET correlates. *Brain* **128**: 1764–1777.

Anderson NE, Budde-Steffen C, Rosenblum MK *et al.* (1988). Opsoclonus, myoclonus, ataxia, and encephalopathy in adults with cancer: a distinct paraneoplastic syndrome. *Medicine* **67**: 100–109.

Antoine JC, Honnorat J, Anterion CT *et al.* (1995). Limbic encephalitis and immunological perturbations in two patients with thymoma. *J Neurol Neurosurg Psychiatry* **58**: 706–710.

Antoine JC, Absi L, Honnorat J *et al.* (1999). Anti-amphiphysin antibodies are associated with various paraneoplastic neurological syndromes and tumors. *Arch Neurol* **56**: 172–177.

Antunes NL, Khakoo Y, Matthay KK *et al.* (2000). Antineuronal antibodies in patients with neuroblastoma and paraneoplastic opsoclonus-myoclonus. *J Pediatr Hematol Oncol* **22**: 315–320.

Aydiner A, Gurvit H, Baral I (1998). Paraneoplastic limbic encephalitis with immune ovarian teratoma. *J Neurooncol* **37**: 63–66.

Bak TH, Antoun N, Balan KK, Hodges JR (2001). Memory lost, memory regained: neuropsychological findings and neuroimaging in two cases of paraneoplastic limbic encephalitis with radically different outcomes. *J Neurol Neurosurg Psychiatry* **71**: 40–47.

Bakheit AM, Kennedy PG, Behan PO (1990). Paraneoplastic limbic encephalitis: clinicopathologic correlations. *J Neurol Neurosurg Psychiatry* **53**: 1084–1088.

Bataller L, Wade DF, Graus F *et al.* (2004). Antibodies to Zic4 in paraneoplastic neurological disorders and small cell lung cancer. *Neurology* **62**: 778–782.

Behin A, Delattre JY (2004). Complications of radiation therapy on the brain and spinal cord. *Semin Neurol* **24**(4): 405–417.

Bell BB, Tognoni PG, Bihrle R (1998). Limbic encephalitis as a paraneoplastic manifestation of renal cell carcinoma. *J Urol* **160**: 828.

Benke T, Wagner M, Pallua AK *et al.* (2004). Long-term cognitive and MRI findings in a patient with paraneoplastic limbic encephalitis. *J Neurooncol* **66**: 217–224.

Bennett JL, Galetta SL, Frohman LP *et al.* (1999). Neuro-ophthalmologic manifestations of a paraneoplastic syndrome and testicular carcinoma. *Neurology* **52**: 864–867.

Bernal F, Graus F, Pifarre A *et al.* (2002). Immunohistochemical analysis of anti-Hu-associated paraneoplastic encephalomyelitis. *Acta Neuropathol* **103**: 509–515.

Bien CG, Schulze-Bonhage A, Deckert M *et al.* (2000). Limbic encephalitis not associated with neoplasm as a cause of temporal lobe epilepsy. *Neurology* **55**: 1823–1828.

Blaes F, Fuhlhuber V, Korfei M *et al.* (2005). Surface-binding autoantibodies to cerebellar neurons in opsoclonus syndrome. *Ann Neurol* **58**: 313–317.

Bloch MH, Hwang WC, Baehring JM, Chambers SK (2004). Paraneoplastic limbic encephalitis: ovarian cancer presenting as an amnestic syndrome. *Obstet Gynecol* **104**: 1174–1177.

Boltshauser E, Deonna T, Hirt HR (1979). Myoclonic encephalopathy of infants, or "dancing eyes syndrome." *Helv Paediatr Acta* **34**: 119–133.

Brierley JB, Corsellis JA, Hierons R, Nevin S (1960). Subacute encephalitis of later adult life mainly affecting the limbic areas. *Brain* **83**: 357–368.

Buckley C, Oger J, Clover L *et al.* (2001). Potassium channel antibodies in two patients with reversible limbic encephalitis. *Ann Neurol* **50**: 73–78.

Candler PM, Dale RC, Griffin S *et al.* (2006). Post-streptococcal opsoclonus-myoclonus syndrome associated with anti-neuroleukin antibodies. *J Neurol Neurosurg Psychiatry* **77**: 507–512.

Chan KH, Vernino S, Lennon VA (2001). ANNA-3 anti-neuronal nuclear antibody: marker of lung cancer-related autoimmunity. *Ann Neurol* **50**: 301–311.

Connolly AM, Pestronk A, Mehta S *et al.* (1997). Serum autoantibodies in childhood opsoclonus-myoclonus syndrome: an analysis of antigenic targets in neural tissues. *J Pediatr* **130**: 878–884.

Cooper R, Khakoo Y, Matthay KK *et al.* (2001). Opsoclonus-myoclonus-ataxia syndrome in neuroblastoma: histopathologic features. *Med Pediatr Oncol* **36**: 623–629.

Corsellis JA, Goldberg GJ, Norton AR (1968). "Limbic encephalitis" and its association with carcinoma. *Brain* **91**: 481–496.

Dalmau J, Graus F, Rosenblum MK, Posner JB (1992). Anti-Hu-associated paraneoplastic encephalomyelitis/sensory neuronopathy: a clinical study of 71 patients. *Medicine* **71**: 59–72.

Dalmau J, Graus F, Villarejo A *et al.* (2004). Clinical analysis of anti-Ma2-associated encephalitis. *Brain* 127: 1831–1844.

Deodhare S, O'Connor P, Ghazarian D, Bilbao JM (1996). Paraneoplastic limbic encephalitis in Hodgkin disease. *Can J Neurol Sci* 23: 138–140.

Dirr LY, Elster AD, Donofrio PD, Smith M (1990). Evolution of brain MRI abnormalities in limbic encephalitis. *Neurology* 40: 1304–1306.

Dorresteijn LD, Kappelle AC, Renier WO, Gijtenbeek JM (2002). Anti-amphiphysin associated limbic encephalitis: a paraneoplastic presentation of small-cell lung carcinoma. *J Neurol* 249: 1307–1308.

Dropcho EJ (2002). Remote neurologic manifestations of cancer. *Neurol Clin* 20 (1): 85–122.

Dropcho EJ (2004). Neurotoxicity of cancer chemotherapy. *Semin Neurol* 24(4): 419–426.

Dropcho EJ (2005). Immunotherapy for paraneoplastic neurological disorders. *Expert Opin Biol Ther* 5(10): 1339–1348.

Duyckaerts C, Derouesne C, Signoret JL *et al.* (1985). Bilateral and limited amygdalohippocampal lesions causing a pure amnestic syndrome. *Ann Neurol* 18: 314–319.

Dyken P, Kolar O (1968). Dancing eyes, dancing feet: infantile polymyoclonus. *Brain* 91: 305–320.

Fakhoury T, Abou-Khalil B, Kessler RM (1999). Limbic encephalitis and hyperactive foci on PET scan. *Seizure* 8: 427–430.

Farrugia ME, Conway R, Simpson DJ, Kurian KM (2005). Paraneoplastic limbic encephalitis. *Clin Neurol Neurosurg* 107: 128–131.

Fauser S, Talazko J, Wagner K *et al.* (2005). FDG-PET and MRI in potassium channel antibody-associated non-paraneoplastic limbic encephalitis. *Acta Neurol Scand* 111: 338–343.

Fisher PG, Wechsler DS, Singer HS (1994). Anti-Hu antibody in a neuroblastoma-associated paraneoplastic syndrome. *Pediatr Neurol* 10: 309–312.

Fujii N, Furuta A, Yamaguchi H *et al.* (2001). Limbic encephalitis associated with recurrent thymoma: a post-mortem study. *Neurology* 57: 344–347.

Gambini C, Conte M, Bernini G *et al.* (2003). Neuroblastic tumors associated with opsoclonus-myoclonus syndrome: histological, immunohistochemical and molecular features of 15 Italian cases. *Virchows Arch* 442: 555–462.

Graus F, Keime-Guibert F, Rene R *et al.* (2001). Anti-Hu-associated paraneoplastic encephalomyelitis: analysis of 200 patients. *Brain* 124: 1138–1148.

Graus F, Delattre JY, Antoine JC *et al.* (2004). Recommended diagnostic criteria for paraneoplastic neurological syndromes. *J Neurol Neurosurg Psychiatry* 75: 1135–1140.

Gultekin SH, Rosenfeld MR, Voltz R *et al.* (2000). Paraneoplastic limbic encephalitis: neurological symptoms, immunological findings and tumour association in 50 patients. *Brain* 123: 1481–1494.

Hammer MS, Larsen MB, Stack CV (1995). Outcome of children with opsoclonus-myoclonus regardless of etiology. *Pediatr Neurol* 13: 21–24.

Hart IK, Maddison P, Newsom-Davis J *et al.* (2002). Phenotypic variants of autoimmune peripheral nerve hyperexcitability. *Brain* 125: 1887–1895.

Hayward K, Jeremy RJ, Jenkins S *et al.* (2001). Long-term neurobehavioral outcome in children with neuroblastoma and opsoclonus-myoclonus-ataxia syndrome: relationship to MRI findings and anti-neuronal antibodies. *J Pediatr* 139: 552–559.

Henson RA, Hoffman HL, Urich H (1965). Encephalomyelitis with carcinoma. *Brain* 88: 449–464.

Hersh B, Dalmau J, Dangond F *et al.* (1994). Paraneoplastic opsoclonus-myoclonus associated with anti-Hu antibody. *Neurology* 44: 1754–1755.

Hirayama K, Taguchi Y, Sato M, Tsukamoto T (2003). Limbic encephalitis presenting with topographical disorientation and amnesia. *J Neurol Neurosurg Psychiatry* 74: 110–112.

Hiyama E, Yokoyama T, Ichikawa T *et al.* (1994). Poor outcome in patients with advanced stage neuroblastoma and coincident opsomyoclonus syndrome. *Cancer* 74: 1821–1826.

Ingenito GG, Berger JR, David NJ, Norenberg MD (1990). Limbic encephalitis associated with thymoma. *Neurology* 40: 382.

Kaniecki R, Morris JC (1993). Reversible paraneoplastic limbic encephalitis. *Neurology* 43: 2418–2419.

Kararizou E, Markou I, Zalonis I *et al.* (2005). Paraneoplastic limbic encephalitis presenting as acute viral encephalitis. *J Neurooncology* 75: 229–232.

Keime-Guibert F, Graus F, Broet P *et al.* (1999). Clinical outcome of patients with anti-Hu-associated encephalomyelitis after treatment of the tumor. *Neurology* 53: 1719–1723.

Kinirons P, Fulton A, Keoghan M *et al.* (2003). Paraneoplastic limbic encephalitis and chorea associated with CRMP-5 neuronal antibody. *Neurology* 61: 1623–1624.

Kinsbourne M (1962). Myoclonic encephalopathy of infants. *J Neurol Neurosurg Psychiatry* 25: 271–276.

Kleopa KA, Elman LB, Lang B *et al.* (2006). Neuromyotonia and limbic encephalitis sera target mature Shaker-type K+ channels: subunit specificity correlates with clinical manifestations. *Brain* **129**: 1570–1584.

Kodama T, Numaguchi Y, Gellad FE *et al.* (1991). Magnetic resonance imaging of limbic encephalitis. *Neuroradiology* **33**: 520–523.

Kohler J, Hufschmidt A, Hermle L *et al.* (1988). Limbic encephalitis: two cases. *J Neurooncology* **20**: 177–178.

Konczak J, Schoch B, Dimitrova A *et al.* (2005). Functional recovery of children and adolescents after cerebellar tumour resection. *Brain* **128**: 1428–1441.

Korfei M, Fuhlhuber V, Schmidt T *et al.* (2005). Functional characterisation of autoantibodies from patients with pediatric opsoclonus-myoclonus syndrome. *J Neuroimmunol* **170**: 150–157.

Kuban KC, Ephros MA, Freeman RL *et al.* (1983). Syndrome of opsoclonus-myoclonus caused by Coxsackie B3 infection. *Ann Neurol* **13**: 69–71.

Lacomis D, Khoshbin S., Schick RM (1990). MR imaging of paraneoplastic limbic encephalitis. *J Comput Assist Tomogr* **14**: 115–117.

Landolfi JC, Nadkarni M (2003). Paraneoplastic limbic encephalitis and possible narcolepsy in a patient with testicular cancer: case study. *Neurooncology* **5**: 214–216.

Lawn ND, Westmoreland BF, Kiely MJ *et al.* (2003). Clinical, magnetic resonance imaging, and electroencephalographic findings in paraneoplastic limbic encephalitis. *Mayo Clin Proc* **78**: 1363–1368.

Lee AC, Ou Y, Lee WK, Wong YC (2003). Paraneoplastic limbic encephalitis masquerading as chronic behavioural disturbance in an adolescent girl. *Acta Paediatr* **92**: 506–509.

Lee EK, Maselli RA, Agius MA (1998). Morvan's fibrillary chorea: a paraneoplastic manifestation of thymoma. *J Neurol Neurosurg Psychiatry* **65**: 857–862.

Liguori R, Vincent A, Clover L *et al.* (2001). Morvan's syndrome: peripheral and central nervous system and cardiac involvement with antibodies to voltage-gated potassium channels. *Brain* **124**: 2417–2426.

Linke R, Schroeder M, Helmberger T, Voltz R (2004). Antibody-positive paraneoplastic neurologic syndromes: value of CT and PET for tumor diagnosis. *Neurology* **63**: 282–286.

Mihara M, Sugase S, Konaka K *et al.* (2005). The "pulvinar sign" in a case of paraneoplastic limbic encephalitis associated with non-Hodgkin's lymphoma. *J Neurol Neurosurg Psychiatry* **76**: 882–884.

Mitchell WG, Snodgrass SR (1990). Opsoclonus-ataxia due to childhood neural crest tumors: a chronic neurologic syndrome. *J Child Neurol* **5**: 153–158.

Mitchell WG, Davalos Y, Brumm VL *et al.* (2002). Opsoclonus-ataxia caused by childhood neuroblastoma: developmental and neurologic sequelae. *Pediatrics* **109**: 86–98.

Mitchell WG, Brumm VL, Azen CG *et al.* (2005). Longitudinal neurodevelopmental evaluation of children with opsoclonus-ataxia. *Pediatrics* **116**: 901–907.

Modrego PJ, Cay A, Pina A, Monge A (2002). Paraneoplastic subacute encephalitis caused by adenocarcinoma of prostate: a case report. *Acta Neurol Scand* **105**: 351–353.

Moe PG, Nellhaus G (1970). Infantile polymyoclonia-opsoclonus syndrome and neural crest tumors. *Neurology* **20**: 756–764.

Mori M, Kuwabara S, Yoshiyama M *et al.* (2002). Successful immune treatment for non-paraneoplastic limbic encephalitis. *J Neurol Sci* **201**: 85–88.

Na DL, Hahm DS, Park JM, Kim SE (2001). Hypermetabolism of the medial temporal lobe in limbic encephalitis on FDG-PET scan: a case report. *Eur Neurol* **45**: 187–189.

Nokura K, Yamamoto H, Okawara Y *et al.* (1997). Reversible limbic encephalitis caused by ovarian teratoma. *Acta Neurol Scand* **95**: 367–373.

Ogata M, Kikuchi H, Satou T *et al.* (2006). Human herpesvirus 6 DNA in plasma after allogeneic stem cell transplantation: incidence and clinical significance. *J Infect Dis* **193**: 68–79.

Okamura H, Oomori N, Uchitomi Y (1997). An acutely confused 15-year-old girl. *Lancet* **350**: 488.

Overeem S, Dalmau J, Bataller L *et al.* (2004). Hypocretin-1 CSF levels in anti-Ma2 associated encephalitis. *Neurology* **62**: 138–140.

Papero PJ, Pranzatelli MR, Margolis LJ *et al.* (1995). Neurobehavioral and psychological functioning of children with opsoclonus-myoclonus syndrome. *Dev Med Child Neurol* **37**: 915–932.

Parisi MT, Hattner RS, Matthay KK *et al.* (1993). Optimized diagnostic strategy for neuroblastoma in opsoclonus-myoclonus. *J Nucl Med* **34**: 1922–1926.

Pelkofer H, Schubart AS, Hoftberger R *et al.* (2004). Modelling paraneoplastic CNS disease: T-cells specific for the onconeuronal antigen PNMA1 mediate autoimmune encephalitis in the rat. *Brain* **127**: 1822–1830.

Petit T, Janser JC, Achour NR *et al.* (1997). Paraneoplastic temporal lobe epilepsy and anti-Yo autoantibody. *Ann Oncol* **8**: 919.

Petruzzi MJ, Alarcon PA (1995). Neuroblastoma-associated opsoclonus-myoclonus treated with intravenously administered immune globulin G. *J Pediatr* **127**: 328–329.

Pittock SJ, Kryzer TJ, Lennon VA (2004). Paraneoplastic antibodies coexist and predict cancer, not neurological syndrome. *Ann Neurol* **56**: 715–719.

Pittock SJ, Lucchinetti CF, Parisi JE *et al.* (2005). Amphiphysin autoimmunity: paraneoplastic accompaniments. *Ann Neurol* **58**: 96–107.

Plonquet A, Gherardi RK, Creange A *et al.* (2002). Oligoclonal T-cells in blood and target tissues of patients with anti-Hu syndrome. *J Neuroimmunol* **122**: 100–105.

Plonquet A, Garcia-Pons F, Fernandez E *et al.* (2003). Peptides derived from the onconeural HuD protein can elicit cytotoxic responses in HHD mouse and human. *J Neuroimmunol* **142**: 93–100.

Pohl KR, Pritchard J, Wilson J (1996). Neurologic sequelae of the dancing eye syndrome. *Eur J Pediatr* **155**: 237–244.

Pozo-Rosich P, Clover L, Saiz A *et al.* (2003). Voltage-gated potassium channel antibodies in limbic encephalitis. *Ann Neurol* **54**: 530–533.

Pranzatelli MR, Hyland K, Tate ED *et al.* (2004a). Evidence of cellular immune activation in children with opsoclonus-myoclonus: cerebrospinal fluid neopterin. *J Child Neurol* **19**: 919–924.

Pranzatelli MR, Travelstead AL, Tate ED *et al.* (2004b). B- and T-cell markers in opsoclonus-myoclonus syndrome: immunophenotyping of CSF lymphocytes. *Neurology* **62**: 1526–1532.

Pranzatelli MR, Tate ED, Dukart WS *et al.* (2005a). Sleep disturbance and rage attacks in opsoclonus-myoclonus syndrome: response to trazodone. *J Pediatr* **147**: 372–378.

Pranzatelli MR, Tate ED, Travelstead AL *et al.* (2005b). Mycophenolate reduces CSF T-cell activation and is a steroid sparer in opsoclonus-myoclonus syndrome (abstract). *Ann Neurol* **58** [Suppl. 9]: S111.

Pranzatelli MR, Tate ED, Travelstead AL *et al.* (2005c). Cyclophosphamide therapy in pediatric opsoclonus-myoclonus syndrome [abstract]. *Ann Neurol* **58** [Suppl. 9]: S90.

Pranzatelli MR, Tate ED, Travelstead AL, Longee D (2005d). Immunologic and clinical responses to rituximab in a child with opsoclonus-myoclonus syndrome. *Pediatrics* **115**: e115–119.

Provenzale JM, Barboriak DP, Coleman RE (1998). Limbic encephalitis: comparison of FDG PET and MR imaging findings. *AJR Am J Roentgenol* **170**: 1659–1660.

Ravizza SM, McCormick CA, Schlerf JE *et al.* (2006). Cerebellar damage produces selective deficits in verbal working memory. *Brain* **129**: 306–320.

Rickman OB, Parisi JE, Yu Z *et al.* (2000). Fulminant autoimmune cortical encephalitis associated with thymoma treated with plasma exchange. *Mayo Clin Proc* **75**: 1321–1326.

Ridley A, Kennard C, Scholtz CL *et al.* (1987). Omnipause neurons in two cases of opsoclonus associated with oat cell carcinoma of the lung. *Brain* **110**: 1699–1709.

Roberts WK, Darnell RB (2004). Neuroimmunology of the paraneoplastic neurological degenerations. *Curr Opin Immunol* **16**: 616–622.

Rojas I, Graus F, Keime-Guibert F *et al.* (2000). Long-term clinical outcome of paraneoplastic cerebellar degeneration and anti-Yo antibodies. *Neurology* **55**: 713–715.

Ronning C, Sundet K, Due-Tonnessen B *et al.* (2005). Persistent cognitive dysfunction secondary to cerebellar injury in patients treated for posterior fossa tumors in childhood. *Pediatr Neurosurg* **41**: 15–21.

Rosenbaum T, Gartner J, Korholz D *et al.* (1998). Paraneoplastic limbic encephalitis in two teenage girls. *Neuropediatrics* **29**: 159–162.

Rosenfeld MR, Eichen JG, Wade DF *et al.* (2001). Molecular and clinical diversity in paraneoplastic immunity to Ma proteins. *Ann Neurol* **50**: 339–348.

Rostasy K, Behnisch W, Kulozik A *et al.* (2005). High-dose pulsatile dexamethasone therapy in children with opsoclonus-myoclonus syndrome [abstract]. *Ann Neurol* **58** [Suppl. 9]: S109.

Rousseau A, Benyahia B, Dalmau J *et al.* (2005). T-cell response to Hu-D peptides in patients with anti-Hu syndrome. *J Neurooncology* **71**: 231–236.

Rudnick E, Khakoo Y, Antunes NL *et al.* (2001). Opsoclonus-myoclonus-ataxia syndrome in neuroblastoma: clinical outcome and antineuronal antibodies: a report from the Children's Cancer Group. *Med Pediatr Oncol* **36**: 612–622.

Russo C, Cohn SL, Petruzzi MJ, Alarcon PA (1997). Long-term neurologic outcome in children with opsoclonus-myoclonus associated with neuroblastoma: a report from the Pediatric Oncology Group. *Med Pediatr Oncol* **29**: 284–288.

Sahashi K, Sakai K, Mano K, Hirose G (2003). Anti-Ma2 antibody related paraneoplastic limbic/brain stem encephalitis associated with breast cancer expressing Ma1, Ma2, and Ma3 mRNAs. *J Neurol Neurosurg Psychiatry* **74**: 1332–1335.

Scheid R, Voltz R, Guthke T *et al.* (2003). Neuropsychiatric findings in anti-Ma2-positive paraneoplastic limbic encephalitis. *Neurology* **61**: 1159–1160.

Scheid R, Honnorat J, Delmont E *et al.* (2004a). A new anti-neuronal antibody in a case of paraneoplastic limbic encephalitis associated with breast cancer. *J Neurol Neurosurg Psychiatry* **75**: 338–340.

Scheid R, Lincke T, Voltz R *et al.* (2004b). Serial FDG positron emission tomography and magnetic resonance imaging of paraneoplastic limbic encephalitis. *Arch Neurol* **61**: 1785–1789.

Shapiro B, Shulkin BL, Hutchinson RJ *et al.* (1994). Locating neuroblastoma in the opsoclonus-myoclonus syndrome. *J Nucl Biol Med* **38**: 545–555.

Sheth RD, Horwitz SJ, Aronoff S *et al.* (1995). Opsoclonus myoclonus syndrome secondary to Epstein-Barr virus infection. *J Child Neurol* **10**: 297–299.

Sillevis Smitt P, Grefkens J, de Leeuw B *et al.* (2002). Survival and outcome in 73 anti-Hu positive patients with paraneoplastic encephalomyelitis/sensory neuronopathy. *J Neurol* **249**: 745–753.

Solomon GE, Chutorian AM (1968). Opsoclonus and occult neuroblastoma. *N Engl J Med* **279**: 475–477.

Stern RC, Hulette CM (1999). Paraneoplastic limbic encephalitis associated with small cell carcinoma of the prostate. *Mod Pathol* **12**: 814–818.

Sutton I, Winer J, Rowlands D, Dalmau J (2000). Limbic encephalitis and antibodies to Ma2: a paraneoplastic presentation of breast cancer. *J Neurol Neurosurg Psychiatry* **69**: 266–268.

Sutton RC, Lipper MH, Brashear HR (1993). Limbic encephalitis occurring in association with Alzheimer's disease. *J Neurol Neurosurg Psychiatry* **56**: 808–811.

Tabarki B, Palmer P, Lebon P, Sebire G (1998). Spontaneous recovery of opsoclonus-myoclonus syndrome caused by enterovirus infection. *J Neurol Neurosurg Psychiatry* **64**: 406–422.

Tattevin P, Schortgen F, Broucker T *et al.* (2001). Varicella-zoster virus limbic encephalitis in an immunocompromised patient. *Scand J Infect Dis* **33**: 786–788.

Taylor RB, Mason W, Kong K, Wennberg R (1999). Reversible paraneoplastic encephalomyelitis associated with a benign ovarian teratoma. *Can J Neurol Sci* **26**: 317–320.

Telander RL, Smithson WA, Groover RV (1989). Clinical outcome in children with acute cerebellar encephalopathy and neuroblastoma. *J Pediatr Surg* **24**: 11–14.

Tersak JM, Safier RA, Schor NF (2005). Rituximab in the treatment of refractory neuroblastoma-associated opsoclonus-myoclonus syndrome [abstract]. *Ann Neurol* **58** [Suppl. 9]: S111.

Thieben MJ, Lennon VA, Boeve BF *et al.* (2004). Potentially reversible autoimmune limbic encephalitis with neuronal potassium channel antibody. *Neurology* **62**: 1177–1182.

Thuerl C, Muller K, Laubenberger J *et al.* (2003). MR imaging of autopsy-proven paraneoplastic limbic encephalitis in non-Hodgkin lymphoma. *AJNR Am J Neuroradiol* **24**: 507–510.

Tomimitsu H, Arimura K, Nagado T *et al.* (2004). Mechanism of action of voltage-gated K$^+$ channel antibodies in acquired neuromyotonia. *Ann Neurol* **56**: 440–444.

Tsukamoto T, Mochizuki R, Mochizuki H *et al.* (1993). Paraneoplastic cerebellar degeneration and limbic encephalitis in a patient with adenocarcinoma of the colon. *J Neurol Neurosurg Psychiatry* **56**: 713–716.

Veneselli E, Conte M, Biancheri R *et al.* (1998). Effect of steroid and high-dose immunoglobulin therapy on opsoclonus-myoclonus syndrome occurring in neuroblastoma. *Med Pediatr Oncol* **30**: 15–17.

Vernino S, Lennon VA (2000). New Purkinje cell antibody (PCA-2): marker of lung cancer-related neurological autoimmunity. *Ann Neurol* **47**: 297–305.

Vernino S, Lennon VA (2004). Autoantibody profiles and neurological correlations of thymoma. *Clin Cancer Res* **10**: 7270–7275.

Vernino S, Eggenberger ER, Rogers LR, Lennon VA (2002). Paraneoplastic neurological autoimmunity associated with ANNA-1 autoantibody and thymoma. *Neurology* **59**: 929–932.

Vincent A, Buckley C, Schott J *et al.* (2004). Potassium channel antibody-associated encephalopathy: a potentially immunotherapy-responsive form of limbic encephalitis. *Brain* **127**: 701–712.

Vitaliani R, Mason W, Ances B *et al.* (2005). Paraneoplastic encephalitis, psychiatric symptoms, and hypoventilation in ovarian teratoma. *Ann Neurol* **58**: 594–604.

Voltz RD, Gultekin HS, Rosenfeld MR *et al.* (1999). A serologic marker of paraneoplastic limbic and brain-stem encephalitis in patients with testicular cancer. *New Engl J Med* **340**: 1788–1795.

Wainwright MS, Martin PL, Morse RP *et al.* (2001). Human herpesvirus 6 limbic encephalitis after stem cell transplantation. *Ann Neurol* **50**: 612–619.

Waragi M, Chiba A, Uchibori A *et al.* (2006). Anti-Ma2 associated paraneoplastic neurological syndrome presenting as encephalitis and progressive muscular atrophy. *J Neurol Neurosurg Psychiatry* **77**: 111–113.

Wingerchuk DM, Noseworthy JH, Kimmel DW (1998). Paraneoplastic encephalomyelitis and seminoma: importance of testicular ultrasonography. *Neurology* **51**: 1504–1507.

Wong AM, Musallam S, Tomlinson RD *et al.* (2001). Opsoclonus in three dimensions: oculographic, neuropathologic and modelling correlates. *J Neurol Sci* **189**: 71–81.

Yiu VW, Kovithavongs T, McGonigle LF, Ferreira P (2001). Plasmapheresis as an effective treatment for opsoclonus-myoclonus syndrome. *Pediatr Neurol* **24**: 72–74.

Younes-Mhenni S, Janier MF, Cinotti L *et al.* (2004). FDG-PET improves tumour detection in patients with paraneoplastic neurological syndromes. *Brain* **127**: 2331–2338.

Yu Z, Kryzer TJ, Griesmann GE *et al.* (2001). CRMP-5 neuronal autoantibody: marker of lung cancer and thymoma-related autoimmunity. *Ann Neurol* **49**: 146–154.

Ziter FA, Bray PF, Cancilla PA (1979). Neuropathologic findings in a patient with neuroblastoma and myoclonic encephalopathy. *Arch Neurol* **36**: 51.

18

Symptomatic therapies and supportive care issues

Alan Valentine and Eduardo Bruera

Introduction

The supportive care of cancer patients routinely involves management of multiple symptoms as well as neuropsychiatric disorders associated with cognitive dysfunction, notably delirium, but also in some instances depression. Cancer therapies themselves (especially medications) can cause or exacerbate cognitive dysfunction. Cognitive disorders of all types are the second most common psychiatric disorders experienced by cancer patients after mood disorders (Derogatis *et al.*, 1983). Patients in particular settings and stages of the disease continuum are at particular risk for cognitive impairment, with potential implications for prognosis. The boundaries between these disorders are not always distinct, which complicates accurate diagnosis and treatment. Co-morbidity is common. The stigma associated with mental illness and the physical burdens of caring for affected patients place family members and other caregivers at increased risk for physical and emotional distress. The common cognitive disorders seen in the oncology setting often respond well to treatment. In other cases, palliation of symptoms is possible and individual patients may respond to creative and unconventional medication interventions. Here we discuss common neuropsychiatric syndromes and clinical settings associated with cognitive dysfunction and altered mental status and behavior, interventions, and potential areas for future research.

Delirium

The American Psychiatric Association defines delirium as a syndrome characterized by rapid onset of impaired cognition, and altered consciousness, and it is presumed to be due to one or more physical or disease-related factors (Table 18.1, American Psychiatric Association, 2000; DSM-IV TR). Other definitions include these criteria but also emphasize altered ability to attend and changes in sleep-wake cycle and behavior (psychomotor agitation or retardation) (Table 18.2, basic psychopathology of delirium). Delirium is a serious complication of medical illness, especially for the hospitalized patient and in geriatric custodial care settings. It is associated with increased length and cost of hospital stay and with increased morbidity and mortality (Caraceni *et al.*, 2000; Franco *et al.*, 2001; Leslie *et al.*, 2005). The prevalence of delirium in oncology varies greatly and ranges from 7%–50% in various inpatient settings to >85% at the end of life (Fann *et al.*, 2002; Lawlor *et al.*, 2000a; Ljubisavljevic & Kelly, 2003; Massie *et al.*, 1983; Prieto *et al.*, 2002). Delirium is often overlooked and is easily misdiagnosed. In intensive care and peri-operative settings, the

Cognition and Cancer, eds. Christina A. Meyers and James R. Perry. Published by Cambridge University Press.
© Cambridge University Press 2008.

Table 18.1. DSM-IV criteria for delirium

1. Disturbance of consciousness (i.e., reduced clarity of awareness of the environment) with reduced ability to focus, sustain, or shift attention
2. Change in cognition (i.e., memory deficit, disorientation, language disturbance) or development of a perceptual disturbance that is not better accounted for by a pre-existing or evolving dementia
3. Development of the disturbance over a short period of time (usually hours–days) with fluctuating course during the day
4. Evidence from this history, physical examination, or laboratory findings that the disturbance is caused by physiological consequences of a medical condition

Source: Reprinted with permission from the *Diagnostic and Statistical Manual of Mental Disorders* (4th edn. Text Revision) (Copyright 2000) (American Psychiatric Association, 2000).

Table 18.2. Basic psychopathology of delirium (Lipowski, 1990)

- Impaired awareness of self and surroundings (also referred to as "reduced level of consciousness")
- Impairment of directed thinking
- Disorder of attention, with hypo- or hyper-alertness
- Impairment of memory
- Diminished perceptual discrimination, with a tendency toward misperceptions, i.e., illusions and hallucinations
- Impairment of spatiotemporal orientation (may be absent in a mild case)
- Disturbance of psychomotor behavior, with hyper- or hypoactivity, both verbal and non-verbal
- Disordered sleep-wake cycle, usually marked by drowsiness and naps during the day, insomnia at night, or both
- Unpredictable fluctuations in alertness and in severity of cognitive impairment during the day and overall exacerbation of symptoms at night and upon awakening
- Acute onset and relatively brief duration (hours to several weeks)
- Laboratory evidence of widespread cerebral dysfunction, especially diffuse changes (slowing or fast activity of background activity on the EEG)

Source: Lipowski ZJ (1990). *Delirium: Acute Confusional States.* New York: Oxford University Press with permission.

misleading term "ICU psychosis" is often used. This implies a functional emotional reaction to the stress of the intensive care setting and discourages or trivializes the need for aggressive search for reversible causes of altered mental status. Because of the fluctuating course and variable presentations of delirium it may be confused with other neuropsychiatric disorders including depression, dementia, and primary thought disorders, leading to inappropriate treatment. The course of delirium often includes lucid intervals characterized by periods in which the patient appears cognitively and behaviorally intact. It may appear that the delirium has resolved only to have the patient return to previous or new abnormal behaviors.

Delirium may be classified by the level and intensity of associated psychomotor activity. Hyperactive, hypoactive, and mixed forms of the syndrome have been described (O'Keeffe & Lavan, 1999; Ross *et al.*, 1991). The hyperactive form with obvious motor agitation, autonomic instability, prominent delusions or hallucinations, and affective lability is usually fairly easy to recognize. The classic model for hyperactive delirium is alcohol withdrawal delirium (*delirium tremens*). The patient in a hyperac-

tive delirium is a potential physical threat to self and others, and will often require treatment with antipsychotic drugs and possibly physical restraint.

Hypoactive delirium presents with slowing of thought processes, speech, and behavior. Affect is minimally reactive. Level of arousal is decreased and attention to the surrounding environment is diminished; this can be difficult to observe during a brief examination. This diagnosis is easily missed, as the initial and prevailing impression may be of a patient who is severely depressed or possibly demented.

A mixed form of delirium is characterized by features of both the hyperactive and hypoactive forms. The behaviors of a patient in a mixed-form delirium may vary from day to day or within a day, often without warning and without any predictability in the variability.

Delirium risk factors in general hospital and geriatric settings are probably relevant in oncology.

These include advanced age, baseline cognitive function, medications (especially anticholinergic drugs and central nervous system depressants), and electrolyte and metabolic dyscrasias (Inouye, 1998, 2000). Recent investigations in cancer patients have produced conflicting data regarding the use of certain common supportive care drugs (benzodiazepines, opioid analgesics) as risk factors for delirium (Gaudreau *et al.*, 2005; Ljubisavljevic & Kelly, 2003).

The cognitive impairment of delirium is such that the patient often (but not always) has no memory of related events afterwards. One sign of improvement in delirium is the patient's realization that perceptual disturbances (illusions and hallucinations) are not real. The patient cannot attend, or does so inconsistently. Short-term memory (and sometimes long-term memory) is impaired. Frequently the patient is disoriented. Thought processes are illogical. Speech may be affected.

Common causes of delirium in cancer patients

Medications may be the most common precipitants of delirium in hospitalized patients, and the list of drugs with any potential to cause altered mental status is extremely long (Brown, 2000; Carter *et al.*, 1996). Geriatric patients are at potentially high risk for drug-induced delirium because of altered (slowed) drug metabolism and because of their relatively high rates of baseline cognitive impairment.

In peri-operative settings, delirium thought secondary to effects of anesthesia is common. Other medications that are routinely associated with altered mental status include opioid analgesics, benzodiazepine sedative-hypnotics, corticosteroids, antiarrhythmics and sympathomimetics (Marcantonio *et al.*, 1994). Anticholinergic drugs have long been associated with a characteristic hyperactive delirium and anticholinergic processes are the best-studied causes of delirium (Trzepacz, 1996; Tune *et al.*, 1981).

Many antineoplastic therapies have been associated with delirium, but there are relatively few that commonly cause the syndrome. These include methotrexate, cytosine arabinoside, ifosfamide and cyclophosphamide (Breitbart & Cohen, 1998). Biological response modifiers especially interleukin-2 and interferon alpha are, especially if used in combination, associated with delirium and sometimes with a prolonged encephalopathic state (Meyers & Valentine, 1995).

Metabolic disturbances are common causes of delirium in this setting. Malignancy-associated hypercalcemia is often implicated, though hypoxia (often related to respiratory failure or anemia or both) is likely a more common cause. Electrolyte disturbances (e.g., significant hyper- or hyponatremia) of any origin and metabolic impairments associated with liver or renal failure (hepatic and renal encephalopathies) are seen frequently. Systemic and central nervous system infections are other common causes. Especially in critically ill patients, it may not be possible to identify a single cause for delirium. The etiology frequently is multifactorial. Figure 18.1 summarizes the most common causes of delirium.

Assessment of delirium

The diagnosis of delirium is clinical and based on history and observation of the patient, review of the medical record and nursing notes, physical examination, and laboratory studies. The delirious patient is often if not always an unreliable historian. It is necessary to rely on family members, nursing staff, and other care providers for details of the onset and characteristics of the clinical presentation. The history of use of medications, use or discontinuation of alcohol and illicit drugs, baseline cognitive function and other events (e.g., falls) is critical in consideration of possible evolving delirium.

Observation and clinical interview of the patient will allow assessment of the level of arousal, psychomotor activity, range and stability of affect, distractibility, and possible illusions, hallucination, and delusions. The formal mental status examination should test attention, orientation, memory, abstract thinking, and speed and dynamics of thought (Lipowski, 1990).

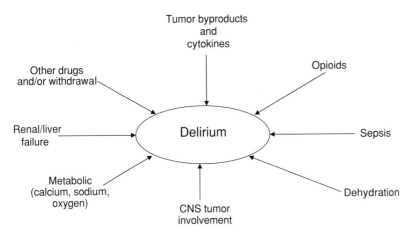

Figure 18.1. Common causes of delirium

Delirium rating scales

The Mini-Mental State Examination (MMSE) may be the most frequently used screen of cognitive function and is often employed to assess delirious patients (Folstein *et al.*, 1975). However, the MMSE does not distinguish delirium from dementia and patients may score poorly on the test for a number of reasons not directly related to delirium (Anthony *et al.*, 1982). The Confusion Assessment Method (CAM) developed by Inouye and colleagues is frequently used and is designed to allow to non-psychiatric clinicians to screen for the presence of delirium (Inouye *et al.*, 1990). Even frequently used instruments such as the CAM have a significant associated error rate and patients who score above threshold levels on these scales should go on to careful clinical evaluation. Other instruments including the Delirium Rating Scale (DRS) and the Memorial Delirium Assessment Scale (MDAS) are used more to assess the severity of delirium and can be used to follow patients over time and assess their response to therapy, and also as research instruments (Breitbart *et al.*, 1997; Trzepacz *et al.*, 1988; Trzepacz, 1994). Physicians, nurses, and other health care professionals with palliative care experience can be trained on the use of the MDAS in a single 2-h review (Fadul, 2007).

Careful physical examination provides information crucial to the search for precipitating and potentially dangerous causes of altered mental status, and will often influence the choice of diagnostic tests. Current and recent vital signs should be assessed. Cardiovascular and pulmonary examinations should be performed. The neurological examination should be emphasized, with assessment for lateralizing signs and increased intracranial pressure.

Laboratory assessment and other tests

Laboratory assessment of possible delirium includes serum chemistries: electrolytes, creatinine, blood urea nitrogen, calcium, magnesium, liver function assays, as well as urinalysis and complete blood count with differential and platelet count. Chest X-ray and electrocardiogram (ECG) should be reviewed or obtained. In appropriate patients, serum drug levels should be obtained; these may include immunosuppressants (e.g., ciclosporin), anticonvulsants, cardiac drugs (e.g., digoxin), and psychotropics (e.g., lithium, tricyclic antidepressants). Especially in the absence of reliable history, urine toxicology screens of prescription and illicit drugs should be obtained. Vitamin B_{12} and serum folate levels should be checked in patients known or suspected to be alcohol-dependent.

Other tests should be considered in certain settings, but are probably not routinely necessary. Neuroimaging (computed axial tomography, magnetic resonance imaging) may be helpful if physical exam reveals focal neurological signs, and in the absence of other obvious causes of delirium, or when delirium persists despite appropriate treatment. The electroencephalogram (EEG) will almost always reveal diffuse, non-specific slowing in the delirious patient. While EEG evaluation is probably not routinely necessary, it should be obtained in cases of suspected seizures. It may also be useful in attempts to distinguish delirium from other causes of similar behavior (e.g., dementia, severe depression, "functional" psychiatric disorders) (Boutros & Struve, 2002).

Management of delirium

Ideally delirium is managed by being prevented. In some settings it is reasonable to anticipate the development of delirium. This is especially true in peri-operative and intensive care settings, the elderly, patients with known cognitive impairment or central nervous system malignancy, patients known to be dependent on alcohol or illicit drugs, and those on complicated medication regimens at baseline. Data from the history, physical examination, and laboratory work-up should guide an aggressive search for potentially reversible or treatable abnormalities that might be responsible for the acute altered mental status.

Behavioral management of delirium includes attention to the physical environment. Ideally the patient is not subjected to excessive light or noise, or other distractions. At the same time, sensory understimulation is probably not helpful. Artificial or natural light should be provided during the day in an attempt to help maintain a normal sleep-wake cycle. Particularly in cases of hypoactive delirium, some physical activity should be encouraged. Low-level background sound and light should be maintained at night. The patient should be reoriented

frequently and assured of his or her safety. The presence of family members is often a source of comfort to the patient. The converse however may not be true: family members are often unprepared for or frightened of behaviors associated with delirium. In such cases and when care requires that the patient be closely monitored, it may be best for all concerned to engage a professional sitter.

Patients in hyperactive delirium are potential threats to themselves or others (e.g., pulled IV lines, self-extubation, violent or impulsive response to perceived threat). The use of physical restraints, while occasionally necessary to aid early management of a patient in a hyperactive delirium, should be avoided if possible and should never be done without pharmacological management.

Pharmacotherapy

Medication management of delirium (especially hyperactive and mixed forms) is usually intended to provide symptomatic control of motor agitation and distressing psychotic symptoms, while attempts are made to identify and correct underlying causes of the disorder. Antipsychotic drugs are the mainstays of such treatment. Of these, haloperidol is generally the agent of choice. The drug may be administered by multiple routes (including intravenously, which is common and effective, though not formally approved), and has comparatively modest anticholinergic and anti-alpha-adrenergic effects. It has been associated with QTc prolongation and ventricular arrhythmia (torsades de pointes) when used at high intravenous doses. Atypical antipsychotic drugs (e.g., risperidone, olanzapine, quetiapine, ziprasidone) have generally favorable safety profiles, though lack of available intravenous administration makes their use potentially problematic in critical care and other special settings (Cassem *et al.*, 2004; Del Fabbro, 2006a; Mazzocato *et al.*, 2000; Valentine & Bickham, 2005).

Benzodiazepines (BZPs) are treatments of choice for alcohol withdrawal delirium because their agonist effects on gamma-aminobutyric acid (GABA) transmission and function directly address one of the primary pathological mechanisms responsible for alcohol withdrawal (Mayo-Smith & Mayo-Smith, 1997). The drugs do not have antipsychotic properties and concomitant use of an antipsychotic may be required. The sedative-hypnotic effects of BZPs are such that they are often used in intensive care and palliative care settings as first-line treatments for delirium not associated with alcohol withdrawal. This approach to management of delirium is problematic. Used alone BZPs will usually not improve cognitive dysfunction associated with delirium and, especially in patients with baseline cognitive impairment (e.g., dementia, elderly patients with mild cognitive impairment), they are likely to exacerbate cognitive dysfunction and may increase psychomotor agitation (Breitbart *et al.*, 1996).

Medication management of hypoactive delirium is less well described in the literature. The patient in a hypoactive delirium is often not obviously psychotic or in emotional distress, and psychomotor retardation is such that the patient is usually not a direct threat to self or others. However, hypoactive delirium is not innocuous and is associated with medical morbidity and adverse outcomes (Kelly *et al.*, 2001; O'Keeffe & Lavan, 1999). Because most antipsychotic drugs are variably sedating, their use in this setting would seem counterintuitive. Classical antipsychotics still may be effective against some symptoms (Platt *et al.*, 1994). Similarly, anticholinergic effects of psychostimulants have the potential to exacerbate some presentations of delirium, but these drugs have been reported effective against the hypoactive form of the syndrome (Gagnon *et al.*, 2005; Morita *et al.*, 2000).

Depression

Cognitive impairment of variable severity is a recognized component of mood disorders, especially major depression (Table 18.3, American Psychiatric Association DSM-IV TR, 2000). In this setting and especially in the elderly, the terms depressive dementia or pseudodementia are used to describe

Table 18.3. DSM-IV major depressive episode

- Depressed mood
- Diminished interest or pleasure in activities
- Significant weight loss/gain or decrease/increase in appetite
- Insomnia or hypersomnia
- Psychomotor agitation or retardation
- Fatigue or loss of energy
- Feelings of worthlessness or excessive guilt
- Diminished ability to think or concentrate, or indecisiveness
- Recurrent thought of death or suicidal ideation

Source: Reprinted with permission from the *Diagnostic and Statistical Manual of Mental Disorders* (4th edn., Text Revision) (Copyright 2000). (American Psychiatric Association, 2000)

significant cognitive impairment. Though major depression and significant adjustment disorders are the most common psychiatric disorders seen in cancer (Derogatis *et al.*, 1983), the pseudodementia construct is likely of less importance in oncology than in general geriatric medicine, where it is a risk factor for development of primary irreversible dementia (Dobie, 2002; Reifler, 2000; Reischies & Neu, 2000; Visser *et al.*, 2000). In our experience, it is uncommon to encounter a patient with depression and significant cognitive impairment without the presence of disease- or treatment-related factors that could also be contributing to the dysfunction, though there are instances in which the diagnosis is in doubt (Pereira & Bruera, 2001). The issue may become more important over time as clinicians encounter and treat increasing numbers of cancer survivors, who are vulnerable to new-onset mood disorders but who have also received neurotoxic therapies.

Anxiety is frequently a co-morbid condition with depression, especially in elderly patients. The chronically anxious patient's complaints of cognitive problems may be a function of impaired attention with subsequent memory registration difficulties. In such instances primary treatment of anxiety may greatly improve day-to-day function.

Disease- and treatment-related factors

Multiple disease- and treatment-related factors may be associated with cognitive impairment in the cancer setting. Often these problems can be palliated, if not completely reversed.

Malignancy-associated metabolic derangements include hypernatremia, hypercalcemia, and other derangements associated with hepatic and renal failure. Acutely and severe dyscrasias are associated with delirium. Chronic and less severe dysfunction is associated with mild encephalopathy. Appropriate primary medical therapies including hydration, pharmacotherapy, and dialysis often will improve cognitive function.

Infectious processes will most often present as delirium that usually will respond to treatment. Viral encephalitis may leave the patient with chronic cognitive impairment, with or without affected sensorium.

Cancer/treatment-related causes of dementia and cognitive impairment

Primary and metastatic brain tumors and some systemic cancers (i.e., small cell lung cancer) are often associated with cognitive impairment, which is usually progressive. Leptomeningeal carcinomatosis and paraneoplastic syndrome may also present with impaired cognition and a clear sensorium. Disease progression and complications may result in nutritional deficiencies, respiratory insufficiency, or anemia that contribute to cognitive impairment. Please see Chapters 7–17 in this book for more indepth discussion of cancer and cancer treatment-related cognitive dysfunction.

Antineoplastic therapies

Several chemotherapy agents and other therapies may cause temporary (occasionally permanent) cognitive impairment. These include antimetabolites (e.g., methotrexate, ifosfamide, cytosine arabinoside), biological response modifiers (e.g., inter-feron, interleukin-2, thalidomide), and brain radiation (late delayed radiation toxicity) (Crossen et al., 1994; New, 2001; Verstappen et al., 2003). Toxicity is in part a function of dose and duration of treatment, and route of administration.

There has been considerable debate about cognitive dysfunction associated with hormonal antineoplastics (e.g., anti-estrogens, aromatase inhibitors). Literature has been mixed regarding the frequency and severity of objective impairment (Ahles & Saykin, 2002; Schagen et al., 2002; Wefel et al., 2004) but these agents are common sources of patient complaints of "chemobrain," and not infrequently of reactive depression given that patients are likely to be on the drugs for years.

Supportive care drugs

Any drug with central nervous system (CNS) depressant properties has potential to cause cognitive impairment, with or without altered sensorium. In the oncology setting, these would include opioid analgesics, benzodiazepine anxiolytics and hypnotics, phenothiazine anti-emetics, anticonvulsants, and some antidepressants.

Palliative care settings

Delirium is the most frequent neuropsychiatric finding in the last days of life. It has been found in approximately 85%–90% of cancer patients in the last hours to days before death (Bruera et al., 1992c; Lawlor et al., 2000a; Massie et al., 1983). Delirium is also associated with increased morbidity and mortality rates. In studies of advanced cancer patients, those with delirium had a median survival of 21 days as compared to 39 days in those without (Caraceni et al., 2000).

Although delirium is one of the most frequent reasons for admission to palliative care units (Lawlor, 2002) it is frequently under-diagnosed. When objective assessment of cognitive function was not performed in patients admitted to a palliative care unit, episodes of delirium went undetected by physicians and nurses in 23% and 20% of cases respectively (Bruera *et al.*, 1992c). In palliative care patient's delirium is frequently misdiagnosed as depression, dementia, or just simply sedation.

In patients admitted to palliative care programs delirium may be reversed through a suitable therapeutic approach in almost 50% of patients (Gagnon *et al.*, 2000; Lawlor *et al.*, 2000b; Sarhill *et al.*, 2001).

Since delirium is extremely frequent and reversible in almost 50% of cases it is very important to use assessment tools for the screening of patients who do not appear to be in delirium. Maintaining a very high index of suspicion and using validated screening instruments will result in earlier detection of this devastating syndrome. This will allow clinicians to conduct immediate investigation of the possible causes, appropriate pharmacological management of symptoms such as agitation, hallucinations, and delusions, and appropriate counseling of caregivers.

Distressed or ill-informed caregivers can exacerbate a patient's distress. Agitated behavior is particularly distressing for families and caregivers (Breitbart *et al.*, 2002). Agitated behavior may be interpreted as a sign of pain and/or suffering. Discussions with family should include a simple explanation of delirium, its increased frequency in advanced illness, potential causes and various clinical presentations, and the efforts made to manage it. In some cases it might be appropriate to conduct specific delirium tests with the family present so as to demonstrate the level of cognitive impairment and disinhibition. This will help families better understand why patients may present increased symptomatic and/or emotional expression as a consequence of disinhibition.

The importance of providing a safe and quiet environment with limited visual and auditory stimulation, surrounded by familiar objects and/or sounds, and avoiding discussions and confrontations should be discussed with caregivers and family members.

Delirium is one of the most common causes of conflict between health care professionals and families in the palliative care setting. It is very important

Table 18.4. Symptom intensity scores upon referral to a multidisciplinary palliative care clinic ($n = 135$)[a]

	Median ESAS Intensity (Inter Quartile Range)
Pain	6 (4, 8)
Fatigue	7 (4.5, 8)
Nausea	1 (0, 5)
Drowsiness	5 (1.5, 8)
Anxiety	5 (1, 8)
Depression	4 (1, 7)
Anorexia	6 (4, 8)
Dyspnea	3 (0, 6)
Sleep	6 (4, 8)
Well-being	6 (5, 8)

[a]Edmonton Symptom Assessment Scores (0; Best, 10; Worst)

to have an established protocol for the evaluation and management of this complex syndrome.

Symptomatic pharmacotherapy

Patients with advanced cancer develop a number of devastating physical and psychosocial symptoms. Table 18.4 summarizes the median (inter quartile range) Edmonton Symptom Assessment Scales (0 = best, 10 = worst) for 135 patients referred to an outpatient palliative care clinic. Since the vast majority of patients develop multiple symptoms they frequently require multiple drug interventions, including opioid analgesics, adjuvant drugs with central effects such as anticonvulsants or antidepressants, anti-emetics, and psychoactive medications. Fatigue and sedation can occur as a consequence of these persistent symptoms but also as a consequence of the pharmacological interventions used for their management.

A temporary impairment in neuropsychiatric tests and increased sedation are frequently observed when patients are started on opioid analgesics or after they undergo a significant dose increase (Bruera *et al.*, 1989). These effects can be reversed by methylphenidate (Bruera *et al.*, 1992a,

1992b). Methylphenidate and other psychostimulants have been used in the management of depression and hypoactive delirium associated with advanced cancer (Gagnon et al., 2005; Homsi et al., 2000; Morita et al., 2000; Olin & Masand, 1996; Rozans et al., 2002; Sood et al., 2006). It has been found to improve both sedation as well as performance on simple tasks such as finger tapping and arithmetic (Bruera et al., 1992a, 1992b). In addition, methylphenidate can allow for increased opioid dose in patients with severe pain who have dose-limiting sedation (Bruera et al., 1992b). A preliminary study observed that patients receiving patient-controlled methylphenidate for the management of cancer fatigue experienced significant relief (Bruera et al., 2003a). However, a randomized controlled trial found that this improvement was not superior to placebo (Bruera et al., 2006).

Patients receiving chronic opioid therapy frequently develop signs of opioid-induced neurotoxicity such as delirium, generalized myoclonus, sedation, or hyperalgesia (Del Fabbro et al., 2006a). In these patients the most important approach is to identify opioids as the likely cause and use opioid rotation to mimimize symptoms (Mercadante & Bruera, 2006).

Fatigue is the most common symptom in patients with advanced cancer. It is a multidimensional syndrome that is frequently associated with cachexia, depression, physical symptoms, and drugs such as opioids and benzodiazapenes (Del Fabbro et al., 2006b). Unfortunately, there is no approved pharmacological treatment for cancer fatigue. A preliminary study found that donepezil was able to improve both sedation and fatigue in patients with advanced cancer receiving opioids (Bruera et al., 2003b). Randomized controlled trials on the role of donepezil for both sedation and fatigue are currently being conducted.

Other psychostimulants such as dextroamphetamine and modafinil have been occasionally used to treat fatigue and decreased arousal in a number of settings including oncology (Ballon & Feifel, 2006). There is limited experience with these drugs in advanced cancer.

Antidepressants with "activating" side-effects (e.g., bupropion, fluoxetine) may be useful in some cases. Some authors have found that antidepressants with adrenergic activity are particularly useful against the cognitive side-effects of interferon therapy (Capuron et al., 2002; Raison et al., 2005).

Future research

Cognitive dysfunction is a problem that requires more research attention from supportive care specialists working in oncology. Potential questions include but are not limited to the following.

Detection and screening

The utility of screening oncology populations at high risk for delirium or other disease-related cognitive dysfunction is not well established. Outcomes research using appropriate endpoints (e.g., quality of life, complication rates, length of survival, cost) would help to determine whether screening is an effective use of health care resources. The role of screening in outpatient/community cancer center settings (and appropriate instruments for this purpose) is largely unaddressed.

Treatment

Aside from treatment of potential alcohol withdrawal delirium, the utility, if any, of prophylactic pharmacotherapy in patients at risk for delirium has not been evaluated. The appropriate role of psychostimulants and other agents (e.g., cholinesterase inhibitors, neuroprotective agents) in management of disease- and treatment-induced chronic cognitive dysfunction is not well established and is worthy of additional investigation. In a setting where haloperidol is the only antipsychotic drug routinely administered intravenously, there is a need to develop new agents that may be given by this route, and to investigate new delivery methods for atypical antipsychotics.

Communication/education

Research into the efficacy of various medical education methods related to cancer-related cognitive impairment would support the goal of improving screening and the treatment of at-risk patients. The impact of patient and caregiver education on this subject is largely unknown.

Conclusion

Symptom management is the primary goal of supportive care for cancer patients. The management of various presentations of cancer-related cognitive impairment will become increasingly important as the general population ages and patients live longer before being diagnosed, or with the disease as a chronic illness. Clinicians should be familiar with various presentations of delirium, its many causes and differential diagnosis, treatment, and the settings in which it is likely to occur. A high index of suspicion is required when evaluating the cognitively impaired cancer patient, and creative pharmacotherapy approaches may be required. Ongoing and future research efforts into the causes, identification, and treatment of cognitive dysfunction have the potential to improve quality of life for cancer patients and caregivers, and possibly to improve the efficacy of primary cancer therapies.

REFERENCES

Ahles TA, Saykin AJ (2002). Breast cancer chemotherapy-related cognitive dysfunction. *Clin Breast Cancer* **3** [Suppl. 3]: S84–S90.

American Psychiatric Association (2000). *Diagnostic and Statistical Manual of Mental Disorders* (4th edn. Text Revision edn. Washington, DC: American Psychiatric Association.

Anthony JC, LeResche L, Niaz U *et al.* (1982). Limits of the mini-mental state as a screening test for dementia and delirium among hospital patients. *Psychol Med* **12**(2): 397–408.

Ballon JS, Feifel MD (2006). A systematic review of modafinil: potential clinical uses and mechanisms of action. *J Clin Psychiatry* **67**(4): 554–566.

Boutros NN, Struve F (2002). Electrophysiological assessment of neuropsychiatric disorders. *Sem Clin Neuropsychiatry* **7**(1): 30–41.

Breitbart W, Cohen KR (1998). Delirium. In Holland JC (ed.) *Psycho-oncology* (pp. 564–573). New York: Oxford University Press.

Breitbart W, Marotta R, Platt MM *et al.* (1996). A double-blind trial of haloperidol, chlorpromazine, and lorazepam in the treatment of delirium in hospitalized AIDS patients. *Am J Psychiatry* **153**(2): 231–237.

Breitbart W, Rosenfeld B, Roth A *et al.* (1997). The memorial delirium assessment scale. *J Pain Symptom Manage* **13**(3): 128–137.

Breitbart W, Gibson C, Tremblay A (2002). The delirium experience: delirium recall and delirium-related distress in hospitalized patients with cancer, their spouses/caregivers, and their nurses. *Psychosomatics* **43**: 183–194.

Brown TM (2000). Drug-induced delirium. *Sem Clin Neuropsychiatry* **5**(2): 113–124.

Bruera E, MacMillan K, Hanson J, MacDonald RN (1989). The Edmonton staging system for cancer pain: preliminary report. *Pain* **37**: 203–209.

Bruera E, Miller MJ, Macmillan K, Kuehn N (1992a). Neuropsychological effects of methylphenidate in patients receiving a continuous infusion of narcotics for cancer pain. *Pain* **48**(2): 163–166.

Bruera E, Fainsinger R, MacEachern T, Hanson J (1992b). The use of methylphenidate in patients with incident cancer pain receiving regular opiates. A preliminary report. *Pain* **50**(1): 75–77.

Bruera E, Miller L, McCallion J, Macmillan K, Krefting L, Hanson J (1992c). Cognitive failure in patients with terminal cancer: a prospective study. *J Pain Symptom Manage* **7**: 192–195.

Bruera E, Driver L, Barnes EA *et al.* (2003a). Patient-controlled methylphenidate for the management of fatigue in patients with advanced cancer: a preliminary report. *J Clin Oncol* **21**(23): 4439–4443.

Bruera E, Strasser F, Shen L *et al.* (2003b). The effect of donepezil on sedation and other symptoms in patients receiving opioids for cancer pain: a pilot study. *J Pain Symptom Manage* **26**(5): 1049–1054.

Bruera E, Valero V, Driver L *et al.* (2006). Patient-controlled methylphenidate for cancer fatigue: a double-blind, randomized, placebo-controlled trial. *J Clin Oncol* **24**(13): 2073–2078.

Capuron L, Hauser P, Hinze-Selch D *et al.* (2002). Treatment of cytokine-induced depression. *Brain Behav Immunol* **16**(5): 575–580.

Caraceni A, Nanni O, Maltoni M *et al.* (2000). Impact of delirium on the short term prognosis of advanced cancer patients. Italian Multicenter Study Group on Palliative Care. *Cancer* **89**(5): 1145–1149.

Carter GL, Dawson AH, Lopert R (1996). Drug-induced delirium. Incidence, management and prevention. *Drug Safety* **15**(4): 291–301.

Cassem NH, Murray GB, Lafayette JM, Stern TA (2004). Delirious patients. In Stern T (ed.) *Massachusetts General Hospital Handbook of General Hospital Psychiatry* (5th edn.). Philadelphia, PA: Mosby.

Crossen JR, Garwood D, Glatstein E, Neuwelt EA (1994). Neurobehavioral sequelae of cranial irradiation in adults: a review of radiation-induced encephalopathy. *J Clin Oncol* **12**(3): 627–642.

Del Fabbro E, Dalal S, Bruera E (2006a). Symptom control in palliative care – Part III: Dyspnea. Dyspnea and delirium. *J Palliat Med* **9**(2): 422–436.

Del Fabbro E, Dalal S, Bruera E (2006b). Symptom control in palliative care – Part II: Cachexia/anorexia and fatigue. *J Palliat Med* **9**(2): 409–421.

Derogatis LR, Morrow GR, Fetting J (1983). The prevalence of psychiatric disorders among cancer patients. *J Am Med Assoc* **249**: 751–757.

Dobie DJ (2002). Depression, dementia, and pseudodementia. *Semin Clin Neuropsychiatry* **7**(3): 170–186.

Fadul N, Kaur G, Zhang T, Palmer JL, Bruera E (2007). Evaluation of the Memorial Delirium Assessment Scale (MDAS) for the screening of delirium by means of simulated cases by palliative care health professionals. *Support Cancer Care* **15**(11): 1271–1276.

Fann JR, Roth-Roemer S, Burington BE *et al.* (2002). Delirium in patients undergoing hematopoietic stem cell transplantation. *Cancer* **95**(9): 1971–1981.

Folstein MF, Folstein SE, McHugh PR (1975). Mini-mental state. A practical method for grading the cognitive state of patients for the clinician. *J Psychiatr Res* **12**(3): 189–198.

Franco K, Litaker D, Locala J, Bronson D (2001). The cost of delirium in the surgical patient. *Psychosomatics* **42**(1): 68–73.

Gagnon B, Allard P, Masse B, DeSerres M (2000). Delirium in terminal cancer: a prospective study using daily screening, early diagnosis, and continuous monitoring. *J Pain Symptom Manage* **19**: 412–426.

Gagnon B, Low G, Schreier G (2005). Methylphenidate hydrochloride improves cognitive function in patients with advanced cancer and hypoactive delirium: a prospective clinical study. *J Psychiatry Neurosci* **30**(2): 100–107.

Gaudreau JD, Gagnon P, Roy MA *et al.* (2005). Association between psychoactive medications and delirium in hospitalized patients: a critical review. *Psychosomatics* **46**(4): 302–316.

Homsi J, Walsh D, Nelson KA (2000). Psychostimulants in supportive care. *Support Care Cancer* **8**(5): 385–397.

Inouye SK (1998). Delirium in hospitalized older patients: recognition and risk factors. *J Geriatric Psychiatry Neurol* **11**(3): 118–125.

Inouye SK (2000). Prevention of delirium in hospitalized older patients: risk factors and targeted intervention strategies. *Ann Med* **32**(4): 257–263.

Inouye SK, van Dyck CH, Alessi CA *et al.* (1990). Clarifying confusion: the confusion assessment method. A new method for detection of delirium. *Ann Int Med* **113**(12): 941–948.

Kelly KG, Zisselman M, Cutillo-Schmitter T *et al.* (2001). Severity and course of delirium in medically hospitalized nursing facility residents. *Am J Geriatric Psychiatry* **9**(1): 72–77.

Lawlor PG (2002). The panorama of opioid-related cognitive dysfunction in patients with cancer: a critical literature appraisal. *Cancer* **94**(6): 1836–1853.

Lawlor PG, Gagnon B, Mancini IL *et al.* (2000a). Occurrence, causes, and outcome of delirium in patients with advanced cancer: a prospective study. *Arch Int Med* **160**(6): 786–794.

Lawlor PG, Gagnon B, Mancini IL *et al.* (2000b). Delirium as a predictor of survival in older patients with advanced cancer. *Arch Int Med* **160**: 2866–2868.

Leslie DL, Zhang Y, Holford TR *et al.* (2005). Premature death associated with delirium at 1-year follow-up. *Arch Intern Med* **165**(14): 1657–1662.

Lipowski ZJ (1990). *Delirium: Acute Confusional States.* New York: Oxford University Press.

Ljubisavljevic V, Kelly B (2003). Risk factors for development of delirium among oncology patients. *Gen Hosp Psychiatry* **25**(5): 345–352.

Marcantonio ER, Juarez G, Goldman L *et al.* (1994). The relationship of postoperative delirium with psychoactive medications. *J Am Med Assoc* **272**(19): 1518–1522.

Massie MJ, Holland J, Glass E (1983). Delirium in terminally ill cancer patients. *Am J Psychiatry* **140**(8): 1048–1050.

Mayo-Smith MF, Mayo-Smith MF (1997). Pharmacological management of alcohol withdrawal. A meta-analysis and evidence-based practice guideline. American Society of Addiction Medicine Working Group on Pharmacological Management of Alcohol Withdrawal. *J Am Med Assoc* **278** (2): 144–151.

Mazzocato C, Stiefel F, Buclin T, Berney A (2000). Psychopharmacology in supportive care of cancer: a review for the clinician: II Neuroleptics. *Support Care Cancer* **(8)**2: 89–97.

Mercadante S, Bruera E (2006). Opioid switching: a systematic and critical review. *Cancer Treat Rev* **32**: 304–315.

Meyers CA, Valentine AD (1995). Neurological and psychiatric adverse effects of immunological therapy. *CNS Drugs* **3**: 56–68.

Morita T, Otani H, Tsunoda J *et al.* (2000). Successful palliation of hypoactive delirium due to multi-organ failure by oral methylphenidate. *Support Care Cancer* **8**(2): 134–137.

New P (2001). Radiation injury to the nervous system. *Curr Opinion Neurol* **14**(6): 725–734.

O'Keeffe ST, Lavan JN (1999). Clinical significance of delirium subtypes in older people. *Age Ageing* **28**(2): 115–119.

Olin J, Masand P (1996). Psychostimulants for depression in hospitalized cancer patients. *Psychosomatics* **37**(1): 57–62.

Pereira J, Bruera E (2001). Depression with psychomotor retardation: diagnostic challenges and the use of psychostimulants. *J Palliat Med* **4**(1): 15–21.

Platt MM, Breitbart W, Smith M *et al.* (1994). Efficacy of neuroleptics for hypoactive delirium. *J Neuropsychiatry Clin Neurosci* **6**(1): 66–67.

Prieto JM, Blanch J, Atala J *et al.* (2002). Psychiatric morbidity and impact on hospital length of stay among hematologic cancer patients receiving stem-cell transplantation. *J Clin Oncol* **20**(7): 1907–1917.

Raison CL, Demetrashvili M, Capuron L, Miller AH (2005). Neuropsychiatric adverse effects of interferon-alpha: recognition and management. *CNS Drugs* **19**(2): 105–123.

Reifler BV (2000). A case of mistaken identity: pseudodementia is really predementia. *J Am Geriatr Soc* **48**(5): 593–594.

Reischies FM, Neu P (2000). Comorbidity of mild cognitive disorder and depression – a neuropsychological analysis. *Eur Arch Psychiatry Clin Neurosci* **250**(4): 186–193.

Ross CA, Peyser CE, Shapiro I, Folstein MF (1991). Delirium: phenomenologic and etiologic subtypes. *Int Psychogeriatr* **3**(2): 135–147.

Rozans M, Dreisbach A, Lertora JJ, Kahn MJ (2002). Palliative uses of methylphenidate in patients with cancer: a review. *J Clin Oncol* **20**(1): 335–339.

Sarhill N, Walsh D, Nelson KA *et al.* (2001). Assessment of delirium in advanced cancer: the use of the bedside confusion scale. *Am J Hospice Palliat Care* **18**: 335–341.

Schagen SB, Muller MJ, Boogerd W (2002). Late effects of adjuvant chemotherapy on cognitive function: a follow-up study in breast cancer patients. *Ann Oncol* **9**(13): 1387–1397.

Sood A, Barton DL, Loprinzi CL (2006). Use of methylphenidate in patients with cancer. *Am J Hospice Palliat Care* **23**(1): 35–40.

Trzepacz PT (1994). A review of delirium assessment instruments. *Gen Hosp Psychiatry* **16**(6): 397–405.

Trzepacz PT (1996). Delirium. Advances in diagnosis, pathophysiology, and treatment. *Psychiatrics Clin North Am* **19**(3): 429–448.

Trzepacz PT, Baker RW, Greenhouse J (1988). A symptom rating scale for delirium. *Psychiat Res* **23**(1): 89–97.

Tune LE, Damlouji NF, Holland A *et al.* (1981). Association of postoperative delirium with raised serum levels of anticholinergic drugs. *Lancet* **2**(8248): 651–653.

Valentine AD, Bickham JG (2005). Delirium and substance withdrawal. In Shaw A (ed.) *Acute Care of the Cancer Patient* (pp. 545–557). New York: Marcel Dekker.

Verstappen CC, Heimans JJ, Hoekman K, Postma TJ (2003). Neurotoxic complications of chemotherapy in patients with cancer: clinical signs and optimal management. *Drugs* **63**(15): 1549–1563.

Visser PJ, Verhey FR, Ponds RW *et al.* (2000). Distinction between preclinical Alzheimer's disease and depression. *J Am Geriatr Soc* **48**(5): 479–484.

Wefel JS, Lenzi R, Theriault RL, Davis RN, Meyers CA (2004). The cognitive sequelae of standard-dose adjuvant chemotherapy in women with breast carcinoma: results of a prospective, randomized, longitudinal trial. *Cancer* **100**(11): 2292–2299.

19

Animal models and cancer-related symptoms

Adrian Dunn

Animal models have frequently been useful in developing treatments for a variety of diseases. Their use permits researchers to ask questions about mechanisms that would be difficult or unethical in humans, and also permits the testing of potential treatments. Models that work in rodents are usually preferred because we know much about their physiology and behavior, and because rodents are relatively inexpensive. Moreover, a host of experimental manipulations have been developed for use in these species. Work with primates that may be more valid is substantially more expensive, and the numbers of subjects that can be used are normally very limited. The development of animal models for behavioral symptoms presents a special challenge, because although many such models and tests exist, they address poorly the symptoms that are of most concern to cancer patients. This chapter will provide a selective overview of animal models and tests, and provide examples of what has been achieved in other areas. The limitations of the use of the non-human animal models and tests will also be addressed.

It is important at the outset to note the distinction between an animal model and an animal test. A *model* is a procedure used to induce a state in the animal that resembles the disease under study. In this context, a *test* is a procedure that reveals symptoms that resemble aspects of the human disease. For example, in the case of depression, most ani- mal models have relied on chronic stress paradigms. However, *tests* for depression would include proce- dures such as the forced swim test or the tail suspen- sion test used to assess depression-like or antide- pressant activity (see below). Cognitive function in animals has been addressed almost exclusively in tests of memory, except in non-human primates. However, other symptoms such as depression and fatigue that are common in cancer patients can also affect cognitive function. Thus this chapter will also address animal models of these symptoms, along with classical cognitive tasks.

Details of animal models of behavior can be found in a number of reviews (e.g., Weiss & Kilts, 1998) and some books; for example, the recently pub- lished *The Behavior of the Laboratory Rat* (Whishaw & Kolb, 2005), *Animal Models of Human Emotion and Cognition* (Haug & Whalen, 1999), and in a book focused on transgenic mice, *What's Wrong with My Mouse?* (Crawley, 2000).

Why use animal models?

The rationales for using animal models of disease states are to identify or determine potential underly- ing mechanisms of the disease, and to test potential treatments. Their use is frequently justified either because certain kinds of experiments are difficult to perform in humans, or because they would be con- sidered unethical. Most often the justification is that

Cognition and Cancer, eds. Christina A. Meyers and James R. Perry. Published by Cambridge University Press.
© Cambridge University Press 2008.

the measurement of some important variable is too intrusive to measure in humans, or because a proposed experimental therapy carries unknown risks. In the most common examples, a drug known to affect a metabolic process may be tested for its efficacy, and/or to reveal unforeseen unacceptable or toxic side-effects.

An obvious problem with the use of animal models is that the drug/treatment may not work in humans the way it does in animals. Conversely, treatments that work in the animal model may induce unforeseen side-effects in humans. It is fair to say that animal models work best when the method for inducing the model is related to the underlying cause of the disease. This may not be too difficult when the underlying cause of the disease is known or suspected, but may be particularly difficult in the case of behavioral symptoms, especially symptoms like those of depression and psychosis. Do we really know that a rat or a mouse can experience depression as humans do? And, what is psychotic behavior in a rat? Can such symptoms be modeled in primates? In such cases, the model can be aimed to have face value, i.e., that it appears to the investigator that the behavior of the rat resembles a human behavior. An example would be the forced swim test developed by Porsolt to assess depression-like behavior. In this test, it is conceived that the animal learns whether a behavioral strategy is useful or not (see below). A "depressed" rat or mouse gives up more rapidly and floats or stays immobile for a longer time. Most often, the test is based on a pharmacological validation, often exclusively. By this is meant that drugs (or other treatments that affect the human disease) similarly affect animals in the model. All drugs that are clinically effective should work in the model, whereas drugs that have no (useful) clinical effect should not work in the model. Moreover, the dose–response relationships should be similar in humans and the animal models.

Animal models

For a model to be useful, the methods used to create it should bear some relationship to the underlying

disease studied. Treatments that are effective in the model are less likely to work in the clinical situation if the method used to induce the model is unrelated to the basic mechanism(s) of the disease. McKinney and Bunney (1969) proposed a set of criteria for animal models of human mental health disorders. The model should resemble the condition it represents in its etiology, biochemistry, symptomatology, and treatment.

An example of the successful use of an animal model is the development of treatments for attention deficit hyperactivity disorder (ADHD). It was observed that methylphenidate, an amphetamine-like drug that stimulates release of the neurotransmitter dopamine (DA), induced a reversal of the hyperactivity observed in 6-hydroxydopamine-treated rats (Shaywitz et al., 1976). This finding was paradoxical, because amphetamine-like drugs normally increase locomotor activity. Thus it was reasoned that methylphenidate might counter the hyperactivity observed in children with ADHD. In practice, methylphenidate treatment has subsequently proven to be very effective for the treatment of ADHD in teenagers (Shaywitz et al., 2001). In this example, the model was almost certainly useful because ADHD in children involves some abnormality in brain catecholaminergic function. However, not all models have proven so useful. For example, the olfactory bulbectomy model mimics depression in several tests, and the effects respond appropriately to many treatments effective in depressed patients (Cryan & Mombereau, 2004; Cryan et al., 2002; Kelly et al., 1997; Song & Leonard, 2005; Willner, 1984). Nevertheless, although the model is of considerable scientific interest, it has failed to provide insight into the mechanism of depression and has so far failed to inspire useful clinical therapies (Willner, 1984).

The most obvious models for cancer patients would be animals bearing tumors. There have been relatively few studies of this type. In an early study, Chance et al. (1983) studied the anorexia associated with inoculation of rats with Walker 256 carcinosarcoma cells and noted increases in brain tryptophan and serotonin (5-hydroxytryptamine,

5-HT) metabolism. The neurochemical changes were reversed when the tumor was resected (Chance *et al.*, 1988). They suggested that the anorexia was associated with changes in hypothalamic 5-HT. Chuluyan *et al.* (2000) studied the neurochemical and pituitary–adrenal effects of inoculating mice with the murine lymphoma cell line AW5E. There were no significant changes after 6 or 8 days, but a sustained increase in hypothalamic norepinephrine (NE) and 5-HT metabolism appeared 10 days after injection. On the last day tested (day 14), plasma corticosterone was slightly elevated, as were the catabolites of DA, NE and 5-HT and concentrations of tryptophan in the brain. The changes in catecholamines were most evident in the hypothalamus. Such changes in brain catecholamines and 5-HT, and in corticosterone are characteristic of stress. In a subsequent study, DBA2 mice were inoculated with L1210 mouse leukemia cells and their behavioral activity was assessed in the tail suspension test (TST) and the Porsolt forced swim test (FST), as well as activity in the open field (OF) (Dunn *et al.*, 2004). No consistent differences from controls were observed in the behavior of these animals on days 8 or 11. However, on day 15, mice inoculated with L1210 cells (5000 or 50 000 cells/mouse) exhibited significant increases in immobility in the TST and the FST (see below). The inoculated mice exhibited increases in plasma corticosterone, as well as significant increases in the metabolism of NE, but not DA, in the hypothalamus, as well as increases in tryptophan and 5-HT metabolism in the cortex and hypothalamus. Vegas *et al.* (2004) recently reported increases in immobility, and changes in social interaction, as well as increases in brain DA and 5-HT metabolism in mice inoculated with B16 melanoma cells.

Models of depression

The most recent reviews indicate that there are some half-dozen rodent models of depression (Cryan & Mombereau, 2004; Cryan *et al.*, 2002;

Porsolt, 2000; Willner, 2005). However, many of these models may not be directly relevant to the clinical situation (Matthews *et al.*, 2005). Most such models have been based on chronic stress (Anisman & Zacharko, 1982). Willner (1984) discussed at length the problems with most of the early models. He proposed that predictive validity should be assessed by whether a model correctly identifies antidepressant treatments of pharmacologically diverse types, without making errors of omission or commission, and whether potency in the model correlates with clinical potency (Willner, 1984).

Stress

Clinical depression is frequently associated with life stress (Anisman & Zacharko, 1982), although stress has not been identified as a factor in all cases of clinical depression (Willner, 1984; van Praag, 2004). Hans Selye (who has the dubious distinction of being known as the father of stress) defined the important distinction between what he called *stress*, which he defined as a state induced by adverse circumstances or treatments, and the *stressor*, the agent responsible for inducing the stress. The most frequently used stress paradigms in rodents are such treatments as chronic electric footshock or restraint. By chronic is meant once or twice daily for 1–2 weeks or more. Needless to say these are not the most common stressors for humans. "Physical" stressors, such as high or low temperature or food deprivation, are seldom used in animal models, because any changes in body temperature and/or metabolism are likely to confound the physiological measures made. However, common stressors in the human condition, such as bereavement, do not appear to affect rodents similarly (although they may do so in primates). Another model commonly used is the chronic mild stress model (CMS) which uses a series of different stressors over an extended time period (4–6 weeks). However, the CMS model promoted by Willner and others has proven to be difficult to replicate in some laboratories, and even in Willner's own laboratory when he moved it from London to Swansea (Willner, 1997). Others have promoted other "cafeteria-style" models in which a variety of different stressors are applied sequentially (e.g., Katz, 1981). Yet another model is learned helplessness (Maier & Seligman, 1976; Overmier & Seligman, 1967). In this model (initially performed in dogs) chronic stressors are used to invoke a state of despair, in which the stressed dogs become immobile and helpless, although whether this is a "learning effect" has been questioned. It has been proposed that the learning merely reflects a decrease in activity associated with the stress-related reduction in brain NE (Weiss & Kilts, 1998). Yet another possibility is to use chronic social stress. When rats are confined in a limited space such as a cage, a dominance hierarchy is created, in which one animal rules over the others. The immediate subordinates are the most stressed in this kind of situation. Social models have been developed by various groups, most notably the Blanchards with the visible burrow system in rats and mice (Blanchard *et al.*, 2001, 2003).

The underlying physiology of stress is similar in animals and humans. The stress response has both central and peripheral components. Peripherally, the principal components are activation of the adrenal gland and the sympathetic nervous system (SNS). Activation of the SNS results in the secretion of substantial quantities of NE and certain peptides (such as substance P and opioid peptides, e.g., the enkephalins), which can act locally and systemically. The adrenal gland also contributes to circulating concentrations of NE, but also adds epinephrine, and still more peptides (again including some opioid peptides). The major effects of catecholaminergic activation are the mobilization of glucose stored as glycogen (principally in the liver, but also in other organs including the brain), and the redirection of blood away from the viscera and towards voluntary muscle (for fighting or fleeing). The adrenal cortex joins the fray as the final component of the so-called hypothalamo–pituitary–adrenocortical (HPA) axis, rapidly increasing circulating glucocorticoids: corticosterone in rodents, and cortisol in humans and many other animals. The glucocorticoids, as their name implies,

divert metabolism towards increasing glucose concentrations in the circulation, and have a host of other physiological actions, including driving lymphocytes from the thymus and spleen into the general circulation, presumably to fight pathogens and to facilitate blood clotting. As its name implies, the HPA axis exists at three levels. In the brain it involves the secretion of corticotropin-releasing factor (CRF) from hypothalamic neurons, which, after secretion into the portal blood supply, acts on the pituitary to elicit the secretion of adrenocorticotropic hormone (adrenocorticotropin, ACTH) into the general circulation which in turn acts on the adrenal cortex stimulating glucocorticoid secretion.

This much is classical physiology, but more recent studies have indicated that the peripheral duality between the HPA and catecholamine components also occurs in the brain. Thus noradrenergic systems within the brain that have cell bodies in the brainstem pour out NE, so that it bathes most if not all of the brain, and certain amounts of endorphins. The global noradrenergic activation in the brain appears to arouse the brain such that it pays special (selective) attention to the novel factors in the environment that have caused the stress. Moreover, CRF is not confined to activation of the pituitary. Hypothalamic and extrahypothalamic CRF-containing neurons exert their own effects on the brain, eliciting fear- and anxiety-like responses, and enhancing other brain functions, presumably to address coping with the effects of the stressor (Dunn & Berridge, 1990). The link between stress and depression becomes obvious when it is recognized that depression appears to be associated with increased activity of brain NE (e.g., Wong *et al.*, 2000), and hyperactivity of the HPA axis (Carroll, 1978; Sachar, 1967).

Animal tests of depression

The Porsolt forced swim test

Currently, the most frequently used test is the FST developed by Porsolt for the rat (Porsolt *et al.*,

1977b) and the mouse (Porsolt *et al.*, 1977a). The test involves placing a rat or a mouse in a tall cylinder of water from which it cannot escape, so that it must either swim or float. Rats are initially placed in the cylinder of water for 15 min. The rats are put back into the cylinder 24 h later for 5 min. An observer records the activity of the rat, especially the time at which the rat stops struggling and floats (i.e., the latency to float), and the duration of the floating, immobile except for the minimal paw movements necessary to keep the nose above water. The concept was that the "depressed" rat would give up struggling or swimming earlier, and float for longer. It has been suggested that the first day session is necessary for the rats to learn that escape is impossible (Borsini & Meli, 1988). Drugs or other treatments are administered immediately after this session and then again 5 h and 1 h before the test on the second day (Porsolt *et al.*, 1977b). However, Porsolt subsequently showed that many antidepressant treatments tested positively with only one or two of the three treatments (Porsolt *et al.*, 1978). Antidepressant treatments increase the latency to float, and reduce the time spent immobile (floating), whereas chronic stress and certain other treatments considered depressogenic increase the time spent floating. This test has been shown to work for many antidepressant treatments, including atypical antidepressants, such as the monoamine oxidase inhibitors (MAOIs) and electroconvulsive therapy (ECT), although the selective serotonin reuptake inhibitors (SSRIs) are less effective and some are ineffective (Cryan & Mombereau, 2004; Porsolt, 2000). Thus the test has been validated pharmacologically, even though the drug treatments work after one, two or three treatments, in contrast to the chronic treatments required in depressed patients. In the test Porsolt developed for mice, they were forced to swim only once, usually with the antidepressant treatments applied shortly before the test. Immobilization is scored during the last 4 min of the 6-min test (Porsolt *et al.*, 1977b). However, some subsequent studies have employed a 2-day test in mice, like that in rats.

The tail suspension test

The TST is conceptually similar to the FST. A mouse is suspended by its tail and the latency to cease struggling and the duration of passive immobility are scored. The duration of immobility displayed by the suspended animals is reduced by antidepressant treatments (Cryan & Mombereau, 2004; Cryan *et al.*, 2002). Although a version of the test for rats has been reported (Chermat *et al.*, 1986), most investigators have had difficulty using the test in rats. The TST has the advantage of eliminating the confounding hypothermic effects of the swimming (Cryan & Mombereau, 2004). It has been suggested that the FST and TST differ in the biological substrates underlying the observed behaviors (Cryan & Mombereau, 2004).

Cognitive tests

In general cognitive tests developed for rodents may be difficult to relate to the cognitive impairments that cancer patients experience. Summarized below are the kinds of tests that are available.

Tests of learning and memory

Many different tests of learning and memory have been devised (Alkon *et al.*, 1991). To review each of them in detail is beyond the scope of this chapter. In general the tests can be divided into appetitive and aversive tests. In aversive tests, the animal is conditioned to learn that a particular stimulus or action is associated with a punishment, most often an electric shock. The advantage of such tests is that they are typically rapidly learned and the memory is retained for a long time. For example, a commonly used task is one-trial passive avoidance in which a rat (or more often a mouse) is placed in a novel apparatus and if it steps through an opening it immediately receives a brief footshock. This test is normally learned in one trial and the memory persists for months (Geller *et al.*, 1970). A common active avoidance task is the shuttle box in which an animal (normally a rat) is trained so that when a light is illuminated it should move to another part of the apparatus within a few seconds, to avoid an electric footshock. Once again in normal animals this conditioning is learned rapidly and the memory is retained for a long time.

Perhaps the most popular task, the Morris water maze employs a different kind of aversive stimulus (Morris, 1984; Schimanski & Nguyen, 2004). The water maze is a circular tank of water that contains a platform which is slightly below the surface of the water onto which the rat can climb and thus avoid swimming. The water is made opaque with a suitable paint or dye, so that the rat cannot see the platform, and the rat is expected to remember the location of the platform.

Appetitive tasks normally rely on a food reward, for example a food pellet, a sugar pill, or perhaps a sweet drink (a sugar solution or sweetened milk). Normally the association is made with a particular location, for example making the correct turn in a "T-maze." The most popular task is the radial arm maze (Alkon *et al.*, 1991; Olton, 1987). The radial arm maze has eight arms, any one of which can be baited with a food reward. Various contingencies can be set up, such as not entering the same arm twice before locating the correct arm; or remembering the location of the reward with respect to the starting position; or, the position of the arm within the room.

Other cognitive tasks

The number of cognitive tests for rodents other than memory tests is quite limited. One such task involves changing stimuli for conditioning. For example, rats and mice can be trained to press a bar to obtain a food reward or to avoid a shock. Once the task is being performed with a high degree of accuracy, the "rules" can be changed. Thus, for example, a food reward that was formerly available when a green light was illuminated may no longer be available when the light is green, but only when the light is red. The rat can then be assessed on its ability to learn the new contingency, a different color of the

light. If the change is only to a different color, this would constitute an *intra*dimensional shift. However, once the rat has learned that the color contingency can be changed, the investigator can play a cruel trick. The contingency can be switched from the color to the *shape* of the illuminated light, so that a light that was formerly circular is now in the form of a triangle, a square, or a cross. This would constitute an *extra*dimensional shift. Rats find it relatively easy to learn the intradimensional shift, but the extradimensional shift is much more difficult. A series of studies in the 1970s showed that certain peptides, especially ACTH and fragments of this molecule, facilitated the learning of the intradimensional shift, but would impair the learning of the extradimensional shift (Sandman *et al.*, 1974). Interestingly, the same peptides that had such opposite effects in rats had similar effects on intra- and extradimensional shifts in humans (Sandman *et al.*, 1975).

Tests for fatigue

Fatigue has been modeled in various ways, but there is some question about whether the models necessarily reflect fatigue as it is observed in cancer patients. First of all, fatigue has different meanings to different specialists. According to Dalakas *et al.* (1998), to a physiologist fatigue is a decrease in the capacity to perform work; to a pathologist, fatigue is an indicator of a neuromuscular or metabolic disorder; and to a psychologist, fatigue is a symptom of depression associated with decreased motivation to engage in mental and physical activities. However, patients report decreased physical performance and muscle weakness, decreased motivation and sadness, and a lack of concentration and decreased ability for problem solving (Glaus *et al.*, 1996).

The animal tests in the literature mostly reflect locomotor activity, such as running in a running wheel or on a treadmill. Takagi *et al.* (1972) studied the activity of mice in a battery of tests on a treadmill and balancing on an oscillating shaker. They observed "fatigue" (failure to keep up with the treadmill) that could be prevented by amphetamine, caffeine and similar stimulants. Chao *et al.* (1992) observed reduced voluntary running and delayed initiation of grooming after swimming associated with infection with *Corynebacterium parvum* antigen or *Toxoplasma gondii*. Ottenweller *et al.* (1998) observed decreased activity in the running wheel and grooming associated with infection with *Brucella abortus*. Davis *et al.* (1997) observed markedly decreased treadmill running following treatment with poly I:poly C (a synthetic double-stranded RNA known to be an effective inducer of interferon-α/β (IFN-α/β). This reduced running correlated with the appearance of IFN-α/β and was prevented by antibodies to IFN-α/β. Consistent with this, IFN-α reduced open field activity and swimming in mice (Dunn & Crnic, 1993). We have also observed that IFN-α administered intracerebroventricularly (icv) to rats increased immobility time in the Porsolt FST (Dunn & Swiergiel, 2004). Kaur and Kulkarni (2000) subjected rats to daily forced swims in the Porsolt swim test for 7 days. Antidepressant treatments provided symptomatic relief. Ayada *et al.* (2002) studied gnawing behavior of mice in a narrow plastic cylinder, which they proposed as a simple system for the study of muscle activity, fatigue, and stress.

Unfortunately, all of these tests were focused on locomotor activity as an indicator of fatigue. Several of them also used infection with pathogens that are known to induce sickness behavior (Kent *et al.*, 1992), thought to be mediated by certain cytokines, such as interleukin-1 (Dunn & Swiergiel, 2005). However, the fatigue experienced by cancer patients appears to be a motivational problem, which may be better assessed with operant tasks, in which an animal has to press a bar or touch an object in order to obtain a reward, or avoid a punishment.

Conclusions

Animal models have proven to be very useful for developing therapies for a number of human diseases. However, the success is probably closely related to the proximity of the model to the underlying causes of the disease. In many cases this may simply reflect luck in the choice of the "right" model. The modeling of psychiatric symptoms in small animals is more difficult, because it is not at all clear that rodents exhibit affective states and emotions like humans. Thus while a number of tests for depression exist, their validity rests largely on the effects of drugs or other therapies known to ameliorate depression in humans. This approach/model was very effective in identifying useful therapies for ADHD, but has not so far been particularly useful for the treatment of such psychiatric diseases as mania, depression, and psychosis. This may be because these diseases are associated with the increased complexity of the primate brain. Thus primate models may be more effective for these kinds of signs.

The neuropsychological symptoms of cancer patients undergoing therapy have additional complexities. Dealing with the symptoms of the cancer itself is one matter, but many of the most bothersome symptoms may be associated with the therapies used to treat the cancer: the radiation therapy, the chemotherapy, and/or the cytokine therapy (e.g., IFN-α). To make matters worse, it is even possible that the unwanted symptoms may reflect interactions between the cancer itself and the therapies used to treat it. Nevertheless, animal models may be able to provide indications of the effects of the cancer and its therapies that may provide clues for novel therapies.

ACKNOWLEDGMENTS

The author's research cited in this article was supported by the U.S. National Institute of Neurological Disorders and Stroke (NS35370).

REFERENCES

Alkon DL, Amaral DG, Bear MF *et al.* (1991). Learning and memory. *Brain Res Rev* **16**: 193–220.

Anisman H, Zacharko RM (1982). Depression: the predisposing influence of stress. *Behav Brain Sci* **5**: 89–137.

Ayada K, Tadano T, Endo Y (2002). Gnawing behavior of a mouse in a narrow cylinder: a simple system for the study of muscle activity, fatigue, and stress. *Physiol Behav* **77**: 161–166.

Blanchard RJ, Yudko E, Dulloog L, Blanchard DC (2001). Defense changes in stress nonresponsive subordinate males in a visible burrow system. *Physiol Behav* **72**: 635–642.

Blanchard DC, Griebel G, Blanchard RJ (2003). The Mouse Defense Test Battery: pharmacological and behavioral assays for anxiety and panic. *Eur J Pharmacol* **463**: 97–116.

Borsini F, Meli A (1988). Is the forced swimming test a suitable model for revealing antidepressant activity? *Psychopharmacology* **94**: 147–160.

Carroll BJ (1978). Neuroendocrine function in psychiatric disorders. In *Psychopharmacology: A Generation of Progress* (pp. 487–497). New York: Raven Press.

Chance W, Von Meyenfeldt M, Fischer J (1983). Changes in brain amines associated with cancer anorexia. *Neurosci Biobehav Rev* **7**: 471–479.

Chance WT, Cao L, Nelson JL, Foley-Nelson T, Fischer JE (1988). Reversal of neurochemical aberrations after tumor resection in rats. *Am J Surg* **155**: 124–129.

Chao CC, DeLaHunt M, Hu S, Close K, Peterson PK (1992). Immunologically mediated fatigue: a murine model. *Clin Immunol Immunopathol* **64**: 161–165.

Chermat R, Thierry B, Steru L, Simon P (1986). Adaptation of the tail suspension test to the rat. *J Pharmacol* **17**: 348–350.

Chuluyan HC, Wolcott RM, Chervenak R, Dunn AJ (2000). Catecholamine, indoleamine and corticosteroid responses in mice bearing tumors. *Neuroimmunomodulation* **8**: 107–113.

Crawley JN (2000). *What's Wrong with My Mouse? Behavioral Phenotyping of Transgenic and Knockout Mice* (pp. 1–368). Wilmington, DE: Wiley-Liss.

Cryan JF, Mombereau C (2004). In search of a depressed mouse: utility of models for studying depression-related behavior in genetically modified mice. *Mol Psychiatry* **9**: 1050–1062.

Cryan JF, Markou A, Lucki I (2002). Assessing antidepressant activity in rodents: recent developments and future needs. *Trends Pharmacol Sci* **23**: 238–245.

Dalakas MC, Mock V, Hawkins MJ (1998). Fatigue: definitions, mechanisms, and paradigms for study. *Semin Oncol* **25**: S48–S53.

Davis JM, Weaver JA, Kohut ML, Colbert LH, Ghaffar A, Mayer EP (1997). Immune system activation and fatigue during treadmill running: role of interferon. *Med Sci Sports Exerc* **30**: 863–868.

Dunn AJ, Berridge CW (1990). Physiological and behavioral responses to corticotropin-releasing factor administration: is CRF a mediator of anxiety or stress responses? *Brain Res Rev* **15**: 71–100.

Dunn AJ, Swiergiel AH (2004). Interferon effects on behavior, corticosterone, catecholamines and indoleamines in mice and rats. *Neuropsychopharmacology* **29**[Suppl. 1]: S120.

Dunn AJ, Swiergiel AH (2005). Effects of interleukin-1 and endotoxin in the forced swim and tail suspension tests in mice. *Pharmacol Biochem Behav* **81**: 688–693.

Dunn AJ, Swiergiel AH, Cork R, Newman RA (2004). Behavior, neurochemical and endocrine responses to leukemia in mice. In *2004 Abstract Viewer/Itinerary Planner* (Vol. 462.13). Washington DC: Society for Neuroscience.

Dunn AL, Crnic LS (1993). Repeated injections of interferon-α A/D in Balb/c mice: behavioral effects. *Brain Behav Immun* **7**: 104–111.

Geller A, Robustelli F, Jarvik ME (1970). Incubation and the Kamin effect. *J Exp Psychol* **85**: 61–65.

Glaus A, Crow R, Hammond S (1996). A qualitative study to explore the concept of fatigue/tiredness in cancer patients and in healthy individuals. *Support Care Cancer* **4**: 82–96.

Haug M, Whalen RE (1999). *Animal Models of Human Emotion and Cognition* (p. 341). Washington DC: American Psychological Association.

Katz RJ (1981). Animal models and human depressive disorders. *Neurosci Biobehav Rev* **5**: 231–246.

Kaur G, Kulkarni SK (2000). Comparative study of antidepressants and herbal psychotropic drugs in a mouse model of chronic fatigue. *J Chronic Fatigue Syndr* **6**: 23–34.

Kelly JP, Wrynn AS, Leonard BE (1997). The olfactory bulbectomized rat as a model of depression: an update. *Pharmacol Ther* **74**: 299–316.

Kent S, Bluthé R-M, Kelley KW, Dantzer R (1992). Sickness behavior as a new target for drug development. *Trends Pharmacol Sci* **13**: 24–28.

Maier SF, Seligman MEP (1976). Learned helplessness: theory and evidence. *J Exp Psychol* **1**: 3–46.

Matthews K, Christmas D, Swan J, Sorrell E (2005). Animal models of depression: navigating through the clinical fog. *Neurosci Biobehav Rev* **29**: 503–513.

McKinney WT, Bunney WE (1969). Animal models of depression. *Arch Gen Psychiatry* **21**: 240–248.

Morris R (1984). Developments of a water-maze procedure for studying spatial learning in the rat. *J Neurosci Methods* **11**: 47–60.

Olton DS (1987). The radial arm maze as a tool in behavioral pharmacology. *Physiol Behav* **40**: 793–797.

Ottenweller JE, Natelson BH, Gause WC *et al.* (1998). Mouse running activity is lowered by *Brucella abortus* treatment: a potential model to study chronic fatigue. *Physiol Behav* **63**: 795–801.

Overmier JB, Seligman MEP (1967). Effects of inescapable shock on subsequent escape and avoidance responding. *J Comp Physiol Psychol* **63**: 28–33.

Porsolt RD (2000). Animal models of depression: utility for transgenic research. *Rev Neurosci* **11**: 53–58.

Porsolt RD, Bertin A, Jalfre M (1977a). Behavioural despair in mice: a primary screening test for antidepressants. *Arch Int Pharmacodyn* **229**: 327–336.

Porsolt RD, Le Pichon M, Jalfre M (1977b). Depression: a new animal model sensitive to antidepressant treatments. *Nature* **266**: 730–732.

Porsolt RD, Anton G, Blavet N, Jalfre M (1978). Behavioural despair in rats: a new model sensitive to antidepressant treatments. *Eur J Pharmacol* **47**: 379–391.

Sachar EJ (1967). Corticosteroids in depressive illness: II. A longitudinal psychoendocrine study. *Arch Gen Psychiatry* **17**: 554–567.

Sandman CA, Beckwith BE, Gittis MM (1974). Melanocyte-stimulating hormone (MSH) and overtraining effects on extradimensional shift (EDS) learning. *Physiol Behav* **13**: 1631–1666.

Sandman CA, George JM, Nolan JD, van Riezen H, Kastin AJ (1975). Enhancement of attention in man with ACTH/MSH4–10. *Physiol Behav* **15**: 427–431.

Schimanski LA, Nguyen PV (2004). Multidisciplinary approaches for investigating the mechanisms of hippocampus-dependent memory: a focus on inbred mouse strains. *Neurosci Biobehav Rev* **28**: 463–483.

Shaywitz BA, Klopper JH, Yager RD, Gordon JW (1976). Paradoxical response to amphetamine in developing rats treated with 6-hydroxydopamine. *Nature* **261**: 153–155.

Shaywitz BA, Fletcher JM, Shaywitz SE (2001). Attention deficit hyperactivity disorder. *Curr Treat Options Neurol* **3**: 229–236.

Song C, Leonard BE (2005). The olfactory bulbectomized rat as a model of depression. *Neurosci Biobehav Rev* **29**: 627–647.

Takagi T, Saito H, Lee C-H, Hayashi T (1972). Pharmacological studies on fatigue I. *Jpn J Pharmacol* **22**: 17–26.

van Praag HM (2004). Can stress cause depression? *Prog Neuropsychopharmacol Biol Psychiatry* **28**(5): 891–907.

Vegas O, Beitia G, Sanchez-Martin JR, Arregi A, Azpiroz A (2004). Behavioral and neurochemical responses in mice bearing tumors submitted to social stress. *Behav Brain Res* **155**: 125–134.

Weiss JM, Kilts CD (1998). Animal models of depression and schizophrenia. In Schatzberg AF, Nemeroff CB (eds.) *The American Psychiatric Press Textbook of Psychopharmacology* (2nd edn.) (pp. 89–131). Washington DC: American Psychiatric Press.

Whishaw IQ, Kolb B (2005). *The Behavior of the Laboratory Rat. A Handbook with Tests.* Oxford: Oxford University Press.

Willner P (1984). The validity of animal models of depression. *Psychopharmacology (Berl)* **83**: 1–16.

Willner P (1997). Validity, reliability and utility of the chronic mild stress model of depression: a 10-year review and evaluation. *Psychopharmacology* **134**: 319–329.

Willner P (2005). Chronic mild stress (CMS) revisited: consistency and behavioural-neurobiological concordance in the effects of CMS. *Psychopharmacology (Berl)* **52**: 90–110.

Wong ML, Kling MA, Munson PJ *et al.* (2000). Pronounced and sustained central hypernoradrenergic function in major depression with melancholic features: relation to hypercortisolism and corticotropin-releasing hormone. *Proc Natl Acad Sci USA* **97**: 325–330.

Interventions and implications for clinical trials

20

Behavioral strategies and rehabilitation

Dona E. C. Locke, Jane H. Cerhan, and James F. Malec

Significant cognitive impairment frequently accompanies cancer and cancer treatment for both adult and pediatric patients. As detailed in previous chapters, common cognitive complaints include cognitive slowing, deficits in attention, and memory inefficiencies. In people with brain tumors, cognitive impairments cause difficulty returning to work or school more often than physical impairments, and caregivers cite cognitive problems as the most difficult problems to manage (Meyers & Boake, 1993). For these reasons, evidence-based cognitive rehabilitation has the potential to meet prevalent needs for improving functional abilities in patients with cancer.

There is considerable focus in the literature on the general concept of quality of life in patients with many different kinds of cancer. Interventions to improve quality of life are often focused on symptoms of the cancer (e.g., physical limitations, decreased activity), physical symptoms related to treatment (e.g., fatigue, nausea, pain), health behavior change, or distress related to the diagnosis of cancer (e.g., Clark *et al.*, 2003; Kuhn *et al.*, 2005; Ronson & Body, 2002). However, very few studies specifically target cognitive symptoms in cancer patients and in fact, many studies exclude patients with cognitive impairment. Thus, the empirical literature on behavioral interventions for cognitive impairments in cancer patients is very limited.

In contrast, there is a long tradition of applying cognitive rehabilitation interventions in cases of acquired brain injury, specifically traumatic brain injury (TBI) and cerebral vascular accident (CVA). A number of studies have addressed the efficacy of various interventions for cognitive impairment, as summarized in recent reviews by Cicerone *et al.* (2000, 2005). Further development, investigation, and application of cognitive rehabilitation was also recommended by an NIH Consensus Conference (NIH Consensus Statement Online 1998 October 26–28). More recently, similar cognitive rehabilitation interventions have been under investigation in neurodegenerative conditions such as Alzheimer's disease (Clare *et al.*, 2005; De Vreese *et al.*, 2001) and mild cognitive impairment (MCI; Chandler & Smith, personal communication, 2005).

The lack of empirical evaluation of behavioral interventions for cognitive difficulties specifically in cancer patients encourages reflection and consideration of the best direction, focus, and methodologies for this research. In the sections below we will: (1) define cognitive rehabilitation and provide a framework for categorizing cognitive rehabilitation techniques; (2) briefly summarize selected behavioral strategies and supporting evidence for use with patients with TBI/CVA; (3) describe how similar behavioral strategies have been applied to patients with a degenerative condition; (4) describe

Cognition and Cancer, eds. Christina A. Meyers and James R. Perry. Published by Cambridge University Press.
© Cambridge University Press 2008.

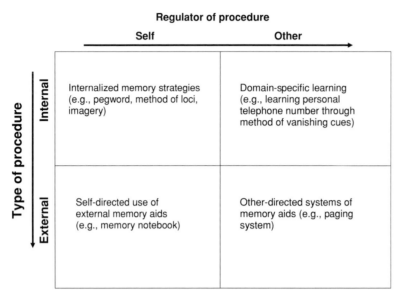

Figure 20.1. Dimensions of rehabilitation. Adapted from Malec & Cicerone (2006)

the limited empirical information on cognitive reha-bilitation with cancer patients; and (5) describe how clinicians may currently apply behavioral interventions to cognitive symptoms in cancer patients by adapting techniques that have been used with other patient populations.

Definition of cognitive rehabilitation

Cognitive rehabilitation has been defined as "a systematic, functionally oriented service of therapeutic activities that is based on assessment and understanding of the patient's brain-behavior deficits" (Cicerone *et al.*, 2000, p. 1596). Cognitive rehabilitation tends to be a highly individualized undertaking in which interventions are closely matched to the patient's specific cognitive impairment profile, severity of impairment, and functional goals. Cognitive rehabilitation techniques may be categorized by the specific type and severity of cognitive impairment that is targeted (e.g., intervention for severe memory impairment). More broadly, however, the wide array of techniques can also be classified as

employing one of two approaches: *strategy training* or *restitution training* (Cicerone *et al.*, 2005).

The goal of strategy training techniques is to *compensate* for cognitive deficits using spared abilities or external devices. Examples of strategy training techniques include using a memory notebook to compensate for memory deficits (Sohlberg & Mateer, 1989) or skill training in Alzheimer's patients using their intact procedural memory while bypassing impaired episodic memory (De Vreese *et al.*, 2001). The goal of restitution training is to *restore* the underlying impaired function, such as through massed practice of sustained attention via computerized tasks. While both approaches may have merit, strategy training enjoys more research support than restitution training as a cognitive rehabilitation model, especially when the deficits involve attention or memory (Cicerone *et al.*, 2000, 2005). Thus, we will focus primarily on strategy training cognitive rehabilitation techniques in this chapter.

Malec and Cicerone (2006) suggest that strategy training cognitive rehabilitation techniques may be further classified along two dimensions (see Figure 20.1). One dimension describes the degree to which the procedure that enhances cognitive functioning is internal or external to the person (e.g., a memory mnemonic versus a memory notebook). The other dimension is the degree to which the procedure is regulated by the person or by the environment, including other people. Figure 20.1 provides examples of cognitive rehabilitation interventions specific to the memory domain defined by these dimensions. In general, a patient's type and severity of cognitive impairment as well as the patient's preserved cognitive abilities, preferences, goals, and amount of family or social support dictate where the specific cognitive rehabilitation technique should fall along these two dimensions. Comprehensive neuropsychological evaluation plays an important role in directing the choice of cognitive rehabilitation technique due to the need to understand areas of deficit as well as areas of preserved functioning.

For example, cognitive rehabilitation strategies that are internal procedures (e.g., a memory mnemonic) and regulated by the patient (e.g., self-applied in the appropriate situation) may depend on some degree of preserved working memory as well as relatively intact executive functions such as the ability to organize and execute such a strategy. That is, internal procedures that are self-regulated by the patient may be most appropriate for patients with relatively mild cognitive impairment and relatively intact cognition in many areas. In contrast, learning an external procedure (e.g., a memory notebook) that is regulated by the patient (e.g., self-applied in the appropriate situation) theoretically may rely more on procedural learning. Thus, an external procedure that is regulated by the patient may be helpful for patients with either a relatively significant cognitive impairment or mild executive functioning difficulty. Domain-specific new learning (an internal procedure) through other-directed overlearning or other specialized procedure may rely entirely on procedural memory and require less self-monitoring than the above techniques. External prompting for implementation of the new learning may still be required. External compensation procedures that are entirely other-directed (such as a paging system) may require minimal ability

to encode new information or procedural memory. These latter two approaches may be appropriate for patients with more severe cognitive impairments. These dimensions are not meant to be inflexible or dogmatic, but rather are meant to provide some guidance to clinicians when choosing a cognitive rehabilitation strategy for the individual patient.

Cognitive rehabilitation in TBI/CVA

Cicerone and colleagues (2000, 2005) recently updated their review of evidence-based cognitive rehabilitation. Based on their findings, they offer Practice Standards, Practice Guidelines, and Practice Options for cognitive rehabilitation of patients with TBI and stroke. These types of recommendations are directly linked to the available empirical evidence. Practice Standards are based on substantive evidence of effectiveness based on the presence of at least one well-designed and adequately powered randomized controlled trial along with additional supportive evidence from less rigorous trials, such as non-randomized cohort studies. Practice Guidelines are offered based on probable evidence of effectiveness obtained from non-randomized or case–control studies. Practice Options are based on evidence of possible effectiveness from uncontrolled case series or case reports. The recommendations of Cicerone and associates for cognitive rehabilitation of attention, executive functioning, memory and learning – the cognitive domains most commonly affected in cancer patients – are summarized in Table 20.1. In the remainder of this section, we will provide more detailed description of specific interventions to serve as examples.

Strategy training for attention deficits

Fasotti *et al.* (2000) reported an empirical trial of compensation for slowed information processing and the experience of "information overload" in daily tasks. Patients in the intervention group received strategy training in the form of Time Pressure Management (TPM). This approach involves

Table 20.1. Recommendations from Cicerone *et al.*
(2000, 2005)

Attention deficits
    1. Practice Standard: strategy training (i.e.,
       compensation strategy)
Executive functioning deficits
    2. Practice Guideline: formal training in problem solving
       with application to everyday situations
    3. Practice Option: strategies including verbal
       self-instruction, self-questioning, and self-monitoring
       to promote self-regulation
Memory and learning deficits
    4. Practice Standard: internalized or external procedures
       for treatment of mild memory impairment
    5. Practice Guideline: external procedures with direct
       application to functional activities for treatment of
       moderate to severe memory impairment

teaching patients strategies for coping with mental slowness utilizing relatively preserved cognitive skills. Examples of specific coping strategies include the following, depending on the patient's relative cognitive strengths: optimizing planning and organization, rehearsing task requirements, or modification of task environment. In general, TPM is a four-step cognitive strategy: (1) recognize time pressure in the task at hand, (2) prevent as much time pressure as possible, (3) deal with time pressure as quickly and effectively as possible, and (4) self-monitor while using these strategies. Thus, in terms of our general cognitive rehabilitation model, TPM is an *internal procedure* that is *self regulated* (Figure 20.1) and would be appropriate for patients with relatively mild cognitive impairment and relatively intact executive functioning.

The control group in Fasotti *et al.* (2000) received four generic suggestions regarding concentration and remembering as much as possible. Participants who received TPM showed significantly greater use of self-management strategies and better performance on behavioral tasks requiring attention and memory (e.g., completing a task according to specific multistep instructions). Specifically, patients in the TPM group were more likely to utilize strategies

such as reiterating information, asking for repetition of information, asking for clarification of information, or asking for a short pause. Patients in the TPM group utilized more of these strategies after receiving training in TPM than they had prior to training, and patients in the TPM group utilized more of these strategies than the generic concentration training group. In addition, TPM appeared to generalize spontaneously over a broader range of tasks than generic advice.

Strategy training for memory and learning inefficiencies: the memory notebook

Sohlberg and Mateer (1989) offered empirical support for compensatory strategy training using a memory notebook for patients with unreliable memory following acquired brain injury. A memory notebook is a portable paper notebook with one or more sections that is personalized to the specific functional needs of the patient. The purpose is to compensate for memory difficulties by teaching patients to store information in the notebook in a manner that facilitates access as well as structuring it to provide cues for tasks to be completed. Thus, this cognitive rehabilitation intervention involves an *external procedure* that is *self regulated* by the patient (Figure 20.1). Because the procedure is external, it serves to cue and prompt self-regulation by the patient. As such it may be useful for patients with more severe memory problems with some executive functioning deficits.

Possible notebook sections could include: orientation, memory log, calendar, things to do, transportation, feelings log, names, and today at work. Patients are trained to use the notebook, for example to remember to complete daily tasks and to document completion of these tasks. Training in the memory notebook system consists of three steps: acquisition, application, and adaptation. The *acquisition* stage consists of introducing the concept of the notebook to the patient and beginning construction of the patient's individualized notebook. The *application* stage involves training and practice in using the notebook daily. The *adaptation* stage involves practicing the use of the notebook in order to make it habitual.

Ownsworth and McFarland (1999) further showed that pairing self-instruction training with use of a memory notebook enhances usage of the notebook. The self-instruction training provided a systematic method to train patients on how to use a memory notebook to compensate for memory problems. The self-instruction specifically involved teaching patients to cue themselves using the following abbreviation: WSTC, where W = what you are going to do; S = select a strategy for the task; T = try out the strategy; C = check out how the strategy is working. In this study, self-instruction training improved subjects' ability to spontaneously access their diaries and make entries in appropriate everyday situations.

Formal problem solving for executive functioning deficits

Ownsworth *et al.* (2000) reported results of the effects of formal training in problem solving on the application of other compensation strategies and on psychosocial functioning in patients with brain injury. The program involved 16 weekly 90-min group sessions. The sessions involved patient education, sharing of patient-developed coping strategies, and teaching of specific strategies recommended in the literature. Formal problem solving was included in the specific strategies taught to the patients to help them decide which of the other compensation techniques should be applied to a problem situation. In many cases, formal problem solving is an *internal procedure* that is *self regulated* by the patient (Figure 20.1). However, for patients with greater cognitive impairment, this type of strategy can be taught in an overlearning procedural paradigm (*other regulated)* and prompted by external materials such as a diagram of the steps of problem solving (*external procedure*).

The results of Ownsworth *et al.* (2000) suggested significant improvements in a patient's anticipatory awareness of deficits, selection of coping strategies, and effectiveness of selected strategies. Patients also improved in psychosocial functioning following training in problem solving. These findings are consistent with those of an earlier trial of similar training in formal problem-solving strategies and application of those strategies to everyday situations and functional activities in patients with acquired brain injury (Von Cramen & Mathes-Von Cramen, 1991). Patients in the latter trial were classified as poor problem solvers on the basis of formal tests of problem solving. Training in problem solving emphasized teaching patients to reduce complex problems into manageable steps (problem orientation, problem definition and formulation, generation of alternative, decision making, and solution verification).

Cognitive rehabilitation in degenerative conditions

Most patients with TBI or CVA are on a stable or improving course when they are referred for cognitive rehabilitation. Some patients with cancer may have a similarly stable course. However, some cancer patients are on a declining course. This brings into question the applicability of the research on patients with TBI or stroke to some patients with cancer. For patients with cancer where decline is expected, behavioral interventions designed or adapted to treat cognitive dysfunction in patients with degenerative conditions such as MCI or Alzheimer's disease may be more appropriate.

In general, limited information suggests that strategy training, or training to compensate for cognitive deficits, may be helpful in neurodegenerative conditions (e.g., De Vreese *et al.*, 2001). In this section, we will offer detailed examples of compensatory cognitive rehabilitation techniques that have been used in people with Alzheimer's disease. Since the primary dysfunction in Alzheimer's disease is memory, the interventions are focused on that type of deficit. The reader is referred to De Vreese *et al.* (2001) for a more comprehensive review of cognitive rehabilitation techniques in Alzheimer's disease.

External memory aids

External memory aids aim to help patients with dementia compensate for memory deficits by providing cues for memory, support for organization and retrieval of information, and prompting initiation of activities. For example, Bourgeois *et al.* (1997) investigated a program for training caregivers in behavioral management strategies aimed at reducing repetitive question-asking in home-dwelling patients with mild to moderate Alzheimer's disease. Behavioral systems were individualized for each patient, but generally consisted of a written cue to help the patients remember the answer to their repetitive question, and a series of instructions to the caregiver including: (1) deliver the cueing system to the patient, (2) refrain from extraneous verbal directions or explanations other than to look at or read the cue, (3) praise the patient for using the written cue, and (4) walk away if an argument occurs related to the cueing. Cards with written cues contained pictures or clock drawings to facilitate understanding. Thus, this type of intervention is an *external procedure* that is *other regulated* and designed for patients with severe cognitive impairment resulting in a very limited capacity for self-regulation.

For example, if a patient repetitively asks about an upcoming outing, an index card with a brief written reminder of the outing and its time is provided to the patient along with a brief explanation, such as, "Today we are going to (location) at (time). Here is a card that tells you this so you can remember when and where we are going. If you forget, look at this card." It is recommended that the patient carry the card in a pocket. If the patient repeats the question about the outing, the caregiver is instructed to say, "Look at your card" and walk away. If the caregiver sees the patient reviewing the card without cueing, the caregiver is instructed to praise the patient and say, "Good, you are looking at that card that says we'll be going to (location) at (time)."

Cues were either simplified [e.g., just a simple orientation statement such as "I have lived at (address) for 30 years"] or broadened (e.g., listing a day's schedule on a dry erase board) depending on the severity of the patient's impairment. The subject sample was small [$N = 7$), but mean rates of repetitive question asking declined from 21.9 per day at baseline to 11.2 per day at the end of 12 weeks of treatment to 8.6 per day at the 6 months follow-up.

Cognitive rehabilitation versus mental stimulation

Other investigations of learning and cueing strategies that may help patients with Alzheimer's disease have identified three promising techniques – spaced retrieval, dual cognitive support, and procedural memory training (Loewenstein *et al.*, 2004). These three cognitive rehabilitation strategies are examples of *internal procedures* that are *other regulated* because of the patient's limited capacity for self-regulation.

Spaced retrieval involves learning associations over multiple trials at progressively longer time intervals and with corrective feedback of any learning errors. Dual cognitive support uses cues and techniques to enhance the saliency of the information to be remembered at both learning and retrieval. Procedural memory training involves eliciting complex motor behaviors during learning in order to activate the presumed intact procedural memory system in Alzheimer's disease patients. For example, Loewenstein *et al.* (2004) compared the efficacy of: (1) a cognitive rehabilitation condition utilizing the above three techniques with a memory notebook and (2) a mental stimulation condition using computer games involving memory, concentration, and problem-solving skills in patients with mild Alzheimer's dementia. All patients were stable on cholinesterase inhibitor medications during the intervention. All patients received 24 individual training sessions of 45 min each over a period of 12–16 weeks.

The cognitive rehabilitation condition utilized a variety of internal and external procedures that varied in the degree of self or other regulation. This broad-spectrum multi-modal approach appeared to provide some benefit to most patients.

Ideally interventions could also be more specifically selected for patient needs. The mental stimulation condition involved computer games requiring patients to match pairs of letters, numbers,
or designs from memory, exercises such as "hang-
man," tasks requiring patients to rearrange sets of
letters to generate as many words as possible, and
asking patients to freely recall information from the
recent or remote past. Results showed that patients
in the cognitive rehabilitation condition, but not
the mental stimulation condition, improved significantly in orientation, learning of new face–name
associations, speed of processing, and specific functional abilities. Patients in the cognitive rehabilitation condition maintained these gains at the
3 months follow-up while the patients receiving the
mental stimulation condition continued to decline.

Cognitive rehabilitation for patients with cancer

In this section, we will extend the discussion of
cognitive rehabilitation interventions by reviewing
research on interventions used specifically with
cancer patients. Several published studies report a
benefit of general inpatient rehabilitation to adult
patients with cancer and brain tumors (Cole *et al.*,
2000; Huang *et al.*, 1998; Marciniak *et al.*, 2001;
O'Dell *et al.*, 1998). However, relatively few cancer patients are referred for rehabilitation services
despite significant need (Davies *et al.*, 2003; Kirshblum *et al.*, 2001; Movsas *et al.*, 2003). Meyers
and Boake (1993) note that at least 34% of non-
CNS cancer patients and essentially all CNS cancer patients develop cognitive deficits during treatment, but that rehabilitation hospitals do not routinely provide cognitive rehabilitation services to
cancer patients and cancer hospitals do not routinely provide cognitive or vocational rehabilitation
services. Empirical studies supporting the effectiveness of specific rehabilitation interventions in this
population could enhance referring oncology practitioners' confidence in rehabilitation services, and
thus increase referrals.

Among the few published studies of cognitive
rehabilitation for patients with cancer, one of the
most elegant is the ongoing rehabilitation research
program with pediatric patients designed by Butler and Copeland (2002). These clinician investigators combine a variety of training techniques in their
Cognitive Remediation Program or "CRP." The program is described as a combination of: (1) drill-
oriented practice, (2) learning skills and strategy
acquisition, and (3) cognitive-behavioral therapy.
These methods combine three disciplines: brain
injury rehabilitation, special education/educational
psychology, and clinical psychology.

The restitution component, utilizing Sohlberg
and Mateer's (1989; Sohlberg *et al.*, 2000) Attention
Process Training, involves massed practice of sustained, selective, divided, and executive attention
skills. The strategy training component includes
teaching a range of metacognitive strategies individualized to the patient's particular needs and abilities. Cognitive-behavioral therapy is also used as
another form of strategy training aimed at teaching patients to resist distraction. A manual for the
complete program is available from the investigators. This combination of strategies is offered across
approximately 50 h of treatment over a 6-month
time period.

Butler and Copeland (2002) reported preliminary
results of 21 patients receiving the intervention with
a comparison group of 10 patients who did not
receive any intervention. Patients who received the
intervention showed significant improvement on
neuropsychological measures of simple attention,
sustained vigilance attention, and memory. These
findings are encouraging, but the authors note that
further research is needed to investigate the ecological validity of this intervention program. The
program developers report that the program is currently being evaluated in a multi-site phase III clinical trial.

Sherer *et al.* (1997) have offered the only published investigation of cognitive rehabilitation for
adult patients. Their trial involved intensive cognitive rehabilitation of a small sample of adults with
primary brain tumors ($N = 13$). All patients were

post-treatment and relatively stable in their disease. Rehabilitation was conducted in an intensive day treatment model that has been empirically supported for patients with TBI. Patients underwent daily cognitive compensation strategy training for an average of 2.5 months in the context of a general day treatment program to improve self-awareness of deficits, behavioral self-regulation, adjustment, and social and vocational participation. The goal was to teach patients techniques to compensate for cognitive difficulties in order to increase independence and productivity. The specific intervention was multidisciplinary in nature and involved strategies from all quadrants of the model in Figure 20.1 depending on the need of the specific patient. The results of that small trial were positive, with six patients increasing their independence and eight patients increasing their productivity; these gains were maintained at the 8 months follow-up.

Nezu and colleagues' (1998, 2003) investigation of problem-solving therapy is also relevant. Their behavioral intervention is primarily aimed to reduce psychological distress, not cognitive dysfunction, in cancer patients. However, the technique they describe is very similar to formal problem-solving therapy recommended as a cognitive rehabilitation treatment for TBI patients with executive dysfunction and therefore might have similar application to a cancer patient population.

Nezu *et al.* (1998) outline a 10-session program to teach patients with cancer effective problem-solving abilities in order to lessen emotional distress and improve quality of life. Sessions involve training in positive problem orientation and in the four rational problem-solving tasks using didactics, in-session practice, and homework assignments. In their book, Nezu *et al.* (1998) provide a detailed manual for the program.

Nezu *et al.* (2003) reported results of a large randomized controlled efficacy trial of problem-solving therapy in distressed adults with cancer. A total of 132 patients were randomized to 1 of 3 groups: (1) problem-solving therapy, (2) problem-solving therapy with a significant other, and (3) wait list control. At post-treatment, both groups who received problem-solving therapy showed decreased distress and increased quality of life. At 1 year, patients who received problem-solving therapy with a significant other were the least distressed and had the highest overall quality of life. No cognitive evaluation or measurement of cognitive symptoms was included in this trial.

At the Mayo Clinic, we are conducting a trial of a brief cognitive rehabilitation intervention for patients with brain tumors. Our primary aim is to determine the feasibility and tolerability of a combined, tailored, cognitive rehabilitation and problem-solving therapy intervention with a sample of patients with brain tumors. The eventual goal of investigating this type of compensation-focused intervention is to increase independence and productivity in patients with brain tumors who are experiencing cognitive difficulties.

In the intervention, patients with primary brain tumors of any kind who have mild to moderate cognitive impairment are given a total of 12 sessions of compensation-focused intervention during the time they are receiving radiation treatment. A support person (e.g., spouse or companion) attends all training sessions with the patient in order to act as a training partner and to have the knowledge to reinforce these strategies outside the treatment sessions. Appendices A and B provide more details of the interventions, which are adapted from evidence-based interventions in other populations.

The memory rehabilitation component involves six training sessions over a 2-week period. The specific intervention involves the development and utilization of the type of memory notebook that has been empirically supported for use in patients with TBI (Sohlberg & Mateer, 1989). The problem-solving component involves six sessions concurrent with the memory rehabilitation sessions. This part of the intervention is an abbreviated adaptation of Nezu *et al.*'s intervention that was empirically supported for use with adults with cancer as described above (Nezu *et al.*, 1998, 2003).

It should be apparent from the brevity of this review that the literature on cognitive rehabilitation in cancer patients is in its infancy. Additional

Table 20.2. Specific research questions. CVA, cerebral vascular accidents; TBI, traumatic brain injury

- Is it feasible to provide cognitive rehabilitation as patients undergo treatment for cancer?
- Do the cognitive impairments in cancer patients differ qualitatively from the cognitive impairments in TBI/CVA patients in nature, localization of dysfunction, and response to treatment?
- How does the feasibility and effectiveness of cognitive rehabilitation vary with respect to cancer type and severity?
- Would brief, compensation-oriented cognitive rehabilitation be feasible and effective for cancer patients?
- For patients where cure is expected, should cognitive rehabilitation be postponed until remission is achieved?
- How does the etiology of the cognitive impairment (e.g., tumor effects vs. radiation effects vs. chemotherapy effects) impact the behavioral intervention plan?

empirical investigations that identify beneficial cognitive rehabilitation interventions are urgently needed. In Table 20.2, we list some research questions that could be addressed as this field of inquiry moves forward.

While a randomized controlled trial may be the gold standard for the most rigorous research trial of a medical or rehabilitation intervention, basic questions of feasibility and appropriate outcome measures would appropriately precede randomized controlled trials at this stage. Furthermore, randomized controlled trials are best applied with interventions that can be strictly standardized for application to very specific deficits. Such strictly controlled scenarios are rare in rehabilitation practice where patients vary greatly in terms of cognitive profiles, goals, and resources such as stamina and social support; and interventions are often combined or adapted. Useful guidelines for researchers designing cognitive rehabilitation experiments are provided by Levine and Downey-Lamb (2002) and in a special supplement to the *American Journal of Physical Medicine and Rehabilitation* (Millis & Johnston, 2003).

Clinical application of cognitive rehabilitation strategies in cancer patients

In the sections above, we have tried to make the case that cognitive rehabilitation with cancer patients requires innovation on the part of practitioners, including adapting the knowledge gained from the literature on other populations including those with TBI, CVA, and Alzheimer's disease. In some cases among patients with cancer, modifications to the cognitive rehabilitation intervention will be appropriate because the patient's disease status, recovery curve, or prognosis differs from that of the original validation group.

Patients with TBI or CVA are expected to have their worst cognitive deficits at the time of injury and to subsequently improve and become stable. However, patients with neurodegenerative conditions are expected to have a worsening of cognitive deficits over time as disease progresses. In patients with cancer, impairments may be improving or stable, similar to TBI/CVA, *or* progressive, similar to a neurodegenerative condition. Prognosis among patients with cancer varies, with some patients cured of disease and others eventually succumbing over varying lengths of time. Thus, the appropriate cognitive rehabilitation technique for the individual cancer patient may be one that has been used with patients with an acquired brain injury *or* a cognitive rehabilitation technique that has been shown useful in cases with progressive deficits as in a degenerative illness. Practitioner flexibility will be required to apply cognitive rehabilitation strategies to cognitive deficits associated with cancer.

The primary impetus for cognitive rehabilitation in cancer patients is a complaint from the patient, a significant other, or from the treating physician that cognitive status is of concern. We first recommend neuropsychological assessment to fully characterize the specific type of impairment, severity of impairment, and areas of retained ability. Fully understanding and objectively quantifying this information is important for selecting an appropriate cognitive rehabilitation approach. For example, for patients with relatively mild cognitive impairment

Table 20.3. Guided application of cognitive rehabilitation for patients with cancer

Patient or significant other complains of cognitive impairment or behavioral problems
- Neuropsychological evaluation to specify type and severity of cognitive behavioral disorder and for recommendations for intervention

Is the patient's cognitive impairment relatively mild?
- If yes, first consider an internal compensation technique such as a memory mnemonic, Time Pressure Management training, or problem-solving training as appropriate to the type of cognitive impairment
- If no, consider an external compensation technique such as a memory notebook or cue card reminders

What is the patient's prognosis?
- <6 months or declining course:
  – External compensation technique
  – Education and coaching for significant other to support, prompt, and cue patient
- >6 months and stable course:
  – Self-directed compensation techniques focused on impaired cognitive domains determined by neuropsychometric evaluation

What is the status of the patient's ability to monitor and regulate his/her own behavior?
- If poor, consider external regulation of cognitive rehabilitation techniques
- If intact, consider internal regulation of cognitive rehabilitation techniques

Is cognitive impairment complicated by lack of self-awareness?
- If yes and prognosis <6 months or declining course:
  – Education and coaching for significant other on managing and coping with patient's cognitive and behavioral problems (i.e., external coping technique that is externally regulated)
- If yes and prognosis >6 months with stable course:
  – Intensive day rehabilitation for brain injury

What are patient's goals?
- Enhanced daily functioning and improved quality of life
  – Environmental modifications only if goals can be achieved without rehabilitation
  – Cognitive rehabilitation if environmental modifications are inadequate or internal control is desired by patient
- Educational or vocational reintegration
  – Consider a cognitive rehabilitation strategy that is internally regulated by the patient
  – In addition to cognitive rehabilitation, specific functional rehabilitation including on-site evaluation, environmental modifications, and coaching with gradual increase in time spent at work or school

Is cognitive impairment complicated by fatigue?
- If yes:
  – Pharmacological treatment for fatigue
  – Coaching for pacing activities
  – Appropriate pacing of rehabilitation intervention

Is cognitive impairment complicated by behavioral problems (e.g., disinhibition, abulia)?
- If yes:
  – Pharmacological interventions for behavioral management
  – Consider externally regulated cognitive rehabilitation techniques and education and coaching for significant other on managing and coping with patient's behavioral disorder

Is cognitive impairment complicated by depression or other emotional disorder?
- If yes:
  – Pharmacological intervention
  – Cognitive behavior therapy

and relatively intact executive functioning (i.e., ability to organize and self-monitor), utilizing an internal compensation strategy that can be applied by the patients themselves may be a place to start with cognitive rehabilitation. If cognitive impairment is more mild to moderate, but the patient's executive functioning is relatively intact, an external compensation strategy may be necessary, but could be applied by the patient without external prompting. For more severely impaired patients, or patients for whom behavioral problems are also significant, an external compensation technique may need to be externally regulated. Sutor *et al.* (2001) suggest some of these types of behavioral management strategies based on their work with patients with dementia.

Another critical consideration, given the differences between patients with cancer and those with TBI or CVA, is the timing of intervention. Many patients with cancer notice cognitive difficulty during the period of diagnosis and treatment. Although delaying cognitive rehabilitation until cancer treatment is complete may reduce the stress and complexity of care for the patient, this must be weighed against the potential benefit of early intervention. In this sense, the goal of cognitive rehabilitation for some types of cancer patients, especially those for whom cure is not expected, may be similar to the goal of cognitive rehabilitation in a neurodegenerative condition; that is, maximizing functional abilities as much as possible in the face of expected decline.

In TBI/CVA rehabilitation, treatment can be very intensive (multiple hours daily) and may last for several months. This model may be necessary and appropriate for a select group of patients with cancer or brain tumors who have multiple cognitive deficits and impaired self-awareness of deficits but who also have relatively low-grade disease with the expectation of disease remission or cure. For many other cancer patients, however, decreased stamina, more limited deficits, busy cancer treatment schedules as well as prognosis issues suggest that less intensive, briefer interventions may be more appropriate.

In general, we recommend that clinicians offer compensation-oriented cognitive rehabilitation approaches to patients with cancer, since this type of technique is most supported by the empirical literature in other areas. In addition, within compensation-oriented techniques, we recommend considering the dimensions outlined in Figure 20.1 and reiterated throughout this chapter. Choosing specific techniques along the dimensions outlined in Figure 20.1 will depend on what is appropriate to the patient's impairments, preserved abilities, cancer prognosis, goals for cognitive rehabilitation, preferences, and available social support.

In Table 20.3, we present a series of questions to guide the clinical application of cognitive rehabilitation in patients with cancer. These guidelines are based on clinical experience as well as on empirical evidence from investigations involving other patient populations. We are optimistic that progress in cognitive rehabilitation for persons with cancer will continue, and that the quality of life for patients and their families will be enhanced.

Appendix A

Cognitive rehabilitation intervention protocol

This intervention is modeled after the techniques described by Sohlberg and Mateer (1989). In each session, some general strategies are used with each patient in order to maximize learning. The patients themselves are encouraged to write in their calendars (instead of the therapist or the support person). Indirect cueing (i.e., a reminder without specific direction) is used whenever possible. Positive feedback is used as much as possible.

Session 1

- Explain the purpose of a memory notebook (to compensate for memory, attention, or organization problems by using this external device)
- Determine if the patient already uses a calendar system

- Introduce our calendar and orient to the format (one page per day, specific times, action list area, date at top)
- Have patient and caregiver verbalize difficulties they notice
- Strategize using the calendar for one difficulty (e.g., remembering medications, entering doctor's appointments, remembering other planned outings, reducing repeated asking or questions) and agree to check off items as they are completed

Session 2

- Review orientation to the calendar with patient leading the way (where the date is located, one day per page, specific times versus action list area)
- Review patient's acquisition of using the calendar for their identified area of difficulty
- Review checking off of completed items
- Agree to expand the calendar for use with other areas (therapist should help indicate what should go in the calendar – upcoming medical appointments, medication schedule, upcoming family events, etc.)

Session 3

- Check with patient and caregiver regarding spontaneous use of the calendar outside the session
- Review calendar for the previous day, today, and next day for: (1) entries and (2) notation of completion
- Ask three questions for the patient to answer (what is today's date, when is your next medical appointment, and did you take your medications yesterday?)

Sessions 4–6

- Review use of calendar and indications of completion since the last session
- Ask three patient-specific questions they would need the calendar to answer
- Ask patient and caregiver for additional difficulties and see if they can be incorporated into using the calendar

At session 6 – seek commitment from the patient and caregiver to using the calendar post-treatment

Appendix B

Problem-solving therapy intervention protocol

This intervention is modeled after the techniques described by Nezu *et al.* (1998, 2003). The intervention is six 50-min sessions over a 2-week period. The patient concurrently receives six sessions of cognitive rehabilitation from another provider.

Session 1

- Explain problem-solving model of stress and a brain tumor as a major life stressor
- Present goals of problem-solving therapy
- Present four components of a positive problem-solving orientation

Session 2

- More detailed development of positive problem-solving orientation using ABC method of constructive thinking, reversed advocacy role play, and using feelings as cues
- Briefly, present the steps of problem solving: defining the problem, generating alternative solutions, decide on a solution strategy, implement the solution, review the outcome of that implementation
- Present categories and specific potential tumor-related problems (e.g., side-effects, psychological distress, marital and family, medical interaction, sexual)

Session 3

- Detailed application of problem-solving steps to example problem
- Patient and support person choose a problem in the session to which they can apply the steps
- Patient and support person will practice the steps on chosen problem outside of the session before session 4

Sessions 4–6

- Review patient's and support person's use of the strategies
- Review positive problem-solving orientation or any of the steps of problem solving if necessary
- Troubleshoot any problems using the steps
- Continued practice of the techniques in session
- Continued refinement of patient's and support person's application of the steps

REFERENCES

Bourgeois MS, Burgio LD, Schulz R, Beach S, Palmer B (1997). Modifying repetitive verbalizations of community-dwelling patients with AD. *Gerontologist* **37**: 30–39.

Butler RW, Copeland DR (2002). Attentional processes and their remediation in children treated for cancer: a literature review and the development of a therapeutic approach. *J Intl Neuropsychol Soc* **8**: 115–124.

Cicerone KD, Dahlberg C, Kalmar K *et al.* (2000). Evidence-based cognitive rehabilitation: recommendations for clinical practice. *Arch Phys Med Rehabil* **81**: 1596–1615.

Cicerone KD, Dahlberg C, Malec JF *et al.* (2005). Evidence-based cognitive rehabilitation: updated review of the literature from 1998–2002. *Arch Phys Med Rehabil* **86**: 1681–1692.

Clare L, Woods RT, Moniz Cook ED, Orrell M, Spector A (2005). Cognitive rehabilitation and cognitive training for early-stage Alzheimer's disease and vascular dementia. *Cochrane Library* **2**.

Clark MM, Bostwick JM, Rummans TA (2003). Group and individual treatment strategies for distress in cancer patients. *Mayo Clin Proc* **78**: 1538–1543.

Cole RP, Scialla SJ, Bednarz L (2000). Functional recovery in cancer rehabilitation. *Arch Phys Med Rehabil* **81**: 623–627.

Davies E, Hall S, Clark, C. (2003). Two year survival after malignant cerebral glioma: patient and relative reports of handicap, psychiatric symptoms, and rehabilitation. *Disabil Rehabil* **25**: 259–266.

De Vreese LP, Neri M, Fioravanti M, Belloi L, Zanetti O (2001). Memory rehabilitation in Alzheimer's disease: a review of progress. *Int J Geriatr Psychiatry*, **16**: 794–806.

Fasotti L, Kovacs F, Eling PATM, Brouwer WH (2000). Time pressure management as a compensatory strategy training after closed head injury. *Neuropsychol Rehabil* **10**: 47–65.

Huang ME, Cifu DX, Keyser-Marus L (1998). Functional outcome after brain tumor and acute stroke: a comparative analysis. *Arc Phys Med Rehabil* **79**: 1386–1390.

Kirshblum S, O'Dell MW, Ho C, Barr K (2001). Rehabilitation of persons with central nervous system cancer. *Cancer Suppl* **92**: 1029–1038.

Kuhn GK, Boesen E, Ross L, Johansen C (2005). Evaluation and outcome of behavioural changes in the rehabilitation of cancer patients: a review. *Eur J Cancer* **41**: 216–224.

Levine B, Downey-Lamb MM (2002). Design and evaluation of rehabilitation experiments. In Eslinger PJ (ed.) *Neuropsychological Interventions: Clinical Research and Practice*. New York: The Guilford Press.

Loewenstein DA, Acevedo A, Czaja SJ, Duara R (2004). Cognitive rehabilitation of mildly impaired Alzheimer's disease patients on cholinesterase inhibitors. *J Geriatr Psychiatry* **12**: 395–402.

Malec JF, Cicerone KD (2006). Cognitive rehabilitation. In Evans RW (ed.) *Neurology and Trauma* (2nd edn.) (pp. 238–261). New York: Oxford University Press.

Marciniak CM, Sliwa JA, Heinemann AW, Semik PE (2001). Functional outcomes of persons with brain tumors after inpatient rehabilitation. *Arch Phys Med Rehabil* **82**: 457–463.

Meyers CA, Boake C (1993). Neurobehavioral disorders in brain tumor patients: rehabilitation strategies. *Cancer Bull* **45**: 362–364.

Millis S, Johnston M (eds.) (2003). Clinical trials in medical rehabilitation: enhancing rigor and relevance. *Am J Phys Med Rehabil* **82** [Suppl. 1].

Movsas SB, Chang VT, Tunkel RS, Vipul SV, Ryan LS, Millis SR (2003). Rehabilitation needs of an inpatient medical oncology unit. *Arch Phys Med Rehabil* **84**: 1642–1646.

Nezu AM, Nezu CM, Friedman SH, Faddis S, Houts PS (1998). *Helping Cancer Patients Cope*. Washington DC: American Psychological Association.

Nezu AM, Nezu CM, Felgoise SH, McClure KS, Houts PS (2003). Project genesis: assessing the efficacy of problem solving therapy for distressed adult cancer patients. *J Consult Clin Psychol* **71**: 1036–1048.

NIH Consensus Statement Online 1998 October 26–28. Rehabilitation of Persons With Traumatic Brain Injury. NIH Consensus Statement 1998 Oct 26–28; **16**(1): 1–41.

O'Dell MW, Barr K, Spanier D, Warnick RE (1998). Functional outcome of inpatient rehabilitation in persons with brain tumors. *Arch Phys Med Rehabil* **79**: 1530–1534.

Ownsworth TL, McFarland K (1999). Memory remediation in long-term acquired brain injury: two approaches in diary training. *Brain Injury* **13**: 605–626.

Ownsworth TL, McFarland K, Young RM (2000). Self-awareness and psychosocial functioning following acquired brain injury: an evaluation of a group support programme. *Neuropsychol Rehabil* **10**: 465–484.

Ronson A, Body JJ (2002). Psychosocial rehabilitation of cancer patients after curative therapy. *Support Care Cancer* **10**: 281–291.

Sherer M, Meyers CA, Bergloff P (1997). Efficacy of post-acute brain injury rehabilitation for patients with primary malignant brain tumors. *Cancer* **80**: 250–257.

Sohlberg MM, Mateer CA (1989). Training use of compensatory memory books: a three stage behavioral approach. *J Clin Exp Neuropsychol* **11**: 871–891.

Sohlberg MM, McLaughlin KA, Pavese A, Heidrich A, Posner MI (2000). Evaluation of attention process training and brain injury education in persons with acquired brain injury. *J Clin Exp Neuropsychol* **22**: 656–676.

Sutor B, Rummans TA, Smith GE (2001). Management of behavioral disturbances in nursing home patients with dementia. *Mayo Clin Proc* **76**: 540–550.

Von Cramen DY, Mathes-Von Cramen MN (1991). Problem solving deficits in brain injured patients: a therapeutic approach. *Neuropsychol Rehabil* **1**: 45–64.

21

Support services

Bebe Guill and Renee H. Raynor

Introduction

Whether the primary treatment approach to cognitive impairment in cancer is remediation/rehabilitation, pharmacotherapy, or a combination, one must not underestimate the importance of comprehensive support services throughout the illness continuum.

Cognitive deficits related to cancer may be primary, related to the disease entity itself, or may be secondary, related to the various methods used to treat the cancer. Such deficits may also be related to direct and indirect co-morbidities of the cancer and treatments. Among the most common co-morbidities are mood disturbances (e.g., depression, anxiety) and fatigue. Fatigue is the most widely reported deleterious symptom in adult cancer patients (Valentine & Meyers, 2001). Additionally, in childhood cancer survivors, fatigue and "aches and pains" are reported as most problematic relative to other symptoms (Zebrack & Chesler, 2002). In this chapter, we will consider cognitive deficits, mood disturbances or emotional distress, and fatigue as highly inter-related symptoms of cancer and will discuss support services that may apply to one or more of these conditions in isolation or in combination.

Support has many definitions, but is generally understood as strengthening the patient's and family's resources by providing emotional, informational, and practical assistance as needed, and by appropriately fostering a sense of hope or optimism. Here, we refer to a wide range of strategies designed to improve emotional and social adjustment and functioning, increase coping, assist with decision-making, and minimize distress. Each individual patient's and family's need for support will be unique, and will depend on a number of factors, including the amount of stress present in the family prior to the illness, the amount of support available from friends and family, and the patient's emotional and medical response to treatment.

Effective support takes place in a variety of contexts and from a variety of sources – both formal and informal. Best support practices have been identified as those that ensure continuity of care, involve all members of the treatment team, and match support services to the unique needs of each patient and family at every phase of the illness continuum (Clinical Practice Guidelines in Oncology, 2008). Support services should be considered a vital component, not an optional extra, of care for persons with cancer.

Sensitivity to the various support needs of patients is the responsibility of all members of the interdisciplinary treatment team – not just those in the mental health fields. Physicians and nurses are important primary sources of support; however, successful management of the cancer patient's health care is best accomplished by a concerted

Cognition and Cancer, eds. Christina A. Meyers and James R. Perry. Published by Cambridge University Press.

interdisciplinary effort, extending far beyond the core medical team. This interdisciplinary team approach requires that team members not only have expertise in their respective disciplines, but must also be able to contribute to the group effort on behalf of the patient and the family.

Numerous studies have demonstrated the importance of effective support in improved quality of life for patients with cancer. The extent to which a person with cancer has support and feels supported has been identified as a major factor in adjustment to the disease. Support services such as psychological therapies have been shown to improve emotional adjustment and social functioning, and reduce both treatment- and disease-related distress in patients with cancer. The efficacy of both supportive and cognitive-behavioral therapies in the treatment of depressive disorders in cancer patients, both in individual and in group therapies, has also been demonstrated (Devine & Westlake, 1995; Sheard & Maguire, 1996, 1999). A meta-analysis of 116 intervention studies found that patients with cancer receiving psycho-educational or psychosocial interventions showed much lower rates of anxiety, depression, mood disorders, nausea, vomiting and pain, and significantly greater knowledge about disease and treatment, than the control group (Devine & Westlake, 1995).

Distinct needs for support for both patients and their families result from cognitive impairment related to cancer and its treatment. By understanding the importance and appropriate use of support services, health professionals can help to reduce patient and family distress, restore a sense of control to patients and caregivers, and improve health-related quality of life. In this chapter, we consider the use of needs assessment, goals for support services across the illness continuum, relevant contexts/settings, modalities for delivery of support services, and identification of appropriate resources.

Needs assessment

A high proportion of people with cancer may have unmet needs, despite expressing satisfaction with their care (Sanson-Fisher *et al.*, 2000). The primary oncology team of oncologist, nurse, and social worker should formally assess and regularly monitor the emotional, informational, and practical needs of patients with cancer and their families. For patients with cognitive impairment, it is essential to check the extent of support available to the patient and family, including ascertaining needs for assistance with practical issues such as transportation, childcare, work, or school, and exploring how the patient and family are coping with any issues related to cognition.

Taking the initiative in inquiring about residual symptoms and concerns is important for health care professionals. Indeed, studies have shown that many patients will not raise their concerns unless this is explicitly invited (Bertakis *et al.*, 1991; Maguire, 1999). In their study of untreated distress in cancer patients, Carlson *et al.* (2004) reported that approximately half of all patients who met distress criteria had not accessed psychosocial support services, despite being aware of their availability. When queried as to their reason for not seeking such services, 44.1% of these patients (who were characterized as distressed) reported a self-perception of not needing any help.

Two assessment tools have proved to be both clinically sensitive and easy to use for early identification of emotional and quality-of-life issues. The Beck Depression Inventory-II (BDI-II) is a 21-item inventory that conforms to the depression criteria of the *Diagnostic and Statistical Manual of Mental Health Disorders* (4th edn.) (DSM-IV). It is a widely used instrument for detecting depression in adults and adolescents and takes approximately 5 minutes to complete. The BDI-II has been demonstrated to be useful in screening for depression in cognitively impaired cancer patients in the clinical setting (Allen *et al.*, 2003). A second instrument, the National Comprehensive Cancer Network's Distress Thermometer and Problem List, uses a scale of 0–10 that can be completed quickly and consists of a list of problems that the patient reads, indicating possible reasons for the distress. Used in conjunction with clinical assessment by the primary oncology team, such tools can be a valuable means for evaluating depression, anxiety, and other quality-of-life symptoms in the clinical setting (NCCN Standards of Care for Distress Management, 2008) and represent a time- and cost-effective method for informing decisions about what support services will be most appropriate.

Being prepared to make recommendations about support services and where these may be available is also important (Ell *et al.*, 1989). Patients frequently request information from their primary oncology team about support and educational services. Matthews *et al.* (2004) surveyed a large multidisciplinary sample of oncology health care professionals and learned that 94% of them had been asked about at least one cancer-related support service by their patients. Of the referrals sought by patients in this study, 72% of inquiries were related to information and education about cancer, 65% were about support groups, and 52% were about hospice referrals. Licensed mental health professionals and certified pastoral caregivers experienced in psychosocial aspects of cancer and cognitive impairment should be readily available as staff members or by referral (Zebrack & Chesler, 2002).

Support needs across the disease continuum

Support needs and targeted outcomes of services will vary depending upon the patient's stage of illness/recovery, type of treatment, and the degree of cognitive deficits experienced. Services should address primary cognitive deficits, psychological/psychiatric distress related to the disease and/or the cognitive deficits, and coping/adjustment challenges related to the losses/changes in the patient's life.

Newly diagnosed/pre-treatment

The newly diagnosed patient may still be in "shock" at the diagnosis of cancer, in denial that they are having cognitive symptoms, or relieved to have an "explanation" for their symptoms. He or she may have cognitive deficits due to the cancer itself, surgical interventions, medications, early radiation/chemotherapy treatment or associated psychological distress related to fear of treatment or death. Psycho-education has been shown to be the most appropriate modality of support in the early stage of the disease, just after diagnosis and pretreatment, when the patient's need for information appears to be at its highest (Carlson *et al.*, 2004).

Additional needs for intervention in this early phase may involve supportive psychotherapy to help cope with diagnosis, to prepare the patient for the treatment road ahead, and/or to begin to process the many changes that the diagnosis and treatment will bring. They may already have appreciable cognitive deficits for which they would benefit from early cognitive rehabilitation, occupational therapy, speech therapy, and/or physical therapy. Emotional lability may be high as a result of situational stress or due to metabolic or medication-related psychiatric symptoms. This sense of emotional upheaval can leave a patient feeling out of control and desperate. Proposing a rehabilitative approach for acutely post-operative brain tumor patients, Gabanelli (2005) points out that, in some cases, medical staff members are not familiar with the common cognitive and emotional sequelae of cancer and may misinterpret psychological distress as evidence of mental deterioration. Such a reaction may leave the patient feeling shamed or patronized.

The newly diagnosed patient may benefit from early exposure to support groups to gain support and insight from fellow patients. Consultation and guidance with a spiritual or religious advisor may provide additional help and perspective. Additionally, the patient may seek out complementary and alternative therapies to treat not only the cancer, but also its associated impacts on quality of life. Goals for support may include crisis intervention, stabilization of the patient's mood, mobilizing support resources including family, friends, and appropriate referrals, and addressing practical concerns such as lodging, childcare, or navigating the challenges of insurance and financial concerns.

Active treatment

During the treatment for cancer, the patient may experience fatigue and cognitive deficits as a result of radiation therapy, chemotherapy, hormonal therapies, or adjuvant medications. This may be the first time the patient realizes the systemic impact of cancer treatment. Cumulative effects of months of therapy may make deficits more pronounced or intolerable. Prolonged changes in cognition, mood, or behavior need to be evaluated and treated.

Rehabilitation services can be critically important for maintaining maximum functioning during the treatment phase for cancer patients. Historically, cancer patients have not been referred to intensive rehabilitation centers because of concerns about reduced life expectancy, pain, and multiple medical complications (DeLisa, 2001). For patients with neurological injury (stroke, traumatic brain injury, or spinal cord injury) and patients with medically related debilitation, rehabilitation services have long been valued by patients and health professionals as the treatment of choice for optimizing function and independence. While cancer patients often have similar needs and capabilities to benefit from rehabilitative therapies, the anticancer treatment has many times remained the sole treatment focus (Cheville, 2001).

However, the benefits of rehabilitation services for cancer patients have been demonstrated in multiple large-scale, well-designed studies. DeLisa (2001) reviewed relevant literature and concluded that there was both a pressing need for rehabilitation in cancer patients and convincing evidence of the value it may have in their functional status and quality of life. Garrard *et al.* (2004) reported on a sample of 21 patients with primary and non-primary central nervous system (CNS) malignancies who underwent inpatient rehabilitation. They found that these patients were responsive to rehabilitative interventions and showed functional improvement regardless of the type of malignancy.

In addition to deficits associated with treatment, many patients will struggle with emotional difficulties during the active phase of treatment. While

there may be a tendency to expect distress levels to reduce once a treatment plan has begun and the "shock" of the cancer diagnosis has passed, evidence suggests that many patients remain distressed throughout the treatment phase and into long-term follow-up. Carlson *et al.* (2004) reported that a significant percentage of a large heterogeneous cancer patient population reported clinically relevant levels of distress across the disease continuum. Symptoms may range from "situational" or "reactive" depression to major depression, a condition characterized by a constellation of signs and symptoms meeting criteria for clinical diagnosis according to accepted psychiatric standards. Angelino and Treisman (2001) refer to "situational" depression as demoralization and describe it as a normal psychological reaction to life stresses that may not imply brain pathology. They characterize major depression, with its impact on the patient's mood and self view, along with its anhedonia and neurovegetative symptoms, as a manifestation of organic brain dysfunction. They recommend antidepressant therapy for major depression in cancer patients and suggest the usefulness of psychotherapy in the treatment of demoralization. Best clinical practice in the management of depression suggests that a combination of psychotherapy and antidepressant drug therapy has shown better treatment outcomes than use of either modality alone (Sutherland *et al.*, 2003). In a meta-analysis of 45 randomized trials of cancer patients receiving psychological interventions, an average of 12% showed significant improvement in measures of emotional adjustment, 10% in social functioning, 14% in treatment- and disease-related symptoms, and 14% in overall quality of life, compared to patients not undergoing psychological therapies (Meyer & Mark, 1995). Goals for supportive therapy may include balancing hope with realistic expectations, addressing fear of recurrence and death, dealing with treatment burnout, and addressing the desire for normalcy.

Additionally, patients may struggle with identity and self-esteem concerns because of changes in their family role (e.g., no longer the breadwinner, no longer the caregiver). Family members and friends may need education on how to identify cognitive and/or mood changes and may need help adjusting and coping with these changes in their loved one.

Further needs for intervention during the active treatment phase may involve practical life concerns. For example, the patient may need assistance as he or she starts to realize that they may not be able to continue work/school during the treatment phase. Many patients have unrealistic expectations for recovery following diagnosis and early interventions and may need help recognizing and accepting that they may not return to work right away. In a recent examination of employment pathways in cancer patients, it was reported that 41% of males and 39% of females who were working at diagnosis stopped during cancer treatment (Short *et al.*, 2005). In a separate review examining return to work practices in cancer patients, Spelten *et al.* (2003) reported a median number of 278 days on sick leave at 12 months follow-up, with a range of 3–652 days. Fatigue levels predicted the return to work in this study.

It may be impossible for the patient to appreciate the large impact that fatigue will have on their functioning until they are well into active treatment. At that point, help in navigating the paperwork required to apply for disability may be required. Similarly, younger patients may need help arranging hospital-based or in-home schooling.

Further practical needs during the active treatment phase might involve assistance with the bureaucracy of health insurance companies, deciding and executing health care and legal powers of attorney, and managing the financial burden that extended cancer therapy invariably causes.

Post-treatment stable disease

In many ways, the end of active cancer treatment, with the outcome of stable disease or remission, is a joyous time. Patients may finally have hope of survival and may begin to return to pre-diagnosis activities. Many will begin to feel healthy again after months or years of aggressive and toxic cancer treatments. Rarely, however, does life after cancer return to pre-diagnosis "normal." Recognition that life may never be the same can be troubling for many patients and families.

Fatigue is an almost universal side-effect of cancer and its related treatment. In many cases, it persists well after treatment is discontinued (Valentine & Meyers, 2001). Disturbances in cognition and mood are frequently seen in post-treatment cancer patients, likely a result of aggressive systemic antineoplastic treatments aimed at combating the cancer, but which may also damage vulnerable CNS tissues (Meyers, 2000). A recent evaluation of 10-year survivors of childhood medulloblastoma showed significant impairment in cognitive abilities and psychosocial domains, including employment, driving, education, independent living, and dating (Maddrey *et al.*, 2005).

Patients may question why they still feel poorly or still have trouble with their thinking and functioning. They may struggle with loss of identity due to an inability to function in the same capacity as they did prior to the cancer diagnosis. Behavioral disturbances may start to wear on family members when treatment is over but the patient does not return to his or her baseline personality. As a result, caregivers and family members may struggle with the loss of their previous relationship with the patient and this may have implications for the future of family roles. The patient may not be able to return to work or may be unable to continue working because of cancer-related disability. Short *et al.* (2005) reported that approximately 13% of a large cohort of cancer survivors had stopped working because of reasons related to their cancer within 4 years of diagnosis. They also found that among survivors who went back to work during the first year, 11% quit due to cancer-related reasons in the next 3 years. Clearly, the impact of cancer on work and career is sometimes long-lasting.

Goals for supportive care during this phase in the cancer patient's life may involve education about the long-term cognitive effects of cancer and its treatments and providing support as the patient learns to adjust to his or her disability and seeks a new normal. The patient may need concrete help with disability or vocational rehabilitation issues. Caregivers may need support in accepting the patient's new post-cancer role and what that means for their future relationship. The goals for intervention may shift from rehabilitation to compensation and acceptance. Modalities for support services in this phase may include vocational rehabilitation services, cancer survivor support groups, and individual/family psychotherapy.

End of life/palliative care

The support needs of the cancer patient who is facing the end of life either because of treatment failure or a conscious decision to discontinue treatment are numerous. They may have physical needs to be addressed by medical intervention (e.g., pain, fatigue) and they may benefit from rehabilitation therapies (e.g., physical, occupational, and speech) to maximize their functioning and communication in the last portion of their life. They may also benefit from supportive psychotherapy, either in individual or group format, to process the many feelings associated with end-of-life issues. Spiritual and existential issues may become paramount to the individual in this stage of the disease continuum and provision of support in these areas of concern may be best provided by members of the clergy or by hospice staff.

Historically, when a patient enters this stage of his or her disease trajectory, interventions to preserve cognition and mood have been seen as superfluous or of lesser importance than the medical elements of comfort care (e.g., pain control). Garrard et al. (2004) make a convincing argument for combining the approaches of rehabilitation and palliation in the care of advanced cancer patients in order to maintain symptom management and to address psychosocial needs related to end of life, while also maximizing the patient's level of functioning during the remaining days of life. In an effort to maximize cognitive and physical functioning in cancer patients, especially those near the end of life, pharmacological interventions, such as the use of psychostimulants, have proven useful. Gagnon et al. (2005) showed improvement in cognitive and psychomotor activities in advanced cancer patients with hypoactive delirium after treatment with low doses of methylphenidate. Similarly, Rozans et al. (2002) found the use of methylphenidate beneficial in combating opioid-induced somnolence and in improving cognitive functioning in late-stage cancer patients.

Hospice agencies are the professional groups most often involved in providing care to patients and families at the end of life. Involvement of a hospice may begin soon after diagnosis or may be initiated later in the disease continuum, when treatment fails or when decisions are made regarding preserving quality of life instead of continuing potentially harsh, invasive anticancer therapies. There is sometimes resistance among patients or families to begin hospice care due to concerns that the patient will just be "waiting to die." On the contrary, the very foundation of hospice care is built on the desire to help patients live out their remaining life with as much vitality and dignity as is possible. Management of symptoms such as pain and mood disturbance is a specialty of hospice care. Hospice staff are dedicated to helping patients remain as alert, engaged, and communicative as possible at the end of life, so that they can have quality time with family and friends. In this regard, hospice staff, working in conjunction with and as an extension of the patient's primary treatment team, can assess and maximize the patient's cognitive abilities in order to provide optimum quality of life in the remaining days of life.

Support settings/contexts

Cancer survivors and their families face specific challenges as they re-negotiate roles and relationships that are necessary for successful integration back into school, work, family, and community settings. Effective support by the primary treatment team can promote optimal coping and adjustment during these transition periods.

Community re-entry/integration

At some point during or after successful cancer treatment, the patient may attempt to move back into their previous life roles. When there are significant changes in cognitive ability, the degree to which patients can realistically do so may be affected. The reactions of others to their different cognitive capabilities may be unexpected and can cause discomfort for the patient, their family, co-workers, friends, and acquaintances. It is vitally important that patients have support in determining if and how they should resume previously held roles. Appropriate support can uncover unrealistic expectations, manage anxiety, ease awkwardness, prevent embarrassment, and monitor progress. In the event that the transition is unsuccessful or incomplete, relevant support can identify appropriate modifications or help the patient begin to accept that the resumption of the previous role is not attainable.

School settings

During the early treatment period, the child with cancer may require some hospital and/or home-bound instruction. However, school attendance should be the goal as soon as the pediatric oncologist considers the child physically able to attend. The continuation of schooling provides the child with hope and stability, because attending school is what normally developing children do daily (Deasy-Spinetta & Spinetta, 1980).

It has been recommended that all pediatric oncology centers have a structured school re-entry program for students who have undergone treatment for cancer (Deasy-Spinetta & Spinetta, 1980). Communication with the student's teachers and counselors is paramount in such programs. One of the greatest dangers in not communicating with the patient's teachers is that if the child has subsequent struggles in the classroom, these can be falsely attributed to attitude problems, daydreaming, a lack of motivation, or emotional maladjustment (Butler & Mulhern, 2005). Components of school

re-entry programs should initially include educating the teachers and/or counselors about the cognitive effects associated with cancer and its treatment, and the specific signs, symptoms, and special needs associated with the patient's treatment and treatment outcome (Leigh & Miles, 2002). Additional components typically include educating the child's peers about cancer and its effects by means of age-appropriate didactic materials and class discussions, and by dispelling myths relating to the disease.

Ongoing liaison with the school at regular intervals is important for many reasons. First, the neuropsychological status of the child may not remain stable after treatment has been completed. The onset of some deficits is delayed and others are not evident until the ability is normally expected (Armstrong *et al.*, 1999). In addition, most children have multiple teachers who will change with each school year.

For the child with cognitive deficits, ongoing support requiring the attention of the interdisciplinary treatment team may include identifying an appropriate educational course (which may be different than what was expected or previously engaged in); negotiating in concert with parents and the school for special services and/or considerations for the child; and referral to specialists who can help the student develop strategies for coping in the educational environment.

Specialists such as pediatric psychologists, speech, occupational, and physical therapists, hospital social workers, and educational consultants and advocates may help the child in a variety of ways. These include: helping the child develop compensatory strategies to minimize effects of lowered energy levels and/or cognitive deficits; providing technological assistance and training; offering special education support; advocating for special needs within the educational system; or focusing on social skill development.

Special education services for children aged 3–21 years who attend public school and have a documented need are mandated (in the US) by the federal Individuals with Disabilities Education Act

(IDEA). Many children undergoing treatment for cancer as well as those who have completed treatment will be classified as "other health impaired" by their local school systems as a means of accessing resources for their special needs. The Individualized Education Plan (IEP) is a legal document that records the determination by school personnel, parents, and members of the health care team of what services the child needs and how those services will be provided. These services can include occupational therapy, physical therapy, speech therapy, a special teacher for visually impaired or hearing-impaired children, placement in a special education resource room for all or part of the school day, and/or an aide to assist the child. Classroom accommodations might include things such as oral tests, reduced workload, extra time for tests or other tasks, and the use of tape recorders or note takers.

The IDEA does not apply to colleges and universities, but other laws (for example, the Americans with Disabilities Act and the Rehabilitation Act of 1973) require these institutions to provide special services to students with disabilities, including cognitive impairment.

Work settings

Although many cancer survivors will return to work after their diagnosis, the rate of employment among survivors is lower than among people without a history of cancer. For working-age cancer survivors, interruption of employment and diminished capacity to work are serious consequences of cancer and treatment that can have economic, psychological, and social implications. Cognitive deficits, including difficulty concentrating, learning new things, analyzing data, and keeping up with the pace set by others (Bradley & Bednarek, 2002), are cited as reasons for reduced work effort and adverse economic outcomes (Chirikos *et al.*, 2002). Job discrimination, difficulties in obtaining work, and subsequent difficulties in obtaining health and life insurance have been reported in studies with childhood cancer survivors (Langeveld *et al.*, 2002).

Once the patient's range of ability and extent of cognitive deficits have been assessed, support should include a liaison with the workplace to ensure informed supervision and the on-site presence of a supervisor who knows how the consequences of cognitive impairment affect the worker's ability to perform duties successfully. Modifications of the job responsibilities, such as alternative work schedules or job restructuring, may also be required. A neuropsychological evaluation can be helpful in making these determinations about abilities and in assisting the employer to identify and implement possible job role modifications to accommodate their employee. On-the-job behavioral counseling by a job coach and education of co-workers are also recommended. Practical issues, such as transportation to and from the workplace (if driving is an issue), should also be addressed. The benefit of support is strongest when combined with supported employment involving a job coach, an interdisciplinary team, and appropriate on- and off-site support (Hall & Cope, 1995).

Family settings

The experience of cancer and cognitive impairment affects not only the patient but also the family (Blueglass, 1991). Research with adult cancer survivors and their families suggests that families are vulnerable to distress in the patient (Compas *et al.*, 1994; Nijboer *et al.*, 2000; Welch *et al.*, 1996; Ybema *et al.*, 2001), that children of patients with cancer may be in particular need of support, and that distress levels of partners of cancer patients may be considerable, sometimes even higher than that of the patients themselves, but they receive less support (Baider & Denour, 1999; Cliff & McDonagh, 2000; Northouse *et al.*, 2000). One study reports that approximately 20%–30% of spouses of cancer patients suffer from psychological impairment and mood disturbance (Blanchard *et al.*, 1997). In addition to increased symptoms of depression, anxiety, and psychosomatic symptoms, research suggests that family caregivers experience restriction of roles and activities, strain in marital relationships, severe sleep problems, and diminished physical health (Carter & Chang, 2000; Johnson, 1988; Northouse, 1988; Oberst et al., 1989). In their study comparing the familial impact of mental illness (including dementia) to other common chronic conditions (including cancer), Holmes and Deb (2003) found that brain-related conditions impose the most significant risk to the psychological well-being of family members.

Caregivers' depression and perceived burden, including financial burden, have been shown to increase as patients' functional status declines (Covinsky, 1994). Alternatively, economic distress not only directly increases the chance that family members will experience emotional distress, but it also appears to reduce the family's ability as a whole to cope psychologically with chronic illness (Holmes & Deb, 2003). Therefore, the family's ability to provide needed care for the patient may be impaired (Cassileth et al., 1985; Given et al., 1993; Nijboer et al., 1999).

Studies of childhood cancer survivors have examined many salient issues, including cognition, social functioning, and post-traumatic stress syndrome. Residual effects of the disease and its treatment, coupled with the potential for newly emerging late effects over time and/or disease recurrence, may continue to be a source of stress not only for the patient but also for the family. Since parents serve as the primary caregivers and decision-makers for their children, parental adaptation to the cancer experience will almost certainly have an impact on the cancer patient's adjustment and quality of life, as well as those of any other siblings or family members. Many families, in fact, report that they never return to where their family was before diagnosis, but instead are forced to find a new "normal" (Van Dongen-Melman et al., 1995). Recognizing that the consequences of chronic or life-threatening illness in childhood concern not only the child, but also the family (Kazak et al., 1997), investigators have begun to focus attention on the impact on parents.

The body of research on parents of childhood cancer survivors has, to date, focused almost exclusively on psychosocial adjustment, and has yielded both limited and conflicting results. Some studies suggest that parents of survivors show adequate levels of adjustment (Frank et al., 2001), while others argue that parents of childhood cancer survivors show high rates of continued distress (Sloper, 2000; Van Dongen-Melman et al., 1995). Studies of parent adjustment and stress have identified such areas as grief, uncertainty, and the experience of post-traumatic stress disorder as being important (Bonner et al., 2006; Brown et al., 2003; Kazak et al., 1997, 2004; Stewart & Mishel, 2000; Van Dongen-Melman et al., 1995, 1998). Other data have suggested that parental stress and distress are ongoing, often lasting well beyond the cancer survivor's childhood and continuing into adulthood (Ressler et al., 2003; Svavarsdottir, 2005).

The ongoing feelings of stress and distress that parents of childhood cancer survivors experience many years after treatment make them a critical group to assist. Indeed, as Butler and Mulhern (2005) have observed, "the family environment might be of equal or greater importance in the treatment and recovery of a chronic life-threatening disease compared with an acute event such as a traumatic brain injury."

Care and support for the family caregiver in conjunction with treatment of the patient has been increasingly acknowledged as essential (Svavarsdottir, 2005). Clinicians are advised that they should not assume that the family is able to offer the patient the support they need and should routinely assess and monitor the support needs of all members of the patient's family. Providers should be especially watchful when their patients with cognitive deficits come from families with limited financial resources and inadequate insurance coverage.

Modalities of support

The delivery of support services to cancer patients may be through any number of modalities, depending upon the nature of the support, the point along the disease continuum at which the support is provided, and the preference/learning style of the patient or caregiver receiving the services. Support services may be provided by any member of an interdisciplinary cancer treatment team, by specialists (e.g., rehabilitation professionals, mental health professionals, complementary and alternative healers) or by members of the community (e.g., family, friends, faith groups, peers). Frequently, in the treatment of cancer patients, the initial support is provided by members of hospitals/medical institutions; as the patient is further along in their treatment/recovery, the emphasis may shift more toward a family and community focus. Ideally, supportive care is provided to patients and families in this manner with a smooth transition back and forth between the various members of these support teams as conditions and needs for support change along the disease trajectory (see Table 21.1). This section addresses psychosocial, rehabilitative, and complementary/alternative modalities.

Psychosocial support

Many studies have shown that psychosocial interventions can have a positive impact on the psychological distress experienced in cancer patients. A meta-analysis of controlled outcome studies demonstrated that psychosocial interventions have a positive impact on quality of life in adult cancer patients and that many different forms of intervention are beneficial (Rehse & Pukrop, 2003). Interestingly, the study found that even more than the specific format of the psychosocial intervention, the duration of the intervention emerged as the most relevant variable. Some of the more common formats are individual psychotherapy or counseling, support groups (professionally facilitated or peer led), and psycho-educational activities. The type of psychosocial intervention selected must be made based on available resources, patient preference, and the nature of the psychosocial stressors being targeted by treatment.

Individual psychotherapy
In one randomized trial, cancer patients with relatively high levels of symptom severity scores who participated in a cognitive-behavioral psychother-

apy intervention experienced a reduction in symptom severity scores as compared to patients receiving conventional care alone (Given et al., 2004). In patients participating in a short course of cancer counseling sessions with a humanist framework, participants reported that the program was helpful in expressing feelings, examining and understanding emotional responses, confronting the fear of death, and working through powerful thoughts and feelings (Boulton et al., 2001). Patients in this program reported overwhelmingly positive attitudes about being in counseling, despite the sometimes difficult subject matter and intense emotions they were asked to consider. The benefits of individual psychotherapy for cancer patients were further evidenced in a European study evaluating the efficacy of short-term face-to-face counseling in self-referred cancer patients (Boudioni et al., 2000). The great majority of patients (>90%) who returned the evaluation of this service reported that their emotional health was better at the end of the counseling sessions. Almost all of the reporting participants expressed a positive view of the service, with more than 95% of them stating that they would return for further counseling if they needed help in the future and would recommend the counseling services to others.

Support groups
In their groundbreaking 1981 study, Spiegel et al. (1981) reported that a group of women with breast cancer, attending a weekly support group, had lower mood disturbance scores, fewer maladaptive coping responses, and lower phobia scores. This was one of the first empirical studies that revealed strong evidence for the benefit of support groups in providing psychological benefit. While there may be multiple benefits for cancer patients sharing their experiences with other patients in similar circumstances, one concept is that the presence of peer support may help to reduce the stigma associated with the diagnosis of cancer and may help to overcome social isolation (Weis, 2003). In their review of several studies on cancer peer support groups, Campbell et al. (2004) found consistent and positive

Table 21.1. Modalities of support across the disease continuum

Modality	Professional staff	Stage of disease	Example goals

Psychosocial support
–Individual
  psychotherapy
–Couples/family
  therapy
–Group therapy
–Support groups
	Neuropsychologist
	Social Worker
	Psychiatrist
	Support Group Leader
	Chaplain
	Pastoral Care Specialist
		Newly diagnosed
		
		Active treatment
		
		Post-treatment –
		  stable
		End of life/palliative
			Coping with "shock" of
			  diagnosis; crisis
			  management
			Dealing with rigors of
			  treatment; adjusting to
			  changes in life
			Learning to live with late
			  effects of treatment
			Death and dying issues;
			  existential concerns

Rehabilitation
–Inpatient unit
–Outpatient center
–Home health
	Physiatrist
	Neuropsychologist
	Physical Therapist
	Occupational Therapist
	Speech Therapist
	Recreational Therapist
	Social Worker
		Newly diagnosed
		
		Active treatment
		
		Post-treatment –
		  stable
		
		End of life/palliative
			Post-operative
			  physical/cognitive
			  deficits
			Managing fatigue;
			  symptom management;
			  cognitive rehabilitation
			Recovery from treatment;
			  facing long-term effects
			  of treatment
			Maximizing/preserving
			  functioning (e.g., treating
			  hypoactive delirium);
			  transitioning to hospice

Community integration
–Work/school
–Family
–Social/recreation
	Voc Rehab specialists
	Education specialists
	Neuropsychologist
	Community members
	Clergy or religious leaders
		Newly diagnosed
		
		Active treatment
		
		Post-treatment –
		  stable
		
		End of life/palliative
			Arranging for short-term
			  disability/sick leave
			Setting up long-term
			  disability or managing
			  symptoms at work
			Returning to work/school;
			  resuming social life;
			  renegotiating family roles
			Preparing for death; final
			  arrangements/legal
			  planning; saying goodbye

benefits from peer support, regardless of the specific manner in which it was delivered and irrespective of the theoretical model on which it was based. Each individual participating in a support group may take away different benefits from the experience, including varying levels of practical information, emotional support, sense of community, and feelings of altruism. Support groups are a very efficient method of providing individualized support services to a number of cancer patients at one time and in an environment that feels safe, friendly, and less intimidating than might individual face-to-face counseling sessions.

Online support groups

The appeal of online cancer support groups is understandable. Online support avoids some of the barriers of traditional support groups, such as inconvenient meeting times, lack of meeting places, and medical complications that make travel to a meeting site challenging. Indeed, there has been a large increase in recent years with respect to the number of cancer support groups that are held exclusively online. In their review of the relevant, but fairly scant, outcome literature on online support groups, Klemm *et al.* (2003) found that most of the studies were small in sample size and were overly homogeneous with respect to gender and disease site. Nonetheless, the authors report that their review of the available literature did seem to suggest a benefit from online support groups for patients with cancer. They found that participants in these studies used the forum primarily to gather information and to give and receive emotional support. Interestingly, the authors did not find that computer inexperience was a barrier to successful use of online groups.

Psycho-educational approaches

Psycho-educational programs have both psychological and educational components. Such programs aim to enhance understanding and knowledge about cancer and associated issues, including symptom management, psychosocial support, and resource identification. Psycho-educational programs have been shown to be effective in increasing knowledge and self-confidence (Braden *et al.*, 1998) and in decreasing depression and anxiety (Johnson, 1982).

Rehabilitation programs

Comprehensive rehabilitation programs for multiple advanced disease populations (e.g., stroke, traumatic brain injury, spinal cord injury) have been in existence for years. Few would argue the benefits of these programs in helping patients to achieve the highest functional status possible, given the limitations created by the disease. These multidisciplinary programs focus on the treatment and management of medical symptoms and complications (physiatrist), improving mobility and level of independence (physical and occupational therapists), enhancing communication (speech language pathologists), improving cognitive functioning (neuropsychologists), and expanding social activities and outlets (recreational therapists). Many participants in such programs make remarkable gains in abilities and achieve levels of increased autonomy and satisfaction that would not be possible without this time- and energy-intensive, formalized approach to restoring impaired patients to the highest level of functioning attainable. See Chapter 20 for an indepth discussion of rehabilitation techniques.

Even though the same principles for rehabilitation as applied to these aforementioned medical populations are appropriate for cancer patients, and even though aggressive cancer therapies have increased survival rates while causing corresponding increases in debilitation, very little attention has been given to rehabilitation of the cancer patient (Cheville, 2001; Kirshblum *et al.*, 2001). Often-cited reasons for not referring cancer patients to rehabilitation programs are life expectancy, pain, and medical co-morbidities. Yet, as Cheville (2001) points out, significant infirmity and poor prognosis for disease improvement in cancer patients should be distinguished from the possibility of improvement in functional abilities. DeLisa (2001) maintains, "rehabilitation for patients with cancer should be no different from rehabilitation for those of other diagnostic conditions, such as cerebrovascular disease, spinal cord injury, or brain injury." Many rehabilitation strategies used in other patient populations have been successful in improving functional status in cancer patients. These include rehabilitation of motor deficits, sensory deficits, cerebellar dysfunction, and deconditioning (Cheville, 2001).

Clinical pathways to cognitive remediation of patients with stroke and brain injury are well documented, but have only recently started to be applied to cancer patients to improve functioning related to deficits due to both neurotoxicity of antineoplastic agents/treatments and direct central nervous system malignancies. Rehabilitation of cognitive deficits related to cancer and cancer treatment can follow the same model that is used with other neurorehabilitative programs where both restorative and compensatory strategies are employed. Restorative efforts attempt to improve the impaired function, whereas compensatory training helps the patient learn to "work around" the deficient area of functioning. Attentional deficits may be improved by helping patients learn to manage distractions and control their environment as much as possible. Memory difficulties may be compensated for by using a memory notebook or by rehearsal and overlearning strategies. Executive dysfunction may be addressed by teaching patients to superimpose organized structure onto tasks and by repetitively stressing the practice of breaking tasks down into their simplest component steps. Communication may be enhanced by using deliberative speech practices and by learning alternative ways to communicate for profoundly aphasic patients (e.g., message boards, gesturing).

The efficacy of comprehensive rehabilitation services for cognitive deficits in cancer patients can be best illustrated by the results of several studies in brain tumor patients. Sherer et al. (1997) demonstrated that six patients with primary malignant brain tumors undergoing an inpatient rehabilitation program showed evidence of increased independence during the time from the start of participation to discharge. In another study with a larger sample size of 40, daily gains in functional abilities in brain tumor patients completing an inpatient rehabilitation program were similar to those made by trau-matic brain injury patients matched by age, gender, and baseline functional status (O'Dell et al., 1998). Interestingly, the length of stay for the brain tumor patients in this study was on average shorter than that for the traumatic brain injury patients. Finally, Marciniak et al. (2001) found that the functional gains made by brain tumor patients in an inpatient rehabilitation program did not differ according to whether the tumor was primary or metastatic. A more important finding from this study was that patients receiving concurrent radiation therapy during the course of rehabilitation made greater functional gains than did those patients not receiving radiation therapy. This result has implications for health care providers who might avoid sending cancer patients to intensive rehabilitation programs for fear that concurrent antineoplastic therapies might make them less amenable to rehabilitation gains.

Complementary and alternative approaches

Interest in complementary and alternative medicine has grown tremendously in recent years; cancer patients in particular have been drawn to unconventional treatments in higher and higher numbers (Ernst & Cassileth, 1998). In a recent study, Bernstein and Grasso (2001) determined that 80% of adult cancer patients in a private non-profit South Florida hospital used some form of complementary and alternative medicine treatment, including vitamins, herbal products, relaxation techniques, massages, and home remedies. In their 2004 evaluation of a complementary and alternative medicine program at the Stanford Center for Integrative Medicine, Rosenbaum et al. (2004) found that over 90% of the patients in the program reported benefit from its services. Those services with the most participants in the program were massage, yoga, and qigong. Other unconventional methods for treating the medical complications and psychological distress that accompany cancer are gaining favor and showing efficacy. In a randomized controlled trial employing a mindfulness-based stress reduction program in cancer outpatients, participants showed a significant reduction in mood disturbances and stress (Speca et al., 2000).

As depression, anxiety, and fatigue are known to impair cognitive functioning, it is reasonable to expect that complementary and alternative medicine therapies that are associated with stress reduction, improved mood, and reduction in fatigue levels may indirectly result in stronger cognitive abilities. Such interventions might include massage, deep muscle relaxation, guided visual imagery, mindfulness, meditation, hypnosis, biofeedback, yoga, reflexology, and qigong. These therapies are most effectively used in combination with conventional therapies for emotional distress and fatigue, such as psychotherapy, antidepressants/anxiolytics, activity-rest cycles, sleep hygiene models, and hematopoietic agents.

Complementary and alternative medicine therapies have gained popularity in the prevention and treatment of dementia. Approaches to preserving or enhancing cognitive functioning, or to minimizing associated functional decline were recently reviewed in an article by Sierpina *et al.* (2005). The authors grouped these complementary and alternative medicine approaches into three categories: (1) mind/body therapies (relaxation, meditation, guided imagery, hypnosis, biofeedback, cognitive-behavioral therapies, and psycho-educational approaches); (2) lifestyle changes/social support (environment, recreation/education, creative expression, music); and (3) nutrients/botanicals (acetylcholinesterase inhibitors, acetylcholine precursors, antioxidants, anti-inflammatory agents, hormonal agents). The authors conclude that mind/body therapies and lifestyle changes/social supports are extremely safe interventions that may show promise in minimizing the negative impact of cognitive decline on quality of life, although they acknowledge that further controlled studies on outcome and efficacy are needed. With respect to nutritional and herbal therapies, they suggest promising links between use of some complementary and alternative medicine agents and improved cognitive functioning in dementia patients, but emphasize that few of these findings are yet supported by empirical evidence. It is of utmost importance that patients discuss the potential use of complementary and alternative medicine agents with all members of their treatment team in order to avoid any drug–herbal interactions or any possible interference in the efficacy of the primary antineoplastic therapies.

The bottom line regarding the role of complementary and alternative medicine therapies in the treatment of cancer-related cognitive deficits is that while many of these approaches may show promise, their empirical efficacy, and, in some cases, their safety in cancer patients are not fully understood and need to be further investigated. It is imperative that medical professionals working with cancer patients be educated and aware of complementary and alternative medicine approaches and prepared to counsel their patients on the risks and benefits of these treatments in the management of cancer and its symptoms: physical, psychological, and cognitive. It is clear from some emerging literature that many of these unconventional approaches are safe and effective in improving cancer patients' quality of life.

ACKNOWLEDGMENTS

The authors wish to thank the following individuals in The Preston Robert Tisch Brain Tumor Center at Duke University Medical Center for their assistance in researching and editing this book chapter:.

Bart Brigidi, Ph.D,
   Assistant Research Professor
Lisa Fornnarino
   Neuropsychological Technician
Pam Clair
   Staff Assistant
Karen Carter
   Clinical Research Associate
Stephen T. Keir, MPH, DrPH
   Assistant Clinical Research Professor
   Quality of Life Research Program

RESOURCES

www.cancer.gov   (National Cancer Institute)
www.cancer.org   (American Cancer Society)
www.cancercare.org (sponsors teleconferences, web-based conferences, has free social work services, etc.)
www.canceradvocacy.org   (National Coalition for Cancer Survivorship)

www.cancersupportivecare.com (dedicated to improving quality of life and reducing morbidity in cancer patients)

http://nccam.nih.gov (National Center for Complementary and Alternative Medicine)

www.ed.gov (Rehabilitation Services Administration)

www.disabilityresources.org (vocational rehabilitation resources)

www.hospicefoundation.org (end of life information and hospice locator guide)

www.chionline.org (information on hospice care specific to pediatric patients)

www.biausa.org (Brain Injury Association of America)

www.epilepsyfoundation.org (information on seizures and disability discrimination policies)

www.candlelighters.org (Candlelighters Childhood Cancer Foundation)

www.acor.org (Association of Cancer Online Resources, Inc. – includes listings of internet support groups)

www.oncolink.upenn.edu (Oncolink)

www.patientcenters.com (Comprehensive listing of resources including first person patient experiences)

www.nichcy.org (National Dissemination Center for Children with Disabilities)

www.livestrong.org (Lance Armstrong Foundation – information and support for survivors)

REFERENCES

Allen DH, Tepper S, Carter K et al. (2003). Use of Beck Depression Inventory II: evaluating quality of life symptoms in glioma patients [Abstract] Society for Neuro-Oncology Eighth Annual Meeting, 13–16 November, 2003. Keystone, Colorado. *Neurooncology* 5: 329.

Angelino AF, Treisman GJ (2001). Major depression and demoralization in cancer patients: diagnostic and treatment considerations. *Support Care Cancer* 9(5): 344–349.

Armstrong FD, Blumberg MJ et al. (1999). Neurobehavioral issues in childhood cancer. *School Psychol Rev* 28: 194–203.

Baider L, Denour AK (1999). Psychological distress and cancer couples: a leveling effect. *New Trends Exp Clin Psychiatry* 15: 197–203.

Bernstein BJ, Grasso T (2001). Prevalence of complementary and alternative medicine use in cancer patients. *Oncology (Huntington)* 15 (10): 1267– 1272; discussion 1272–1278, 1283.

Bertakis KD, Roter D, Putnam SM (1991). The relationship of physician medical interview style to patient satisfaction. *J Fam Pract* 32(2): 175–81.

Blanchard CG, Albrecht TL, Ruckdeschel JC (1997). The crisis of cancer: psychological impact on family caregivers. *Oncology* 11: 189–194.

Blueglass K (1991). Care of the cancer patient's family. In Watson M (ed.) *Cancer Patient Care: Psychosocial Treatment Methods* (pp. 159–189) Cambridge: British Psychological Society and Cambridge University Press.

Bonner MJ, Hardy KK et al. (2006). Development and validation of the parent experience of illness (PECI) questionnaire. *J Pediatr Psychol* 31: 310–321.

Boudioni M, Mossman J et al. (2000). An evaluation of a cancer counselling service. *Eur J Cancer Care* 9: 212–220.

Boulton M, Boudioni M et al. (2001). "Dividing the desolation": clients views on the benefits of a cancer counselling service. *Psychooncology* 10: 124–136.

Braden CJ, Mishel MH et al. (1998). Self-help intervention project: women receiving breast cancer treatment. *Cancer Pract* 6(2): 87–98.

Bradley CH, Bednarek HL (2002). Employment patterns of long-term cancer survivors. *Psychooncology* 11: 188–198.

Brown RT, Madan-Swain A et al. (2003). Posttraumatic stress symptoms in adolescent survivors of childhood cancer and their mothers. *J Trauma Stress* 16: 309–318.

Butler RW, Mulhern RK (2005). Neurocognitive interventions for children and adolescents surviving cancer. *J Pediatr Psychol* 30(1): 65–78.

Campbell H, Phaneuf M et al. (2004). Cancer peer support programs – do they work? *Patient Educ Counsel* 55: 3–15.

Carlson LE, Angen M, Cullum J et al. (2004). High levels of untreated distress and fatigue in cancer patients. *Br J Cancer* 90(12): 2297–2304.

Carter PA, Chang BL (2000). Sleep and depression in cancer caregivers. *Cancer Nurs* 23: 410–415.

Cassileth BR, Lusk EJ et al. (1985). A psychological analysis of cancer patients and their next-of-kin. *Cancer* 55: 72–76.

Cheville A (2001). Rehabilitation of patients with advanced cancer. Rehabilitation in the New Millennium. *Cancer* 92 [4 Suppl.]: 1039–1048.

Chirikos TN, Russell-Jacobs A et al. (2002). Functional impairment and the economic consequences of female breast cancer. *Women Health* 36(1): 1–20.

Cliff AM, McDonagh RP (2000). Psychosocial morbidity in prostate cancer II; a comparison of patients and partners. *Br J Urol Int* 86: 834–839.

Clinical Practice Guidelines in Oncology. Version 1.205 Available at: http://www.nccn.org. Accessed 11 April, 2008.

Compas BE, Worsham NL *et al.* (1994). When mom or dad has cancer: markers of psychological distress in cancer patients, spouses, and children. *Health Psychol* **13**: 507–515.

Covinsky KE (1994). The impact of serious illness on patients' families. SUPPORT investigators study to understand prognoses and preferences for outcomes and risks of treatment. *J Am Med Assoc* **272**(23): 1839–1844.

Deasy-Spinetta P, Spinetta JJ (1980). The child with cancer in school: teacher's appraisal. *Am J Pediatr Hematol Oncol* **2**: 89.

DeLisa JA (2001). A history of cancer rehabilitation. Cancer Rehabilitation in the New Millennium. *Cancer* **92** [4 Suppl.]: 970–974.

Devine EC, Westlake SK (1995). The effects of psychoeducational care provided to adults with cancer: meta-analysis of 116 studies. *Oncol Nurs Forum* **22**(9): 1369–1381.

Ell KO, Mantell JE, Hamovitch MB, Nishomoto RH (1989). Social support, sense of control, and coping among patients with breast, lung, or colorectal cancer. *J Psychosocial Oncol* **7**: 63–89.

Ernst E, Cassileth BR (1998). The prevalence of complementary/alternative medicine in cancer: a systematic review. *Cancer* **83**(4): 777–782.

Frank NC, Brown RT *et al.* (2001). Predictors of affective responses of mothers and fathers of children with cancer. *Psychooncology* **10**: 293–304.

Gabanelli P (2005). A rehabilitative approach to the patient with brain cancer. *Neurol Sci* **26**: S51–S52.

Gagnon B, Low G, Schreier G (2005). Methylphenidate hydrochloride improves cognitive function in patients with advanced cancer and hypoactive delirium: a prospective clinical study. *J Psychiatry Neurosci* **30**(2): 100–107.

Garrard P, Farnham C, Thompson AJ, Playford ED (2004). Rehabilitation of the cancer patient: experience in a neurological unit. *Neurorehabil Neural Repair* **18**(2): 76–79.

Given CW, Stommel M *et al.* (1993). The influence of cancer patients' symptoms and functional states on patients' depression and family caregivers' reaction and depression. *Health Psychol* **12**: 277–285.

Given C, Given B *et al.* (2004). Effect of a cognitive behavioral intervention on reducing symptom severity during chemotherapy. *J Clin Oncol* **22**(3): 507–516.

Hall IM, Cope DN (1995). The benefit of rehabilitation in traumatic brain injury: a literature review. *J Head Trauma Rehabil* **10**: 1–13.

Holmes AM, Deb P (2003). The effect of chronic illness on the psychological health of family members. *J Mental Health Policy Econ* **6**(1): 13–22.

Johnson J (1982). The effect of a patient education course on persons with a chronic illness. *Cancer Nurs* **5**(2): 117–123.

Johnson J (1988). Cancer: a family disruption. *Recent Results Cancer Res* **108**: 306–310.

Kazak AE, Barakat LP *et al.* (1997). Posttraumatic stress, family functioning, and social support in survivors of childhood leukemia and their mothers and fathers. *J Consult Clin Psychol* **65**: 120–129.

Kazak AE, Alderfer M *et al.* (2004). Posttraumatic stress disorder (PTSD) and posttraumatic stress symptoms (PTSS) in families of adolescent childhood cancer survivors. *J Pediatr Psychol* **29**: 211–219.

Kirshblum S, O'Dell M *et al.* (2001). Rehabilitation of persons with central nervous system tumors. *Cancer Suppl* **92**(4): 1029–1038.

Klemm P, Bunnell D *et al.* (2003). Online cancer support groups: a review of the research literature. *Computers Infomatics Nursing* **21**(3): 136–142.

Langeveld NE, Stam H *et al.* (2002). Quality of life in young adult survivors of childhood cancer. *Support Care Cancer* **10**(8): 579–600.

Leigh LD, Miles MA (2002). Educational issues for children with cancer. In Pizzo PA, Poplack DG (eds.) *Principles and Practice of Pediatric Oncology* (pp. 1463–1476). Philadelphia, PA: Lippincott Williams & Wilkins.

Maddrey AM, Bergeron JA, Lombardo ER (2005). Neuropsychological performance and quality of life of 10 year survivors of childhood medulloblastoma. *J Neurooncol* **72**(3): 245–253.

Maguire P (1999). Improving communication with cancer patients. *Eur J Cancer* **35**: 1415–1422.

Marciniak C, Sliwa J *et al.* (2001). Functional outcomes of persons with brain tumors after inpatient rehabilitation. *Arch Phys Med Rehabil* **82**: 457–463.

Matthews B, Baker F, Spillers RL (2004). Oncology professionals and patient requests for cancer support services. *Support Care Cancer* **12**(10): 731–738.

Meyer TJ, Mark MM (1995). Effects of psychosocial interventions with adult cancer patients: a meta-analysis of randomized experiments. *Health Psychol* **14**(2): 101–108.

Meyers CA (2000). Neurocognitive dysfunction in cancer patients. *Oncology* **14**(1): 75–85.

NCCN Standards of Care for Distress Management, DIS-3. Version 1.205 Available at: http://www.nccn.org. Accessed 9 April, 2008.

Nijboer C, Triemstra M *et al.* (1999). Determinate of caregiving experiences and mental health of partners of cancer patients. *Cancer* **86**: 577–588.

Nijboer C, Gtriemstra M *et al.* (2000). Patterns of caregiver experiences among partners of cancer patients. *Gerontologist* **40**: 738–746.

Northouse LL (1988). Social support in patients' and husbands' adjustment to breast cancer. *Nurs Res* **37**: 91–95.

Northouse LL *et al.* (2000). Couples' patterns of adjustment to colon cancer. *Soc Sci Med* **50**: 271–284.

Oberst MT, Thomas SE *et al.* (1989). Caregiving demands and appraisal of stress among family caregivers. *Cancer Nurs* **12**: 209–215.

O'Dell M, Barr K *et al.* (1998). Functional outcome of inpatient rehabilitation in persons with brain tumors. *Arch Phys Med Rehabil* **79**: 1530–1534.

Rehse B, Pukrop R (2003). Effects of psychosocial interventions on quality of life in adult cancer patients: meta analysis of 37 published controlled outcome studies. *Patient Educ Counsel* **50**: 179–186.

Ressler IB, Cash J *et al.* (2003). Continued parental attendance at a clinic for adult survivors of childhood cancer. *J Pediatr Hematol Oncol* **25**: 868–873.

Rosenbaum E, Gautier H *et al.* (2004). Cancer supportive care, improving the quality of life for cancer patients. A program evaluation report. *Support Care Cancer* **12**: 298–301.

Rozans M, Dreisbach A, Lertora JJ, Kahn MJ (2002). Palliative uses of methylphenidate in patients with cancer: a review. *J Clin Oncol* **20**(1): 335–339.

Sanson-Fisher R, Girgis A, Boyes A *et al.* (2000). The unmet supportive care needs of patients with cancer. Supportive Care Review Group. *Cancer* **88**(1): 226–237.

Sheard T, Maguire P (1996). The effect of psychological interventions on anxiety and depression in oncology; results of two meta-analyses. Paper presented at Third World Congress of Psycho-Oncology. New York.

Sheard T, Maguire P (1999). The effect of psychological interventions on anxiety and depression in cancer patients: results of two meta-analyses. *Br J Cancer* **80**(11): 1770–1780.

Sherer M, Meyers CA, Bergloff P (1997). Efficacy of post-acute brain injury rehabilitation for patients with primary malignant brain tumors. *Cancer* **80**(2): 250–257.

Short PF, Vasey JJ, Tunceli K (2005). Employment pathways in a large cohort of adult cancer survivors. *Cancer* **103**(6): 1292–1301.

Sierpina V, Sierpina M *et al.* (2005). Complementary and integrative approaches to dementia. *South Med J* **98**(6): 636–645.

Sloper P (2000). Predictors of distress in parents of children with cancer: a prospective study. *J Pediatr Psychol* **25**: 79–92.

Speca M, Carlson L *et al.* (2000). A randomized, wait-list controlled clinical trial: the effect of a mindfulness meditation-based stress reduction program on mood and symptoms of stress in cancer outpatients. *Psychosomatic Med* **62**: 613–622.

Spelten ER, Verbeek JH, Uitterhoeve AL *et al.* (2003). Cancer, fatigue and the return of patients to work – a prospective cohort study. *Eur J Cancer* **39**(11): 1562–1567.

Spiegel D, Bloom JR *et al.* (1981). Group support for patients with metastatic cancer. A randomized outcome study. *Arch Gen Psychiatry* **38**(5): 527–533.

Stewart JL, Mishel MH (2000). Uncertainty in childhood illness: a synthesis of the parent and child literature. *Sch Inq Nurs Pract* **14**: 299–319.

Sutherland JE, Sutherland SJ, Hoehns JD (2003). Achieving the best outcome in treatment of depression. *J Fam Prac* **52**(3): 201–209.

Svavarsdottir EK (2005). Caring for a child with cancer: a longitudinal perspective. *J Adv Nurs* **50**: 153–161.

Valentine AD, Meyers CA (2001). Cognitive and mood disturbance as causes and symptoms of fatigue in cancer patients. *Cancer Supplement* **92**(6): 1694–1698.

Van Dongen-Melman JEWM, Pruyn JFA *et al.* (1995). Late psychosocial consequences for parents of children who survived cancer. *J Pediatr Psychol* **20**: 567–586.

Van Dongen-Melman JEWM, Van Zuuren FJ *et al.* (1998). Experiences of parents of childhood cancer survivors: a qualitative analysis. *Patient Educ Couns* **34**: 185–200.

Weis J (2003). Support groups for cancer patients. *Support Care Cancer* **11**: 763–768.

Welch AS, Wadsworth ME *et al.* (1996). Adjustment of children and adolescents to parental cancer. Parents' and children's perspectives. *Cancer* **77**: 1409–1418.

Ybema JF, Kuijer RG *et al.* (2001). Depression and perceptions of inequity among couples facing cancer. *J Psychosocial Oncol* **27**: 3–13.

Zebrack BJ, Chesler MA (2002). Quality of life in childhood cancer survivors. *Psychooncology* **11**(2): 132–141.

22

Pharmacological interventions for the treatment of radiation-induced brain injury

Edward G. Shaw, Jerome Butler, L. Douglas Case, Ralph d'Agostino, Jr., John Gleason, Jr., Edward Ip, Mike E. Robbins, Paul Saconn, and Stephen R. Rapp

Introduction

Neoplasms of the central nervous system (CNS) are a pathologically diverse group of benign and malignant tumors for which a variety of management strategies, including observation, surgery, radiation therapy (RT), and/or chemotherapy, are employed. Shown in Table 22.1 are the primary and metastatic brain tumors treated with RT, and the usual radiation doses employed for each (Shaw, 2000). Regardless of the type of brain tumor treated, radiation-treated patients will experience acute side-effects of therapy and be at risk for late sequelae. Chapter 7 outlined the biological basis of radiation-induced CNS injury. This chapter will focus on the treatment and prevention of radiation-induced brain injury, with an emphasis on pharmacological therapies.

Symptoms and symptom clusters in brain tumor patients

The symptoms of primary and metastatic brain tumors are dependent on tumor location (Table 22.2) (Shaw, 2000). Besides location-dependent symptoms, patients with brain tumors may experience symptoms related to their physical, emotional, and cognitive functions. Often, these symptoms occur in clusters. In newly diagnosed brain tumor patients, two symptom clusters typically occur: a mood cluster including anxiety, depression, and sadness, and an expressive language cluster including difficulty reading, writing, and finding the right words (Gleason et al., 2006). In long-term survivors, three symptom clusters are more common, including a physical function cluster (decreased energy, fatigue, and frustration), mood cluster (anger, anxiety, confusion, and depression), and a cognition cluster (difficulty concentrating, reading, remembering, and finding the right words) (Saconn et al., 2006). The severity of these symptoms changes over the lifespan of the brain tumor patient, from initial diagnosis to treatment, into the post-treatment follow-up or survivorship period. Although quality of life interventions for cancer patients tend to focus on single symptoms such as fatigue (Dodd et al., 2001, 2004), as with other types of brain pathologies (stroke, trauma, neurodegenerative diseases), a multidisciplinary approach, including pharmacological, behavioral, and rehabilitative therapies, is needed to optimize quality of life in the brain tumor patient.

Management of radiation-induced brain injury

Acute reactions

The most common acute reactions associated with brain radiation include fatigue, hair loss, and skin

Cognition and Cancer, eds. Christina A. Meyers and James R. Perry. Published by Cambridge University Press.
© Cambridge University Press 2008.

Table 22.1. Usual treatment volumes and doses for primary and metastatic brain tumors treated with radiation therapy

Pathological type	Treatment volume	Total dose (Gy/no. fractions)
Glioblastoma (WHO IV)		60/30
Initial field	Edema and enhancing tumor	46/23
Boost field	Enhancing tumor	14/7
Anaplastic astrocytoma, oligoastrocytoma (WHO III)		59.4/33
Initial field	Edema and enhancing tumor	50.4/28
Boost field	Enhancing tumor	9/5
Astrocytoma (WHO II)	Edema (and enhancing tumor if present)	50.4/28 to 59.4/33
Pilocytic astrocytoma (WHO I)	Enhancing tumor	50.4/28 to 55.8/31
Pituitary adenoma	Enhancing tumor	45/25 to 50.4/28
Meningioma (WHO I)	Enhancing tumor	52.2/29
Medulloblastoma and anaplastic ependymoma		55.8/31
Initial volume	Entire brain and spine	36/20
Boost volume	Enhancing tumor	19.8/11 to 23.4/13
Ependymoma	Enhancing tumor	50.4/28 to 59.4/33
Brain metastases	Whole brain	30/10 to 50.4/28

erythema. The onset of fatigue is generally within several weeks of the first radiation treatment. It is usually mild to moderate in severity. Typically, the fatigue persists for 1–2 months after the completion of treatment but may be chronic (lasting ≥3 months) in some patients. One characteristic of the fatigue associated with RT is a lack of improvement by rest. Methylphenidate (Ritalin®), a CNS stimulant, can be used to treat the fatigue that usually occurs in patients receiving whole-brain radiation. It also improves the depression and cognitive dysfunction that often accompanies fatigue in these patients (Weitzner *et al.*, 1995b). The usual dose of methylphenidate is 10 mg twice per day, escalating to 20–30 mg twice per day in 1-week increments as tolerated. Methylphenidate can also be used in children, usually at half the dose recommended for adults (Mulhern *et al.*, 2004). The dose-limiting toxicities are usually anxiety, insomnia, and tachycardia. Butler *et al.* (2005) recently reported the results of a Phase III prospective, randomized, double-blind, placebo-controlled clinical trial of d-methylphenidate (d-MPH) in adults undergoing curative or palliative partial- or whole-brain RT. Patients received d-MPH or placebo during brain RT and for 8 weeks afterward. The prophylactic use of d-MPH in this study was not associated with an improved overall or brain-specific quality of life, or reduction in fatigue, as measured by the Functional Assessment of Cancer Therapy (FACT) including both the brain and fatigue subscales (Butler *et al.*, 2005; Weitzner *et al.*, 1995a; Yellen *et al.*, 1997).

Hair loss occurs in the same time frame as fatigue, about 2–3 weeks into a course of fractionated whole- or partial-brain radiation. Complete or near-complete hair regrowth is the rule, though it may take 6 months to a year. There are no known interventions to prevent radiation-induced hair loss, nor are there any effective treatments to accelerate or maximize hair regrowth. Skin erythema is managed symptomatically with anti-inflammatory and moisturizing creams, typically 1% hydrocortisone or Aquaphor®, which are applied two to four

Table 22.2. Common brain tumor symptoms

Aphasia (including dysphasia) (T)
Ataxia (including truncal and limb) (BS, CB)
Bowel/bladder continence problems (F)
Deafness (BS, CPA, CN VIII)
Dementia (T)
Diplopia (BS, CS, CN III, IV, VI)
Dizziness (BS, CB, CPA, CN VIII)
Dysarthria (BS, CN IX/X)
Dysphagia (BS, CN IX/X)
Facial numbness (BS, CN VII, CPA)
Facial pain (BS, CS, CN VII)
Headache (G, 3/4V, HC)
Memory impairment (T)
Nausea (G, CB, BS, 3/4V, HC)
Neck pain (CB, BS)
Personality changes (including
   mood/mentation/concentration) (G, F, T)
Seizures (G)
Sensory changes (including numbness, tingling,
   paresthesias) (P, BS)
Visual field deficits (including blindness) (T, P, S/PIT, SS)
Vomiting (G, CB, BS 3/4V, HC)
Weakness (F, BS)

Key: 3/4V, 3rd or 4th ventricle; BS, brainstem; CB, cerebellum; CN, cranial nerve; CPA, cerebellopontine angle; CS, cavernous sinus; F, frontal lobe; G, general cerebral (including any intracranial location); HC, symptoms associated with hydrocephalus; P, parietal lobe; PIT, pituitary gland; S, sellar; SS, suprasellar; T, temporal lobe.

times daily or as needed for patient comfort. Moist desquamation behind the ears and in the external auditory canals may develop following whole brain radiation. Treatment usually involves skin creams and Cortisporin otic suspension (i.e., neomycin, polymyxin B, and hydrocortisone). Rarely, debridement of the external auditory canals by an otolaryngologist may be necessary. Radiation-induced otitis media may also occur. Symptomatic treatment with oral decongestants is usually adequate. Occasionally, a tympanic membrane tube may be necessary.

Early delayed reactions

There are no known interventions or therapies to prevent or treat early delayed reactions involving the brain, which are thought to occur because of transient demyelination. Somnolence syndrome in children is an example of an early delayed reaction involving the brain. The symptoms of somnolence syndrome include somnolence, irritability, anorexia, and sometimes an exacerbation of underlying tumor-associated symptoms or signs. Prior to or concomitant with the treatment of somnolence syndrome, a careful history and exam as well as re-imaging of the brain (usually with magnetic resonance imaging) should be done, to rule out a bleed, stroke, or tumor recurrence. Steroids are usually initiated with the onset of somnolence syndrome, 2–4 mg dexamethasone bid to qid orally (higher doses perhaps with intravenous administration if the symptoms are severe or life-threatening), with a rapid taper if no symptomatic improvement occurs (which is usually the case), or a slower taper over 1–2 months if the symptoms are responsive to steroids. Somnolence syndrome is transient, though it may last for several weeks to months, and does not predict for subsequent radiation-induced brain injury (Halperin *et al.*, 1994).

Late delayed reactions

Although edema and necrosis of the white matter are usually classified as late delayed reactions, brain edema can occur as an early or late effect of radiation. The treatment of radiation-induced brain edema is more of an art than a science and typically involves the use of steroids (Wen & Marks, 2002). Oral dexamethasone is usually used in initial doses of 2–4 mg bid for mild symptoms and 4–6 mg qid for moderate to severe symptoms. Oral doses in excess of 10 mg qid (40 mg daily) usually do not increase the likelihood of clinical benefit. The initial dexamethasone dose is usually maintained for 2–4 weeks, with a slow taper (2–4 mg per day reduction every 5–7 days) as tolerated thereafter. For patients with life-threatening edema, intravenous dexamethasone

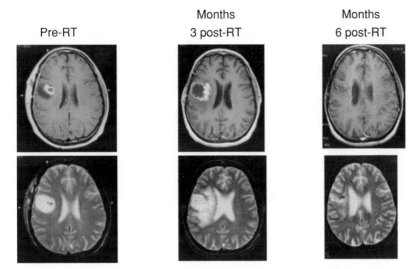

Figure 22.1. MRI scans of a 30-year-old man with a WHO grade II oligodendroglioma of the right posterior frontal lobe. The images on the left (T2-weighted images on top, T1-weighted images with contrast on bottom) were obtained before 64.8 Gy in 36 fractions radiation therapy (RT) was given to a localized treatment field (tumor plus margin 1–2 cm). Three months following RT, the patient developed headaches and left-sided weakness and had a repeat MRI scan (center images), which demonstrated radiation necrosis. Note increase in enhancement and surrounding edema in the absence of much mass effect. The patient was treated with a 3-month course of dexamethasone. A follow-up MRI scan 3 months later showed resolution of the imaging changes associated with the radionecrosis (right images). The patient's MR imaging remained stable for over a decade, by which time he had tumor progression

is used, 10–25 mg as a bolus followed by 4–10 mg qid. If these patients do not respond to dexamethasone, intravenous mannitol may be required. Patients on dexamethasone should receive gastritis prophylaxis (with H2 blockers or proton pump inhibitors) and appropriate treatments for hyperglycemia (oral hypoglycemic agents or insulin) and oral thrush (fluconazole 200 mg day 1 then 100 mg daily for 6 days) should they arise. Prophylaxis for pneumocystis pneumonia using one double-strength trimethoprim/sulfamethoxazole (Bactrim®) tablet daily three times per week is commonly used in children as well as adults also taking temozolomide (Temodar®) chemotherapy (Stupp et al., 2002). Patients taking dexamethasone chronically (1 month or longer) usually become cushingoid, characterized by fatigue, weight gain, facial swelling, central obesity, muscle wasting (particularly in the extremities), striae, and arthral-gias. Treatment is symptomatic. The physical manifestations of chronic dexamethasone administration use can take months to resolve after its discontinuation.

Necrosis of the brain can be difficult to clinically and radiographically differentiate from tumor recurrence (Figure 22.1) (Forsyth et al., 1995). Since cerebral radiation necrosis is always accompanied by varying degrees of edema, the initial management of clinically suspected or pathologically proven radionecrosis is with steroids, as previously described. Several adjunctive medical treatments for brain radiation necrosis have been anecdotally described as being helpful to arrest or reverse the process, such as hyperbaric oxygen, warfarin (Coumadin®), pentoxifylline (Trental®), and antioxidant vitamins such as vitamin E (Leber et al., 1998; Liu et al., 2001; Nieder et al., 2005). One recent report of 50 patients with biopsy-proven

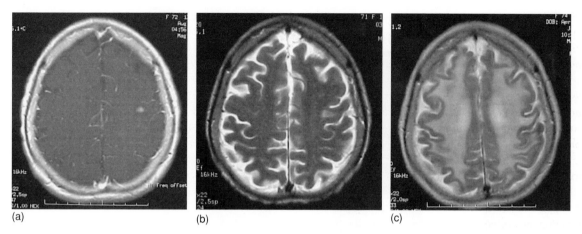

(a)   (b)   (c)

Figure 22.2. MRI scans of a 72-year-old woman with ovarian cancer metastatic to the brain. (a) and (b) were obtained before 37.5 Gy in 15 fractions whole-brain radiation therapy (WBRT) was administered. A subcentimeter left posterior frontal metastasis is seen on the T1-weighted image with contrast (a). There are minimal surrounding T2 changes in the white matter (b), and no other white matter abnormalities present. Two years following WBRT, the patient has diffuse white matter demyelination and atrophy, as seen on the T2-weighted image (c). The patient died 1 year later of a progressive Alzheimer's-like dementia

brain radionecrosis suggested benefit in the use of pentoxifylline 400 mg tid and vitamin E 1000 IU daily (Rogers, 2006). In medically unresponsive patients, surgical resection of the necrotic lesion, providing it can be safely performed, will often allow the dexamethasone dose to be reduced and also provide relief from the symptoms and signs of mass effect associated with the cerebral edema (Rogers, 2006). While the various interventions cited have no proven preventive role in the development of brain radionecrosis, very little research has been conducted in this area, pre-clinically or clinically. One animal model of radiation-induced injury to the optic nerves even suggested an increased incidence of optic neuropathy with "preventive" hyperbaric oxygen (Kim *et al.*, 2004), in addition to or instead of dexamethasone.

Cognitive dysfunction, a late delayed effect of whole-brain and large-field partial-brain radiation, can occur with total doses as low as 20 Gy in adults and 24 Gy in children given with conventional fractions of 1.8–2 Gy (Armstrong *et al.*, 2002; Crosson *et al.*, 1994; Mulhern *et al.*, 1992; Ochs *et al.*, 1991; Ris & Noll, 1994), and is more com-

mon with larger fraction sizes (>2Gy) (DeAngelis *et al.*, 1989). Symptoms range from cognitive slowing, poor attention and concentration, difficulty multi-tasking, decreased short-term (and eventually long-term) memory, word finding problems, and decreased IQ (in children), to a progressive Alzheimer's-like dementia, which is also characterized by urinary incontinence and gait disturbance (Figure 22.2). Changes in energy and mood, particularly fatigue, anxiety, and depression, often accompany the cognitive changes that occur in long-term survivors of brain radiation (Shaw *et al.*, 2006). Like brain radionecrosis, there are no proven preventive interventions for radiation-induced cognitive dysfunction. However, there are several therapies that have been reported as beneficial, one of which, methylphenidate (Ritalin®), is described in the section on acute reactions. Methylphenidate is particularly useful when fatigue is one of the symptoms, or the prominent symptom experienced by a particular patient.

The Wake Forest University School of Medicine Comprehensive Cancer Center, through its Community Clinical Oncology Program (CCOP) Research

Base, has recently completed two sequential open-label Phase II clinical trials utilizing novel interventions for the treatment of symptomatic late radiation-induced brain injury in adults. Eligibility criteria included partial- or whole-brain radiation to a dose of >25 Gy for a primary or metastatic brain tumor completed 6 months or more prior to study entry and no radiographic evidence of tumor progression in the 3 months prior to study entry. Endpoints included quality of life (measured by the brain subscale of the FACT) (Weitzner *et al.*, 1995a), mood (measured by the Profile of Mood States, POMS) (McNair *et al.*, 1992), and cognitive function (measured by a neurocognitive test battery including assessment of attention and concentration, verbal and visual memory, verbal fluency, and executive function) (Benton & Hamsher, 1983; Delis *et al.*, 1987; Fastenau *et al.*, 1999; Kaplan *et al.*, 1978; Reitan, 1958; Wechsler, 1981). Both studies utilized a 24-week intervention with quality of life, mood, and cognitive function evaluations occurring at baseline and at weeks 6, 12, and 24 of treatment. The first study utilized donepezil (Aricept®) 5 mg daily for 6 weeks followed by 10 mg daily for 18 weeks, whereas the second study utilized *Ginkgo biloba* 40 mg three times a day. Both interventions were based on data from previously reported randomized trials in dementia (Bryson & Benfield, 1997; Le Bars *et al.*, 1997; Rogers *et al.*, 1998a, 1998b). Of patients who completed the 24-week study, significant improvements were seen in quality of life (increase in FACT brain subscale score), mood (decrease in POMS score), and cognitive function (improved attention and concentration and memory) with both donepezil and *Ginkgo biloba*. In addition, *Ginkgo biloba* patients had significant improvement in executive function. Patient dropout for lack of efficacy or toxicity was greater in those taking *Ginkgo biloba* than donepezil (Shaw *et al.*, 2006). An open-label Pilot study of donepezil is currently being conducted in children at Wake Forest. A Phase III randomized double-blind placebo controlled trial of donepezil is being conducted by Wake Forest Cancer Center with its CCOP Research Base in conjunction with the M. D.

Anderson Cancer Center and its CCOP Research Base. Other neuroprotective and neurotherapeutic strategies, particularly single drugs or combinations of agents, are being studied in this patient population, including therapies that target the presumed pathophysiology of radiation-induced injury (Fike *et al.*, 1994; Hopewell *et al.*, 1993; Hornsey *et al.*, 1990; Lynch *et al.*, 2002; Nakagawa *et al.*, 1996; Nieder *et al.*, 2000; Sminia *et al.*, 2003; Spence *et al.*, 1986) and newer approaches using neural stem cells (Rezvani *et al.*, 2002) or new agents that stimulate neurogenesis (Monje *et al.*, 2002).

ACKNOWLEDGMENT

Supported by NCI grant CA81851.

REFERENCES

Armstrong CL, Hunter JV, Ledakis GE *et al.* (2002). Late cognitive and radiographic changes related to radiotherapy: initial prospective findings. *Neurology* **59**: 40–48.

Benton AL, Hamsher K (1983). *Multilingual Aphasia Examination*. Iowa City, IA: AJA Associates.

Bryson HM, Benfield P (1997). Donepezil. *Drug Aging* **10(3)**: 234–243.

Butler J, Case D, Atkins J *et al.* (2005). A phase III double blind placebo controlled prospective randomized clinical trial of the effect of d-threo-methylphenidate HCL (d-MPH) on quality of life in brain tumor patients receiving radiation therapy. *Int J Radiat Oncol Biol Physics* **63** [Suppl.]: 80.

Crossen JR, Garwood D, Glatstein E, Neuwelt EA (1994). Neurobehavioral sequelae of cranial irradiation in adults: a review of radiation-induced encephalopathy. *J Clin Oncol* **12**: 627–642.

DeAngelis LM, Delattre J, Posner JB (1989). Radiation-induced dementia in patients cured of metastases. *Neurology* **39**: 789–796.

Delis DC, Kramer JH, Kaplan E, Ober BA (1987). *California Verbal Learning Test-Research Edition*. San Antonio, TX: The Psychological Corp.

Dodd MJ, Miaskowski C, Paul SM (2001). Symptom clusters and their effect on the functional status of patients with cancer. *Oncol Nurs Forum* **28**(3): 465–470.

Dodd MJ, Miaskowski C, Lee KA (2004). Occurrence of symptom clusters. *J Natl Cancer Inst Monographs* 32: 76–78.

Fastenau PS, Denburg NL, Hufford BJ (1999). Adult norms for the Rey-Osterrieth Complex Figure Test and for supplemental recognition and matching trials from the Extended Complex Figure Test. *Clin Neuropsychol* 13: 30–47.

Fike JR, Goebbel GT, Martob LJ, Seilhan TM (1994). Radiation brain injury is reduced by the polyamine inhibitor alpha-difluoromethylornithine. *Radiat Res* 138: 99–106.

Forsyth PA, Kelly PJ, Casano TL *et al.* (1995). Radiation necrosis or glioma recurrence: is computer assisted stereotactic biopsy useful? *J Neurosurg* 82(4): 36–44.

Gleason J, Case D, Rapp S *et al.* (2006). Symptom clusters in newly-diagnosed brain tumor patients [Abstract]. In 2006 ASCO Annual Meeting Proceedings Part I. *J Clin Oncol* 24(18S) [June 20 Suppl.]: 8587.

Halperin EC, Constine LS, Tarbell NJ, Kun LE (eds.) (1994). *Pediatric Radiation Oncology* (2nd edn.). New York: Raven Press.

Hopewell JW, Van Den Aardweg GJMJ, Morris GM *et al.* (1993). Unsaturated lipids as modulators of radiation damage in normal tissues. In Horrobin DF (ed.) *New Approaches to Cancer Treatment* (pp. 88–106). London: Churchill Communications Europe.

Hornsey S, Myers R, Jenkinson T (1990). The reduction of radiation damage to the spinal cord by postirradiation administration of vasoactive drugs. *Int J Radiat Oncol Biol Phys* 18: 1437–1442.

Kaplan EF, Goodglass H, Weintraub S (1978). *The Boston Naming Test*. Boston, MA: E. Kaplan & H. Goodglass.

Kim JH, Brown SL, Kolozsvary A *et al.* (2004). Modification of radiation injury by Ramipril, inhibitor of the angiotensin-converting enzyme, on optic neuropathy in the rat. *Radiat Res* 161: 137–142.

Le Bars PL, Katz MM, Berman N, Itil TM, Freedman AM, Schatzberg AF (1997). A placebo-controlled, double-blind, randomized trial of an extract of ginkgo biloba for dementia. *J Am Med Assoc* 278: 1327–1332.

Leber KA, Eder HG, Kovac H, Anegg U, Pendl G (1998). Treatment of cerebral radionecrosis by hyperbaric oxygen therapy. *Stereotact Funct Neurosurg* 70 [Suppl. 1]: 229–236.

Liu CY, Yim BY, Wozniak AJ (2001). Anticoagulation therapy for radiation-induced myelopathy. *Ann Pharmacother* 35: 188–191.

Lynch CD, Sonntag WE, Wheeler KT (2002). Radiation-induced dementia in aged rats: effects of growth hormone and insulin-like growth factor 1 [Abstract]. *Neurooncology* 4: 354.

McNair DM, Lorr M, Droppleman LF (1992). *Profile of Mood States Manual*. San Diego, CA: Educational and Industrial Testing Service.

Monje ML, Mizumatsu S, Fike JR, Palmer TD (2002). Irradiation induces neural precursor-cell dysfunction. *Nat Med* 8: 955–962.

Mulhern R, Hancock J, Fairclough D, Kun L (1992). Neuropsychological status of children treated for brain tumors: a critical review and integrative analysis. *Med Pediat Oncol* 20: 181–191.

Mulhern RK, Khan RB, Kaplan S *et al.* (2004). Short-term efficacy of methylphenidate: a randomized, double-blind, placebo-controlled trial among survivors of childhood cancer. *J Clin Oncol* 22: 4795–4803.

Nakagawa M, Bellinzona M, Seilhan TM *et al.* (1996). Microglial responses after focal radiation-induced injury are affected by alpha-difluoromethylornithine. *Int J Radiat Oncol Biol Phys* 36: 113–123.

Nieder C, Price RE, Rivera B, Ang KK (2000). Both early and delayed treatment with growth factors can modulate the development of radiation myelopathy (RM) in rats. *Radiother Oncol* 56 [Suppl. 1]: S15.

Nieder C, Zimmerman FB, Adam M, Molls M (2005). The role of pentoxifylline as a modifier of radiation therapy. *Cancer Treat Rev* 31: 448–455.

Ochs J, Mulhern R, Fairclough D *et al.* (1991). Comparison of neuropsychologic functioning and clinical indicators of neurotoxicity in long-term survivors of childhood leukemia given cranial radiation or parenteral methotrexate: a prospective study. *J Clin Oncol* 9: 145–151.

Reitan RM (1958). Validity of the Trail Making Test as an indicator of organic brain damage. *Percept Motor Skills* 8: 271–276.

Rezvani M, Birds DA, Hodges H, Hopewell JW, Milledew K, Wilkinson JH (2002). Modification of radiation myelopathy by the transplantation of neural stem cells in the rat. *Radiat Res* 156: 408–412.

Ris M, Noll R (1994). Long-term neurobehavioral outcome in pediatric brain-tumor patients: review and methodological critique. *J Clin Exp Neuropsychol* 16: 21–42.

Rogers LR (2006). Natural history and results of therapy in 50 patients with histologically confirmed cerebral radiation necrosis [Abstract]. *Neurooncology* 8(4): 489.

Rogers SL, Doody RS, Mohs RC, Friedhoff LT, Donepezil Study Group (1998a). Donepezil improves cognition and global function in Alzheimer's disease. *Arch Int Med* **158**: 1021–1031.

Rogers SL, Farlow MR, Doody RS, Mohs R, Friedhoff LT, Donepezil Study Group (1998b). A 24-week, double-blind, placebo-controlled trial of donepezil in patients with Alzheimer's disease. *Neurology* **50**(1): 136–145.

Saconn PA, Ip E, Rapp S, D'Agostino RB Jr, Naughton MJ, Shaw EG (2006). Symptom clusters in irradiated brain tumor survivors [Abstract]. In 2006 ASCO Annual Meeting Proceedings Part I. *J Clin Oncol* 24 (18S) [June 20 Suppl.]: 8581.

Shaw EG (2000). Central nervous system overview. In Gunderson LL, Tepper JE (eds.) *Clinical Radiation Oncology*. Philadelphia, PA: Churchill-Livingstone.

Shaw EG, Rosdhal R, D'Agostino RB Jr *et al.* (2006). A phase II study of donepezil in irradiated brain tumor patients: effect on cognitive function, mood, and quality of life. *J Clin Oncol* **24**: 1415–1420.

Sminia P, van der Kleij AJ, Carl UM, Feldmeier JJ, Hartmann KA (2003). Prophylactic hyperbaric oxygen treatment and rat spinal cord irradiation. *Cancer Lett* **191**: 59–65.

Spence AM, Krohn KA, Edmonson SW, Steele JE, Rasey JS (1986). Radioprotection in rat spinal cord with WR-2721 following cerebral lateral intraventricular injection. *Int J Radiat Oncol Biol Phys* **12**: 1479–1482.

Stupp R, Dietrich PY, Ostermann Kraljevic S *et al.* (2002). Promising survival for patients with newly diagnosed glioblastoma multiforme treated with concomitant radiation plus temozolomide followed by adjuvant temozolomide. *J Clin Oncol* **20**: 1375–1382.

Wechsler D (1981). *Wechsler Adult Intelligence Scale – Revised Manual*. New York: Psychological Corp.

Weitzner MA, Meyers CA, Gelke CK, Byrne KS, Cella DF, Levin VA (1995a). The Functional Assessment of Cancer Therapy (FACT) scale: development of a brain subscale and revalidation of the general version (FACT-G) in patients with primary brain tumors. *Cancer* **75**: 1151–1161.

Weitzner MA, Meyers CA, Valentine AD (1995b). Methylphenidate in the treatment of neurobehavioral slowing associated with cancer and cancer treatment. *J Neuropsychiatry Clin Neurosci* **7**: 347–350.

Wen PY, Marks PW (2002). Medical management of patients with brain tumors. *Curr Opin Oncol* **14**: 299–307.

Yellen SB, Cella DF, Webster K, Blendowski C, Kaplan E (1997). Measuring fatigue and other anemia-related symptoms with the Functional Assessment of Cancer Therapy (FACT) measurement system. *J Pain Symptom Manage* **13**: 63–67.

23

Neurocognitive testing in clinical trials

Jennifer A. Smith and Jeffrey S. Wefel

Importance of formal neurocognitive testing

Since the early 1990s it has been recognized that the "net clinical benefit" of a therapy includes not only traditional survival endpoints but also benefits in terms of symptoms and quality-of-life endpoints (O'Shaughnessy *et al.*, 1991). With increasing awareness that it is often inadequate to measure survival without consideration of the "quality" of that survival, there has been a call to develop and include neurocognitive and patient-reported outcome (PRO) measures into modern trial design. Members of the Food and Drug Administration (FDA), National Cancer Institute (NCI), American Association for Cancer Research (AACR), and American Society of Clinical Oncology (ASCO) met in 2006 to discuss endpoints for drug registration trials in primary brain cancer. The recommendations generated from this meeting were provided for the Oncology Drug Advisory Committee's (ODAC) consideration and included a *composite progression endpoint* in which radiographical, neurocognitive, neurological, and PRO are jointly considered (http://www.fda.gov/cder/drug/cancer_endpoints/brain_summary.pdf; accessed 10 April, 2008). The FDA has recently opined that a therapeutic agent may be approvable if preservation of neurocognitive function can be demonstrated even if survival endpoints are equivalent (minutes of an end-of-phase-II meeting regarding a novel radiation sensitizing agent, October 21, 1998).

Impaired neurocognitive functioning occurs in the majority of patients with central nervous system (CNS) tumors and has been shown to be impaired by cancer therapies for tumors arising outside the brain (Meyers *et al.*, 1995; Wefel *et al.*, 2004b). Magnetic resonance imaging (MRI) abnormalities may not always be clinically symptomatic (Fleissbach *et al.*, 2003) and patients with deteriorating neurocognitive function may not always show concomitant structural brain changes on imaging. In fact, Meyers and Hess (2003) demonstrated that, in patients with primary brain tumors, neurocognitive dysfunction occurred in advance of MRI evidence of tumor progression. The addition of measures of neurocognitive function also predicts survival better than clinical prognostic factors alone in patients with primary brain tumors, leptomeningeal disease, and parenchymal brain metastases (Meyers *et al.*, 2000, 2004; Sherman *et al.*, 2002; Taphoorn & Klein, 2004).

Neurocognitive measures can be utilized in clinical trials to monitor patient function and to determine if a therapeutic strategy results in: (1) improvement or stability in neurocognitive function associated with better tumor control; (2) less rapid decline in neurocognitive function associated with the disease; or (3) increased or decreased acute or late neurotoxicity (Meyers & Brown, 2006). In the

Cognition and Cancer, eds. Christina A. Meyers and James R. Perry. Published by Cambridge University Press.
© Cambridge University Press 2008.

case of CNS disease, serial monitoring may demonstrate improved neurocognitive function secondary to better tumor control or a reduced rate of expected neurocognitive decline. Similar outcomes may be measured in disease outside the brain (Wefel et al., 2004b) and can separate adverse disease effects from treatment-related neurotoxicity (Meyers et al., 1995; Wefel et al., 2004a).

It is important to choose psychometrically sound, objective, and standardized measures of neurocognitive function. It has been routinely demonstrated that mental status screening measures such as the Mini-Mental State Examination (MMSE), intended to detect extreme changes in neurocognitive function such as delirium or significant dementia, are inadequate (Meyers & Wefel, 2003). Patient-reported outcomes (PROs) and subjective complaints of neurocognitive dysfunction have been demonstrated to have little relationship with formal, objective assessment (Cull et al., 1996; van Dam et al., 1998). Moreover, serial monitoring of PRO may be susceptible to biases such as patient response shift, such that these measures offer insights into patient preferences and adjustment rather than changes in the actual level of function. Clinician-determined performance status, measures of symptoms (i.e., fatigue, pain, etc.), and activities of daily living (ADL) have been thought to better capture important aspects of patient well-being. However, they are also inappropriate as proxy measures of cognitive function and frequently appear insensitive to meaningful changes in patient function during longitudinal trials (Meyers & Hess, 2003).

Choice of neurocognitive tests

As discussed previously, neurocognitive testing provides direct, objective evidence of patient cognitive function that often corresponds to the structural and functional integrity of the brain. An advantage of neurocognitive testing is the standardized administration and scoring procedure coupled with normative data adjusted for age, education, gender,

and handedness, when appropriate, against which a patient's performance can be referenced. Decisions regarding which tests to include in a trial must consider a myriad of issues including the psychometric properties of the measures, the population and treatment under study, and their expected effect on neurocognitive function, frequency of testing, and the study design.

Psychometric properties

When selecting tests for a clinical trial it is important to establish that the tests are psychometrically sound. Preferably the tests will have been validated in the population of interest and have adequate test-retest reliability to permit serial monitoring and meaningful determination of change. Tests should also be chosen to avoid ceiling and floor effects, such that the majority of patients are able to complete the testing and the tests have sufficient sensitivity and range to detect serial improvement or deterioration in patient performance.

Focal versus diffuse function

Measures of neurocognitive function can measure discrete processes such as expressive language function or right upper-extremity strength. For each of these tests, regional damage located outside the area specifically assessed by these tests is likely to exert relatively little influence on test performance. In contrast, some tests (e.g., information processing speed) will reveal performance deficits following damage to any one of a number of areas in the brain due to the more distributed nature of these cognitive processes. If the goal is to identify where the damage is occurring then these tests are less than ideal. They will identify that something is wrong but not where it is wrong.

There are tradeoffs associated with the test choice. If the desire is to detect any damage then a single test sensitive to activity in a number of brain regions may be preferable. Benefits of such a choice include decreased time for both test administration and data processing. If the desire is to narrow down the damage to a particular locus of functioning then it would often be necessary to employ multiple tests that specifically target discrete brain areas or functional domains. However, even in this case, a single test could suffice if damage to a specific brain area is suspected and the neural network underlying the neurocognitive function of interest is not widely distributed. If, however, the study is more exploratory, a greater number of tests would be needed. As discussed below, selection of tests that can localize discrete versus distributed functions will be predicated on the expected treatment or disease effect on the brain.

Impact of disease and treatment

In selecting a test battery it is critical to consider the expected impact of the disease or treatment on neurocognitive function. In some cases, the mechanisms of action of a therapy may be well understood and hypothesized to potentially disrupt a specific neurocognitive domain (e.g., memory dysfunction). For example, Meyers *et al.* (1997) studied CI-980 in a Phase II trial as a potential therapy for individuals with ovarian and colorectal cancer. This agent is a synthetic mitotic inhibitor that shares structural and functional similarities with colchicine, binds to tubulin at the colchicine-binding site, and crosses the blood–brain barrier. Cognitive testing, including monitoring of memory function, was a component of this protocol because of the ability of colchicine to selectively damage cholinergic neurons in and around the hippocampus and basal forebrain, structures critical to learning and memory functions. Serial testing demonstrated declines in memory function using standardized neuropsychological measures.

However, often either the mechanism of the potential neurocognitive toxicity of a therapeutic strategy is not well understood or the expected brain lesions are not homogeneous enough (i.e., right parietal, left frontal, etc.) to permit selection of tests based on known brain–behavior relationships.

These considerations are illustrated in two recent trials conducted by Pharmacyclics, Inc. assessing the effect of motexafin gadolinium on the neurocognitive functioning in patients with brain metastases. As brain metastases arise in a number of regions and as the effect of any one metastasis could be quite subtle, the study design group chose a number of tests that measured neurocognitive domains sensitive to the functioning of specific and distinct brain regions. The desire was to capture the effect of a single lesion but at the same time allow for sensitivity to functioning throughout the brain. Additionally, the trial was designed to describe the functional deficits due to brain metastases, not simply to catalogue the presence or absence of any deficit.

Frequency of testing

The frequency of testing depends, in part, on the rate of functional change and the goal of the follow-up assessments. If the rate of change is slow or the goal is to characterize performance months or years after initiation of treatment then infrequent or delayed follow-up would suffice. Similarly, if memory for particular test information plays a large role in subsequent test performance (practice effect) and alternative validated versions of the test are not available, then the scores may be biased if testing is too frequent.

Additional factors may dictate test frequency, such as the monetary burden of testing or patient compliance. Patients having regular study visits are often willing to submit to additional neurocognitive testing (Herman *et al.*, 2003; Mehta *et al.*, 2002). In a large multisite Phase III trial in patients with brain metastases (Meyers *et al.*, 2004) the protocol specified monthly visits for 6 months and then every third month thereafter. Frequent testing was necessary due to the sharp decline in functioning observed in these patients as well as their short overall life expectancy; 98% of patients completed testing at baseline and 87% completed the 6 months follow-up testing.

Study design: baseline versus repeated testing

Aspects of the study design can greatly influence test selection. Baseline, pre-treatment assessments are sometimes performed to serve as a predictor of later functioning (e.g., Meyers *et al.*, 2000). Again, the tradeoffs are apparent. There can be less emphasis on the feasibility of the number of tests as they will be given only at baseline and not at repeated visits. A variety of tests may be included to provide a comprehensive picture of functioning. Performance on these tests can be used to predict later functioning or can aid the development of prognostic categories (Meyers *et al.*, 2000, 2004; Sherman *et al.*, 2002; Taphoorn & Klein, 2004). Baseline performance can also be used to divide people into groups at baseline for stratification purposes in the analysis of related endpoints. Correlations between performance on neurocognitive tests and other standard tests can be computed.

Repeated measurement of neurocognitive performance is required if it is to be used as an endpoint; measures of both baseline and follow-up performance are needed. The baseline measurement ensures balance across treatment arms or describes the incoming level of functioning of patients on the trial. Performance is then assessed over time for change, especially due to treatment.

Measurement of patient performance over time may be confounded by the effects of repeated practice. Test performance often improves despite the absence of underlying change or even a decline in neurocognitive function. This improvement can be divided into two broad categories: general improvement as the patient learns the task demands or relaxes in the presence of the examiner, and more specific improvement that results from learning of the unique information presented in a test, such as the particular words presented in a memory test. Procedures can be introduced to reduce the effects of both general and specific learning. Practice tests can be given prior to formal testing to reduce the effects of the general testing situation on later test performance. However, for measures that assess performance in response to novel situations, such as measures of abstract reasoning or problem solving, this procedure may inadvertently alter the nature of the test and thus invalidate the findings. The effects of specific learning on future performance may be reduced by choosing tests that have minimal practice effects or multiple versions that can be alternated over time. These alternative versions should be standardized and externally validated.

Implementation in clinical trials

There are several challenges to the successful implementation of neuropsychological testing. In addition to the issues surrounding the choice of tests and frequency of testing as summarized above, one must consider the personnel required for testing, the training of such personnel, the data collection procedures and the particulars of data analysis.

Required personnel and training

During study planning, a neuropsychologist should be consulted to discuss potential treatment benefits and toxicities in terms of cognitive function, the frequency of testing, the choice of appropriate tests (i.e., tests that assess cognitive processes of interest and that have adequate psychometric properties for the purpose of the study), and inclusion or exclusion criteria for the study population given properties of the tests to be used (e.g., certain tests are not appropriate for patients over/under a certain age or those not fluent in English). Additionally, a neuropsychologist can train the study personnel and ensure quality control of the data collection process across the entire trial.

Neuropsychological testing offers the ability to objectively assess neurocognitive functions using standardized procedures that limit the variability between examiners. However, this requires careful training and monitoring when personnel without formal education in neuropsychology are conducting the tests. The feasibility of multinational repeated administration of testing by trained study personnel was demonstrated in a recent Phase III trial in brain metastases (Meyers *et al.*, 2004). Our experience suggests that the process of training and certifying study personnel to administer standardized neuropsychological tests is most effective when the following components are included in the study procedures:

1. All individuals administering the tests undergo training including review of a training manual designed by the neuropsychologist that includes standardized instruction sets and administration procedures.
2. Review of a training video demonstrating and explaining each test, accompanied by a post-test that is reviewed by the neuropsychologist to ensure trainee comprehension of key procedural elements.
3. Administration of a practice test to a non-patient colleague by the trainee that is reviewed for accuracy by the consulting neuropsychologist and followed up to discuss administration errors or concerns.

The successful completion of all of these components was required before a trainee was deemed certified to administer the cognitive test battery to any protocol patient. Ideally, this training and certification will occur close in time to when the first protocol patient is seen for their baseline evaluation to minimize the chance of examiner drift (i.e., the tendency to forget prior training or deviate from standardized procedures). From a pragmatic standpoint as well, a neuropsychologist may need to be consulted in trials involving cognitive testing as test publishers often will not sell or permit use of these instruments by individuals without appropriate training.

Data collection

Modifications to the test forms such as including the standardized instruction set on each form can facilitate consistent, accurate test administration. Additional formatting may also be undertaken to ensure proper test administration and data capture. For example, we have generated a space on our modified memory test forms where the certified test administrator is required to record the time at which the learning trials were completed and the time at which the delayed recall portion of the test was begun, to ensure that the standardized delay interval is adhered to for each patient. Similarly, it is important to include indicator statements on each form that the certified test administrator completes, which specify whether the test was completed or not completed due to issues such as patient non-compliance, neurological deficit (e.g., hemiparesis) or altered mental status (e.g., confusion). This information greatly assists the determination of whether the missing data represent informative (i.e., progression of neurocognitive dysfunction) or non-informative (i.e., patient refusal/non-compliance, examiner error) trial information, which has an impact on the data analyses.

Early and regular feedback regarding test administration and data collection is recommended. Unforeseen practices in the administration, timing, or scoring of tests may arise, especially in international, multicenter trials. For instance, if the study endpoint is a measure of change from baseline, then incorrect baseline test administration for a number of patients would invalidate both their baseline and their subsequent change-from-baseline measurements; this could compromise the integrity of the endpoint results. Two of the more common administration and scoring issues include failing to stop at the specified time for timed tests and failing to distinguish between a score of zero (for instance remembering zero words on a memory test) and an incomplete or missing test score; the two should be handled quite differently in the statistical analysis. Ideally, the neuropsychologist will review all test results to ensure standardized procedures were followed and patient response errors were appropriately marked. Similarly, the neuropsychologist may calculate the final scores for each test to provide a blinded, central review that eliminates potential bias in assessing outcomes.

Statistical and interpretive considerations

Confounding variables and missing data

The interpretation of the neurocognitive data depends in part on the context of the overall trial results. Information regarding possible confounders of neurocognitive function (e.g., concomitant medications such as steroids, medical complications such as seizures, and depression or other mood disorders) should be collected throughout the trial. Performance of neurocognitive testing at the same time as other physical examinations or staging evaluations (e.g., neurological exams, MRI scans) provides contextual information for analyzing the neurocognitive outcomes over time.

Missing data, often not at random, can occur when patients who are experiencing diminished neurocognitive capacity become unable to complete the neurocognitive testing. It is possible, as described previously, to collect information on the reason for such missing values and to then incorporate this information into the analysis. For instance, inability to perform the test due to a new impairment of comprehension, such that the person cannot understand test instructions as they could before, might rightfully be considered an indication of neurocognitive decline.

Analytical approaches

Reliable change index

The reliable change index (RCI) is a method for determining if and when a patient has deteriorated. According to the RCI method (Jacobsen & Truax, 1991), a distribution of change scores is created under the null hypothesis of no change. The distribution parameters can be generated from published normative data or can be generated from previous study data. Consider a hypothetical distribution of follow-up (Time 2) minus baseline (Time 1) scores for 100 normal individuals or control patients tested soon after baseline. Barring practice effects, the scores are not predicted to change over time and the differences in the follow-up minus baseline scores reflect measurement errors. Thus the distribution is centered approximately at zero and 90% of the scores are within 1.65 standard deviations (SD) of the center. Taking this distribution as the reference distribution for future trials, an observed patient with a follow-up minus baseline

score of less than $-1.65 \times$ SD from this distribution is said to have deteriorated (assuming higher scores indicate improved performance) as it is unlikely to have occurred by chance (under the null hypothesis only 5% of patients decline by that much or more). Note that calculating the SD of the change scores is mathematically equivalent to calculating the RCI according to the formula presented by Jacobsen and Truax, using the correlation between Time 1 and Time 2 scores and the SD of the Time 1 scores.

Since its introduction, the RCI has been subject to improvements and some criticisms (Chelune et al., 1993; Crawford & Garthwaite, 2006; Maassen, 2004; Tempkin, 2004; Tempkin et al., 1999). Despite this, it remains a common and frequently justifiable method for analysis. Probably the most helpful improvement is an adjustment for practice effects introduced by Chelune et al. (1993). Practice effects are also estimated from the reference data and manifest as a positive shift in the reference distribution. This can be conceptualized as a distribution that is not centered at zero but instead at some increased delta indicating a mean effect of practice. Analysis of patient data in the trial then incorporates this practice effect such that a smaller decrease is now considered indicative of decline ($-1.65 \times$ SD + delta).

A criticism of the RCI method is that the parameters from the reference data are treated as fixed values not subject to measurement error themselves. This topic is addressed in an article that promotes regression-based methods to predict change scores (Crawford & Garthwaite, 2006). The authors performed simulations that varied the size of the reference dataset and found that the regression-based method outperformed the RCI at small reference dataset sizes (e.g., n values of 5, 10, or 20), but for moderate ($n = 50$) to large ($n = 100$ or more) reference datasets the RCI performed well, in that the predicted number of declines was within 1% of the actual number. In fact, for reference datasets as small as 20 the predicted number of declines was within 2% of the actual number.

As mentioned above the parameters from the reference distribution can be obtained from actual previous study data (calculate the SD of the change scores directly or use the correlation of Time 1 and

Time 2 data, and Time 1 SD to calculate the SD of the change scores) or from published test-retest reliability (correlation) coefficients and baseline SDs. It's important in the latter case that the reliability coefficients and the Time 1 SDs are calculated from the same study population. It is not recommended, for instance, to use a published correlation coefficient and the baseline SD from another source. This will not result in an accurate estimate of the SD of the change score distribution because the published correlation coefficient is dependent on the baseline spread of data from which it was derived, a phenomenon known as "range restriction."

Regression-based methods for predicting change scores

These methods are similar to the RCI as they predict follow-up scores under the null hypothesis of no treatment effect; if a patient's score is beyond the limits of the prediction interval the patient is determined to have deteriorated (Crawford & Garthwaite, 2006). For large reference datasets the RCI can be considered a subset of this method where the predictor (X) is the Time 1 data and the outcome value (Y) is the Time 2 score in the reference dataset. The spread of the residuals around Y forms the reference distribution to which the observed follow-up Y values are compared. A strength of these methods is the ability to incorporate additional predictor variables such as baseline demographics (e.g., age and education) in addition to the Time 1 data. In addition, these methods do not treat the parameters from the reference sample as fixed values but instead treat them as having random variation. They incorporate potential regression to the mean effects and allow for greater variation in outcome variables for patients with extreme values on the predictor variables.

A comparison of RCI and regression-based methods was conducted by Tempkin *et al.* (1999) using simulations. They concluded that although the additional demographic variables were related to performance, they had relatively little impact on the number of patients incorrectly classified as having deteriorated; the best predictor of Time 2 scores was the Time 1 score. The prediction intervals based on the regression techniques were on a par with the intervals from the practice-corrected RCI; relatively similar misclassification rates were observed. Before choosing between these methods it would be advisable to read the relevant literature as many authors have weighed in on the pros and cons of these methods (Chelune *et al.*, 1993; Crawford & Garthwaite, 2006; Maassen, 2004; Tempkin, 2004; Tempkin *et al.*, 1999).

The above discussions center on the statistical properties of a single follow-up minus baseline score. In practice there are often repeated follow-up measurements. Without any correction for multiple comparisons it is likely that more than the nominal level of patients will be misclassified as declined. Researchers have thus tried to control the effect of multiplicity by requiring confirmation of the suspected decline, by either requiring decline in more than one measure (often from a similar domain of functioning), or maintenance of that decline on a subsequent follow-up test.

Time-to-event analyses

The RCI and regression-based methods result in a categorization of decline, yes or no, at a given time. This leads nicely to a time-to-event analysis in which the endpoint is transformed from one of repeated continuous measurements to a single time variable representing time to neurocognitive decline. One advantage of this analysis is that sporadically missing values that are followed by test scores indicating preserved functioning no longer require compensation in the analysis. In addition, patients who exit the study early or have differential follow-up can contribute to the estimate of time to progression in an unbiased manner because of the ability to include censoring in time-to-event analyses. Lastly, the time-to-event analysis confers an advantage over a repeated measures analysis of the continuous outcome: the endpoint offers an interpretation of the proportion of patients with clinically meaningful neurocognitive decline (events) or change in the timing of such events.

Repeated measures analyses

The models discussed above turn a continuous outcome measure into a dichotomous variable indicating decline (yes/no). It is also possible to analyze the outcome measures directly using generalized linear mixed effects modeling. These models estimate and incorporate the correlations induced by multiple testing over time and avoid the multiplicity issues present in the RCI and regression-based methods. They are powerful and flexible and allow for random and fixed effects, varying functions of decline, and a variety of distributions for the outcome measures. For example a skewed outcome could be modeled with a gamma distribution. Although they can incorporate missing values, there are most often assumptions about the random nature of the missing variables that would need to be justified. More generally, the strength of (and the liability of) these models lies in the ability to (and need to) specify the form of the relationship between treatment, time, and outcome. These models generally require parametric assumptions about the data.

Growth mixture modeling

Growth mixture modeling has garnered some attention recently for the ability to estimate decline (growth) curves separately for latent classes of patients. The models can be modified to allow for separate control arm curves but similar treatment effects across the latent classes, or for differential treatment effects across the classes as well. These models have been successfully used to identify subgroups of patients that have unique trajectories across time (Muthen *et al.*, 2002). Although these models allow for discovery of subgroups of patients whose performance over time is distinguished from the rest, the same issues of multiplicity arise as might be expected in the case of post-hoc subgroups. These models may be better tools for exploratory analyses and studies rather than confirmatory Phase III studies where it is necessary to pre-specify effects.

Q-TWiST methods

Statistical methodologies have been developed to analyze a combined endpoint of more traditional measures, such as survival, with neurocognitive and PRO measures. Techniques include quality-adjusted survival (Glasziou *et al.*, 1990) and quality-adjusted time without symptoms of disease or toxicity of treatment (Q-TWiST) methodologies (Gelber *et al.*, 1993).

Conclusions

In recent years, regulatory agencies have emphasized the importance of clinical trial endpoints that directly measure clinical benefit, in contrast to surrogate measures of benefit such as tumor response. They have also emphasized the importance of "net clinical benefit" that captures not just survival but the quality of that survival. Neurocognitive endpoints consist of objective, standardized tests that directly measure a patient's cognitive function. The information obtained with these measures is not captured through patient self-report (e.g., quality of life questionnaires), mental status screening instruments, or a general neurological exam. Thus, they provide a unique and direct assessment of patient benefit.

Several theoretical and logistical issues must be considered to successfully incorporate neurocognitive testing into clinical trials. The expected impact of disease and treatment on neurocognitive functioning, choice of test, and frequency of testing must be determined. In addition, successful implementation includes personnel training, management of practice effects, early and frequent data review, and appropriate statistical methodologies. Despite these challenges, the feasibility of neurocognitive testing and analysis has been demonstrated in recent large randomized multinational Phase III trials in oncology.

REFERENCES

Chelune GJ, Naugle RI, Luders H *et al.* (1993). Individual change after epilepsy surgery: practice effects and base-rate information. *Neuropsychology* **7**: 41–52.

Crawford JR, Garthwaite PH (2006). Detecting dissociations in single-case studies: type I errors, statistical power and the classical versus strong distinction. *Neuropsychologia* **44**: 2249–2258.

Cull A, Hay C, Love SB *et al.* (1996). What do cancer patients mean when they complain of concentration and memory problems? *Br J Cancer* **74**: 1674–1679.

Fliessbach K, Urbach H, Helmstaedter C *et al.* (2003). Cognitive performance and magnetic resonance imaging findings after high-dose systemic and intraventricular chemotherapy for primary central nervous system lymphoma. *Arch Neurol* **60**: 563–568.

Gelber RD, Goldhirsch A, Cole BF (1993). Evaluation of effectiveness: Q-TWiST. *Cancer Treat Rev* **19** [Suppl. A]: 73–84.

Glasziou PP, Simes RJ, Gelber RD (1990). Quality-adjusted survival analysis. *Stat Med* **9**: 1259–1276.

Herman MA, Tremont-Lukats I, Meyers CA *et al.* (2003). Neurocognitive and functional assessment of patients with brain metastases: a pilot study. *Am J Clin Oncol* **26**: 273–279.

Jacobson NS, Truax P (1991). Clinical significance: a statistical approach to defining meaningful change in psychotherapy research. *J Consult Clin Psychol* **59**: 12–19.

Maassen GH (2004). What do Temkin's simulations of reliable change tell us? *J Int Neuropsychol Soc* **10**: 902–903.

Mehta MP, Shapiro WR, Glantz MJ *et al.* (2002). Lead-in phase to randomized trial of motexafin gadolinium and whole-brain radiation for patients with brain metastases: centralized assessment of magnetic resonance imaging, neurocognitive and neurologic end points. *J Clin Oncol* **20**: 3445–3453.

Meyers CA, Brown PD (2006). Role and relevance of neurocognitive assessment in clinical trials of patients with CNS tumors. *J Clin Oncol* **24**: 1305–1309.

Meyers CA, Hess KR (2003). Multifaceted end points in brain tumor clinical trials: cognitive deterioration precedes MRI progression. *Neurooncology* **5**: 89–95.

Meyers CA, Wefel JS (2003). The use of the Mini-Mental State Examination to assess cognitive functioning in cancer trials: no ifs, ands, buts, or sensitivity. *J Clin Oncol* **21**: 3557–3558.

Meyers CA, Byrne KS, Komaki R (1995). Cognitive deficits in patients with small cell lung cancer before and after chemotherapy. *Lung Cancer* **12**: 231–235.

Meyers CA, Kudelka AP, Conrad CA *et al.* (1997). Neurotoxicity of CI-980, a novel mitotic inhibitor. *Clin Cancer Res* **3**: 419–422.

Meyers CA, Hess KR, Yung WK *et al.* (2000). Cognitive function as a predictor of survival in patients with recurrent malignant glioma. *J Clin Oncol* **18**: 646–650.

Meyers CA, Smith JA, Bezjak A *et al.* (2004). Neurocognitive function and progression in patients with brain metastases treated with whole-brain radiation and motexafin gadolinium: results of a randomized phase III trial. *J Clin Oncol* **22**: 157–165.

Muthen B, Brown CH, Masyn K *et al.* (2002). General growth mixture modeling for randomized preventive interventions. *Biostatistics* **3**: 459–475.

O'Shaughnessy JA, Wittes RE, Burke G *et al.* (1991). Commentary concerning demonstration of safety and efficacy of investigational anticancer agents in clinical trials. *J Clin Oncol* **9**: 2225–2232.

Sherman AM, Jaeckle K, Meyers CA (2002). Pretreatment cognitive performance predicts survival in patients with leptomeningeal disease. *Cancer* **15**: 1311–1316.

Taphoorn MJ, Klein M (2004). Cognitive deficits in adult patients with brain tumours. *Lancet Neurol* **3**: 159–168.

Tempkin NR (2004). Standard error in the Jacobson and Truax reliable change index: the "classical approach" leads to poor estimates. *J Int Neuropsychol Soc* **10**: 899–901.

Tempkin NR, Heaton RK, Grant I *et al.* (1999). Detecting significant change in neuropsychological test performance: a comparison of four models. *J Int Neuropsychol Soc* **5**: 357–369.

van Dam FS, Schagen SB, Muller MJ *et al.* (1998). Impairment of cognitive function in women receiving adjuvant treatment for high-risk breast cancer: high-dose versus standard-dose chemotherapy. *J Natl Cancer Inst* **90**: 210–218.

Wefel JS, Lenzi R, Theriault R *et al.* (2004a). "Chemobrain" in breast cancer? A prologue. *Cancer* **101**: 466–475.

Wefel JS, Lenzi R, Theriault R *et al.* (2004b). The cognitive sequelae of standard dose adjuvant chemotherapy in women with breast cancer: results of a prospective, randomized, longitudinal trial. *Cancer* **100**: 2292–2299.

Index